Handbook of
Oncology Nursing

Jones and Bartlett Series in Oncology

Handbook of Oncology Nursing

THIRD EDITION

Edited by

BONNY LIBBEY JOHNSON, RN, MSN
Oncology Research Coordinator
University of Connecticut Health Center
Farmington, Connecticut

JODY GROSS, RN, MSN, OCN®
Director of Clinical Services
Hospice of the Florida Keys and the Visiting Nurse Association
Key West, Florida

Jones and Bartlett Publishers
Sudbury Massachusetts
Boston   Toronto   London   Singapore

World Headquarters
Jones and Bartlett Publishers
40 Tall Pine Drive
Sudbury, MA 01776
1-800-832-0034
978-433-5000
info@jbpub.com
www.jbpub.com

Jones and Bartlett Publishers Canada
P.O. Box 19020
Toronto, ON M5S 1X1
CANADA

Jones and Bartlett Publishers International
Barb House, Barb Mews
London W6 7PA
UK

Copyright © 1998 by Jones and Bartlett Publishers, Inc.

PRODUCTION CREDITS
ACQUISITIONS EDITOR Karen McClure
PRODUCTION EDITOR Lianne B. Ames
MANUFACTURING BUYER Jane Bromback
DESIGN University Graphics
EDITORIAL PRODUCTION SERVICE University Graphics
TYPESETTING University Graphics
COVER DESIGN Dick Hannus
PRINTING AND BINDING Malloy Lithographing
COVER PRINTING Malloy Lithographing

Library of Congress Cataloging-in-Publication Data
Handbook of oncology nursing / edited by Bonny Libbey Johnson, Jody Gross.—3rd ed.
     p.   cm.
   Includes bibliographical references and index.
   ISBN 0-7637-0624-8
   1. Cancer—Nursing—Handbooks, manuals, etc.   I. Johnson, Bonny L.   II. Gross, Jody.
   RC266.H36   1998
   610.73'698—dc21   98-14512
                                                                        CIP

The selection and dosage of drugs presented in this book are in accord with standards accepted at the time of publication. The authors and publishers have made every effort to provide accurate information. However, research, clinical practice, and government regulations often change the accepted standard in this field. Before administering any drug, the reader is advised to check the manufacturer's product information sheet for the most up-to-date recommendations on dosage, precautions, and contraindications. This is especially important in the case of drugs that are new or seldom used.

Printed in the United States of America

02 01 00 99 98   10 9 8 7 6 5 4 3 2 1

Contents

Contributors   vii
Preface to the Third Edition   xi
Abbreviations and Symbols   xii

UNIT I PRINCIPLES OF CANCER CARE

1. Behavior of Malignancies   3
2. Cancer Treatment   21
   A. Surgery   22
   B. Radiation Therapy   36
   C. Chemotherapy   66
   D. Biotherapy   105
3. Special Treatments   127
   A. Marrow and Peripheral Stem Cell Transplantation   127
   B. Parenteral Therapy: Access and Delivery   171
4. Principles of Clinical Research   219

UNIT II COMMON CLINICAL PROBLEMS

5. Prevention and Early Detection   241
6. Information and Resources   263
   A. Information   263
   B. Resources   277
7. Coping   289
8. Comfort   305
   A. Pain   305
   B. Sleep   336
   C. Fatigue   360
9. Nutrition   377
10. Protective Mechanisms   417
    A. Bone Marrow   417
    B. Mucous Membranes   440
    C. Skin   459
11. Neurologic Complications   495
12. Elimination   527
    A. Anatomical Alterations   527
    B. Functional Alterations: Bowel   545
    C. Functional Alterations: Bladder   557

13. Sexuality   585
14. Pulmonary Function   599

UNIT III ONCOLOGIC EMERGENCIES

15. Obstructive Emergencies   617
    A. Increased Intracranial Pressure   617
    B. Spinal Cord Compression   631
    C. Superior Vena Cava Syndrome   645
    D. Tracheal Obstruction   655
    E. Bowel Obstruction   661
    F. Cardiac Tamponade   673
16. Metabolic Emergencies   687
    A. Hypercalcemia   687
    B. Tumor Lysis Syndrome   703
    C. Syndrome of Inappropriate Antidiuretic Hormone Secretion   711
    D. Anaphylaxis   721
    E. Septic Shock   729
    F. Coagulopathies   737
17. Infiltrative Emergencies   751
    A. Carotid Artery Erosion and Rupture   751
    B. Leukostasis   762

UNIT IV APPENDICES

Appendix A: Tumor Type and Common Sites of Metastatic Spread   773
Appendix B: Tumor Type and Potential Oncologic Emergency   775
Appendix C: Staging of Cancer   777

Index   789

Contributors

Paula R. Anderson, RN, MN
Research Specialist
Nursing Research and Education
City of Hope National Medical
  Center
Duarte, California

Alice Basch, RN, MSN, ET
Ostomy and Wound Care
  Consultant
San Rafael, California

Anne R. Bavier, RN, MN, FAAN
Special Assistant to the Dean
Nell Hodgson Woodruff School of
  Nursing
Emory University
Atlanta, Georgia

Jennifer Dunn Bucholtz, RN, MS, OCN®
Clinical Specialist
Division of Radiation Oncology
The Johns Hopkins Oncology
  Center
Baltimore, Maryland

Patricia C. Buchsel, RN, MSN
Marrow and Stem Cell Transplant
  Consultant
University of Washington
Seattle, Washington

Patricia Manda Collins, RN, MSN, OCN®
Clinical Nurse Specialist,
  Oncology/Pain
Baptist Health Systems of South
  Florida
Miami, Florida

Reidun Juvkam Daeffler, RN, MS, OCN®
Clinical Nurse Specialist, Oncology
Scottsdale Healthcare
Scottsdale, Arizona

Lyn Sturdevant Davis, RN, MSN
Goshen, Connecticut

Grace E. Dean, RN, MSN
Research Specialist
Nursing Research and Education
City of Hope National Medical
  Center
Duarte, California

Sharon Dellinger, RN, MSN, CS, OCN®
Oncology Nurse Clinician
University of Connecticut Health
  Center
Farmington, Connecticut

Susan A. DiStasio, RN, MS, OCN®
Clinical Research Nurse
Yale Cancer Center
Clinical Assistant Professor
Yale School of Nursing
New Haven, Connecticut

Lynne M. Early, RN, BSN, CETN
Master's Candidate
University of California at Los
  Angeles
Los Angeles, California

Contributors

Jeanne M. Erickson, RN, MSN, OCN®
Clinician III
University of Virginia Cancer Center
Charlottesville, Virginia

Betty R. Ferrell, RN, PhD, FAAN
Research Scientist
Nursing Research and Education
City of Hope National Medical Center
Duarte, California

Annette L. Galassi, RN, MA, AOCN, CANP
Oncology Nurse Practitioner
Lombardi Cancer Center
Georgetown University Medical Center
Washington, DC

Marcia Grant, RN, DNSc, FAAN
Director and Research Scientist
Nursing Research and Education
City of Hope National Medical Center
Duarte, California

Mikel Gray, PhD, CUNP, CCCN, FAAN
Nurse Practitioner
Department of Urology
Associate Professor
School of Nursing
University of Virginia
Charlottesville, Virginia

Susan L. Groenwald, RN, MS
Assistant Professor, Complemental
Rush University College of Nursing
Rush-Presbyterian St. Luke's Medical Center
Chicago, Illinois

Jody Gross, RN, MSN, OCN®
Director of Clinical Services
Hospice of the Florida Keys and Visiting Nurse Association
Key West, Florida

Douglas Haeuber, RN, MSN, JD
Biotechnology Licensing Attorney
Cooley Godward LLP
Palo Alto, California

Susan Molloy Hubbard, RN, BS, MPA
Director, International Cancer Information Center
Acting Director, Office of Cancer Information, Communication, and Education
National Cancer Institute
National Institutes of Health
Bethesda, Maryland

Patricia Jassak, RN, MS, AOCN
Administrative Director
Creticos Cancer Center
Illinois Masonic Medical Center
Chicago, Illinois

Bonny Libbey Johnson, RN, MSN
Oncology Research Coordinator
University of Connecticut Health Center
Farmington, Connecticut

Diahann Kazierad, RN, MSN, CCRN, APRN
Nurse Practitioner
University of Connecticut Health Center
Farmington, Connecticut

Sharon Sebold Kilbride, RN, BSN, OCN®
Formerly Oncology Nurse
  Clinician
University of Connecticut Health
  Center
Farmington, Connecticut

M. Tish Knobf, RN, MSN, PhD(©), FAAN
Associate Professor, Yale School
  of Nursing
Oncology Clinical Nurse
  Specialist
Ambulatory Service
Yale New Haven Hospital
New Haven, Connecticut

Kristen Kreamer, RN, MSN, CRNP, AOCN
Nurse Practitioner
Ambulatory Oncology
Fox Chase Cancer Center
Philadelphia, Pennsylvania

Deborah K. Mayer, RN, MSN, AOCN, FAAN
Advanced Practice Nurse and
  Oncology Consultant
South Easton, Massachusetts

Karen Kane McDonnell, RN, MSN
Director, Hunterdon Regional
  Cancer Program
Hunterdon Medical Center
Flemington, New Jersey

Johanna LaRoss Meehan, RN, MSN, CS, AOCN
Oncology Nurse Practitioner
University of Connecticut Health
  Center
Farmington, Connecticut

Suzanne Mellon, RN, PhD
Assistant Professor
University of Detroit Mercy
Detroit, Michigan

Joan Martin Moore, MN, RN, AOCN
Oncology Clinical Nurse Specialist
Department of Patient Care Services
Saint Francis Hospital and Medical
  Center
Hartford, Connecticut

Marion E. Morra, MA, ScD
Director of Health Informatics
Morra Communications
Milford, Connecticut

Laurel L. Northouse, RN, PhD, FAAN
Associate Professor
Wayne State College of Nursing
Detroit, Michigan

Linda Celentano Norton, RN, MSN
formerly Assistant Professor
Yale University School of Nursing
New Haven, Connecticut

Mary Ropka, RN, PhD, FAAN
Associate Professor of Research
Department of Health Evaluation
  Sciences
School of Medicine
Research Associate Professor
Center for Survey Research
University of Virginia
Charlottesville, Virginia

S. Katharine Sandstrom, RN, BSN, OCN®
Clinical Research Nurse
Experimental Therapeutics Program
Cleveland Clinic Cancer Center
Cleveland, Ohio

Ellen Sitton, RN, MSN, OCN®, RT(T)
Advanced Practice Nurse
Ambulatory Care
USC/Kenneth Norris Jr. Cancer
    Hospital
Los Angeles, California

Dorothy B. Smith, RN, MS, OCN®, CETN, FAAN
Director of Clinical Relations
Deschutes Medical Products, Inc.
Bend, Oregon

Rebecca Stockdale-Woolley, RN, MSN, APRN
Program Manager
LungLife Pulmonary Rehabilitation
    Program
Hospital of Saint Raphael
New Haven, Connecticut

Cheryl McCullen Tafas, RN, MSN, OCN®
Oncology Clinical Nurse Specialist
University of Connecticut Health
    Center
Farmington, Connecticut

Myra Woolery-Antill, RN, MN, CPON
Pediatric Clinical Nurse Specialist
Adult and Pediatric Nursing Service
Department of Nursing
National Institutes of Health
Bethesda, Maryland

Preface

In the four years that have elapsed since the publication of the 2nd edition of the *Handbook of Oncology Nursing*, we have been reminded on many occasions of the utility of this book, both professionally and personally. Our colleagues frequently tell us of the use they make of it, and we too have referred to it in the course of our work. As one of the contributors has said, ". . . it is a standard, and so many nurses rely on it . . ." Both of us have had recourse to its pages on several occasions over the past year: BLJ, whose father remains chronically ill, and JG, in caring for her father who died in May 1997 of metastatic colon cancer.

While the majority of the material will be familiar to readers of the previous two editions, we have included in this edition a chapter on fatigue, and new content throughout related to spirituality and quality of life. The chapter on bone marrow transplantation has been expanded to cover peripheral stem cell transplantation, and the section on radiation therapy includes expanded information about both internal and external radiation therapy techniques. All other chapters have been updated with relevant current information.

We continue to envision this book as an aid to the nurse at the bedside, wherever that may be in our changing healthcare environment: the hospital, outpatient clinic, physician office, extended care facility, home, or hospice. An understanding of the pathophysiology of problems commonly encountered by nurses in caring for patients with cancer assists in the provision of compassionate, appropriate care, regardless of practice setting. The problems encountered by cancer patients have remained constant in the fifteen years since we published the first edition of the handbook. The innovative focus on common clinical problem areas is designed to avoid the fragmentation that results from the more common disease-oriented approach to nursing care. By focusing on these areas, care for a particular problem may be performed in a uniform fashion for patients with different tumor types, different stages of disease, and in different care settings. Our experiences, and those of our colleagues, confirm for us the validity of approaching care from this perspective, and the universal and consistent nature of nursing practice.

Unlike the prior editions, here we wish to thank our contributors, for sharing their knowledge of cancer nursing practice with us and our readers, our colleagues in cancer nursing who have taught us and shared their experiences with us, and our patients and our fathers, who continually remind us that good nursing care is vital to their well being.

BLJ and JG

Abbreviations and Symbols

ABG	arterial blood gas	IV	intravenous
ADL	activities of daily living	kg	kilogram
AIDS	acquired immunodeficiency syndrome	L	liter
		LDH	lactic dehydrogenase
ATC	around the clock	LFT	liver function test
BID	twice per day	m^2	meter squared
BMD	bone marrow depression	mcg	microgram
BP	blood pressure	mEq	milliequivalent
BSA	body surface area	mg	milligram
BUN	blood urea nitrogen	MI	myocardial infarction
CBC	complete blood count	ml	milliliter
cGy	centigray	MRI	magnetic resonance imaging
cc	cubic centimeter	N/V	nausea/vomiting
CHF	congestive heart failure	ng	nanogram
CNS	central nervous system	NG	nasogastric
COPD	chronic obstructive pulmonary disease	NPO	nothing by mouth
		NS	normal saline
CSF	cerebrospinal fluid	NSAID	non-steroidal antiinflammatory drug
CV	cardiovascular		
CVP	central venous pressure	OOB	out of bed
CXR	chest x-ray	OT	occupational therapy
D/C	discontinue	OTC	over the counter
D5W	5% dextrose/water	PE	physical exam
dl	deciliter	PFT	pulmonary function test
EKG	electrocardiogram	PO	oral
g	gram	PRN	as needed
GI	gastrointestinal	PT	physical therapy
GIT	gastrointestinal tract	q	every (each)
GU	genitourinary	QID	four times per day
H_2O	water	RBC	red blood count
HCG	human chorionic gonadotropin	ROM	range of motion
		RT	radiation therapy
Hct	hematocrit	SC	subcutaneous
Hgb	hemoglobin	SL	sublingual
HIV	human immunodeficiency virus	TID	three times per day
		TIW	three times per week
I&O	intake and output	U	unit
IA	intra-arterial	UTI	urinary tract infection
IM	intramuscular	VS	vital signs
IU	international unit	WBC	white blood count

U N I T

I

PRINCIPLES OF CANCER CARE

Chapter 1 The Behavior of Malignancies   1

Chapter 2 Cancer Treatment   2

       A. Surgery   2A

       B. Radiation Therapy   2B

       C. Chemotherapy   2C

       D. Biotherapy   2D

Chapter 3 Special Treatments   3

       A. Marrow and Peripheral Stem Cell Transplantation   3A

       B. Parenteral Chemotherapy   3B

Chapter 4 Principles of Clinical Research   4

The Behavior of Malignancies

Susan L. Groenwald

INTRODUCTION

For many years, the scientific community has known that organisms regulate their cells by the expression of genes and that an alteration in cell division is central to the development of cancer cells. However, the advances in molecular biology and biochemistry in the 1980s catapulted our knowledge about cancer into a whole new arena. Through the discovery of oncogenes and, later, proto-oncogenes and anti-oncogenes, we now understand not only *how* cancer cells differ from normal cells, but *why*. Research now focuses on exactly how normal cells become malignant and how to correct abnormal mechanisms and eradicate the cancer cell population.

Changes in knowledge of basic science lead to changes in cancer treatment. Therefore, it is critical for nurses to understand the scientific principles underlying the behavior of malignancies in order to anticipate needed changes in clinical practice and to bring new scientific information and knowledge to a level where patients can derive direct benefit.

WAYS IN WHICH CANCER CELLS DIFFER FROM NORMAL CELLS

Differences in Growth

A primary feature of the cancer cell is loss of control over its growth. Control of cell division is carefully maintained by two opposing sets of genes, one set promoting growth (oncogenes), and the other set inhibiting growth (cancer suppressor genes). Although these are normal genes involved in the natural growth process of a cell, their names reflect the fact that they were discovered initially as "cancer" genes.

For normal cells, the stimulus for cellular proliferation is the need for cell renewal or replacement. The growth of normal cells is rigidly regulated so that new cells equal the number of cells lost by cell death or injury. In cancer cells, this growth control mechanism is lost or altered, causing cancer cells to divide continuously and without regard for the tissue requirements of the host. The number of new cells is greater than the number of cells lost, resulting in a tumor mass. There are several properties that contribute to the changes in growth patterns of cancer cells.

Most normal cells are limited to a certain number of divisions before they die, usually about 50. This programmed death is called *senescence*. Senescence is controlled by the cell's normal "biological clock," called a *telomere*, located at the ends of chromosomes. Telomeres protect the chromosomal ends of the DNA from damage. With each cell replication, the telomere is not copied completely. The result is that with age, the telomere grows progressively shorter. When it shrinks below a certain level, a signal is sent to the cell to enter senescence. If the cell continues to divide, it will die. Normal germ cells in the testis and ovary have an enzyme, telomerase, that prevents aging by duplicating the telomeres. Many cancers contain this enzyme, which replaces the segments lost during cell division, enabling the cell to replicate indefinitely.

The body has a mechanism called *apoptosis* to deal with abnormal cells early in their development. Each human cell has the capacity to program itself for cell death in the event of serious damage or loss of regulation. The process of apoptosis is defective in cancer cells.

In culture, normal cells spread out in a uniform monolayer. If a cut is made through the single layer of cells, the damaged cells disintegrate and other cells develop to restore the integrity of the monolayer. This phenomenon was thought to be due to contact inhibition of growth; that is, cells would cease to grow when they touched each other. However, it is now thought that normal cells develop in a monolayer because such a structure facilitates optimal utilization of nutrients. Accordingly, the term *density-dependent growth* has replaced the term *contact inhibition*.

In contrast, cancer cells, when placed in the same culture medium, continue to divide, crowding the space they occupy until the cells are piled on each other in an unorganized mass. Cancer cells are held less firmly to each other, move about more freely than normal cells, and also have less requirement for nutrients. Therefore, they have a different density dependence than normal cells.

Substances found in the serum, known as *growth factors,* are known to be necessary for the growth of normal cells. In normal cells, growth factors produced by one cell type bind to specific receptors on the cell membrane of the target cell, initiating a series of events that lead to mitosis. Cancer cells are able to grow and divide either in the absence of serum growth factors or in serum in which the concentration of growth factors is significantly reduced. This lack of dependence on growth factors means that cancer cells are independent of the body's normal control systems that keep cell division and cell loss in balance. Some cancer cells even make their own growth factors.

Cellular proliferation occurs as a result of two coordinated events: the duplication of DNA within the cell, and mitosis, the division of the cell into two daughter cells with identical complements of DNA. Together the two events make up the *cell cycle* (see Figure 1–1). Control of the cell cycle resides in the cell's nucleus. The phases of the cell cycle are G_0, G_1, S, G_2, and M.

G_0, a resting or quiescent state, describes those cells not actively in the cell cycle. This category includes cells that will never divide (such as mature brain cells) and cells that are dormant but capable of being stimulated to reenter the cell cycle in times of physiologic need (such as hepatocytes).

The G_1 phase is a period of decreased metabolic activity. During this period, the cell carries out its designated physiologic functions and synthesizes proteins in preparation for copying its DNA in the S phase of the cell cycle.

The S phase is the portion of the cell cycle in which DNA is duplicated. Normal cellular replication depends on the orderly synthesis of genetic material. Structural damage or disarray of the DNA molecule during its reproduction can result in cell death. Cells are most vulnerable to damage in this phase, and it is thought that many cell-cycle–specific chemotherapeutic agents exert their cytotoxic effects during this period.

The G_2 phase immediately follows the S phase and is characterized by another period of decreased activity. Cells entering this stage possess the duplicated genetic material synthesized in the S phase. Although some production of RNA and protein production occurs during G_2, cells in this stage are primarily awaiting entry into the mitotic phase.

The M phase, or mitosis, is the portion of the cell cycle in which the actual division of the cell occurs. The parent cell segregates the duplicated chromosomes and divides into two daughter cells. After mitosis, the two new cells either pass into G_1 to reenter the cell cycle or enter the resting state of G_0.

A cell in G_0 or G_1 receives a signal that determines whether the cell proceeds through the cell cycle or remains or returns to G_0. The point at

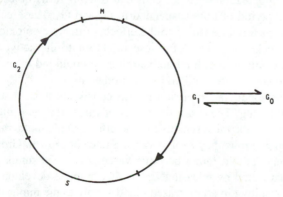

Figure 1–1. Phases of the cell cycle. (See text for discussion.)

which this determination is made is called the *restriction point*. When a cell passes this point, it must continue through all phases of the cell cycle and return to G_1. It is likely that the transformation of normal cells to cancer cells involves a recruitment of cells from G_0 to G_1.

The durations of the M, S, and G_2 phases are relatively constant, but the length of the G_1 phase varies widely and determines the overall length of the cell cycle. Rapidly dividing cells, such as renewing cells and neoplastic cells, are able to complete the cell cycle faster by reducing the length of G_1.

Normal tissues can be described in terms of three major categories of cell proliferation: static, expanding, and renewing. Normal cells of *static* tissues, such as the brain, do not retain the capacity to divide after the postembryonic period. Because of this inability to divide, cells of this type that are damaged or destroyed cannot be replaced. Normal cells of *expanding* tissues in the body temporarily cease proliferating when the tissue reaches its normal adult size but remain capable of reentering the cell cycle and dividing in times of physiologic need, such as cell injury or death. The liver, kidneys, and endocrine glands contain cells with this potential to repair or replace damaged cells. *Renewing* cell populations have the most proliferative activity. Cells in this category have a finite lifespan and continuously replace cells lost to injury or death. Blood cells, epithelial cells of the gastrointestinal mucosa, and germ cells are examples of renewing cell populations. Renewing cell populations most closely resemble actively proliferating cancer cells in their degree of proliferative activity.

Tumors, like normal tissues, contain mixtures of cells in various stages of proliferation. Some cells within a tumor are actively proliferating, some are temporarily dormant, and others are permanently nondividing. As the mass enlarges, some cells are pushed away from the vascular supply. Because of this distance, these cells receive inadequate regional nutrition, which leads to cell death and tissue necrosis. Dead cells add only mass to the tumor and are of little concern for treatment purposes.

The subpopulation of tumor cells that is temporarily quiescent spends an extended period of time suspended in G_1 and G_0. These cells are partially or completely insensitive to the effects of many cytotoxic drugs. Attempts to synchronize entry of quiescent cells into the active part of the cell cycle by administering an activating drug could aid in increasing the number of malignant cells killed by chemotherapy.

A third subpopulation of cancer cells consists of those that remain actively proliferating. These are the target of most treatment interventions, because they are the most sensitive to the effects of chemotherapy.

As tumors grow, they exhibit varying rates of growth. Growth is slow or nonexistent until the tumor becomes vascularized. The tumor provides its own vascularization by releasing agents that promote development of new capillaries, resulting in an increased blood supply to the tumor. A period of exponential growth follows vascularization. Cell growth continues at the periphery of the tumor mass, with the center becoming increasingly dormant and ultimately necrotic. Finally, the tumor reaches a critical mass when cell death approximates new cell formation and a plateau phase is reached. By the time a tumor has grown to the size where it can be clinically detected, it has probably already reached the plateau phase and growth has slowed.

Doubling time is the time required for a mass to double its volume. A mass must achieve the size of at least one centimeter to reach the lower limit of sensitivity for most clinical methods of detection. In general, this represents approximately 30 doublings.

The doubling times of various tumors have been examined in *in vitro* systems and vary greatly. The actual tumor growth rate in humans is difficult to ascertain because of the number of variables that influence doubling times. For example, *in vivo* tumor growth can be retarded by hormonal and immunologic factors. Information about doubling times of tumors is applied to clinical situations to predict possible therapeutic responses. In general, rapidly growing tumors are more responsive to chemotherapy and radiation therapy than slow-growing cancers.

Because not all cells within a tumor are dividing simultaneously, growth fraction is an important variable in determining a tumor's doubling time. *Growth fraction* refers to the portion of a tumor mass that is actively proliferating. Tumors with larger growth fractions expand their mass more rapidly. Growth fractions have been estimated at 100 percent in some germ-cell tumors and as low as 10 percent in slow-growing adenocarcinomas. Responsiveness to drugs has been directly correlated with the growth fraction of tumors.

As tumors grow, they tend to undergo an evolution in their histologic patterns. This evolution, referred to as *tumor progression,* is the tumor's change from a very low degree of malignancy, or preneoplastic state, to a rapidly growing, virulent neoplasm. It is characterized by changes in the growth rate, invasive potential, metastatic frequency, morphologic traits, and responsiveness to therapy. Progression is thought to occur as a result of the natural selection of a cell type that becomes dominant within the tumor because it proliferates more rapidly than other cells. In addition, cancer treatments could actually facilitate tumor progression through mutagenic effects that hasten the appearance of more malignant cellular variants. For example, certain lymphomas commonly undergo progression to a more malignant cell type.

Differences in Appearance

Normal cells have a well-organized and extensive cytoskeleton that causes the cells of specific tissues to be consistent in size and shape. In contrast, transformed cells are *pleomorphic,* or of variable sizes and shapes. In addition, the nuclei of cancer cells are *hyperchromatic*—they stain darker than normal cells—and are disproportionately larger. Finally, cancer cells exhibit a variety of abnormal mitotic figures (see Figure 1–2).

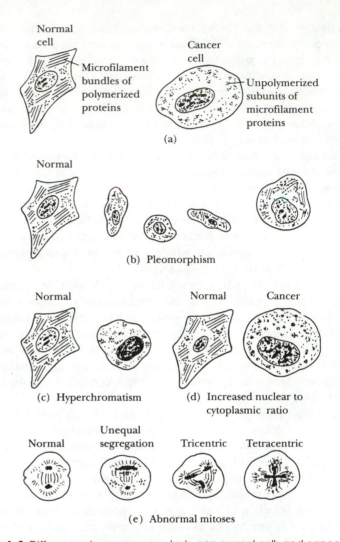

Figure 1-2. Differences in appearance between normal cells and cancer cells.

Reprinted with permission from Groenwald, S. L., M. H. Frogge, M. Goodman, et al., eds. Cancer nursing: Principles and practice. 3rd ed. Jones and Bartlett, Boston. p.51. 1993.

Differences in Differentiation

The turning on and off of genes that characterizes *differentiation* of cells from human embryo to mature adult results in a human being with cells specialized for various structural and functional purposes. Cancer cells can arise at any point during differentiation. In addition, genes that were active in embryos but suppressed during differentiation can be reactivated by carcinogenic agents.

Cancer cells tend to be less differentiated than cells from surrounding normal tissue. The spectrum of proliferative growth patterns ranges from benign to increasingly malignant. *Hyperplasia* is an increase in the number of cells of a certain type in a tissue. Although hyperplasia can be a characteristic of neoplasia, it also occurs commonly as a normal physiologic response during episodes of rapid growth and development, such as those occurring during the prenatal and adolescent periods. It is also a common feature of bone marrow cells and epithelial cells of the gastrointestinal mucosa.

Metaplasia occurs when a change is initiated in the differentiation of a stem cell and results in the replacement of one normal adult cell type with another. Vitamin deficiency and various chemical agents can induce these changes.

Dysplasia is a disturbance in the usual distinct histologic pattern of a group of cells within a tissue. Microscopically, cells within tissues are readily characterized by their intracellular features and their relationship to one another in the architecture of the tissue. Both the cell-to-cell regularity and the arrangement of cells within a tissue can be altered in this type of proliferation. This pattern can be an early characteristic of neoplasms or can result from chronic inflammation.

The difference between dysplasia and *anaplasia* is a matter of degree. Anaplastic cells lack any normal characteristics of cellular differentiation and are associated almost exclusively with neoplasia. Some cancer cells are so poorly differentiated that the tissue of origin cannot be identified.

Neoplasia is a proliferative abnormality characterized by an autonomous uncontrolled growth pattern. Neoplasms are classified as either benign or malignant. Benign neoplasms are encapsulated, highly differentiated, and noninvasive; they generally grow slowly and do not metastasize. Malignant neoplasms are nonencapsulated, invasive, poorly differentiated to varying degrees, and generally metastatic and rapidly growing.

Differences in Cell Surface

Research has shown that a variety of changes occur in the surface of a cancer cell. Some new molecules appear, some molecules that are usually present are lost, and other molecules are changed. Fibronectin, responsible for the integrity of the extracellular matrix, is present in lower concentrations or in a defective form, contributing to lowered adhesiveness of cancer cells and increased propensity to metastasize. Transformed cells have also been shown to secrete a variety of protein-degrading enzymes, called *proteases,* that contribute to metastasis by invading the extracellular matrices of tissues surrounding the tumor. Finally, new molecules, called *tumor-associated antigens,* form on the surface of cancer cells and can be detected by immunological assay. Tumor-associated antigens are used clinically as markers for detection of tumors, evaluation of patient prognosis, and monitoring of response to treatment.

Differences in Biochemistry

Several biochemical substances are altered, missing, abnormally secreted, or secreted in increased amounts by tumor cells. These biochemical alterations can affect cell growth and cell-to-cell interactions. Examples of biochemical alterations in cancer cells include lowered levels of cyclic adenosine monophosphate (cAMP), which affects availability of nutrients to the cell; increased uptake of nutrients such as amino acids and sugars; decreased concentration of chalone responsible for inhibition of cell division in homeostasis; and alterations in the quality and quantity of growth factors, leading to a lack of responsiveness to inhibitory controls.

Differences in Genes

Cells of a tumor originate from a single cell altered through genetic mutation. The initial change in the cell is the alteration of a regulatory gene (called a *proto-oncogene)* providing the cell with a heritable and selective growth advantage over other cells. The altered regulatory gene is an oncogene. As the cell divides and produces offspring, each daughter cell inherits the genetic defect that provides the capacity to invade, metastasize, and grow without regard to inhibitory growth controls. Although tumor cells originate from a single cell, the characteristics of cells within a tumor vary considerably and differ significantly from the original cell. This diversity, or *heterogeneity,* of cells within a tumor is established early in the tumor's development and results from additional mutations in cells within the clone. The result is the sequential appearance within the tumor of subpopulations of heterogeneous cells with varying degrees of invasiveness, metastatic potential, morphologic traits, and responsiveness to treatment. Heterogeneity is the most significant reason that cancer treatment fails, as cells resistant to therapy survive and metastasize. A goal of cancer therapy is to design treatments that will succeed despite a tumor's heterogeneity.

In addition to the heritable genetic alterations, tumor cells are genetically unstable when compared with normal cells. Tumor progression results when continual mutations of cells within the clone produce more and more virulent tumor cells.

CAUSES OF CANCER

Carcinogenesis

Carcinogenesis is the process during which normal genes are damaged so that cells lose normal control mechanisms of growth and proliferate out of control. When the genes of a single cell are altered by a carcinogenic event, the offspring of that single cell continue to mutate and divide, producing ever more virulent mutant clones. This process has many steps, each of which activates an oncogene or inactivates a cancer-suppressor gene. The process of carcinogenesis has been described as occurring in three phases: initiation, promotion, and progression.

The conversion of normal cell to latent tumor cell is called initiation. An *initiator* is an agent capable of permanently and irreversibly altering the DNA structure within a cell. Initiation can occur after a single exposure to the agent. Chemical compounds, radiation, and viruses are examples of agents that can initiate carcinogenesis.

The process of promotion is dose-related and has a distinct, measurable threshold. A *promoter* is thought to alter the genetic expression of a cell, increasing DNA synthesis, increasing the number of copies of a particular gene, and altering intercellular communication. The effects of promoting agents are transitory and potentially reversible. Repeated, frequent application of or exposure to a promoter is necessary to stimulate latent tumor cells to form tumors and complete the neoplastic transformation. Hormones and growth-stimulating factors are examples of agents that can function as promoters. For example, estrogen has been linked to breast cancer and endometrial cancer. Many promoting agents, such as tobacco, alcohol, and dietary fat, are related to lifestyle and can be controlled by the individual.

The third stage of carcinogenesis, *tumor progression,* is irreversible and leads to morphologic changes and malignant behavior.

Both initiation and promotion are necessary for the complete transformation of the cell, but the sequence of these events is of critical importance. A cell must be transformed by an initiating agent before further neoplastic changes can occur. In laboratory models, the change induced by an initiator is permanent and results in the cell being forever susceptible to further neoplastic transformation by a promoter. In experimental systems, tumors can be induced even when there is a prolonged interval between the change produced by exposure to an initiating agent and the application of a promoter. Promoters can cause neoplasia only if preceded by the appropriate initiating effects. A single exposure to the promoter and/or prolonged intervals between exposures will not result in actual tumor development in animal systems.

These phases were derived from a series of experiments in skin carcinogenesis in animals. In human beings, carcinogenesis is much more complex. The distinction among the three stages is blurred, and there are many more steps. There is most likely more than one type of initiating event. Carcinogens act as either initiators or promoters; in some cases, initiators act as their own promoters—that is, they are complete carcinogens. An agent's ability to act as a complete carcinogen could be dose-related or vary with other environmental influences. Tobacco is thought to be a complete carcinogen. However, in humans, unlike the laboratory model in which initiation is irreversible, the smoker who quits returns in 10 to 15 years to the normal low-incidence pattern for the development of cancer.

The carcinogens that damage genes are classified as familial, viral, bacterial, dietary, chemical, and physical.

Familial Carcinogenesis

It is estimated that up to 15 percent of all human cancers might have a hereditary component. For example, breast cancer is estimated to have a familial component in up to 13 percent of cases.

Familial carcinogenesis is based in part on *cancer-suppressor genes* that seem to prevent cancer when they are functioning normally and, when mutated, cause cancer by their absence. The list of familial syndromes has increased significantly in recent years as new genes have been discovered that, when inherited, increase the risk of cancer. Genes have now been isolated for the following classic familial syndromes: retinoblastoma; Wilms' tumor; neurofibromatosis; familial polyposis associated with colon cancer; syndromes of multiple endocrine neoplasias, associated with tumors of the pituitary, parathyroid, and thyroid and with pheochromocytoma and islet cell tumors; von Hipple-Lindau syndrome, associated with hemangioblastoma, pheochromocytomas and renal cell cancers; Fanconi's anemia associated with leukemia and other malignancies; ataxia telangiectasia associated with leukemia, lymphoma, and breast and ovarian cancer; Bloom syndrome associated with leukemia and several other tumors; Li Fraumeni syndrome associated with multiple cancers; xeroderma pigmentosum associated with skin cancer and leukemia; hereditary nonpolyposis colorectal cancer; and dysplastic nevus syndrome associated with melanoma.

In addition, two new growth-suppressor genes have been isolated that are associated with a lifetime risk of breast cancer of up to 80 percent. There is a 50 percent chance of passing these gene mutations on to a child. This gene can be diagnosed with blood testing, which will allow identification of families at risk. Particularly at risk are individuals in families with a prominent history of early bilateral breast cancer and ovarian cancer.

Most chromosomal disorders that increase susceptibility to cancer involve extra chromosomes, loss of chromosomes, or translocation of specific arms or areas of the chromosomes within the gene structure. Persons with chromosomal abnormalities are at a much higher risk than the general population for the development of specific neoplasms.

In only a small proportion of cancers is the presence of the genetic factor alone sufficient to induce tumors. In most cases, hereditary neoplasia results from a complication of an inherited defect that predisposes the person to cancer upon exposure to specific environmental influences. For example, in xeroderma pigmentosum, there is an enzyme deficiency that impedes repair of DNA in skin damaged by ultraviolet light. This unrepaired damage to genetic material results in the development of multiple skin cancers of various histologies.

Certain tumors and tumor syndromes are transmitted by heredity in a pattern of Mendelian dominance. One tumor at a single site might be the only manifestation of a syndrome, or it could be accompanied by the development of multiple primary tumor sites and other congenital abnormalities.

For example, familial medullary carcinoma of the thyroid can occur by itself or in combination with other benign and malignant neoplasms such as neurofibromas, mucosal neuromas, or pheochromocytomas. Mendelian dominant diseases are often characterized by onset at an early age and site multiplicity (e.g., bilateral development of tumors in paired organs). Retinoblastoma occurs bilaterally much more commonly in children with a family history of the disease than in cases that arise spontaneously.

Some inherited premalignant conditions are in the form of a severe intrinsic immunologic deficiency that could contribute to the increased risk of developing cancer. Persons with these syndromes are prone to develop malignancies of the lymphatic tissues; however, other sites, such as brain and stomach, can also be affected. These syndromes include ataxia-telangiectasia, the Wiskott-Aldrich syndrome, and "late onset" or "common variable" immunodeficiency. Each disorder has defects of both cellular and humoral immunity.

Viral Carcinogenesis

Although evidence of viral-induced cancers in animal systems has existed for many years, viruses associated with specific human cancers have been identified in only a small number of cases.

Epidemiological evidence for the viral etiology of cancer is strongest between human T-cell leukemia-lymphoma virus (HTLV-1) and human T-cell leukemia or lymphoma, and between hepatitis B virus (HBV) and hepatocellular carcinoma, endemic in Asia and Africa. Several tumors have been associated with DNA viruses, including human papillomaviruses (HPV) associated with cervical carcinomas, and the Epstein-Barr virus (EBV) associated with Burkitt's lymphoma, some cases of Hodgkin's disease, and nasopharyngeal carcinoma, especially in the Chinese population.

Bacterial Carcinogenesis

An exciting new discovery is the relationship between the bacteria *Helicobacter pylori* and the mucosa-associated lymphoid tissue (MALT) lymphoma, unique to the gastric mucosa. *H pylori* grows in the stomach and is responsible for gastric and duodenal ulcers. In early stages, the lymphoma is reversible with antibiotic treatment to eradicate the bacteria. Later stages of tumor development require conventional chemotherapy.

Dietary Carcinogenesis

Several dietary factors have been implicated in the development of human cancer, including high levels of dietary fat, nitrosamines, alcohol, and deficiencies of certain micronutrients. Ingestion of dietary fat increases the secretion of bile. The metabolites of bile acids can act as tumor-promoting agents in the colon. Cells that have been initiated by some other agent or an intrinsic genetic defect can be transformed with repeated exposure to consistently high levels of these metabolites. In addition, increased fat intake can modify the endocrine status of the host by increasing the synthesis of hormones. This can affect the induction of cancer in endocrine-dependent sites. Studies have correlated an increased incidence of cancers of the breast, colon, and prostate to high levels of dietary fat intake.

Dietary deficiencies of vitamins and other trace elements have been linked with the development of cancers of the head and neck. These findings have prompted investigations of the anticarcinogenic potential of various micronutrients. It has been proposed that adding to the diet such elements as vitamins A and C, riboflavin, and selenium can protect the host by inhibiting oxidation and the release of free radicals from mutated cells. The anticarcinogenic role of these "antioxidant" dietary components is under investigation.

Although it is clear that dietary chemicals play a role in carcinogenesis, changes in diet would have to be made in early life to have a significant impact on the incidence of cancer. However, a diet low in animal fat, high in fiber, and high in fruits and cruciferous vegetables could offer minimal protection against certain types of cancer, especially colon cancer.

Chemical Carcinogenesis

Chemicals exert their effects by biochemical interaction with cellular DNA. During the metabolism of the carcinogen, free radicals can be formed that carry no charge but possess a single unpaired electron, making them extremely reactive with macromolecules that are rich in electrons, such as DNA. Compounds called *antioxidants* inhibit carcinogenesis because they react with free radicals before the free radicals damage the DNA.

During recent years, more and more chemicals have been implicated as possible carcinogens. However, there are very few chemicals that have been proven to cause cancer in humans.

Although deaths from cancers caused by industrial carcinogens are rare, a handful of industrial chemicals have been identified as carcinogens, including 2-naphthylamine, vinyl chlorides, metals, and benzene.

Cancer chemotherapeutic agents, especially alkylating agents, are known to be carcinogenic. The most common cancers that develop after cancer chemotherapy are lymphoproliferative cancers such as leukemia and lymphoma.

The association of tobacco with lung cancer is well established. As alarming as are the rates of lung cancer in smokers are the statistics on lung cancer related to passive or involuntary smoking. Nonsmoking spouses of smokers can have three times the lung cancer mortality of spouses of nonsmokers. Smoking tobacco makes lung cancer the most prevalent and the most preventable of cancers.

Physical Carcinogenesis

Physical carcinogens are those that affect genes by physical rather than chemical means. Ionizing radiation is a physical carcinogen that causes breaks in DNA strands. If there are many breaks in DNA, cell death occurs. If the injury is minimal, repair could occur. If repair does not take place, the result is mutation, which can lead to the development of a neoplasm.

Ultraviolet radiation from the sun also causes injury to DNA. If the injuries are not repaired, basal cell and squamous cell carcinomas of the exposed areas of the skin can result.

Asbestos is another physical carcinogen that is thought to act as a promoter to tobacco smoke, because lung cancer is rare in asbestos workers who do not smoke. The carcinogenic potential of asbestos depends on its particle size and crystal type; not all types of asbestos are carcinogenic.

CANCER METASTASIS

The ability of a malignant cell to metastasize and invade nonadjacent tissues is its most virulent property, because metastatic lesions, not primary tumors, account for the majority of deaths related to cancer. Knowing the pathogenesis of invasion and metastasis enables the nurse to understand the rationale behind the design of effective therapies for preventing or controlling the spread of disease, to appreciate the clinical implications of current research findings, and to interpret clinical changes in patients with disseminated disease.

Metastasis is a highly organized series of sequential, interdependent steps that lead to the establishment of one or more secondary tumors at a site apart from the primary tumor. The metastatic sequence has been described in terms of six steps:

1. Tumor growth and neovascularization;
2. Tumor cell invasion of the basement membrane and other extracellular matrices;
3. Detachment and embolism of tumor cell aggregates;
4. Arrest in distant organ capillary beds;
5. Extravasation;
6. Proliferation within the organ parenchyma.

Tumor Growth and Neovascularization

As described earlier, cancer starts from the genetic transformation of a single cell. Subsequent alterations in the cellular DNA lead to autonomy from normal growth regulatory mechanisms, uncontrolled proliferation, and growth advantages over adjacent host tissues. Because the cells of the primary tumor are heterogeneous, not all are metastatic, and those that are have varying degrees of metastatic potential. However, research has shown that the subpopulation of cells with metastatic potential dominates the primary tumor mass early in its growth. Cells with metastatic potential seem to have a survival advantage over other cells in the tumor, and they are more aggressive, even from the start.

When a tumor has begun, any subsequent increase in the tumor cell population must be preceded by an increase in blood supply. The tumor initiates its own blood supply through the release of *angiogenic factors*, which stimulate the growth and development of new capillaries that arise from preexisting capillaries or venules. When the blood supply to the tumor has been established, local shedding of cancer cells into the tumor's venous drainage can begin.

Invasion of the Basement Membrane and Extracellular Matrices

Metastasis begins with the local invasion of the surrounding host tissue by either single cells or clumps of cells from the primary tumor. The mechanism of this local invasion has been described in terms of three distinct biochemical events: (1) attachment of the tumor cell to the vascular basement membrane; (2) degradation of the basement membrane by proteolytic enzymes secreted by the tumor cells; and (3) locomotion, the ability of the tumor cell to move itself into surrounding tissues.

Cell-surface molecules that anchor to the basement membrane are called *integrins*. If normal cells do not attach to a surface via these molecules, the cells will not be able to reproduce and will eventually undergo apoptosis. In order for normal cells to survive, they must have the right matrix code and the correct integrin. Cancer cells develop mechanisms to survive away from their normal position along a basement membrane, contributing to their metastatic potential.

Tumor cells must penetrate the basement membrane that exists between parenchymal cells and connective tissue before they can invade adjacent tissue and enter the capillary system. A strong correlation has been established between the invasive and metastatic capabilities of tumor cells and the intracellular levels of specific enzymes. For example, because type IV collagen is the primary structural protein of basement membrane, the higher the level of collagenase in a tumor cell, the greater the tumor cell's ability is to invade tissue and metastasize.

Dissemination

When the tumor cells penetrate the vascular or lymphatic channels, they either grow at the site of penetration or detach and circulate as emboli of individual cells or cell aggregates through the lymphatic or circulatory systems.

Proliferation of cells will cause pressure within a contained space, forcing projections of cells into nearby tissues and body cavities. These cells can attach to the serosal surfaces of viscera within the cavity, leading to *serosal seeding,* a common occurrence in lung and ovarian tumors. Although tumor cells might implant on the surface of organs within the pleural and peritoneal cavity, infiltration into the parenchyma of the organ is uncommon. However, the clinical syndromes of pleural effusion and ascites result, causing major challenges in patient care.

An expanding tumor can also cause damage to local tissue, resulting in pain, bleeding, bone fractures, and loss of function. Tumor cells that enter the lymphatic system are transported passively from the site of the primary tumor to the first draining lymph node. Some tumors pass quickly through the lymph node; others are arrested in the node and either proliferate to form a tumor, die, remain dormant, or enter the bloodstream. A mass in a regional lymph node could be the first clinical sign of metastasis.

Several factors can determine where tumor cells first seed within the lymphatic system. Initially, regional lymph nodes might exert a barrier effect to impede the passage of tumor cells into the lymphatic system. In addition, there is an initial immunologic response to the presence of tumor cells that occurs in the regional lymph nodes and is characterized by the release of immunocompetent cells. It is unknown whether this early immunologic response has any effect on the ultimate progression of disease. At some point, the local lymph nodes lose their ability to filter and destroy tumor cells, and they become infiltrated with malignant cells. The cause of this transformation in their capabilities is unclear. Tumor growth itself might reduce the efficacy of filtration. In addition, chronic inflammation within the node or fibrosis resulting from radiation can alter the barrier effect of lymph nodes. The presence of malignant cells in the lymph nodes can also occur as a result of some overall change in the host's immunocompetence. When the barrier effect of the lymph nodes changes as a result of these factors, passage of neoplastic cells throughout the lymphatic system is unhindered.

Because of the numerous connections between the lymphatic and the vascular systems, most tumor cells that enter the lymphatic system eventually find their way into the vascular system. When there, tumor cells face many threats, including injury or death from blood turbulence and death from attack by immunologic cells. Therefore, entry to the vascular system alone is not sufficient to produce a metastatic deposit. In fact, fewer than 1 percent of tumor cells that enter the circulation survive. To minimize injury and increase the likelihood of arresting in a target organ, tumor cells frequently travel throughout the vascular system attached to each other or to other blood cells, especially platelets. These tumor cell–platelet aggregates form a fibrin-platelet clot, which helps protect the tumor cells from the hostile host environment and facilitates their adherence to the capillary walls of the target organ.

Arrest

Eventually, tumor cells arrest in capillaries and attach to endothelial cells and/or vascular basement membrane by the same process by which they first invade local tissue at the primary tumor site.

Recent experimental studies have supported clinical observations that certain tumors consistently metastasize to particular organs. Although lung, liver, bone, and brain are the most common sites of metastasis, many tumors have been observed to have unique patterns of metastasis that include not only these common target organs but some more unusual sites as well. The usual sites of metastasis for common tumors are listed in Appendix A.

Tumor cells reach many organs. Some tumors metastasize to the first organ linked anatomically to the site of the primary tumor. It is estimated that 50 percent to 60 percent of metastatic distribution can be predicted from the anatomic route followed by the disseminating tumor cell.

In the other 40 percent of tumors, however, the distribution of metastases cannot be predicted by anatomic proximity alone. The distribution seems to be selective and to depend on a match between the tumor cell and the target organ. Certain properties on the surfaces of tumor cells are probably responsible for the organ specificity of metastatic cells. Cell-surface glycoproteins could create "organ-honing" tendencies that allow neoplastic cells to migrate to specific organs and attach themselves to tissues. In addition, it is thought that, although tumor cells can lodge in the capillary beds of multiple organs, certain microenvironmental characteristics determine whether tumor growth will be supported.

Specific and predictable patterns of lymphatic and/or hematogenous spread have been identified clinically for many tumors. For example, testicular tumors generally favor the lymphatic system as an initial route. When entry into the lymphatic channels has occurred, vascular spread follows, and the lungs are the most common distant target organ for this particular tumor.

Knowledge of the expected tissue distribution of metastasis is important to the clinician, who must accurately identify the stage of cancer in the patient at the time of diagnosis, plan appropriate therapy, and monitor progress. Only through knowledge of the natural history of an individual tumor can the specific routes and sites of metastasis be anticipated.

Extravasation

When implanted into the vessel wall of the affected organ, the tumor cell must exit the circulatory system of the organ and penetrate the organ tissue in order to proliferate. Approximately 1 in 10,000 circulating tumor cells will successfully reach this point. The process of extravasation is the same process as invasion, which began the metastatic sequence. Degradative enzymes produced by the tumor cell break down the capillary basement membrane, allowing the tumor cell to penetrate the capillary and move into the tissue of the target organ.

Neovascularization and Growth of Metastasis

The last major step in the metastatic process is the vascularization of the new tumor implant. As in the growth and development of the primary tumor, the cells of the metastatic deposit remain dormant and harmless if they do not have adequate blood supply. New blood vessels, again induced

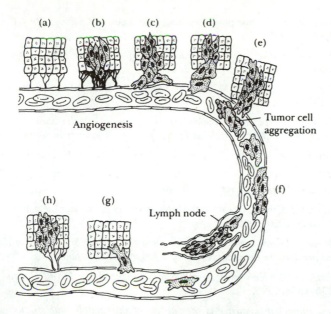

Figure 1-3. The metastatic sequence. (a) Normal tissue; (b) angiogenesis and growth of tumor; (c) attachment of tumor cells to epithelial basement membrane; (d) invasion of the basement membrane by tumor cells; (e) tumor cell dissemination into lymphatic and circulatory systems; (f) arrest of tumor cells on capillary wall or in lymph node; (g) extravasation of tumor cells from capillary into target tissue; (h) angiogenesis and growth of the secondary tumor into a clinically detectable mass.

by the release of tumor angiogenesis factor, are required for the continued growth of the newly established metastasis. Subsequent proliferation of the tumor within the tissue completes the metastatic process. The cycle can begin again as cells from the metastatic tumor invade the basement membrane of the organ tissue, penetrate blood vessels, and enter the circulation to produce secondary metastases. The metastatic sequence is depicted in Figure 1–3.

Researchers continue to look for means to interrupt metastasis at any point in its sequence. In the meantime, the fact that many cancers are metastatic at diagnosis still persists. We still need to know how to detect tiny amounts of disease, how to predict the metastatic potential of a tumor at diagnosis, the degree of silent metastasis, and how to tell when a tumor is completely eradicated. The search continues.

BIBLIOGRAPHY

1. Ameisen, J. C. The origin of programmed cell death. *Science* 272: 1278–1279. 1996.

   A timely review of the phenomenon of apoptosis is presented.

2. Clark, W. H. Tumor progression and the nature of cancer. *Br J Cancer* 64: 631–644. 1991.

   This is a good review of the biology of cancer and the mechanisms of malignant transformation.

3. Clurman B. E., and J. M. Roberts. Cell cycle and cancer. *J Natl Cancer Inst* 87:1499–1501. 1995.

   This editorial introduces the reader to a group of articles about genetic mutations affecting the cell cycle and subsequent malignant transformations.

4. Doll, R., and R. Peto. *The Causes of Cancer*. Oxford University Press, New York. 1981.

   This is a classic work on carcinogenesis.

5. Fidler, I. J. Critical factors in the biology of human cancer metastasis. *Am Surg* 61: 1065–1066. 1995.

   This well-known expert on cancer metastasis describes stages of metastasis and presents an excellent review of years of research findings.

6. Holzman, D.: New view of metastasis is spreading. *J Natl Cancer Inst* 88: 1336–1338. 1996.

   How tumors metastasize is the subject of this article with discussion of research on tumor cells after they have extravasated from vessels into organ tissue.

7. LeMarbre, P. J., and S. L. Groenwald. Biology of Cancer. In Groenwald, S. L., M. H. Frogge, M. Goodman, and C. H. Yarbro, eds. *Cancer Nursing: Principles and Practice*, 4th Ed. 17–37. Jones and Bartlett, Boston. 1997.

   A comprehensive review is presented of the biology of cancer.

8. Vogelstein, B. Cancer: A deadly inheritance. *Nature* 348: 681–682. 1990.

   This is an interesting account of the heritable nature of cancer.

9. Weinberg, R. A. Oncogenes, tumor-suppressor genes and cell transformation: Trying to put it all together. In Brugge, J., T. Carron, E. Harlow, and F. McCormick, eds. *Origins of Human Cancer*. 1–16. Laboratory Press, Cold Springs Harbor, NY. 1991.

   A good review is given of knowledge about oncogenes and their relationship to cancer causation.

10. Weinberg, R: How cancer arises. *Sci Am* 275: 62–70. 1996.

    This is a beautifully illustrated highly readable, comprehensive and up-to-date review of the biology of cancer.

11. Yarbro, J. W. Carcinogenesis. In Groenwald, S. L., M. H. Frogge, M. Goodman, and C. H. Yarbro, eds. *Cancer Nursing,* 4th Ed. 39–49. Jones and Bartlett, Boston. 1997.

    This is a sophisticated presentation of the several possible mechanisms for malignant transformation of a cell. It includes current controversies and colon cancer as a model for carcinogenesis in humans.

Cancer Treatment

It is a striking fact that cancer is the disease that people fear most. The word is often used in our society as a metaphor for death. Actually, this is paradoxical, because cancer is now one of the more curable diseases when the principles of cancer surgery, radiation, chemotherapy, and biotherapy are applied in a well-integrated, multidisciplinary treatment approach. Current estimates of the five-year relative survival rate for persons with cancer in the United States have risen from the 1980–1982 rates of 52 percent for whites and 40 percent for African Americans to the 1986–1993 rates of 60 percent and 44 percent respectively. These figures exclude persons who develop basal or squamous cell cancer of the skin or in situ cancers other than in situ bladder cancer. If these easily cured cancers were included in these figures, many more persons with cancer would be considered long-term survivors. Moreover, these estimates do not reflect the improvements in survival that will undoubtedly be realized when the impact of current treatment becomes widely observed.

Whereas the rate of cancer mortality is falling in all persons under age 55, the most dramatic increases in survival rates have occurred in children. In children, five-year survival rates have increased from 65 percent in 1980–1982 to 72 percent in 1986–1993. These rates indicate that advances in cancer treatment being developed at research centers are being applied widely throughout the country.

The reason that the likelihood of complete cure and prolonged survival for cancer patients is steadily improving is that fundamental changes have occurred in our understanding of the biology of cancer, and this information has proven to have practical applications.

A key consideration in the treatment of cancer is the therapeutic intent. When cure is the goal, the initial management of the patient is often the most critical period and can determine the ultimate outcome. The development of an individualized treatment plan for a patient must take into consideration the following factors: (1) the biology and natural history of the cancer; (2) the extent of disease dissemination (including specific sites of involvement); and (3) the potential of surgery, radiation, chemotherapy, and biotherapy to eradicate all viable cancer cells. Surgery and radiation alone are generally curative in cancers that are truly localized; and they play a major role in palliation when the neoplasm has disseminated throughout the body.

In contrast, cancer chemotherapy and biotherapy can be curative even when the disease is widespread, because drugs can, at least theoretically, destroy cancer cells in all parts of the body. Modern treatment programs are designed to maximize the curative potential of each modality by utilizing each to exploit the different biological characteristics of each cancer. Today, surgery and radiation are often integrated with chemotherapy and biotherapy in order to preserve bodily function and to prevent distant metastases.

A. Surgery

M. Tish Knobf

INTRODUCTION

Surgery as the primary and definitive approach to cancer treatment has changed considerably over the past several decades. Surgical intervention continues to have a substantial impact on the curability of cancer as a primary treatment approach, specifically in patients with localized solid tumors. Although surgery remains the primary treatment for many newly diagnosed patients, it has increasingly become an integrated modality in oncology. The interdisciplinary, multimodality approach to cancer management has fostered the contribution and advances of each discipline in the management of specific malignancies. In addition, the current health care environment has further stimulated such collaborative efforts, resulting in the generation of interdisciplinary clinical practice guidelines (Winn, Botnick, and Dozier 1996). Such guidelines provide a consensus for treatment approaches and the opportunity for evaluating care of specific cancers and the associated therapeutic outcomes.

EVOLUTION OF SURGICAL ONCOLOGY

The introduction of general anesthesia and the principles of antisepsis in the mid-1800s was a significant development in surgery, particularly for the treatment of cancer. Historic milestones in the late 1800s include the first gastrectomy by Bilroth, thyroid surgery by Kocher, radical mastectomy by Halsted, and oophorectomy for breast cancer by Beatson. In the early 1900s, the surgical expertise in the treatment of major cancers, such as tumors of the prostate, uterus, and colon, continued to expand, and major advances were made in thoracic surgery.

Innovative surgical developments have continued in the late 20th century, such as microsurgery, stapling devices, lasers, and advances in laparascopic and endoscopic procedures. These developments have increased surgical options and can result in better physical and psychological outcomes for the patient. Salient examples include advances in colorectal surgery, which have dramatically altered the need for colostomy; nerve-sparing prostatectomy, which minimizes the risk of impotency; and surgical placement of prosthetics or bone grafts, which can allow limb preservation in patients with sarcoma.

The most significant advance, however, is related to the multidisciplinary approach to management. Several factors have facilitated this collaborative approach and expanded the role of each treatment modality: an increased understanding of the biology of cancer; improved recognition of the patterns of failure, particularly in solid tumors; identification of important prognostic factors; technological advances in surgery and radiation therapy; new chemotherapeutic agents; molecular and genetic developments; increased emphasis on the importance of participation in clinical trials; an expanding nursing research base; and a greater emphasis on quality-of-life issues.

2A

THE ROLE OF SURGERY IN CANCER

Surgery has a major role across the spectrum of the cancer experience, including prophylactic surgery for high-risk populations, diagnosis, staging, primary treatment, supportive and palliative procedures, resection of metastases, and rehabilitative surgery (Table 2A–1).

Table 2A–1
Approaches of Oncologic Surgical Management

Approach	Example
Prophylactic	Excision of premalignant lesions
Primary/Definitive	Local excision En bloc dissection
Supportive	Insertion of access devices Radiation implants
Palliative	Cytoreduction Oncologic emergencies Neurosurgical procedures/pain control Nutritional support
Resection of metastases	Pulmonary Liver
Rehabilitative	Cosmetic and functional restoration

Prophylaxis

The role for *prophylactic* surgery in preventing invasive carcinoma is limited, though it is well established for *in situ* cervical cancer and selected conditions with a high risk for malignant transformation. Surgical treatment for *in situ* cervical cancer produces a high cure rate that appears durable in long-term follow-up. Familial diseases (e.g., polyposis coli, familial breast, and ovarian and colon cancers) and selected underlying medical conditions (e.g., cryptorchidism, ulcerative colitis) represent premalignant diseases for which surgery might be considered. The degree of risk varies and must be evaluated carefully based on the patient's medical and family history. In addition, the patient's psychological status and perception of risk, as well as the effectiveness and morbidity of the procedure, must be taken into account.

Diagnosis

The diagnosis of cancer largely depends on tissue for pathologic examination. Common surgical techniques for obtaining a tissue sample include needle aspiration, core needle biopsy, and incisional and excisional biopsies (see Table 2A–2). Historically, incisional or excisional biopsies have been the most commonly performed biopsy techniques. Advances in technology combined with knowledge of the biology and behavior of specific malignancies has generated new approaches to obtaining tissue diagnosis. Examples include stereotactic core needle breast biopsy and endoscopic biopsy approaches. Prior to choosing a specific biopsy technique, the surgeon must consider the suspected diagnosis, the adequacy of tissue sample for the pathologist, and whether the tissue will require any special preparation (e.g., staining). Regardless of which technique is chosen, there are several important principles to observe: (1) carefully planning needle or incision placement so that tracks or scars will not compromise subsequent treatment or definitive resection; (2) avoiding contamination of uninvolved tissue planes; (3) avoiding excessive bleeding and hematomas; and (4) using separate instruments to obtain more than one tissue sample.

Staging

Staging provides a description of the cancer according to its local, regional, and distant extent. It is important to evaluate prognosis and treatment outcome and to determine primary treatment. The American Joint Committee on Cancer (AJCC) describes five methods for determining disease stage (Table 2A–3); the most commonly used are the clinical and the surgical evaluative/pathologic.

Table 2A–2
Surgical Techniques for Biopsy

Type	Method	Advantages	Disadvantages
Aspiration	Aspirate cells using a needle	Easily available materials Little or no local anesthesia required Inexpensive Minimal time	Margin of error Limitations of cytologic diagnosis Risk of injury to adjacent tissue
Core needle	Specially designed needle pulls out a core of tissue	Local anesthesia Minimal time Histologic diagnosis	Requires accessible target tissue Tissue specimen not adequate for all tumors
Incisional	Resection of part of a tumor	Local anesthesia often possible Histologic diagnosis Preferred for large masses	Potential sampling error Potential contamination of new tissue planes with tumor
Excisional	Removal of entire tumor	Local anesthesia often possible Histologic diagnosis Adequate tissue sample	Indicated for relatively small tumors

The most widely recommended system to stage cancer is TNM. T refers to the primary tumor, N to regional nodes, and M to distant metastases. This has been promoted by the International Union against Cancer (UICC) and the American Joint Committee on Cancer. Other systems are disease specific, such as FIGO (International Federation of Gynecologists and Obstetricians), for gynecological malignancies, and the Dukes' classification for colon cancer. Appendix C provides staging criteria for specific common cancers according to these systems. Surgical expertise is essential for pathologic staging to obtain knowledge of the disease's spread. This is critical because of the influence of staging on therapeutic decisions and patient outcome.

Treatment

The goal of *primary* or *definitive* surgical treatment is cure, by complete resection of all disease. The surgeon must know the natural history of the disease and be able to predict, with reasonable certainty, the feasibility

Table 2A–3
Staging of Cancer

Type	Method	Data Base	Comment
1. Clinical diagnostic	Physical exam X-rays and scans Biopsy	All information available prior to definitive treatment	Almost all cancers are clinically staged. Accuracy limited.
2. Surgical evaluation	Biopsy Exploratory surgery with intraoperative palpation ± biopsies	All clinical information Histology from biopsies	More information is required to make definitive treatment decision. Examples include exploratory laparotomy for Hodgkin's disease; mediastinoscopy for lung primary.
3. Postsurgical pathologic	Resection of tumor	Histologic information on all resected tissues	Comprehensive histologic information of the tumor ± regional nodes or organs.
4. Retreatment	Biopsy Blood studies X-rays and scans Tumor markers, where appropriate	Clinical information and histology, where available	Restaging indicated for additional or secondary treatment, e.g., Hodgkin's disease, testicular cancer. In ovarian cancer, "second-look" operations to determine presence or absence of disease are now less common with diagnostic imaging advances.
5. Autopsy	Evaluation of all tissues	Pathologic	Very accurate. May provide useful information to clinicians but value somewhat limited.

of a curative resection. In addition, the surgeon must consider the mortality and morbidity associated with the specific operative procedure and the general status of the patient (e.g., functional status, preexisting conditions, nutritional status, rehabilitation potential). The age of patients should not influence the decision to operate unless it is associated with advanced disease or co-morbid conditions that would compromise the potential outcome.

Local excision and en bloc dissections are definitive surgical interventions for resectable solid tumors. *Local excision,* with or without wide margins (sufficient to ensure normal margins free of tumor), is commonly used for basal cell carcinomas of the skin and primary melanomas. *En bloc dissection* refers to more extensive resection with total removal of the tumor with or without regional lymphatics, such as for colon, lung, or gynecologic cancers. Over the past decade, there has been an increasing effort to decrease the invasiveness and complications of surgical intervention. The goal is to conserve tissues or structures, function, and cosmesis without compromising cure. Technological advances in surgery alone or advances in multimodality approaches, which can achieve the same or an improved curability outcome, have made significant contributions to the quality of life for patients with cancer in the past decade. Examples include limb preservation in sarcoma, breast-preserving surgery with radiation therapy for breast cancer, nerve-sparing prostatectomy, and sphincter-sparing surgery for colorectal malignancies. In addition, newer surgical techniques, such as Mohs micrographic surgery for skin cancer, produces high cure rates and better conservation of tissue and skin. This technique is particularly useful in areas such as the eyelid and lips, where skin conservation is critical. For large tumors that either are unresectable or associated with a very poor prognosis if resected, the multimodality approach using chemotherapy as initial treatment (referred to as neoadjuvant) has resulted in tumor shrinkage to permit surgical resection. Encouraging results thus far include Stage III breast cancer and more advanced staged gynecologic cancers.

Supportive Care

The *supportive* role of surgery has become an integral part of oncology practice. Insertion of devices such as implanted vascular access ports and central venous catheters provide the means for delivery of systemic or regional cytotoxic therapy and supportive therapy (e.g., blood products, antibiotics). Insertion of devices can also provide access for palliative therapy with greater safety, convenience, and symptom control (e.g., via the Ommaya reservoir for the administration of treatment for CNS disease).

Palliation

The goal of *palliative* surgical treatment for cancer is optimal quality of life for the patient for whom cure is not possible. The indications for surgery vary widely. Some procedures might prolong survival, such as cytoreductive surgery in ovarian cancer followed by chemotherapy. Other more common palliative procedures focus on relief of symptoms, maintenance of organ function, and prevention of significant or fatal complications. Examples include surgery to repair damage from oncologic emergencies, such as hemorrhage, perforation, or spinal cord compression; bypass surgery for intestinal obstruction; lysis of adhesions; feeding jejunostomy for an altered upper gastrointestinal tract; neurosurgical procedures to relieve or reduce pain; tracheostomy for airway obstruction; debridement and grafting for wound or skin complications; and urological procedures such as insertion of stents to maintain renal function.

Treatment of Metastases

The indications for *resection* of metastases are limited but can provide improved survival in selected patients. Resection of pulmonary metastases in patients with sarcoma, testicular cancer, and melanoma have been reported to significantly improve five-year survival rates, and selected patients with colon cancer could similarly benefit from resection of hepatic metastases. In addition to prolonging survival, these procedures enhance quality of life by providing a symptom-free period. The morbidity of the surgical procedure, type and length of recovery, and the likely time until recurrence are critical factors to weigh in order to determine the risks and benefits of any procedure.

Rehabilitation

The goal of *rehabilitative* surgery is restoration of function and cosmesis. Physical, psychological, and sexual rehabilitation is expected for patients receiving cancer therapy. Advances in surgery, especially in the field of plastic and reconstructive surgery, have increased rehabilitative options for patients. There have been dramatic improvements in existing procedures as well as new techniques (e.g., microsurgical tissue transfer) in reconstructive surgery for head and neck and breast cancers.

Laser Surgery

The role of laser surgery in cancer treatment is evolving. The word *laser* stands for light amplification of stimulated emission of radiation. Lasers produce thermal and nonthermal effects. The thermal effect is a result of heat that is generated by the laser beam, which in turn destroys the tissue. Laser heat is powerful and highly selective, concentrating its energy on a small surface. Laser therapy for cervical carcinoma *in situ* produces similar cure rates to cryosurgery or cold-knife conization and has the advantage of preserving more normal tissue. The disadvantages are cost and the need for experienced personnel.

Lasers can produce nonthermal effects through photodissociation, creation of shock waves, fluorescence, and induction of chemical reactions. Well-known examples include treatment of cataracts, kidney stones, and gallstones. The energy from the laser beam creates an ionized plasma, producing shock waves that break apart the stones or the opaque posterior membrane of the secondary cataract. In cancer treatment, the role of lasers in photochemical reactions is under investigation. Patients are injected with a photosensitizing dye, which tumors retain. This is followed by laser treatment, which produces a chemical reaction that destroys the tumor cells. Although there are reported successes in the palliative treatment of a variety of tumors, this photodynamic therapy remains under investigation. A major disadvantage thus far has been prolonged photosensitivity (one to two months after injection) to the dye. Other disadvantages include equipment expense and the need for specially trained personnel (physician, nurse, technician). Although their role in treatment continues to be evaluated, the use of lasers combined with fiber optics could have exciting diagnostic potential for the future.

QUALITY OF LIFE

Quality of life is a multidimensional construct. Although there are multiple definitions of the concept of quality of life, there appears to be consensus on the following dimensions as key components to one's quality of life: physical, psychological, social, and spiritual. All dimensions are affected by a cancer diagnosis and primary therapy. Surgery, as a primary therapy, can dramatically alter the physical dimension of one's quality of life, possibly compromising function, comfort, cosmesis, and body image. Advances in surgical techniques combined with an emphasis on conserving tissues and function (Table 2A–4) have contributed to the goal of curative cancer therapy with an optimal quality of life. Quality of life is also a dynamic concept and requires assessment over time. Long-term side effects of therapy can compromise quality of life, as do short-term or immediate surgical sequelae. Alterations in sexual potency and bladder function in men after surgery for prostate cancer, living with a stoma following colorectal surgery, and changes in sexuality and bladder function for women with gynecologic cancer secondary to surgical intervention highlight a few examples of therapy outcomes that have an impact on the physical dimension of quality of life in cancer survivors. Because quality of life is complex and multidimensional, the impact of physical alterations related to cancer treatment will most likely affect other dimensions, such as the psychological and social, including sexual, aspects of one's perceived quality of life. Therefore, evaluation of the patient should be sufficiently broad-based to capture dimensions of quality of life as well as treatment outcome indicators, such as response and survival.

NURSING CONSIDERATIONS

Providing high-quality nursing care to cancer patients who require surgical intervention is a significant challenge. Factors that influence care delivery and patient outcome are the transition from primary care provider to multiple specialists in different settings in a relatively short period of time, the high percentage of care occurring in ambulatory settings, length of hospital stay, and model of nursing care delivery. Surgical nursing care is typically described according to the timing of a surgical event: diagnos-

Table 2A–4
Evolution of Therapies for Management of Solid Tumors

Past Treatment	Present Treatment	Future Treatment
Radical surgery	Conservation surgery	Ultraconservation surgery
Chemotherapy for advanced disease	Adjuvant/neoadjuvant chemotherapy	Advanced neoadjuvant/ adjuvant chemotherapeutic/ pharmacologic therapies
Nonselective external-beam radiotherapy	Selective external-beam radiotherapy with or without brachytherapy irradiation	Selective external-beam and brachytherapy irradiation
	Focused application of biologic tumor modifier/immunotherapy	Biologic response modifiers
		Antiangiogenesis tumor induction
		Metalloprotease inhibitors
		Immunotherapies/tumor vaccines (active)
		Gene therapy
Examples	**Examples**	**Examples**
Halsted radical mastectomy	Conservation breast surgery	Selective tumor cytoreductive neoadjuvant therapies/irradiation
	Sphincter-sparing anorectal resections	
Radical limb amputations	Limb-sparing surgery	Conservation/ ultraconservation breast/ colon/neck resection
Radical neck lymph-node dissection	Modified neck lymph-node dissection	Postoperative selective biologic or antiangiogenesis therapies

Reprinted with permission from Bland, K. I. *Quality of life management of cancer patients. CA A J Clin* 47(4): 194–196. 1997.

tic (biopsy), preoperative, postoperative, and discharge planning. The dramatic decrease in length of hospital stay and shift to short-stay surgery (less than 24 hours) have significantly challenged nurses who provide care to surgical patients. Preoperative classes by appointment with caregivers in attendance, caregiver demonstration of proficiency prior to discharge for postoperative care, and preprinted order forms during the perioperative phase to facilitate timely discharge for 23-hour short-stay patients are examples of creative strategies to maintain quality nursing care delivery with optimal patient outcomes. Collaboration among nurses in various health care settings (inpatient, ambulatory, home care) is necessary to communicate patient information, and to reduce repetitive, redundant assessments; help patients negotiate the system with the least amount of distress; and implement a plan of care that is progressive and continuous. One strategy is to identify generic components of nursing practice in surgical oncology—i.e., assessment, teaching/learning, emotional support, physical care, and rehabilitation—considering each for its essential contribution to a patient at a given time as well as over the course of the illness.

Assessment

Basic data must be collected on patients whether the purpose is preoperative assessment or discharge planning. A detailed physiologic assessment can be adapted for acute, critical, and outpatient care. The goal of assessment is maintenance of a current data base on the patient so that the plan of care and interventions are appropriate. Building on an initial assessment, rather than reassessing patients as they move from setting to setting, should be a goal. Coordination and communication among nurses in the various settings are the first steps in developing guidelines for assessment and evaluation of interventions as the patient moves through the health care system. The use of computerized data systems for patient information and care delivery greatly facilitates the transfer of data, reduces the burden on the patient and health care providers, and promotes continuity of care.

Teaching/Learning

Assessment of learning needs and provision of information occurs throughout a patient's illness but is likely to be of paramount importance in surgical oncology at the time of initial biopsy, between diagnosis and definitive treatment, and at discharge (see Chapter 6A). The time periods between suspicion of cancer and biopsy, and between biopsy and definitive treatment have been reported by patients as highly stressful, characterized by anxiety, fear, and overall emotional distress. Patients are often overwhelmed by information and need time and professional help to consider the impact of the diagnosis and prognosis and to make decisions for definitive therapy. It is important to assess what level of participation in the decision making process is desired by the patient, because that will help direct the nurse's informational interventions and can reduce anxiety and psychological distress. This is particularly important for patients who have a choice between two treatment options (e.g., mastectomy versus wide excision/axillary dissection/radiation therapy) or are deciding between participating in a clinical trial or receiving standard therapy.

Accurate preparation for surgical procedures, preferably oral and written, for the patient, family, and/or significant others is essential. Sensory information and visual depiction are good strategies to enhance the patient's understanding and expectations. Nursing research published 20 years ago on the value of sensory preparatory information continues to be confirmed in today's practice. Visual depiction of procedures and description of common sensations experienced by patients are helpful in reducing anxiety and emotional distress.

Discharge is a critical time, as length of hospital stay shortens and expectations for self-care and family involvement in care escalate. Referral for postoperative home care needs is common for the patient discharged from hospital to home, but less routine is *communication* among nurses in ambulatory settings such as clinics and physician offices. Whom to call (e.g., the home care nurse, the surgeon, the primary oncologist) for which symptoms, when to resume certain activities, and what to expect emotionally are important, often lingering questions for patients. Written discharge instructions to supplement oral information is strongly recommended. Telephone follow-up after discharge (e.g., the next day) and a postoperative home or office/clinic visit by a nurse to assess status and self-care management are additional approaches to maximize recovery, minimize urgent care visits for complications, and promote optimal quality of life.

Emotional Support

Identifying the patient's need for emotional support begins with baseline assessment of the patient, particularly self-concept and coping skills/styles. Other important variables include the existing support system, disease status, prognosis, treatment options, and functional status (see Chapter 7). The patient's need for emotional support will also depend on where he or she is in the course of the disease. One survey of gynecological cancer patients by Corney and colleagues (1992) showed that two-thirds of the respondents were alone when the diagnosis was given, and many reported the time between diagnosis and surgery as the most stressful period. Nursing intervention during this time is imperative yet often lacking.

Physical Care

Care required to meet physical needs related to surgical intervention can be delivered by either a nurse, the patient, a family member or significant other, or ancillary personnel. Nursing care for the surgical oncology patient follows generic surgical nursing principles and focuses on physiologic maintenance: cardiovascular, pulmonary, renal, integumentary, gastrointestinal, nutrition, and mobility. Trends in ambulatory surgery, express admissions, and shortened hospital stays have shifted care significantly to the home. Regardless of agency referrals and support, the patient is integrally involved and often responsible for elements of self-care. This shift reemphasizes the importance of assessment of learning needs and of the ability of the patient and family to manage the physiologic aspects of care and to assess the psychosocial response in order to provide timely and effective interventions.

Rehabilitation

Rehabilitation begins following diagnosis and initially consists of teaching, providing emotional support, and preparing the patient for surgical intervention. Following surgery, rehabilitation is focused on meeting the patient's basic needs: physical, psychological, social, sexual, financial, occupational, and informational. Baseline assessment will provide information to identify potential problem areas, and the type of cancer surgery will predict specific needs. For example, alterations in body image and sexual functions are predictable issues for patients who undergo gynecological surgery, prostate surgery, or colon resection that requires a colostomy. Difficulty with such issues might surface immediately after surgery, but it is more common to observe concerns a few months after physical recovery. It is critical that patients know whom to call and that they are encouraged to maintain contact with health care providers. The timing and frequency of routine postsurgical follow-up does not necessarily coincide with the peak times of need for the patient. This dilemma provides another opportunity for nurses to creatively and innovatively develop models that promote ongoing patient access to care during a critical rehabilitation period.

SUMMARY

Surgical oncology is a rapidly expanding subspecialty that offers varied and exciting roles for nurses. Like the surgical oncologist, the surgical oncology nurse must be knowledgeable about other disciplines, participate in multidisciplinary conferences, and take a leadership role in coordinating care, communicating with nursing colleagues in other settings, and teaching general surgical nurses as well as oncology nurses from other disciplines.

BIBLIOGRAPHY

1. Barrere, C. C. Breast biopsy support program: Collaboration between the oncology clinical nurse specialist and the ambulatory surgery nurse. *Oncol Nurs Forum* 9(19): 1375–79. 1992.

A collaborative approach to address the pre- and postoperative psychosocial needs of women undergoing breast biopsy is reviewed. The interaction between ambulatory surgery nurses and the oncology clinical specialist is discussed, as well as the use of goal-directed communication in meeting the emotional and information needs of women prior to biopsy and after, when diagnosis is established.

2. Bassett, L., D. P. Winchester, B. Caplan et al. Stereotactic core-needle biopsy of the breast: a report of the Joint Task Force of the American College of Radiology, American College of Surgeons and College of American Pathologists. *CA A J Clin* 47(3) 171–190. 1997.

   This article provides a comprehensive review of stereotactic core needle biopsy for breast lesions including indications, contraindications, informed consent, specimen handling, communication of results, patient management and follow-up, and quality assurance issues.

3. Burke, C. C., C. L. Zabka, K. J. McCarver, and S. E. Singletary. Patient satisfaction with 23 hour "short stay" observation following breast cancer surgery. *Oncol Nurs Forum* 24(4): 645–51. 1997.

   This article reviews a programmatic approach to the transition of a 23-hour hospital stay for patients who undergo breast cancer surgery. Preoperative preparation, perioperative system issues related to practice, and postoperative discharge standards are described in detail.

4. Corney, R., H. Everett, A. Howells, and M. Crowther. The care of patients undergoing surgery for gynecological cancer: The need for information, emotional support and counseling. *J Adv Nurs* 17: 667–71. 1992.

   This is a report of a study of 105 patients who had undergone gynecological surgery. The psychosocial and psychological adjustment of this group was investigated by means of data collected during semi-structured interviews.

5. Davison, B. J., and L. F. Degner. Empowerment of men newly diagnosed with prostate cancer. *Canc Nurs* 20(3): 187–96. 1997.

   This article reported on a study that provided men with newly diagnosed prostate cancer a self-efficacy intervention (written information, with discussion, questions to ask and audiotape of the medical consultation) or written information alone. Men who received the self-efficacy intervention assumed a more active role in decision making and had lower levels of state anxiety at six weeks following the intervention.

6. DeCosse, J. J., and W. J. Cennerazzo. Quality of life managment of patients with colorectal cancer. *CA A J Clin* 47(4): 198–206. 1997.

   This article reviews quality of life issues for the patient diagnosed and treated for colorectal cancer, including coping with the side effects of surgery.

7. Dobkin, K. A., and D. C. Broadwell. Nursing consideration for the patient undergoing colostomy surgery. *Semin Oncol Nurs* 4(2): 249–55. 1986.

   This article describes the types of colostomies created, psychosocial and sexual issues facing patients with colostomies, and nursing care needs for patients with newly created colostomies, including preoperative and postoperative and colostomy care.

8. Donegan, W. L. Operative treatment of cancer in the older patient by general surgeons. In Balducci, A., G. H. Lyman, and W. B. Ershler, eds. *Geriatric Oncology.* 151–159. J. B. Lippincott, Philadelphia. 1992.

This chapter, in a text covering treatment of the older patient with cancer, reviews the frequency of minor and major cancer surgeries in a community teaching hospital, postoperative complications, and mortality in older patients.

9. Dziurbejko, M. M., and J. C. Larkin. Including the family in preoperative teaching. *Am J Nurs* 11: 1892–94. 1978.

This early nursing research article describes the benefits of preoperative teaching to female patients undergoing gynecologic surgery with respect to reducing anxiety, increasing cooperation, and reducing length of hospital stay and number of opioid injections. The greatest positive effect was seen for the experimental group that included both the patient and family.

10. Frogge, M. H., and B. H. Kalinowski. Surgical Therapy. In Groenwald, S. L., M. H. Frogge, M. Goodman, and C. H. Yarbro, eds. *Cancer Nursing Principles and Practice*, 4th ed. 229–246. Jones & Bartlett, Boston. 1997.

A comprehensive overview of surgical oncology is presented with special considerations for nursing care.

11. Herr, H. W. Quality of life in prostate cancer patients. *CA A J Clin* 47(4): 207–217. 1997.

This author reviews the treatment options for prostate cancer, the clinical outcomes over the past decade and results of quality of life studies with patients and spouses.

12. Kelly, P., and E. H. Winslow. Needle wire localization for nonpalpable breast lesions: Sensations, anxiety levels and informational needs. *Oncol Nurs Forum* 23(4): 639–45. 1996.

A descriptive study was conducted to determine the sensations experienced during needle wire localization for nonpalpable breast lesions and the level of preprocedure anxiety. A moderate to high level of anxiety and a variety of sensations experienced by women were reported. Providing sensory information before the procedure was the recommendation by the authors.

13. McCaughan, L. Lasers in photodynamic therapy. *Nurs Clin North Am* 3(25): 725–38. 1990.

This article is a review of the uses of laser treatment for malignant diseases. It provides information on the treatment process, equipment and personnel requirements, patient selection, and nursing care requirements prior to, during, and after the procedure.

14. McHugh, N. G., N. J. Christman, and J. E. Johnson. Preparatory information: What helps and why. *Am J Nurs* 5: 780–82. 1982.

This article discusses the nature of information that contributes to decreased distress during and after procedures. Though brief, it provides excellent guidelines to assist in identifying information needed by individual patients.

15. Northouse, L. L., K. M. Tocco, and P. West. Coping with a breast biopsy: How healthcare professionals can help women and their husbands. *Oncol Nurs Forum* 24(3): 473–480. 1997.

A study was conducted to examine the types of information women received from their physicians prior to breast biopsy and to describe the concerns of women and their husbands during this time. A high degree of concern was associated with breast biopsy in women and their husbands regardless of whether the woman was told that she probably did not have cancer. The need for information and support, involving husbands, was recommended.

16. Polomano, R., F. N. Weintraub, and A. Wurster. Surgical critical care for cancer patients. *Semin Oncol Nurs* 10(3): 165–176. 1994.

   The authors provide a review of the potential problems experienced by surgical oncology patients and associated nursing care.

17. Steginga, S. K., and J. Dunn. Women's experiences following treatment for gynecologic cancer. *Oncol Nurs Forum* 24(8): 1403–1408. 1997.

   A descriptive study of women previously treated for a variety of gynecologic cancers was carried out to identify psychological and physical difficulties; informational, emotional, and practical support; and coping strategies. Women described a wide range of physical and psychosocial difficulties and reported family as providers of emotional support.

18. Winn, R. J., W. Botnick, and N. Dozier. The NCCN Guidelines development program. *Oncology* 10(11): 23–28. 1996.

   The National Comprehensive Cancer Network (NCCN) is described with its program for development of clinical practice guidelines. Definitions, goals, and steps in the guideline development are presented. This article is part of a special supplement issue that reviews the eight adult cancer guidelines developed thus far in addition to articles that address quality of life, guideline implementation and evaluation.

19. Yasko, A. W., G. P. Reece, T. A. Gillis, and R. E. Pollack. Limb-salvage strategies to optimize quality of life: The M.D. Anderson Cancer Center experience. *CA A J Clin* 47(4): 226–238. 1997.

   This article reviews the multidisciplinary approach to management of sarcomas, preoperative and operative strategies, limb salvage, and rehabilitation. Discussion is enhanced by the inclusion of selected case studies.

B. Radiation Therapy

Cheryl McCullen Tafas
Jennifer Dunn Bucholtz

INTRODUCTION

Radiation therapy employs ionizing radiation to treat disease. Although it can be used to treat specific benign diseases—such as hyperthyroidism, benign brain tumors, and heterotopic bone formation—it is most commonly used to treat malignant tumors. Approximately 60 percent of all persons with cancer will receive radiation therapy during some stage of their illness. In general, radiation is considered a local therapy utilizing external beam x-rays or gamma rays as well as radioactive sources that are strategically placed in close proximity to a tumor located in a specific area of the body. However, unsealed radioactive isotopes can also be given systemically: orally, intravenously, or by instillation.

GOALS OF TREATMENT

The goals of radiation therapy in the oncology patient care setting are similar to treatment goals for other cancer therapies and include (1) cure of disease, (2) control of disease locally or limitation of its growth, (3) palliation of distressing symptoms, and (4) prophylaxis or prevention of disease recurring in a particular body site. Table 2B–1 lists examples of diagnoses commonly treated with these four goals. It might be the sole treatment for some cancers but is often combined with other treatment modalities such as surgery, chemotherapy, or biotherapy to achieve the desired goal of tumor eradication or palliation. Nurses might be most familiar with the use

2B

Table 2B–1
Examples of Cancer Diagnoses Treated with Radiation Therapy Classified by Potential Therapeutic Intent

Intent	Example
Cure (stage dependent)	Basal cell cancer
	Hodgkin's disease
	Seminoma of testes
	Thyroid cancer
	Cervical cancer
	Head/neck cancer
	Breast cancer
	Prostate cancer
	Medulloblastoma
	Non-Hodgkin's lymphoma
	Anal cancer
	Lung cancer (early stage)
Control (stage-dependent)	Lung cancer (advanced stage)
	High-grade glioma
	Head and neck cancer (advanced stage)
Palliation	Spinal cord compression
	Brain metastases
	Bone metastases
	Superior vena cava syndrome
	Tracheal obstruction
	Uncontrolled bleeding from tumor
Prophylaxis	Small cell lung cancer in CNS
	Acute lymphoblastic leukemia in CNS

CNS—central nervous system.

of radiation for palliation, especially for bone pain or oncologic emergencies. Approximately 50 percent of people who receive radiation, however, are treated with the intent of cure.

THE BIOLOGY OF RADIATION THERAPY

The challenge of radiation therapy is to deliver a precisely measured dose of ionizing radiation to a specific tumor volume resulting in maximum tumor cell kill while causing minimal injury to the structure and function of adjacent normal tissues and organs. Radiation causes cellular damage when high energy electromagnetic photons, electrons, or nuclear particles interact with the atoms and molecules of cells. The process of ionization involves the interaction of radiation with the target atoms causing the ejection of orbital electrons. This leads to biological changes in DNA, which can cause death of both normal and malignant cells. The mechanism of action of radiation therapy is not by "burning," as many people think, but by permanent damage to the DNA molecule inside the tumor cell either directly or indirectly, in such a way that the tumor cell can no longer divide and will eventually die.

The interaction of ionizing radiation with target cell DNA can lead to cell death by a variety of mechanisms. If the ionizing radiation interacts with DNA directly, the process is referred to as a *direct effect*. This includes double- or single-strand breaks and base pair damage or deletions in DNA's double helix structure and is the dominant damaging process caused by neutrons and alpha particles. The dominant mechanism of cellular damage for photons and electrons, the most common forms of radiation used clinically, involves an *indirect effect*. In this process, the ionizing radiation interacts with cellular water producing free radicals. These reactive substances subsequently disrupt molecular bonds within DNA and can cause cellular death.

There are various forms of ionizing radiation that can be used clinically to treat specific disease processes. These forms are chosen on the basis of how and where the radiation needs to be delivered inside the body. Ionizing radiation is divided into two categories: electromagnetic and particulate. *Electromagnetic radiation* is high-frequency, high-energy waves called *photons,* which include x-rays and gamma rays. X-rays are electrically produced by specially designed equipment such as linear accelerators, betatrons, or orthovoltage units. They have the ability to penetrate to deeply seated tumors and produce ionization in living cells by interacting with matter through which they pass. Gamma rays are produced by emission of energy from the decay of an unstable atomic nucleus, which is attempting to become more stable. They are emitted by radioactive materials such as cobalt 60, which can be housed in a treatment machine, or sources such as cesium, iridium, iodine, or gold, which can be used for internal radiation applications. Despite their sources, x-rays and gamma rays are identical in all other respects, have similar biologic effects, and damage cells largely through an indirect effect.

Other types of radiation used clinically include *particulate radiation,* which does not have the penetrating distance of x-rays and gamma rays, and differs from electromagnetic waves in that these particles have measurable mass and might or might not be electrically charged. Although particulate radiation can be directed to precise body sites, the machinery needed to produce some forms of it is complex and expensive. Specific particles that can be used for therapy are alpha and beta particles, protons, neutrons, and electrons. Electrons are the most frequently used form of particulate radiation and can be accelerated to high speeds through the use of electrical devices such as a linear acclerator.

Radiation kills some cancer cells more effectively than others. Factors influencing cellular radiosensitivity include cell cycle phase, tissue oxygenation, and cell type. The actual total dose of radiation required to eradicate a tumor is a function of tumor size. Normal cells and tissues have a specific amount of radiation that they can safely tolerate, which is determined by the most radiosensitive cell population of a specific organ and the volume of the organ radiated. This largely determines the maximum dose of radiation that can be given, the side effects of treatment, as well as the treatment outcome. Although some tumors could be classified as radiosensitive, they might not be considered curable by radiation due to normal adjacent tissue tolerance and other factors. In other words, the amount of radiation needed to eradicate a tumor might not be tolerated by normal cells in close proximity. If, however, the dose of radiation required to kill a specific tumor can be delivered without causing significant irreversible injury to normal tissues, eradication of the tumor can be attained. Tables 2B–2 and 2B–3 list the radiosensitivity of certain tumors and normal tissues.

Table 2B–2
Relative Radiosensitivity of Tumors

Sensitivity	Tumor
High	Lymphoma
	Leukemia
	Seminoma
	Dysgerminoma
	Squamous cell cancers of the head and neck and anus
Medium	Astrocytoma
	Lung cancer (non–small cell)
	Colon cancer
	Salivary gland tumors
Low	Hepatoma
	Osteogenic sarcoma
	Renal cell cancer
	Pancreatic cancer
	Sarcoma

Table 2B–3
Relative Radiosensitivity of Normal Tissues

Sensitivity	System	Normal
High	Reproductive	Fetus Ovary Testes
	Gastrointestinal	Intestines Liver
	Genitourinary	Kidney
	Other	Bone marrow Lymphoid organs Head and neck mucosa Cornea Optic lens Lung Immature brain
Medium	Endocrine	Thyroid Pituitary
	Cardiopulmonary	Lung Heart
	Gastrointestinal	Stomach Pancreas Esophagus
	Other	Growing bone and cartilage Skin Bladder Spinal cord
Low	Connective	Mature Bone Cartilage Muscle
	Genitourinary	Cervix Vagina
	Other	Mature brain Adrenals Rectum

Note: Each organ/tissue has a maximal tolerated dose of radiation before acute or permanent injury occurs.

The International Commission on Radiological Units has proposed the adoption of the Gray (Gy) or centigray (cGy) as the unit of measure of the dose of radiation that is prescribed. The rad, which reflects the radiation absorbed dose, was the unit of measure used until the mid 1980s. One Gray is equal to 100 rads and one centigray is equal to one rad. Daily doses of radiation can range from 180 to 400 cGy. The total dose of conventionally fractionated radiation can range from 2,000 cGy to 7,000 cGy and is determined by many factors, including treatment goals (i.e., cure or palliation) and the type and bulk of tumor being treated.

Fractionation, or the dividing of a total dose of radiation into equal daily fractions, reduces normal tissue damage and improves the biological effectiveness of treatment in several ways:

1. It allows the normal tissues to repair damage between daily doses, something tumor cells are theoretically less capable of doing as treatment progresses;
2. It allows repopulation of normal tissues after repair of injury from radiation;
3. It redistributes tumor cells in their cell cycle, potentially making more tumor cells radiosensitive;
4. It allows time for tumor cells to reoxygenate.

Standard fractionation in the United States involves the delivery of 180–200 cGy once daily, Monday through Friday. In Europe and Canada, fraction sizes of 250 cGy are commonly used. When radiation is given on a continuous basis, as with internal methods, more complex radiobiological effects involving tissue damage and repair occur.

In addition to single daily treatment fractions, alternative fractionation schedules are being used to achieve greater cell kill by either allowing higher total doses to be given or decreasing the opportunity for tumor cell regeneration during the radiation therapy course. These include *hyperfractionation,* which uses smaller than standard doses given more than once per day to approximate a standard daily treatment dose or a slightly greater than standard treatment dose, and *accelerated fractionation,* which refers to giving a much shorter overall course of treatment by using close to standard doses per fraction and increasing the number of fractions per day. For instance, instead of using a single standard daily dose of 200 cGy for treatment of a head and neck tumor, a hyperfractionation schedule might administer 120 cGy twice per day; an accelerated schedule might administer 160 cGy twice per day completing the treatment course in a shorter number of days. (For special techniques in radiation therapy see Table 2B–4.)

Other efforts intended to improve tumor cell kill without increasing damage to normal cells include the development of chemical modifiers used concurrently with radiation therapy. These compounds are called *radiosensitizers* and *radioprotectors,* and they either enhance the damaging effects of ionizing radiation on tumor cells or protect normal cells and tissues against

Table 2B-4
Special Techniques In Radiation Therapy

Technique	Description	Side Effects

Stereotactic Radiosurgery (SRS)	A method of administering a precise beam of radiation to a discrete intracranial lesion (more than one lesion can be treated)
	Can be delivered by a gamma knife, a modified linear accelerator, a linear accelerator designed for radiosurgery, or charged particle beams
	Involves giving one or more large fractions of high dose radiation
	Linear accelerator systems deliver treatment in an arc fashion, administering the target dose to the tumor while sparing normal brain
	Requires sophisticated computerized treatment planning
	Uses special head immobilization devices to ensure precise target
	Treatment times are often lengthy and can last an hour or longer
	Doses vary; the single dose fraction ranges from 1,200 cGy to 3,000 cGy
	Common tumors treated: gliomas, meningiomas, craniopharyngiomas, accoustic neuromas, arteriovenous malformations, pituitary adenomas, and metastatic lesions
	Potential exists to treat other body sites when immobilation devices are developed to ensure precise localization of the tumor
		Potential infection or discomfort from head frame or screw placed in the skull
		Cerebral edema, which might be present for months after treatment, can cause increased intracranial pressure manifested as headaches, visual disturbances, nausea, vomiting, seizures, personality and cognitive changes, changes in level of consciousness and other neurological symptoms, such as limb weakness (see Chapter 15A)
		Alopecia
		
		Long term effects:
		  cerebral edema
		  brain necrosis
		  permanent cranial nerve damage
		  decreased hormone production
		  secondary neoplasms (rare)

Stereotactic Radiotherapy (SRT)	Multiple fractions are given with stereotactic technique and head immobilization Noninvasive head fixation is used (i.e., masks) Fractionated doses up to 6,000 cGy can be used	Same as for SRS

Total Body Irradiation (TBI)	A preparative regimen given prior to bone marrow transplantation, particularly for leukemias and lymphomas
	Objective is to eradicate tumor cells and suppress the immune response allowing engraftment to occur
	Radiation is given to the entire body 2 to 3 times per day for 3 days
	Doses vary but standard protocols deliver a total of 1,200 cGy
	Lead blocks can be used to reduce the dose to the lungs
	Patient will be placed in a side lying position or lie prone/supine
		Multi-organ effects:
		  alopecia
		  parotiditis
		  xerostomia
		  ocular dryness
		  nausea and vomiting
		  oral mucositis
		  diarrhea
		  fatigue
		  fever
		  skin erythema
		  pancreatitis (possible)

Technique	Description	Side Effects

	Treatment time often takes an hour, including set-up time	Long term effects:
		  cataracts
		  pneumonitis and fibrosis
		  veno-occlusive disease
		  sterility
		  myelodysplasia
		  delayed growth and development for children
		  secondary malignancies

	Total skin low energy electron radiation can be given for the treatment of cutaneous T-cell lymphoma and Kaposi's sarcoma Treats the entire skin surface while sparing deeper tissues (i.e., GI tract, bone marrow) Usually given with patient in a standing position Eyes and nail beds are shielded Total dose ranges from 3,000 cGy to 3,600 cGy and is fractionated over several weeks	Skin erythema Desquamation Generalized skin edema Temporary alteration in sweat gland function
Hyperthermia	The application of heat to tumors in the temperature range of 41–45 degrees C to improve local and regional tumor control Heat kills cells in a resting or radioresistant phase, inhibits the repair of radiation damage, and can work synergistically with radiation and chemotherapy (usually given in combination) Can be local, regional, or whole body Various radiofrequency and ultrasound applicators are used Procedure lasts 60–90 minutes Presence of any metallic objects in the body might be a contraindication Can be utilized in a number of cancers including brain, breast, esophageal, vaginal, and rectal	Skin reactions are most common and can include blisters and complete skin breakdown; discomfort from heat and placement of microwave heating devices; infection or irritation at cannula site Site specific: temporary or permanent sterility, cataracts, hyperthermia With whole body: nausea, vomiting, diarrhea, fatigue, electrolyte disturbances, cardiac arrythmias, and drug enhancement can occur
Intraoperative Radiotherapy (IORT)	The delivery of a large single dose of a high energy electron beam to a surgically exposed tumor or resected tumor bed with the goal of improving local tumor control and minimizing radiation exposure to normal tissues Used most commonly in cancers of the stomach, pancreas, colon, and rectum, and less commonly to sarcomas and recurrent GU and GYN cancers Common dose given: 1,500–2,000 cGy	Anastamotic leaks Wound infections Hemorrhage Postoperative complications

Continued

Special Techniques In Radiation Therapy

Technique	Description	Side Effects
	Can be performed in a dedicated operating room or in a radiation therapy department after transporting the anesthetized, surgically prepared patient from the operating room Adjuvant treatment with external beam radiation or chemotherapy is common	
Radiosensitizers	Chemicals administered intravenously or intraarterially to increase the effect of radiation when given concurrently **Hypoxic cell sensitizers** replace oxygen and make tumor cells more radiosensitive Types: *Oxygen mimetic sensitizers* like SR 2508 (etanidazole) and nimorazole; administered intravenously and followed by RT	Peripheral neuropathy, nausea, vomiting, rash, cramping; arthralgias can occur but are unusual; nimorazole is less toxic
	Glutathione modulators cause depletion of this tripeptide, which normally detoxifies cytotoxic agents by scavenging free radicals and competing with oxygen; includes an agent called BSO	
	Non-hypoxic cell sensitizers Includes halogenated pyrimidines IUdR (iododeoxyuridine) and BUdR (bromodeoxyuridine); both have thymidine and are taken up by and incorporated into the DNA making it more radiosensitive; depend on actively dividing tumor cells to work, therefore thymidine metabolism modulation is being explored	Dose limiting toxicities are myelosuppression and mucositis
	Hypoxic cytotoxic agents have independent cytotoxic activity and can work to enhance radiation cytotoxicity; include SR4233 (tirapazamine) and analogues of Mitomycin (EO9), which both have selective toxicity for hypoxic cells; dual function agents like RB 6145 being researched Erythropoietin increases the oxygen carrying capacity of the blood; nicotinamide produces alterations in blood flow	
Radioprotectors	Chemicals that protect cells from the normal tissue injury caused by radiation by acting as a free radical scavenger Includes WR-2721 (amifostine) which is given intravenously before radiation (or chemotherapy)	Drug-dependent toxicities Dose limiting toxicities are emesis and hypotension; can include sneezing and somnolence

Table 2B-4 (*Continued*)
Special Techniques In Radiation Therapy

Technique	Description	Side Effects
Altered Fractionation Schedules	*Hyperfractionation:* smaller than standard radiation doses per fraction, given more than once per day, total dose is increased *Quasi-hyperfractionation:* same as above except that total dose is not increased *Accelerated fractionation:* shorter treatment course and reduced total dose, while increasing the number of daily fractions *Quasi-accelerated fractionation:* same as accelerated except the overall time is not reduced between the accelerated segments Time between treatments should be at least four to six hours to allow repair of sublethal damage Two to three fractions per day may be given Used in head and neck cancer and medulloblastoma	Patient may experience more significant acute and late site-specific toxicity
Radioimmunotherapy (RIT)	The use of monoclonal antibody-labeled radioactive isotopes to selectively implant specific tumors and tumor proteins Radiation can enhance effectiveness of antibody uptake Iodine 131, iodine 125 and yttrium 90 can be used Administered intravenously, intraarterially, intrathecally, or intraperitoneally (see Chapter 3B) Used primarily for Hodgkin's and non-Hodgkin's lymphoma and leukemia, also utilized in glioma, hepatoma, ovarian cancer, and melanoma Radiation isolation might be required, depending on which radioisotope is used	Dose limiting toxicity is myelosuppression and with high dose immunotherapy might require rescue with autologous bone marrow transplant Headaches or seizures can occur for patients with gliomas
Remote Afterloading Brachytherapy	Radioactive sources are loaded into an applicator that has been inserted into a patient, by using a remotely activated system Used for interstitial and intracavitary brachytherapy applications May be low-dose-rate (LDR) and high-dose-rate (HDR) LDR systems use cesium 137 or iridium 192 HDR systems commonly use iridium 192 giving a greater cGy per hour than LDR; HDR given in shielded treatment room Can be an outpatient procedure, and applicator insertion and treatment might be given in a treatment room Can be used in GYN and bronchial cancers, and sarcomas	Patients do not require hospitalization or bedrest, complications are decreased Site specific side effects might / might not be increased

C—Celsius; GI—gastrointestinal; GU—genitourinary; GYN—gynecologic

the damaging effects. Radiosensitizers act by diffusing into hypoxic tissue and potentiating free radical–induced DNA damage by mimicking the effects of oxygen. Radioprotectors, alternatively, act by scavenging free radicals before they interact with and damage normal tissue DNA. Although the use of these agents occurs generally in the context of a clinical trial at this time, this is an area of active research and potential benefit for the patient.

Antineoplastic agents can be given concurrently during a radiation therapy course to enhance locoregional disease control and prevent future distant metastases. Although still under investigation, it could also allow organ preservation such as with head and neck tumors. Other common disease sites where concomitant chemotherapy is used include rectal and anal cancer. In addition, chemotherapy can be given prior to radiation therapy, referred to as *neoadjuvant chemotherapy,* or after, called *adjuvant chemotherapy.* Chemotherapy enhances cell kill of the tumor by potentiating the DNA damage caused by the radiation. The use of combined modality approaches, however, is limited by the increase in side effects for the patient caused by the enhancement of normal tissue damage. New drugs and different treatment doses and schedules are being studied to improve the therapeutic ratio, which refers to the percentage difference between tumor control and major complications.

METHODS OF TREATMENT

Radiation can be delivered to tumors or disease by two basic methods, externally or internally. When it is delivered from outside the body by a radioactive source or from a machine generating electromagnetic or particulate energy placed at a distance from the target, it is called *external radiation,* teletherapy, or external beam radiation therapy. This is the most common method of delivery. *Internal radiation* includes the use of temporary or permanent radiation sources placed inside the body near a tumor (implant therapy), by using sealed or unsealed forms of radioisotopes. Sealed-source applications are usually referred to as *brachytherapy.* The prefix *brachy* is derived from a Greek word that means "short" and in this context refers to the proximity of the radiation source transmitting energy to the tumor. Unsealed sources called radiopharmaceuticals are given systemically. The radiation oncologist selects the method of treatment on the basis of a person's tumor type, size, and location, dosage needed, potential side effects, factors related to the person, and the availability of resources for the particular method. For some tumors, a combination of external and internal radiation is needed, taking advantage of the complementary physical and biological effects of both modalities. Women who have a cancer of the cervix, for example, usually require both external pelvic radiation and one or two gynecologic implants to "boost" the dose to the tumor for curative intent. Patients with a squamous cell carcinoma of the head and neck might also require both internal and external radiation therapy.

External Radiation

External radiation can be delivered by a variety of machines that emit energy in the form of high-energy x-rays and gamma rays (photons), as well as electron particles. Linear accelerators are used most commonly in a clinical setting to deliver x-rays ranging from 4 million electron volts to 20 million electron volts (4MeV–20MeV). The radiation beam comes out of the machine in an exact path, giving off very little scatter. Cobalt 60 machines deliver gamma rays from a radioactive source located in the head of the machine. The average energy of cobalt gamma rays is 1.25 million electron volts (1.25MeV). A source of cobalt 60 decays over time; it has to be replaced every five to seven years as the activity of the source decreases. Because of its versatility, high photon energy, speed with which treatments can be given, precision of dose distribution, and other factors, the linear accelerator is the machine predominantly used for external treatment in most centers today.

External radiation machines are chosen on the basis of the energy needed to penetrate to the tumor. Both the linear accelerator and the Cobalt 60 machine have the advantage of delivering penetrating energy to treat deep-seated tumors. For example, a 4MeV machine is well suited for tumors located in the head and neck region, whereas a higher energy machine, a 15MeV accelerator, is able to reach deep-seated tumors in the pelvis. Megavoltage or supervoltage machines, like linear accelerators and the Cobalt 60 machine, are said to be skin sparing because they can deliver doses deep in the body with relatively lower doses to the skin surface.

When tumors are located close to or directly below the skin surface, a superficial form of radiation such as electrons can be used. Electron energies range from 6MeV to 20MeV, and due to the limited depth of penetration, deeper tissues are spared significant radiation exposure. This superficial radiation is useful in treating skin lesions such as basal cell cancers and Kaposi's sarcoma, for delivering a "boost" to a surgical site such as for breast cancer, and for treating chest wall breast cancer recurrences or superficial lymph nodes. Because electron therapy often results in a higher dose to the skin, it characteristically produces a more intense skin reaction. Electron therapy is most commonly given by linear accelerators, which can be equipped to allow use of the electron beam. An older machine called the *betatron* can also deliver electron therapy.

Special treatment machines such as cyclotrons are presently used in some treatment centers. These machines deliver protons and neutrons at higher energies than linear accelerators and can be advantageous for this reason. Protons are useful for tumors located near critical structures, such as base of skull tumors, as they deliver a high dose to the tumor with less radiation to normal tissues outside the tumor volume. Neutrons have shown an advantage in the control of salivary gland and prostate cancers. Treatment with protons and neutrons is used for select cases but is not commonly available; with future investigation, it might become a more prevalent option.

Equipment

Treatment Planning

After a patient is evaluated by a radiation oncologist and the choice is made to use external beam therapy, an informed consent is signed stating that the treatment benefits and risks have been explained and that all of the patient's questions have been answered. Additional diagnostic studies needed to determine the extent of disease or to help define normal tissues in proximity to the radiation beam are done prior to the development of the treatment plan. Each plan is unique and depends on the specific details of an individual patient's anatomy, tumor location and medical condition.

The majority of patients require a special treatment planning session called a *simulation,* which helps determine the exact area of the body to be treated. The *simulator* is a special x-ray unit that assists the radiation oncologist and radiation therapist to map or design the shape of the radiation field or port. An exact treatment volume is determined with the use of x-rays, computerized tomography scans, magnetic resonance imaging scans, surgical clips, and other diagnostic studies that point to the location of the tumor.

X-rays called simulator films are taken to identify the treatment area. Permanent small ink dots, or tattoos, are often placed on the skin corresponding to the treatment area and are used to position the patient under the machine for each treatment, usually with laser lights. During this time, a physicist or dosimetrist might make a contour of the area of the body in the treatment field using plaster, wire, or thermoplastic tubing. Other measurements required for dosimetric calculations might be taken. The radiation oncologist might also design customized shielding or alloy "blocks" to protect normal tissues in the treatment area. These blocks can then be mounted on a lucite tray and placed directly between the beam and the patient (into the treatment head of the machine) so that normal tissue can be shielded from radiation. An alternative method of custom blocking is achieved with multileaf collimators, which are available in newer generation accelerators. Multileaf collimators consist of 20–40 thin lead leaves that are mounted into the head of the treatment machine and are used to precisely shape the radiation field.

Because the patient's position needs to be reproducible for each treatment, special immobilization devices such as custom casts, plastic masks, or polyurethane molds can be fabricated for use during the simulation and subsequent treatment. The patient can also be positioned using tape or bite blocks. These immobilization devices allow the radiation to be administered more accurately. Devices such as wedges or tissue compensators are used to distribute the dose more evenly to the treatment field, improving the desired dose distribution. Tissue equivalent material called *bolus* can be applied to the treatment field if a higher dose of radiation to the skin is needed.

In addition, computer plans are used to optimize the delivery of the radiation therapy. A computer plan, expressed as isodose curves, specifies the amount of radiation that will be delivered to the tumor and to all of the normal tissues inside the radiation field. The computer planning process helps the radiation oncologist determine how to aim the radiation beams to maximize the dosage of radiation to the tumor and minimize the dosage of radiation to normal tissues. Some patients may need to have the radiation aimed from multiple directions while others may need the machine set up with only one to two fields. The entire simulation procedure takes from one half to two hours; the entire treatment planning process may take several days.

Treatment

After the treatment plan is complete, the patient will begin radiation treatments. The treatments are usually given five days per week over two to eight weeks. For example, a woman being treated with lumpectomy followed by radiation for early-stage breast cancer would require daily, Monday through Friday, treatment for approximately five to six weeks. A common daily dose of 180–200 cGy might be administered to a breast dose of 4,500–5,000 cGy. This is often followed by an additional boost of five to seven treatments with electrons to the lumpectomy site. This can be given at 200 cGy per day to a dose of 1,400 cGy, bringing the total treatment dosage to 5,900–6,400 cGy. A woman being treated for a metastatic lesion to a femur or brain from breast cancer however, might only need ten treatments, given five days per week for two weeks, to palliate her symptoms. The daily dose in this case might be 300 cGy, with a total treatment dose of 3,000 cGy to either the femur or whole brain.

External beam treatments require a patient to lie still on a hard table or couch. Because the radiation is painless and invisible, the actual radiation beam causes no discomfort. The treatment table, however, can be uncomfortable for some people, and measures to ensure comfort might be needed. Should a patient require pain medication on a regular basis or have pain when lying in the treatment position, analgesic administration prior to simulation or treatment is advisable. Although the radiation beam is actually on for only a few minutes, the period needed for positioning and technical checks could increase the total daily time in the treatment room to 10 to 30 minutes. The first treatment generally takes longer than subsequent treatments because x-rays, called "port films," are taken to verify the accuracy of positioning and blocks. These films are not diagnostic quality and therefore in most cases do not provide an accurate measure of the tumor's response to treatment.

The patient is alone in the treatment room during treatment but is constantly monitored by a closed-circuit television screen and audio intercom. It is important for the patient on the treatment table to know that the machine can be turned off at any time by the technologist administering and monitoring the treatment if the patient moves or indicates that treatment needs to be stopped. A few persons, mainly children under the age of three, will need to be sedated or anesthetized each day for treatment.

Patients who receive external beam therapy, their clothing and personal items in the treatment room, are never radioactive. Patients are only aware of a faint buzzing noise when the treatment machine is being activated. Radiation is only present in the room when the treatment machine is in the "on" position.

Internal Radiation

Internal radiation is an excellent way to deliver a concentrated dose of radiation to a desired area over a short period of time with relative sparing of normal tissues. The choice of method used for internal radiation is based on the size, location, and type of tumor. Factors relating to the specific radioisotopes also play a significant role.

The two basic ways of delivering internal radiation are (1) through brachytherapy or mechanically positioning sealed radioactive sources with one of two placement methods: interstitial or intracavitary, and (2) administering an unsealed source or radiopharmaceutical systemically, that can be metabolized or absorbed by body tissues. Table 2B–5 gives examples of each method.

Interstitial implants involve the placement of radioactive sources contained in needles, wires, seeds or catheters directly into or adjacent to the tumor, either permanently or temporarily. When an intracavitary implant is performed, the radioactive source is placed directly into the body cavity and held in place by an applicator. These implants are temporary. For example, a vaginal implant using an applicator might be used for a woman with endometrial cancer, while an interstitial implant using catheters and radioactive seeds might be used for a squamous cell carcinoma of the head and neck. Both of these methods usually require hospitalization for the surgical placement of the intracavitary applicator or interstitial implant device that will house the radioisotope. Local or general anesthesia might be needed for placement. The radioisotope can be loaded during the surgical procedure, as with some prostate implants, or postoperatively, as with gynecologic implants, either in the radiation therapy department or in the patient's hospital room. Verification films are obtained to identify where the applicator or implant device and/or seeds are located. When the radioisotope has not been loaded during the surgery, as with many gynecologic or head and neck implants, "dummy" seeds can be used during the verification process to identify future seed placement. Determining the exact location of each radioisotope source will assist in determining the radiation dose to the site. As with external radiation, a computerized plan is generated to identify the dose distribution and length of time the radioisotope must be implanted to achieve the desired dose. A standard length of time for an implant placement ranges from 24 to 72 hours, and total doses can range from 1,000 cGy to 4,500 cGy.

A more recent technology, remote afterloading brachytherapy, both low-dose-rate and high-dose-rate, allows interstitial and intracavitary implants to be administered on an outpatient basis. A special applicator or catheter is placed in proximity to the tumor similar to conventional

Table 2B-5
Examples of Internal Radiation Therapy

Tumor Location	Type	Source	Half-life	Duration/ Application
Mechanically Positioned Sealed Sources:				
Cervix	Intracavitary (Afterloading or remote afterloading)	Cesium 137	30 years	Temporary
		Iridium 192	74.2 days	Temporary
Head and neck (lip, tongue, neck)	Interstitial (after loading)	Gold 198	2.696 days	Permanent
		Cesium 137	30 years	Temporary
		Iridium 192	74.2 days	Temporary
Breast	Interstitial (afterloading or remote afterloading)	Iridium 192	74.2 days	Temporary
Lung	Intracavitary (remote afterloading)	Iridium 192	74.2 days	Temporary
	Interstitial	Iodine 125	60.2 days	Permanent
Prostate	Interstitial	Iodine 125	60.2 days	Permanent
		Palladium 103	16.96 days	Permanent
		Iridium 192	74.2 days	Temporary
Brain	Interstitial	Iridium 192	74.2 days	Temporary
		Iodine 125	60.2 days	Permanent
Unsealed Sources:				
Thyroid		Iodine 131	8.04 days	Ingested
Malignant ascites or malignant pleural effusion		Phosphorus 32	14.24 days	Instilled
Metastatic bone lesions		Strontium 89	50.5 days	Injected
		Samarium 153	46.7 hours	Injected

(Recommendations from the International Commission on Radiological Protection publication #38, 1983, Radionuclide Transformations)

brachytherapy techniques. A remote afterloading system mechanically loads and unloads the radioactive sources and utilizes built-in safety mechanisms that verify placement of the applicator or catheter and the position of the radioactive isotope. Personnel are not exposed to the radioactive source.

Systemic or radiopharmaceutical therapy can be used for the palliative management of pain from metastatic bone disease in breast, lung, and prostate cancers such as with strontium 89 (Metastron®) or samarium 153

(Quadramet®). These are given intravenously, usually on an outpatient basis by a radiation oncologist or a nuclear medicine physician. Another systemic radioisotope employs radioactive iodine (iodine 131) administered orally for the treatment of benign and malignant thyroid diseases. Depending on the dosage given, the patient might need to be hospitalized for the period of greatest activity, the first several days after administration.

The safety practices needed when internal radiation is used depend on many factors. Many hospitals have lead-lined rooms for patients receiving internal radiation or designate a room at the end of a hallway to provide the least radiation exposure to others. Nurses working with patients receiving radioisotopes should request appropriate information by the radiation safety officer, to understand how to reduce their exposure to radiation while providing safe patient care.

The type of radiation emitted from the isotope is the first factor that must be considered. Whether gamma rays or beta particles are used will determine the amount of radiation exposure and risk to medical personnel. Beta-particle radiation can be blocked by the thickness of plastic and can be shielded by the body's own tissue. When the source of beta radiation is inside the human body, the recipient is not a direct radiation hazard to others. Body fluids such as urine and blood are themselves radioactive after radiopharmaceutical administration. High-energy gamma-emitting isotopes, on the other hand, are extremely penetrating and present the greatest external hazard. They require a significant thickness of lead to prevent the radiation from being absorbed by others. Patients receiving high doses of gamma-emitting systemic radioisotopes or implants often require radiation isolation in the hospital; pure beta-emitting isotope procedures can generally be performed in an outpatient setting.

The second factor in radiation safety practice is the dosage or activity of the radioisotope used. The activity refers to the number of disintegrations or nuclear transformations per unit of time. Low doses of radioisotopes yield less radiation than higher doses of the same isotope. The dosage is expressed in curies, abbreviated Ci, the unit of activity measuring the total number of disintegrations per second. A person treated with 10 millicuries of iodine 131 for hyperthyroidism would not require radiation isolation, but a person who is given 150 millicuries for thyroid cancer would. Guidelines for regulating the doses and necessary radiation safety practices are determined by the federal government and/or state radiation safety organizations.

Two factors that are helpful in determining radiation safety practices include the radioisotope's unique energy and the half-life. For example, the gamma radiation exposure from the same amount of millicuries of an iridium 192 source is greater than from a gold 198 source at the same distance, because iridium 192 has a greater photon energy than gold 198. The half-life of a radioisotope refers to the measurement of the isotope's rate of decay, which is predictable, and equals the time required for the number of atoms in a particular source to decay by one-half or the source to lose 50 percent of its radioactivity. Radioisotopes have a wide range of half-lives. Generally, isotopes with lower photon energy and short half-lives are used for permanent implants, whereas isotopes with high photon energy and long half-lives are used in temporary implants. For example, an isotope, such as iodine 125 (which has a half-life of 60 days and low energy), can be used as a permanent implant, as for a prostate cancer; but cesium 137, which has a half-life of 30 years and is high energy, can be used as a temporary implant, as for a gynecological cancer. Table 2B–5 identifies half-lives of commonly used radioisotopes.

Finally, the method of radioisotope delivery must also be considered. Persons receiving sealed radioactive sources are not themselves radioactive. With sealed sources, all radiation safety practices are based upon the source itself, which is radioactive. Nurses should follow the basic principles of time, distance, and shielding to reduce their exposure. In other words, they should minimize the time they spend in contact with the radioactive source, maximize their distance from the source, and use proper shielding from it. When the source is removed, no radiation is present. Unsealed sources of radiation require different safety precautions. If radiation is swallowed or injected, the person's body fluids will be radioactive for a period related to the physical and biological half-life of the isotope. Table 2B–6 outlines specific radiation safety practices for sealed and unsealed radioactive sources. Radiation safety practices are based on guidelines established by each state, or by the Nuclear Regulatory Commission.

Adhering to the principles of time, distance, shielding, and contamination control when dealing with any source of radioactivity will keep occupational exposure "As Low As Reasonably Achievable" (ALARA). The ALARA guideline is recommended by the National Council on Radiation Protection, a federal agency that has also established recommended radiation dose limits for the general public and for occupational exposure (see Table 2B–7).

NURSING CARE ISSUES

The nursing care of persons receiving internal or external radiation therapy encompasses many activities, including patient and family education and advocacy, counseling, and direct care. Assessing a patient's knowledge about radiation, providing information about the acute and long-term side effects of treatment, monitoring the patient for side effects, and assisting the patient and family with self-care measures to manage those side effects are important responsibilities for nurses.

Factors that predict side effects include the following: (1) the size of the treatment field; (2) the exact body tissues being treated within the treatment field; (3) the daily and total dose to be given; (4) the particular

Table 2B–6
Radiation Safety Practices

Radioactive Source	Specific Radiation Safety Practice
Sealed gamma source Temporary (cesium 137, iridium 192) Examples: Cervical, breast, brain, sarcoma or head and neck implants	Assign patient to a private room; the patient must remain there at all times until radioactive source(s) removed Identify the patient with a radiation caution sign on door and medical record. Do not allow pregnant staff or ancillary personnel in room Wear a radiation dosimeter (film badge, thermoluminescent dosimeter detector (TLD) or ring badge, or electronic pocket dosimeter (EPD)) when entering patient room, to measure personnel exposure Place lead shields in room Keep lead container, long handled forceps in room in case of dislodged radioactive source(s) Utilize univeral precautions, however, only the source is radioactive, not the patient or body fluids Allow visitors per institutional policy, except pregnant women and children under 18 are not allowed in patient room Do not exceed regulatory limits for visitor time in room; many institutions limit each visitor to one-half hour per day Allow visitors brief physical contact with the patient; instruct visitor to spend the majority of the visit at least 6 feet away from the patient Limit nursing time to one-half hour per nurse per shift, or as determined by radioisotope characteristics and exposure rates around the patient Provide routine nursing care, but bed baths are usually omitted. Provide patient with necessary items in close proximity to maximize self-care Keep dressings that have covered the area of radioactive implant in a basin to be checked by the radiation safety officer for any dislodged source Notify the radiation safety officer and radiation oncologist immediately if source(s) is dislodged, emergency measures (CPR, emergency surgery) are required, or if the patient expires Survey the patient to certify that no sources are left behind after the implant has been removed Survey the patient room for any possible source dislodgment; following this procedure, no further radiation measures are required
Sealed gamma source Permanent (iodine 125, palladium 103) Examples: Prostate, head and neck, brain implants	*If patient is hospitalized:* Assign patient to a private room; the patient must remain there at all times unless/until instructed otherwise Identify the patient with a radiation caution sign on door and medical record Do not allow pregnant staff or ancillary personnel in room Wear a radiation dosimeter (film badge, TLD or ring badge, or EPD) when entering patient room, to measure personnel exposure Utilize universal precautions, however, only the sources are radioactive, not the patient or body fluids, unless a seed breaks internally during or after the interstitial insertion procedure Allow visitors per institutional policy, except pregnant women and children under 18 are not allowed in patient room Do not exceed regulatory limits for visitor time in room; many institutions limit each visitor to one-half hour per day Allow visitors brief physical contact with the patient Limit nursing time to one-half hour per nurse per shift, or as determined by radioisotope characteristics and exposure rates around the patient Provide routine nursing care, but bed baths are usually omitted. Provide patient with necessary items in close proximity to maximize self-care

Table 2B–6 *(Continued)*
Radiation Safety Practices

Radioactive Source	Specific Radiation Safety Practice
	Strain all urine for patients who have prostate implants, to capture any excreted radioactive seeds. Patient may have a Foley catheter in place initially
	Notify the radiation safety officer and radiation oncologist immediately if sources are excreted in urine, emergency measures (CPR, emergency surgery) are required, or if the patient expires
	Survey the patient prior to discharge to certify that radiation levels fall below regulatory limits
	Survey the patient room for any possible source contamination; following this procedure, no further radiation measures are required
	On discharge from the hospital:
	Educate patient/family that
	radioactive seeds will decay over a period of a few months
	pregnant women and children under 18 should maintain a distance of at least 3 feet from patient for approximately 1 month
	sexual intercourse is allowed but a condom should be used for 3 months by patients with prostate implants, to capture any excreted seeds
Unsealed permanent source (Gamma: oral iodine 131 when greater than 33 millicuries is given Beta: strontium 89 Beta and gamma: samarium 153) Examples: Iodine 131: thyroid cancer Strontium 89 or samarium 153: metastatic bone disease from prostate, breast and lung cancers	*If patient is hospitalized, usually for other medical reasons:*
	Assign patient to a private room; the patient must remain there at all times unless/until instructed otherwise
	Identify the patient with a radiation caution sign on door and medical record
	Do not allow pregnant staff or ancillary personnel in room
	Wear a radiation dosimeter (film badge, TLD or ring badge, or EPD) when entering patient room, to measure personnel exposure
	Prepare the room for possible contamination of contents by radioactive patient body fluids: place plastic cover on mattress, pillow, and bathroom floor, call button, etc
	Wear a gown, disposable gloves and shoe protectors at all times while attending the patient
	Leave all items in patient room (e.g., patient linens, disposable food trays, and gowns, gloves, and shoe protectors worn by staff)
	Utilize universal precautions, patient body fluids (urine, perspiration, saliva, blood and feces) are temporarily radioactive. Wash hands well after gloves are removed
	Do not exceed regulatory limits for visitor time in room; many institutions limit each visitor to one-half hour per day
	Do not allow visitors physical contact with the patient
	Visitors should remain at least 6 feet away from patient
	Limit nursing time to one-half hour per nurse per shift, or as determined by radioisotope characteristics and exposure rates around the patient
	Provide routine nursing care, but bed baths are usually omitted. Provide patient with necessary items in close proximity to maximize self-care
	Instruct patient to double flush the toilet after use
	Notify the radiation safety officer immediately if patient vomits or there is a spill of body fluids in the room; survey personnel who may have stepped in or touched the spill at the doorway for any possible contamination of shoes or clothing
	Notify the radiation safety officer and radiation oncologist immediately if emergency measures (CPR, emergency surgery) are required, or if the patient expires

Continued

Table 2B-6 *(Continued)*
Radiation Safety Practices

Radioactive Source	Specific Radiation Safety Practice
	Survey the patient prior to discharge, to certify that radiation levels fall below regulatory limits Survey the patient room and contents for any possible source contamination; following this procedure, no further radiation measures are required

Iodine 131 falls below 33 millicuries and/or dose rate falls below 7 mrem/hr at 1 cm, or strontium 89 or samarium 153 injection	*On discharge from the hospital or if patient does not require hospitalization:*
	For one week after an administration of oral iodine 131 or injection of strontium 89 and for 3 days after an injection of samarium 153
	    encourage patient to use toilet rather than urinal, bedpan or bedside commode; double flush toilet after use
	    encourage patient to sit to urinate
	    reinforce good handwashing by patient after urinating or defecating
	    rinse urinals, bedpans or commodes twice after each use, double flush excrement and rinse water
	Educate patient/family
	    that patient body fluids (urine, perspiration, saliva, blood and feces) are temporarily radioactive, handling body fluids by others should be avoided, to utilize universal precautions and good handwashing when handling is necessary
	    to notify the radiation safety officer if there is direct contact of caregiver's skin with the patient's body fluids
	    to clean clothes or linens contaminated with blood, feces or urine immediately, separating these items from other clothing/articles
	    to avoid intimate/personal contact, especially with pregnant women and children under 18

Table 2B-7
Maximum Dose Limits for Radiation Exposure Excluding Doses from Natural Sources and Any Medical Administration

Exposures	Dose Limits
Occupational exposures Effective dose equivalent limit:	
Annual	50 mSv (5 rem)
Cumulative	10 mSv × age
Annual public exposures Effective dose equivalent limit:	
Continuous or frequent exposure	1 mSv (0.1 rem)
Infrequent exposure	5 mSv (0.5 rem)
Embryo–fetus exposures Total dose equivalent limit:	5 mSv (0.5 rem)
Dose equivalent monthly limit:	.5 mSv (0.05 rem)

mSv—milliSievert.
(Recommendations of the National Council on Radiation Protection and Measurements, Report No. 116, 1993)

method of radiation delivery (i.e., internal versus external or both); (5) the type of equipment used; (6) whether other modalities (chemotherapy and/or surgery) are being utilized; and (7) individual patient factors, including age and other active medical problems. A child's developing tissues could sustain permanent or long-term effects above and beyond what an adult might experience. For example, radiation delivered to the growth plate of a young child's leg for a Ewing's sarcoma could prevent growth of the limb to a normal length. Because the adult's leg is no longer growing, this would not be a potential side effect. Radiation carcinogenesis effects are also more pronounced in children.

Table 2B–8 outlines general and site-specific side effects of radiation and the nursing management of those toxicities. The majority of patients will experience skin erythema and irritation as well as fatigue during treatment and for a period of time after treatment is completed. Factors that might enhance the severity and hasten the occurrence of these general and site-specific side effects include higher dose (curative intent); high dose rate (accelerated fractionation); large treatment fields; fields with significant amounts of radiosensitive tissues; concurrent chemotherapy; recent surgery or chemotherapy; and use of low energy machines. Nutritional problems prior to diagnosis and treatment along with potential treatment related toxicity make significant weight loss a serious concern in patients both during and after treatment. This is particularly important when radiation is directed to the head and neck, lung, esophagus, and abdomen. Identifying these factors prior to treatment will help the nurse recognize those patients at risk for greater toxicity, and plan for their care accordingly.

Several innovative radiation delivery techniques and experimental radiation modalities are now available in some radiation therapy departments, including hyperthermia, intraoperative radiation therapy, use of radiosensitizers and radioprotectors, radioimmunotherapy, hyperfractionation, total body irradiation, particle radiation therapy, and stereotactic radiosurgery. These technologies are offered in some centers in an attempt to improve response to treatment and/or reduce toxicity. Table 2B–4 gives a description, purpose, and possible side effects for these modalities.

SUMMARY

Radiation therapy has changed dramatically since it began in the late 1890s. The nursing care of persons receiving radiation has evolved into a specialty in oncology nursing with its own set of standards for nursing practice and education. Nurses are instrumental members of the radiation treatment team; they work in collaboration with the radiation oncologist to prepare a patient and family for radiation, monitor and manage subsequent side effects, and assist patients and families in coping with this phase of the cancer experience.

Table 2B–8
Nursing Management of Radiation Therapy Side Effects

Treatment Site	Description	Intervention
General: *Fatigue*	Fatigue might not occur but if present, can range from mild to severe fatigue Can occur 1–2 hours after treatment but might be more noticeable in the afternoon and evening Peak incidence generally from 3rd week to end of treatment and may last for 2–12 weeks after completion May be expressed as increased irritability in children	Encourage planning, prioritizing and balancing of activities and rest periods Encourage social, diversionary and physical activities to tolerance (e.g., walking, aerobic activity) Monitor performance status throughout treatment course Encourage maintenance of well balanced diet Nutrition consult as needed See Chapter 8C

Skin	During treatment, reaction can include
	  erythema often noticeable after 2–3 weeks of treatment; varies in intensity
	  dry desquamation
	  moist desquamation: peaks 4–6 weeks into treatment
	  epilation (alopecia): begins 3–4 weeks into treatment and occurs only in the treatment field
	  decreased sebaceous and sweat gland function
	  ulceration, hemorrhage and necrosis (rare)
	Healing time varies but may range from 2–8 weeks
	Hair regrowth usually begins within 2–3 months after treatment and might be a different color or consistency and potentially more sparse
	Late effects:
	Can appear 10 weeks after treatment but might not be evident for years and include atrophy, hypo- and hyperpigmentation, xerosis, telangectasia, permanent epilation (associated with higher doses), and rarely, ulceration and necrosis
	Reactions might be enhanced during concurrent treatment or after radiation is completed (radiation recall) with chemotherapy such as doxorubicin, dactinomycin
		Identify additional factors that might enhance skin reaction (e.g., skin folds in treatment site, alterations in skin integrity at start of treatment, poor nutritional status, use of skin irritants, concomitant illnesses, e.g., diabetes mellitus, circulatory problems)
		Promote good hygiene, and reduce friction and impact of irritants (e.g., sun exposure, mechanical and thermal irritants, chemicals, perfumes, powders, or alcohol)
		Provide education to patient/family regarding proper skin care during treatment
		Monitor skin changes throughout treatment
		Promote well-balanced diet and adequate fluid intake
		Provide skin care products and comfort measures that promote a moist healing environment; this can include topical agents and dressings
		Provide treatment breaks if necessary depending on severity of reaction
		
		See Chapter 10C

Blood and Bone Marrow	Ultimate effect is dependent on the percentage or volume of active bone marrow or lymphoid tissue in the field and total radiation dose given Radiation therapy might not be as effective in the anemic patient due to the radioresistance of hypoxic cells in solid tumors	Identify patients at risk for hematopoietic suppression Monitor blood counts for patients at risk (often weekly) Monitor patient for signs and symptoms of infection, bleeding and anemia

Table 2B–8 *(Continued)*
Nursing Management of Radiation Therapy Side Effects

Treatment Site	Description	Intervention
	Late effects: Occurring several months after treatment include chronic hypoplasia or aplasia of the marrow when greater than 25 percent of it is irradiated or greater than 3,000 cGy is given in a fractionated schedule; recovery of lymphoid tissue is considerably better than in the bone marrow	Instruct patient/family in: observation and reporting of signs and symptoms of infection, bleeding and anemia; maintenance of optimum nutrition (and neutropenic diet if necessary) Instruct measures to prevent infection and bleeding and assist patient to cope with symptoms of anemia Provide treatment breaks, blood product support, and/or hematopoietic growth factors as necessary for patients with low counts See Chapter 10A
Brain and Spinal Cord	Cerebral edema (which might be present prior to radiation) could occur following even one fraction, could cause increased intracranial pressure manifested as headaches, visual disturbances, nausea, vomiting, seizures, personality and cognitive changes, changes in level of consciousness and other neurological symptoms, such as limb weakness Alopecia (see Skin) Somnolence syndrome, which includes excessive sleepiness, drowsiness, lethargy, and anorexia, can occur 6–12 weeks after radiation and last for up to 2 weeks Craniospinal fields place patient at significant risk for hematopoietic suppression (see Blood and Bone Marrow) Late effects: Radiation necrosis occurs in approximately 1%–5% of patients given high dose brain radiation, is usually progressive and potentially fatal (often requires corticosteroids and surgery) Neurocognitive and emotional changes are more noticeable in children post treatment and are expressed as potentially decreased IQs and behavioral difficulties Decreased hormone production can occur several years after treatment for hypothalmic or pituitary tumors Secondary neoplasms are rare, but more common in children Transient myelopathy (Lhermitte's sign) 2–4 months following radiation to the spine, as with mantle field radiation for Hodgkin's disease, can occur and will usually resolve within 2–6 months untreated Permanent paralysis and chronic myelopathy are rare	Monitor and reinforce adherence to medication regimen (dexamethasone, anti-seizure medications) Monitor for side effects of medications and educate patient/family regarding side effects to observe for and report (e.g., oral moniliasis, labile mood swings, GI disturbances, nystagmus, altered gait) Monitor drug levels of anti-seizure medication and discuss dose adjustments with physician as needed Monitor for and educate patient regarding signs and symptoms of increased intracranial pressure (see Chapter 15A) Instruct family regarding seizure precautions Monitor for signs and symptoms of thromboembolic disease in patients with brain tumors Assess effect of hair loss on body image Provide information regarding prosthetic support (wigs, scarves, turbans, and hats) Encourage patient who has received treatment to hypothalamic or pituitary tumor to receive follow-up with physician to monitor hormone levels Educate patient/family regarding potential for Lhermitte's sign post mantle field radiation See Chapter 11

Continued

Table 2B–8 *(Continued)*
Nursing Management of Radiation Therapy Side Effects

Treatment Site	Description	Intervention
Oral Cavity and Neck	Xerostomia could be present within one week and can progress throughout the treatment course; increases risk of dental and gum disease, stomatitis, and taste changes Altered and/or loss of taste is most noticeable after 2–3 weeks of radiation Mucositis and pharyngitis with associated oral and throat pain, dysphagia, and odynophagia typically occur 2–3 weeks after radiation is initiated; this can cause progressive symptoms, and result in ulceration and bleeding Oral moniliasis, which can progress to esophagus Anorexia and weight loss are common Late Effects: Osteoradionecrosis can occur (rarely) to mandible (less common with higher energy machines and more common with higher doses) Taste changes or lack of taste can persist for months and might not resolve for up to a year or longer after treatment ends Dysphagia, pharyngitis, and odynophagia persist for up to 6 months after treatment Some degree of xerostomia is likely to be a permanent problem Dental caries and periodontal disease might occur without proper dental and gum care and regular dental follow-up Trismus might occur and is progressive unless treated; might require surgery or use of dynamic bite openers	Provide pretreatment dental consult for potential extraction of diseased teeth or gum surgery, and fluoride gel trays Provide nutrition consult; patient might need feeding tube placement Provide nutritional supplements as necessary during treatment and potentially for months after treatment (see Chapter 9) Obtain frequent weights (at least weekly during treatment) Encourage avoidance of oral irritants (e.g., alcohol, chewing tobacco, smoking cigarettes, hard-bristled toothbrushes, poor fitting dentures, acidic and spicy foods) Provide comfort measures as needed (e.g., topical anesthetics, opioid analgesics, nonsteroidal anti-inflammatory drugs, antacids) Patient might benefit from saliva substitutes, pilocarpine tablets, humidified air, soft bland moist diet, foods at moderate temperatures, blenderized foods, and small frequent meals Encourage good oral hygiene; saline mouth rinses prior to and after meals, and use of foam toothbrush (see Chapter 10B) Monitor for and instruct patient regarding signs and symptoms of oral infection and dehydration Promote adequate fluid intake Refer to NCI Booklet: "Eating Hints" Encourage long-term follow-up care with dentist, radiation oncologist, and surgeon after treatment course Educate patient/family regarding prevention of trismus with exercise (e.g., chewing, mouth opening)
Lung/Esophagus	Esophagitis and pharyngitis can lead to sore throat, dysphagia, esophageal reflux and heartburn, epigastric pain and odynophagia within 2–3 weeks after radiation is initiated; can last for several weeks after treatment is completed Anorexia and weight loss are common Occasionally, nausea and/or vomiting occur	Obtain baseline assessment of gastrointestinal and pulmonary symptoms and medications used to manage them Monitor for and instruct patient to report signs and symptoms of dehydration, infection, and pulmonary compromise

Table 2B–8 *(Continued)*
Nursing Management of Radiation Therapy Side Effects

Treatment Site	Description	Intervention
	Patient is at risk for herpetic or monilial infections of the esophagus	Promote coughing and deep breathing
	Dyspnea and nonproductive cough can occur during treatment to the lung	Encourage smoking cessation and avoidance of alcohol
	Pneumonitis—which might be manifested by significant cough (sometimes productive), tachycardia at rest, dyspnea, and fever—can occur 1–3 months after radiation is completed. Volume of lung treated, dosage given, and dose rate will determine likelihood of occurrence. If it occurs, future pulmonary fibrosis is common	Promote adequate fluid intake
		Obtain nutrition consult
		Obtain frequent weights (at least weekly during treatment)
		Encourage soft bland diet, high calorie supplements, small frequent meals, and foods at moderate temperatures; thick beverages might be easier to tolerate than thin liquids (e.g., milkshakes)
	Carmustine or bleomycin prior to or during radiation can increase the severity of these side effects	Provide use of comfort measures as needed (i.e., topical anesthetics, opioid analgesics, stool softeners and laxatives, antacids, cough suppressants, bronchodilators, antiemetics and oxygen)
	Late Effects:	
	Pulmonary fibrosis can occur without an episode of previous pneumonitis and occurs after 6 months post treatment	Provide humidified air and relaxation techniques if appropriate
	Esophageal fibrosis and stenosis leading to fistula are rare but more common if prior surgery to esophagus has occurred	Instruct patient/family regarding signs and symptoms of pneumonitis, pulmonary fibrosis, esophageal fibrosis and stenosis
		Administer/instruct medication (steroids) for pneumonitis
		See Chapters 9, 14
Abdomen	Stomach field can cause gastritis with indigestion/dyspepsia, and ulceration with hematemesis and melena	Obtain baseline assessment of gastrointestinal symptoms and medications used to manage them
	Nausea/vomiting possible several hours after the first treatment to abdomen	Monitor for and instruct patient to report gastrointestinal signs and symptoms during and after treatment completion
	Abdominal cramps, excess flatus, and diarrhea from effect of radiation on bowel in field can occur early but are usually noticeable after 2–3 weeks of radiation and can last several weeks to months after RT	Promote adequate fluid intake; monitor fluid/electrolyte balance as indicated by symptoms
	Anorexia and weight loss are common	Obtain nutrition consult
	Fluorouracil prior to or during radiation can increase the severity of these side effects	Obtain frequent weights (at least weekly during treatment)
	Late Effects:	Use nutritional supplements
	Decreased acid secretion, fibrosis with gastric outlet obstruction and atrophy, and ulceration of the gastric mucosa can occur with treatment to the stomach	Avoid caffeine and alcohol
		Provide low-residue diet, rest after meals
	Veno-occlusive disease can occur within several months of treatment to liver with progression to fibrosis, cirrhosis, and liver failure	Provide comfort measures: antiemetics (may be needed prior to treatment each day), antacids, and antidiarrheals (see Chapter 9)

Continued

Table 2B–8 *(Continued)*
Nursing Management of Radiation Therapy Side Effects

Treatment Site	Description	Intervention
	Decreased pancreatic enzyme secretion with radiation to pancreas, requiring replacement enzymes Multiple effects on the kidney can occur up to many years after treatment and include radiation nephropathy and progressive renal failure, which can result in death Small bowel adhesions, obstruction, atrophy and alterations in absorption, perforation, and fistulas are possible	
Pelvis (includes anal/rectal fields)	Abdominal cramps, excess flatus, and diarrhea from effect of radiation on bowel in field can occur early but are usually noticeable after 2–3 weeks of radiation and can last several weeks to months after RT Anorexia and weight loss can occur Proctitis with increased mucus secretion, tenesmus, perianal pruritis and discomfort, and ulcerations with bleeding can occur and might take several weeks to months to resolve post treatment Cystitis might be noticeable within 3 weeks; symptoms include urinary frequency, hesitancy, urgency, a feeling of incomplete emptying of the bladder, incontinence, hematuria (rare), and dysuria Patient is at risk for urinary tract infection; gradual resolution usually occurs several weeks to months after treatment is completed Large pelvic fields place patient at significant risk for nausea/vomiting and hematopoietic suppression (see Blood and Bone Marrow) Fluorouracil and/or levamisole or mitomycin might increase the severity of these side effects Late Effects: Small bowel adhesions, obstruction, atrophy and alterations in absorption, perforation, and fistulas are possible Decreased colon absorption and rarely obstruction are possible Rectal fibrosis with loss of rectal compliance and chronic proctitis might occur Chronic cystitis might persist, bladder atrophy might occur, and rarely incontinence	Obtain baseline assessment of gastrointestinal and urologic symptoms and medications used to manage them Monitor for and instruct patient to report gastrointestinal and urologic signs and symptoms during and after treatment completion Promote adequate fluid intake; monitor fluid/electrolyte balance as indicated by symptoms Obtain nutrition consult if needed Patient could benefit from use of supplements, avoidance of caffeine and alcohol, low-residue diet, and rest after meals Obtain frequent weights (recommended weekly during treatment) Instruct regarding comfort measures as indicated: antiemetics for large fields (might be needed prior to treatment each day); urinary analgesics, alpha-1 adrenergic blockers and antispasmodics; anal/rectal analgesics and anti-inflammatories, sitz baths, and antidiarrheals

Table 2B–8 (Continued)
Nursing Management of Radiation Therapy Side Effects

Treatment Site	Description	Intervention
Reproductive organs: *Prostate*	See Pelvic field Possible burning with ejaculation during treatment period; decreased libido, and dysfunction with erections, orgasm, and ejaculation might or might not be permanent (30%–40% risk of impotence post-radiation)	See Chapter 13 Provide support and counsel regarding effects of radiation on sexual functioning/impotence during and after treatment Provide information regarding surgical and medical techniques to improve sexual function (i.e., prostheses, injection devices, hormones)
Testes	Decreased libido, dysfunction with erections, orgasm, and ejaculation might or might not be permanent Temporary or permanent sterility	Support and counsel regarding effects of radiation on sexual functioning/infertility Patient might want to consider sperm-banking prior to treatment Provide information regarding surgical and medical techniques to improve sexual function (i.e., prostheses, injection devices, alpha adrenergic stimulating drugs, and hormones)
Ovaries	Temporary or permanent sterility (early menopause might be induced)	Provide support and counsel regarding effects of radiation on sexual functioning/infertility Instruct patient regarding egg banking if available prior to radiation
Cervix/Vagina	Acutely, vaginitis (mucositis) can occur along with and can last up to several weeks after treatment is completed Loss of libido and potential burning from semen after ejaculation from intercourse Less commonly, vaginal infections Late Effects: Vaginal dryness and permanent stenosis are common and can cause painful intercourse and pelvic exams Vaginal ulceration and necrosis Vesicovaginal fistulas and ureteral strictures that might require surgical intervention	Monitor for and instruct patient regarding signs and symptoms of vaginal infections Instruct on use of estrogen cream if appropriate Provide instruction in use of vaginal lubricants and dilators (encourage use at least 2–3 times per week for 10–15 minutes; might be needed indefinitely) Provide support and counsel regarding effects of radiation on sexual functioning and decreased libido during and after treatment Provide information regarding strategies to improve sexual dysfunction (i.e., Kegel exercises, position changes)

GI—gastrointestinal; IQ—intelligence quotient

BIBLIOGRAPHY

1. Altman, G. B., and C. A. Lee. Strontium-89 for treatment of painful bone metastases from prostate cancer. *Oncol Nurs Forum.* 23(3): 523–527. 1996.

   This article discusses clinical studies of strontium 89, indications, action, side effects, and nursing management of a patient who will receive this treatment.

2. Brandt, B. Informational needs and selected variables in patients receiving brachytherapy. *Oncol Nurs Forum* 18(7): 1221–1235. 1991.

   This article describes research on the informational needs of brachytherapy patients. The findings provide good content for educational programs and counseling of brachytherapy patients. This is the first published brachytherapy patient education study.

3. Bucholtz, J. Implications of radiation therapy for nursing. In Clark, J., and R. F. McGee, eds. *Core Curriculum in Oncology Nursing.* 319–328. W. B. Saunders, Philadelphia. 1992.

   The updated chapter on radiation therapy is useful in studying for the Oncology Nursing Certification Exam. There is less emphasis on the technical aspects of radiation therapy than in the first edition, and more concentration on nursing care issues.

4. Dunne-Daly, C. F. External radiation therapy self-learning module. *Cancer Nursing.* 17(2): 156–169. 1994.

   ———Nursing care and adverse reactions of external radiation therapy: A self learning module. *Cancer Nursing.* 17(3): 236–256. 1994.

   ———Brachytherapy. *Cancer Nursing.* 17(4): 355–364. 1994.

   ———Education and nursing care of brachytherapy patients. *Cancer Nursing.* 17(5): 434–445. 1994.

   ———Radiation therapy for oncologic emergencies. *Cancer Nursing.* 17(6): 516–527. 1994.

   ———Potential long-term and late effects from radiation therapy. *Cancer Nursing.* 18(1): 67–79. 1995.

   ———Skin and wound care in radiation oncology. *Cancer Nursing.* 18(2): 144–162. 1995.

   This series of programmed instruction in radiation therapy provides significant information regarding the topics identified in the titles and includes a pre-test, content information with learning objectives, and a post-test. These instructional units can be useful for nursing staff education and for those attempting to understand the basics of radiation therapy.

5. Hassey, K. Demystifying care of patients with radioactive implants. *Am J Nurs* 85(7): 788–792. 1985.

   This excellent article describes sealed brachytherapy procedures and radiation safety concerns. It is also available from the American Cancer Society as a reprint in booklet form.

6. Hassey, K. Principles of radiation safety and protection. *Semin Oncol Nurs* 3(1): 23–29. 1987.

This is a comprehensive, helpful article on the issues involved in radiation safety. It assists nurses in understanding the factors involved in reducing their radiation exposure. It is found in a Seminars in Oncology Nursing *issue that is exclusively devoted to brachytherapy.*

7. Hassey-Dow, K., J. D. Bucholtz, R. R. Iwamoto, V. K. Fielar, L. J. Hilderly, eds. *Nursing Care in Radiation Oncology,* 2d Ed. W. B. Saunders, Philadelphia. 1997.

This excellent nursing textbook written by radiation oncology nurses covers all aspects of radiation therapy. Specific content includes the history and science of radiation therapy; common clinical radiation therapy problems; age-related concerns; radiation for oncologic emergencies; innovative radiation therapy techniques and future trends; late effects and uncommon complications of radiation therapy; and dimensions of nursing practice in radiation oncology.

8. Hilderley, L. Radiotherapy. In Groenwald, S., M. Frogge, C. Yarbro, and M. Goodman, eds. *Cancer Nursing: Principles and Practice,* 4th Ed. 247–282. Jones & Bartlett Publishers, Inc., Boston. 1997.

This excellent chapter on radiation therapy is found in a large oncology nursing textbook. It provides an easy-to-understand discussion of radiation science, equipment used in radiation therapy, and radiation oncology nursing issues.

9. Iwamoto, R. Radiation therapy. In Varricchio C, ed. *A Cancer Source Book for Nurses.* 91–102. Jones & Bartlett, Inc., Boston. 1996.

An overview chapter on radiation therapy for nurses is found in this free American Cancer Society nursing publication. It provides concise, helpful guidelines.

10. Jordan, L., and R. Mantravandi. Nursing care of the patient receiving high dose rate brachytherapy. *Oncol Nurs Forum* 18(17): 1167–1174, 1235–1238. 1991.

This is the best nursing resource article on high-dose-rate, remote afterloading brachytherapy. An added plus is the author's patient information pamphlet on this therapy, found on pages 1235–1238, which gives thorough explanations and photographs.

11. Perez, C. A. and L. W. Brady, eds. *Principles and Practice of Radiation Oncology,* 3d Ed. J. B. Lippincott, Philadelphia. 1997.

This textbook will provide the reader with comprehensive information regarding the science and medical practice of radiation oncology. Specific content addresses the biology of treatment, acute and late tissue effects, specific information regarding all methods of treatment including innovative treatments, and site-specific treatment information.

12. Sitton, E. Early and late radiation-induced skin alterations. Part I: Mechanisms of Skin Changes. *Oncol Nurs Forum* 19(5): 801–807. 1992.

This excellent article explores skin anatomy and physiology and describes the early and late effects of radiation on the skin and factors influencing the effects of radiation on the skin.

13. Sitton, E. Early and late radiation-induced skin alterations. Part II: Nursing care of irradiated skin. *Oncol Nurs Forum* 19(6): 907–912. 1992.

This excellent article details radiation skin reactions and the nursing care interventions. It compares various skin care products and is a very helpful guide for nurses who are evaluating skin care protocols.

14. Strohl, R. The nursing role in radiation oncology: Symptom management of acute and chronic reactions. *Oncol Nurs Forum* 15: 429–434. 1988.

This article is the 1988 Schering Clinical Lectureship award presentation by the author at the 1988 Oncology Nursing Society Congress. It provides an excellent description of the nurse's role in radiation oncology and also vividly describes the patient's perspective. Radiation side effects and their management are well presented.

15. Watkins-Bruner, D., J. Bucholtz, R. Iwamoto, R. Strohl, eds. *Manual for Radiation Oncology Nursing Practice and Education.* The Oncology Nursing Press, Pittsburgh. 1998.

This second edition of the ONS sponsored manual outlines the content necessary for the up-to-date education and practice for radiation oncology nurses. It also provides all nurses caring for radiation oncology patients with basic information relating to radiation therapy principles, side effect management, specialized radiation therapy, modalities, radiation protection, and quality assurance.

C. Chemotherapy

Annette L. Galassi
Susan Molloy Hubbard

INTRODUCTION

By the early 1950s, scientists discovered that drugs could selectively kill the microorganisms that caused malaria and tuberculosis. This discovery led to the successful development of broad spectrum antibiotics and the modern management of infectious disease and also stimulated research to develop drugs that would selectively kill cancer cells. The discovery of the anticancer effects of two chemicals, mechlorethamine and methotrexate, provided the impetus to stimulate the systematic development of cancer drugs.

The anticancer effects of mechlorethamine were discovered during World War II after an explosion of mustard gases in Naples, Italy. Physicians observed that, after this explosion, many of the soldiers exposed to these gases died with atrophy of the lymph glands and bone marrow hypoplasia. Based on these observations, mechlorethamine, a similar chemical, was administered to patients with widely disseminated lymphomas;

transient but impressive antitumor responses were observed. In 1947, research on folic acid, a form of vitamin B, led to the discovery of the antitumor activity of methotrexate in acute leukemia. This breakthrough followed the observation that folic acid accelerated the production of abnormal white blood cells by the bone marrow in patients with acute leukemia. Administration of folic acid antagonists, which inhibited the metabolic effects of folic acid, proved to be cytotoxic to leukemic cells, and methotrexate was identified as the most useful compound. In the mid-1950s, methotrexate was also tested in women with widely disseminated choriocarcinoma, a rare but inevitably fatal cancer of the placenta. Much to the surprise of skeptics, the administration of methotrexate as a single agent produced complete cures in a significant fraction of women with pulmonary metastases.

These early successes with chemotherapy eventually led to a national program for drug development established in 1955 by the National Cancer Institute (NCI). Although many of the techniques used in new drug development have changed over time, the process has remained relatively constant. It begins with the procurement of substances from many different sources, including microbes and plant and marine life. These substances are then screened for activity against panels of *in vitro* human tumor cell lines. Substances that demonstrate activity in this *in vitro* system are then screened *in vivo* using mice implanted with tumors from the same cell line. Small amounts of active substance are then formulated for use in toxicology studies. During formulation, information such as the stability and solubility of the agent is obtained. Unfortunately, active agents cannot always be produced in usable forms.

When formulated, the agent is investigated in preclinical toxicology studies. During this phase, the agent is administered to mice, rodents, and dogs at various doses and schedules. These studies are done to determine a safe starting dose to be used in the first phase of human clinical trials and to predict organ toxicity.

When toxicology studies are completed, an investigational new drug (IND) application is filed with the Food and Drug Administration (FDA). A research protocol is developed outlining how the agent is to be administered and the criteria for selection of participants. When the IND and the research protocol are approved, clinical trials of the agent commence (see Chapter 4). From the time a substance is screened for potential anticancer activity until it becomes commercially available often takes many years. Fortunately, this process has become more expedient in the past decade due to a "fast track" review process which has been put in place at the FDA for promising new drugs.

Since 1992, several exciting new drugs have become commercially available for the treatment of a variety of cancers bringing the number of commercially available antineoplastic agents to over 50. Several of these recently approved drugs represent new categories of chemotherapeutic agents, the taxanes and topoisomerase inhibitors. Chemotherapy is now the

2c

Table 2C–1
Cancers Responsive to Chemotherapy in Advanced Stages

Choriocarcinoma
Acute lymphocytic leukemia in children
Hodgkin's disease
Non-Hodgkin's lymphoma
Testicular carcinoma
Ovarian carcinoma
Acute myelogenous leukemia
Wilms' tumor
Burkitt's lymphoma
Embryonal rhabdomyosarcoma
Ewing's sarcoma

primary treatment modality used to cure the 12 disseminated cancers listed on Table 2C–1. Table 2C–2 lists cancer chemotherapeutic agents by class, including the new catagories. Tables 2C–3 and 2C–4 alphabetically list cancer chemotherapeutic agents and hormonally active agents, including data on dosage, schedule, and major toxicities. Table 2C–5 lists other drugs that are used in cancer treatment.

AGENTS USED IN CHEMOTHERAPY

Alkylating Agents

Alkylating agents are an important class of chemotherapeutic drugs. They occupy a central place in conventional combination chemotherapy regimens as well as in high-dose regimens used in bone marrrow or peripheral blood stem cell transplantation. These drugs kill cells by interfering with the structure of DNA. The alkyl groups attach to DNA, causing misreading of the DNA code, breaks in the DNA molecule, and cross-linking of the DNA strands. The result is disruption of DNA replication and transcription. Because synthesis of other cellular components continues, growth becomes unbalanced and cell death results. Because alkylating agents act on preformed nucleic acids, they are effective in killing cells in all phases of the cell cycle. Therefore, their antitumor activity is not cell cycle specific. However, they do produce a greater antitumor effect in rapidly dividing cells.

The long-term toxicities associated with alkylating agents are due to their effects on hematopoietic stem cells. Alkylating agents can produce delayed and prolonged bone marrow depression. They can also cause amenorrhea in women and oligospermia or azoospermia in men, or permanent infertility. This class of drugs can be mutagenic and ultimately carcinogenic to bone marrow stem cells. This can result in the development of secondary malignancies, such as acute myelogenous leukemia.

Table 2C-2
Cancer Chemotherapeutic Agents by Class

Alkylating Agents	Platinum Analogues	Antimetabolites
Busulfan	Carboplatin	Cytidine Analogues
Chlorambucil	Cisplatin	Azacytidine
Cyclophosphamide		Cytarabine
Ifosfamide		Gemcitabine
Mechlorethamine		Folic Acid Antagonist
Melphalan		Methotrexate
Prednimustine		Fluorinated Pyrimidines
Streptozocin		Fluorouracil
Thiotepa		Ribonucleotide Reductase
Nitrosoureas		Inhibitor
Carmustine		Hydroxyurea
Lomustine		Purine Analogues
Nonclassic Alkylating		Azathioprine
Agents		Mercaptopurine
Dacarbazine		Thioguanine
Hexamethylmelamine		Adenosine Analogues
Procarbazine		Cladribine
		Fludarabine
		Pentostatin

Antimicrotubule Agents	Topoisomerase Inhibitors	Antitumor Antibiotics	Miscellaneous Agents
Estramustine	Topoisomerase I	Bleomycin	Asparaginase
Vinca Alkaloids	Inhibitors	Dactinomycin	
Vinblastine	Irinotecan	Mitomycin	
Vincristine	Topotecan	Plicamycin	
Vindesine	Topoisomerase II	Anthracyclines	
Vinorelbine	Inhibitors	Daunomycin	
Taxanes	Amsacrine	Doxorubicin	
Docetaxel	Etoposide	Anthracenediones	
Paclitaxel	Teniposide	Mitoxantrone	
		Anthracycline	
		Analogues	
		Epirubicin	
		Idarubicin	

Nitrosoureas

Nitrosoureas are considered a subset of alkylating agents because of their similar mechanism of action. Unlike alkylating agents, nitrosoureas are lipid soluble, which enables them to cross the blood-brain barrier following systemic administration. This property makes them active in brain tumors. Nitrosoureas lack cross-resistance with other alkylating agents. Tumors that are resistant to treatment with alkylating agents will occasionally respond to therapy with nitrosoureas. The most impressive toxicity of this class is delayed and cumulative myelosuppression, which develops three to four weeks after administration. As a result, the interval between each treatment is usually six weeks.

Table 2C-3
Cancer Chemotherapy Agents

Drug (Synonym)	Dose, Route & Schedule When Used As Single Agent	Side Effects	Comments & Precautions for Safe Administration
Amsacrine (AMSA, m-AMSA) [NSC 249992]	90–120 mg/m^2 IV q21–28d 120 mg/m^2 IV qd × 5d	BMD. Severe pain and burning in vein. N/V, mucositis (all uncommon).	Tissue vesicant. Chemical thrombophlebitis. Increase diluent to 500 ml D5W and decrease rate to decrease venous spasm and pain. Do not infuse in less than 1 hr. Do not use chloride containing solutions. Orange urine; yellow skin discoloration. Administer only if serum potassium is normal as cardiac arrests during infusion have been reported.
Asparaginase (Elspar®, Crasnitin, L-ASP, Asnase, Colaspase)	200 IU/kg IV qd × 28d 6,000–10,000 IU/m^2 IM 3 × wk × 3 wks	Hypersensitivity reactions. Risk increases with repeated use. Moderate–severe N/V, anorexia, abdominal cramps, weight loss, mucositis. Hepatotoxicity common. Coagulation abnormalities. CNS abnormalities: personality changes, fatigue, seizures, irritability, somnolence, confusion, lethargy. Azotemia, hyperglycemia, proteinuria. Pancreatitis.	Give IV dose over 30 mins. IM route recommended. Test dose of 2 units intradermally recommended prior to first dose and should be repeated if >1 week since last dose. Observe patient for 1 hr prior to administering full dose and for at least 1 hr after full dose. Patients who develop hypersensitivity reaction to *E. coli* product may tolerate PEG-asparaginase or the *Erwinia* preparations. Use only clear solutions.
Azacytidine [NSC-102816]	150–300 mg/m^2 IV qd × 3–5d q21d 150–200 mg/m^2 2×/wk for 2–8 wks	BMD. Dose- and schedule-dependent N/V, diarrhea, stomatitis. Alopecia, rash, pruritis.	Short stability (2–3 hrs) in solution. Can be given SC but is painful and causes brown skin discoloration. Neurologic toxicity (weakness, lethargy, confusion, coma) reported but rare. Hepatotoxicity rare but serious complication. Hypotension with rapid infusion.
Bleomycin (Bleo, Blenoxane®)	10–20 units/m^2 IV, IM, or SC qwk (or intralesional) 15–20 units/m^2/d IV as CI over 3–7d	Mild BMD. Anorexia; mild N/V. Chills and fever to 103–105°F within 10 hrs. Hypersensitivity reactions, anaphylaxis. Cutaneous toxicities common including hyper-pigmentation, hyperkeratosis, erythema, peeling, rash, stomatitis, alopecia.	Anaphylactic reactions noted in patients with lymphoma. Test dose of 1–5 units is recommended followed by observation for at least 1 hr prior to administration of remainder of dose. Total cumulative dose should not exceed 400 units due to risk of interstitial pneumonitis and pulmonary fibrosis. This toxicity is increased by radiation therapy, especially to the lung, and concomitant drug therapy. Acetaminophen can decrease febrile reactions. Reduce dose if creatinine is >1.5 mg/dl. Radiation recall reactions. Sensitivity to sunlight; use of sunscreen is recommended.

Table 2C–3 *(Continued)*
Cancer Chemotherapy Agents

Drug (Synonym)	Dose, Route & Schedule When Used As Single Agent	Side Effects	Comments & Precautions for Safe Administration
Busulfan (Myleran®)	4–8 mg PO qd continuous; dose titration based on WBC Higher doses (8–16 mg/kg) given in bone marrow transplantation	Cumulative and prolonged BMD. Mild N/V. Mucositis and diarrhea with high dose therapy. Hyper-pigmentation, dry skin, alopecia, rash, urticaria. Gonadal suppression, amenorrhea, azoospermia, gynecomastia. Cataracts (rare). Dizziness, confusion, seizures with high dose therapy.	Hydration and allopurinol necessary to avoid hyperuricemia if WBC is high. Pulmonary fibrosis can occur after prolonged use. Symptoms include dry cough, fever, rales, and dyspnea.
Carboplatin (CBDCA, Paraplatin®)	400–500 mg/m^2 IV q4 wks Higher doses given in bone marrow transplantation	Mild N/V. BMD (thrombocytopenia dose-limiting).	Minimal nephrotoxicity; hydration and diuresis unnecessary. Mild neurotoxicity and ototoxicity.
Carmustine (BCNU, BiCNU®)	150–200 mg/m^2 IV q6 wks 75–100 mg/m^2 IV × 2d q6 wks	Severe N/V in 2–4 hrs. Facial flushing, vein irritation. Alopecia. Delayed and cumulative BMD.	Irritant. Marked facial flushing and venous spasm due to alcohol diluent. Increase volume, decrease rate of infusion, and apply ice above injection site to decrease pain. Chemical thrombophlebitis often occurs in several days. Pulmonary fibrosis seen after cumulative doses of 900 mg/m^2 or after 6 months of therapy or with concomitant bleomycin or radiation therapy to chest. Hepatotoxicity in 20%. Nephrotoxicity. Avoid direct contact with skin and eyes. Enters CSF; CNS disturbances (dizziness and ataxia). Venous discoloration.
Chlorambucil (Leukeran®)	0.1–0.2 mg/kg PO qd continuous; 16 mg/m^2 PO qd × 5d q28d; dose titration based on WBC	Well tolerated. BMD (dose related). Occasional alopecia. Exfoliative dermatitis (rare).	Interstitial pneumonitis and pulmonary fibrosis can occur after prolonged use. GI distress only at high dosages.

Continued

Table 2C–3 *(Continued)*
Cancer Chemotherapy Agents

Drug (Synonym)	Dose, Route & Schedule When Used As Single Agent	Side Effects	Comments & Precautions for Safe Administration
Cisplatin (Platinol®, CDDP)	20–120 mg/m² IV q3–4 wks 20–40 mg/m² IV qd 3–5d q3–4 wks	Severe N/V in 1 hr lasting up to 96 hrs. Hypersensitivity reactions (rare). Nephrotoxicity. Ototoxicity (cumulative). Peripheral neuropathy, neurologic toxicity (dose-limiting). Ophthalmic toxicity. Mild to moderate BMD.	Irritant. Nephrotoxicity can be avoided with adequate hydration and diuresis. Check BUN, serum creatinine, and estimated creatinine clearance prior to administration. For doses <40 mg/m², hydration of 1000 ml NS IV is often given. For doses ≥40 mg/m², prehydration with 1000–2000 ml NS IV is often used. Cisplatin can be admixed in 3% saline solution or with mannitol 12.5–25 gm to ensure diuresis. Urinary output should be 100–150 ml prior to the administration of cisplatin. Post cisplatin hydration of 1000–2000 ml NS is also often given. Treat hypersensitivity reactions with antihistamines and steroids, then pretreat with same for future doses. Post treatment check. Magnesium wasting requiring magnesium sulfate (IM/PO) replacement to manage neuromuscular irritability.
	90 mg/m² intraperitoneally in 2L dialysate q3 wks	N/V. Abdominal discomfort. Sterile ascites.	Nephrotoxicity dose-limiting at 90 mg/m². Administration of mannitol and sodium thiosulfate (7.5 gm/m² loading dose and 2.13 gm/m² q 12 hrs) permits IP administration of CDDP at 270 mg/m² without nephrotoxicity; N/V is dose-limiting. Dwell time 4 hrs. Strict catheter asepsis is essential. Fullness and abdominal discomfort commonly seen due to increased intra-abdominal pressure.
Cladribine (2-CdA, Leustatin®)	0.09 mg/kg IV qd as Cl × 7d	BMD. Fever. Nausea. Fatigue, headache. Rash.	Patients with large tumor burden should also receive allopurinol to decrease hyperuricemia from tumor lysis syndrome.

Table 2C–3 (Continued)
Cancer Chemotherapy Agents

Drug (Synonym)	Dose, Route & Schedule When Used As Single Agent	Side Effects	Comments & Precautions for Safe Administration
Cyclophosphamide (CTX, Cytoxan®, Neosar®, Endoxan®)	500–1500 mg/m² IV q3 wks 50–200 mg/m² PO qd × 14d q28d 60–120 mg/m² PO qd continuous; dose titration based on WBC	BMD. Dose-related N/V in 3–12 hrs, can last 8–10 hrs. Anorexia common. Dizziness, nasal congestion, watery eyes, rhinorrhea, sneezing can occur with rapid IV infusion. BMD. Alopecia, hyperpigmentation of skin and nailbeds. Gonadal suppression.	Vigorous hydration with oral or intravenous fluids (>3 liter/d) to maintain adequate urine output in order to decrease risk of hemorrhagic cystitis. D/C if dysuria or hematuria develops. Chronic nausea can occur with daily oral CTX. Divided doses taken with meals can help. Inappropriate antidiuretic hormone (ADH) secretion can occur at doses >50 mg/kg. Interstitial pneumonitis and pulmonary fibrosis and acute pericarditis (rare). Potentiation of anthracycline cardiotoxicity reported. Barbiturates and phenytoin may increase toxic effects by affecting activation by hepatic microsomal enzymes.
Cytarabine (cytosine arabinoside, Ara-C, Cytosar-U®)	100 mg/m² q12 hrs IV or SC × 7–21d 60–200 mg/m² IV qd as CI × 5–10d 3 gm/m² q12 hrs IV × 3–6d (high-dose therapy) 10–30 mg/m² IT up to 3 ×/wk	Dose- and schedule-dependent N/V. Marked BMD. Anorexia, stomatitis, diarrhea. Skin rash, alopecia. Flu-like syndrome (fever, arthralgias, myalgias, malaise). Conjunctivitis, keratitis, photophobia.	Prophylactic glucocorticoid eye drops may reduce keratitis. Sensitivity to sunlight: use of sunscreen recommended. Cerebellar toxicity and peripheral neuropathy seen in high-dose therapy. Use with caution if hepatic or renal dysfunction exists. Systemic toxicity from IT use includes mild N/V, fever, HA.
Dacarbazine (Imidazole carboxamide, DTIC)	50–250 mg/m² IV qd × 5d q3–4 wks 375 mg/m² IV d 1 and 15 (ABVD) 650–1450 mg/m² IV q3–4 wks	BMD. Severe N/V in 1–3 hrs; anorexia. Vein irritation. Facial flushing, rash, alopecia (uncommon).	Irritant. Decrease rate of infusion and apply ice above injection site to decrease pain from venous spasm. Flu-like syndrome with fever, headache, myalgia, and malaise occurring 1 wk after treatment lasting 7–10 d (rare). Sensitivity to sunlight; use of sunscreen recommended.
Dactinomycin (Actinomycin-D, Act-D, Cosmegen®)	0.25–0.6 mg/m² IV qd × 5d q3–4 wks—not to exceed 0.5 mg/d for children	BMD. Moderate–severe N/V in 2 hrs lasting 12–24 hrs. Acneiform rash, erythema, desquamation, hyperpigmentation, alopecia. Stomatitis, glossitis, anorexia, diarrhea, proctitis.	Tissue vesicant. N/V tends to increase with daily use. Severe radiation recall reactions with necrosis can occur. Sensitivity to sunlight; use of sunscreen is recommended.

Continued

Table 2C-3 (Continued)
Cancer Chemotherapy Agents

Drug (Synonym)	Dose, Route & Schedule When Used As Single Agent	Side Effects	Comments & Precautions for Safe Administration
Daunorubicin (Daunomycin, Rubidomycin, Cerubidine®)	30–60 mg/m^2 IV qd × 3d	BMD. Moderate–severe N/V. Allergic and hypersensitivity reactions. Diarrhea, stomatitis. Alopecia, rash, nail changes. Chemical phlebitis. Gonadal suppression.	Tissue vesicant. Local venous irritation. Cardiotoxicity—limit total dose to 550 mg/m^2. Dose reduction with hepatic dysfunction (bilirubin >1.2). Red urine. Radiation recall reactions.
Daunorubicin citrate liposome (DaunoXome®)	40 mg/m^2 q2 wks	Similar to daunorubicin; severity might be decreased.	Infuse over 60 min. Not a known vesicant. Liposomal preparation has a low plasma level and a shorter half-life than daunorubicin.
Diaziquone (aziridinylbenzo-quinone, AZQ) [NSC 104800]	6–8 mg/m^2 IV qd × 5d q4 wks 15 mg/m^2 IV qd × 3d q4 wks	Mild N/V. BMD, especially thrombocytopenia. Stomatitis, diarrhea, anorexia.	Penetrates CSF. Do not administer unless solution is clear. Dissolution of particles in IV preparation is extremely slow. Given as IV infusion over 20 mins or as continuous infusion. Transient hepatotoxicity (increased LFTs).
Docetaxel (Taxotere®)	60–100 mg/m^2 IV q3 wks	Hypersensitivity reactions. Fluid retention. BMD. Peripheral neuropathy (paresthesias, burning). Fatigue, weakness, lethargy. Rash, nail changes.	Premedication with steroid such as dexamethasone 8 mg po bid is recommended beginning one day prior to treatment and continuing for a total of 3–5 d to reduce hypersensitivity reactions and the severity of fluid retention. Patients with elevated bilirubin, SGOT, SGPT and alkaline phosphatase are at an increased risk of developing significant toxicities.
Doxorubicin (Adriamycin®, Rubex)	60–75 mg/m^2 IV q3–4 wks 20 mg/m^2 IV weekly	BMD. Dose-related N/V occurring in 1–3 hrs and lasting 24 hrs. Allergic and hypersensitivity reactions. Anorexia, diarrhea, stomatitis. Complete alopecia, hyperpigmentation, nail changes. Gonadal suppression.	Tissue vesicant. Local venous irritation with pain, erythema, urticaria, and pruritus along vein during administration. Dose reduction with hepatic dysfunction (bilirubin >1.2). Cardiotoxicity—limit total dose to 550 mg/m^2. Prolonged infusion of dose over several days may reduce cardiotoxicity. Red urine. Radiation recall reactions. Sensitivity to sunlight; use of sunscreen recommended.

Table 2C–3 (Continued)
Cancer Chemotherapy Agents

Drug (Synonym)	Dose, Route & Schedule When Used As Single Agent	Side Effects	Comments & Precautions for Safe Administration
Doxorubicin liposome (Doxil®)	20 mg/m^2 q3 wks	Similar to doxorubicin.	Irritant. Infuse over 30 min. Doxorubicin is encapsulated in liposomes with surface-bound methoxypolyethylene glycol. Results in prolonged half-life. Dose reduction for hepatic dysfunction (bilirubin >1.2). Cardiotoxicity—maximum dose same as doxorubicin.
Epirubicin (4′-Epidoxorubicin, 4′-Epiadriamycin) [NSC-256942]	60–100 mg/m^2 IV q3 wks	BMD. N/V. Arrhythmias (transient and reversible). Mucositis, alopecia.	Tissue vesicant. Less cardiotoxic than doxorubicin at equivalent myelosuppressive doses.
Estramustine (estracyte, Emcyt®)	15 mg/kg PO qd in three divided doses	Severe N/V (dose limiting). Anorexia, diarrhea. Nipple tenderness and gynecomastia. Decreased libido, impotence. Hypercalemia.	Take on empty stomach. N/V usually decrease with continued use. Hepatotoxicity (transient increased LFTs). Thromboembolic disorders. Sodium retention. Use cautiously in patients with history of CHF or previous MI, CV disease.
Etoposide (VP-16, VePesid®, epipodophyllo-toxin)	200–250 mg/m^2 IV qwk 100 mg/m^2 IV qd × 5 q3 wks 50 mg/m^2 PO qd × 21d	Hypersensitivity reactions—fever, chills, hypotension, dyspnea, bronchospasm (rare). BMD. Mild N/V, anorexia. Alopecia. Rarely, peripheral neuropathy, fatigue, headache, somnolence.	Irritant. Chemical phlebitis. Infuse drug over 30–60 min to prevent hypotension and bronchospasm. Oral formulation causes N/V, diarrhea. Oral dose is twice the IV dose. Divide oral dose if it exceeds 400 mg total. Dose reduction with impaired renal function.
Floxuridine (fluo-rodeoxyuridine)	0.2–0.3 mg/kg/d intra-arterial × 7–14d	BMD. Diarrhea, stomatitis. N/V. Dermatitis.	Used in patients with metastatic disease confined to the liver to provide high local drug concentration. Hepatic toxicity usually is dose-limiting in this setting. Includes chemical hepatitis, cholestatic jaundice, biliary sclerosis.
Fludarabine (Fludara®)	25 mg/m^2 IV qd × 5d q28d	BMD (moderate to severe). Mild N/V, anorexia. Diarrhea, mucositis are rare. Somnolence, fatigue, peripheral neuropathy.	Tumor lysis syndrome can occur.

Continued

Table 2C–3 *(Continued)*
Cancer Chemotherapy Agents

Drug (Synonym)	Dose, Route & Schedule When Used As Single Agent	Side Effects	Comments & Precautions for Safe Administration
Fluorouracil (5-FU, Adrucil®), Fluoroplex® (topical), Efudex® (topical)	300–450 mg/m² IV qd × 5d q28d 1 gm/m² IV qd as CI × 4–5d q28d 2.6 gm/m² IV as CI × 24 hr weekly Topical for malignant keratoses	BMD. Stomatitis, esophagitis, pharyngitis, diarrhea, and proctitis may be severe. Anorexia, N/V. Hyperpigmentation, nail changes, skin rash, dermatitis, hand-foot syndrome, partial alopecia. Conjunctival irritation; excessive lacrimation, blurred vision, photophobia.	BMD less common with CI. Interrupt therapy when GI toxicity appears as it often precedes serious myelotoxicity. Decreased myelotoxicity with intra-arterial use. Sensitivity to sunlight; use of sunscreen recommended. MTX or leucovorin administered prior to 5-FU to enhance effectiveness. Cerebellar syndrome (HA, ataxia, confusion, nystagmus) with high doses. Toxicities more common and more severe in patients with dihydropyrimine dehydrogenase deficiency.
Gemcitabine (Gemzar®)	1000 mg/m² IV qwk, 3 wks on & 1 wk off	BMD. Flu-like syndrome (fever, headache, fatigue). N/V, diarrhea. Rash, alopecia. Fluid retention (peripheral edema).	Skin rash, usually maculopapular and pruritic, occurs within 72 hrs of treatment. Rash resolves with discontinuation of drug or dose reduction.
Hexamethylmela-mine (HMM, HXM, Hexalen®, altretamine)	4–12 mg/kg PO qd × 14–21d or continuous 6–8 mg/kg PO qd × 21d q6 wks	BMD. Moderate-severe N/V, abdominal cramps, anorexia, diarrhea. Peripheral neuropathy, agitation, somnolence, lethargy, confusion, hallucinations, depression, petit mal seizures, coma. May exacerbate vincristine-related neuropathy.	Nausea and vomiting may be dose-limiting. Give in divided doses, with meals or at bedtime.
Hydroxyurea (Hydrea®)	25 mg/kg PO qd continuous; dose titration based on WBC. IV preparation investigational	BMD. Minimal N/V; anorexia, diarrhea, mucositis are rare. Rash, erythema, hyperpigmentation, pruritis.	Renal toxicity. Neurologic disturbances—headache, drowsiness, dizziness, disorientation are rare. Radiation recall can occur.
Idarubicin (Idamycin®)	12 mg/m² IV qd × 3d 8–15 mg/m² IV q3 wks	BMD. Mild N/V, diarrhea, stomatitis, anorexia. Alopecia (partial).	Tissue vesicant. Radiation recall (uncommon). Hepatotoxicity. Probably less cardiotoxic than doxorubicin and daunorubicin. Evaluate cardiac function as cumulative dose approaches 135 mg/m².

Table 2C–3 *(Continued)*
Cancer Chemotherapy Agents

Drug (Synonym)	Dose, Route & Schedule When Used As Single Agent	Side Effects	Comments & Precautions for Safe Administration
Ifosfamide (Ifex®, isophosphamide)	1,200 mg/m² IV qd as CI × 5d q3–4 wks 2,000 mg/m² IV qd × 5d q3 wks 2,400 mg/m² IV qd × 3d	Dose-related N/V in 2–10 hrs, often persists several days; anorexia, constipation, diarrhea, stomatitis. BMD. Alopecia. Transient hepatotoxicity. At high doses, acute tubular necrosis and neurotoxicity (somnolence, lethargy, confusion).	More toxic to urinary tract than cyclophosphamide. Hemorrhagic cystitis reduced by concomitant administration of 2-mercaptoethane sulfonate sodium (Mesna) as uroprotection. Fluid intake must be at least 2 liters/m²/d to maintain adequate urine output. Neurotoxicity occurs more frequently in setting of low serum albumin and with concomitant administration of sedatives. Hepatic microsomal enzyme activation affected by phenytoin and barbiturates. Chemical thrombophlebitis.
Irinotecan (CPT-11, Camptosar™)	125 mg/m² IV qwk, 4 wks on, 2 wks off	BMD. Diarrhea, abdominal cramping, N/V. Alopecia.	Diarrhea is dose-limiting. It must be treated early and aggressively. Can use loperamide 4 mg at onset then 2 mg q2 hr until diarrhea has stopped for 12 hrs.
Lomustine (CCNU, CeeNU®)	130 mg/m² PO q6 wks	Delayed and cumulative BMD. Moderate–severe N/V in 2–6 hrs, diarrhea, anorexia, stomatitis, alopecia (mild).	N/V may be reduced if taken at bedtime with antiemetics. GI absorption in 30–60 min. Give on empty stomach. Anorexia often lasts several days. Renal & pulmonary toxicity with prolonged use (cumulative dose >1100 mg). Enters CSF.
Mechlorethamine (HN₂, nitrogen mustard, Mustargen®)	0.4 mg/kg IV q3–4 wks 6 mg/m² IV d 1 & 8 q4 wks (MOPP)	Severe N/V in ½–2 hrs, lasting 2–8 hrs. Metallic taste. Fever, chills. Diarrhea; anorexia lasting several days. BMD. Gonadal suppression. Stomatitis, alopecia, maculopapular rash (rare).	Tissue vesicant. Chemical thrombophlebitis and venous discoloration common. Administer promptly after reconstitution. Allergic and anaphylactic reactions (rare).
	0.2–0.4 mg/kg intracavitary for malignant effusions	Fever, chills, malaise, mild N/V.	Pain common due to intense inflammatory reaction. Reposition patient q15 mins × 1 hr to maximize drug distribution.

Continued

Table 2C–3 (Continued)
Cancer Chemotherapy Agents

Drug (Synonym)	Dose, Route & Schedule When Used As Single Agent	Side Effects	Comments & Precautions for Safe Administration
Mechlorethamine (Continued)	10 mg dissolved in 50 ml aqueous solution applied topically TIW then qwk for mycosis fungoides	Erythema, hyperpigmentation, urticaria, and pruritus.	Gloves should be worn during application. Aqueous solution is applied topically and intralesionally for mycosis fungoides. Hypersensitivity reactions occur frequently with topical use. Desensitization is generally effective.
	10 mg in petrolatum-based ointment		Ointment greatly simplifies application and appears to increase absorption into the skin. Associated with a lower incidence of hypersensitivity reactions. Decreases dry skin problems created by aqueous preparation.
Melphalan (Alkeran®, L-phenylalanine mustard, L-PAM, L-sarcolysin)	0.25 mg/kg PO qd × 4d q6 wks 6 mg/m² PO qd × 5d q6 wks 0.05–0.1 mg/kg PO qd × 2–3 wks then 2–4 mg qd when BM recovered IV preparation investigational Higher IV doses given in bone marrow transplantation (140 mg/m²)	BMD (delayed and cumulative). Nausea uncommon with oral route, severe with high doses given IV. Occasional dermatitis, rash, alopecia. Stomatitis, diarrhea uncommon.	Take on empty stomach. Serious hypersensitivity reactions have been reported with IV use. Pulmonary fibrosis can occur after prolonged use.
Mercaptopurine (6-MP, Purinethol®)	2.5 mg/kg PO qd continuous; dose titration based on WBC. IV preparation investigational	BMD. N/V, anorexia, diarrhea, mucositis. HA, fever.	Dose reduction to 75% if allopurinol is given concurrently. Allopurinol inhibits 6-MP degradation by xanthine oxidase. Hepatic or renal dysfunction requires dose reduction. When combined with doxorubicin, risk of hepatotoxicity may be increased. Cholestatic jaundice and hepatic encephalopathy associated with hepatic necrosis.

Table 2C-3 *(Continued)*
Cancer Chemotherapy Agents

Drug (Synonym)	Dose, Route & Schedule When Used As Single Agent	Side Effects	Comments & Precautions for Safe Administration
Methotrexate (MTX, amethopterin, Folex®, Mexate®)	20–80 mg/m^2 IV, IM, PO	BMD. Mild–moderate N/V, stomatitis, diarrhea. Alopecia; skin rash; hyperpigmentation. Gonadal suppression. Hypersensitivity reactions.	Renal impairment delays excretion and increases systemic toxicity. Renal function (BUN, creatinine) must be checked prior to each dose. GI ulceration can develop along all of GI tract, requiring discontinuation of therapy.
	10–15 mg/m^2 IT qwk	Chemical arachnoiditis, vomiting, fever, headache.	Pulmonary and serious hepatic toxicity can occur. MTX is protein-bound; avoid sulfonamides, aspirin, tetracycline, phenytoin, and chloral hydrate, which displaces MTX from plasma proteins. Avoid folic acid containing vitamins since they may alter response to MTX. Radiation recall reactions. Sensitivity to sunlight; use of sunscreen is recommended. MTX levels in CSF should be monitored carefully.
	"High-dose" MTX 1–10 gm/m^2 plus leucovorin rescue	Mild–moderate N/V.	Renal tubular necrosis. Maintain urinary pH$>$7.0 and ensure high urinary output to prevent precipitation of MTX in renal tubules. Adjust urinary pH with IV NaHCO$_3$ to maintain urine alkalinity and check pH q void during therapy. Check BUN, serum creatinine, creatinine clearance, LFTs prior to each dose. Use only preservative-free MTX for "high dose" or IT therapy. Monitor serum MTX levels and continue leucovorin rescue until serum MTX $<10^{-8}$ molar (0.45 µg/100 ml). Pneumothorax can occur within 48 hrs after "high dose" therapy in patients with pulmonary mets.

Continued

Table 2C–3 (Continued)
Cancer Chemotherapy Agents

Drug (Synonym)	Dose, Route & Schedule When Used As Single Agent	Side Effects	Comments & Precautions for Safe Administration
Mitomycin (Mutamycin®; Mitomycin-C)	2 mg/m^2 IV qd × 5d 10–20 mg/m^2 IV q6–8 wks	Delayed and cumulative BMD. Mild-moderate N/V lasting up to 2–3d. Anorexia, stomatitis (uncommon), diarrhea (uncommon). Fatigue, lethargy, weakness.	Tissue vesicant. Erythema and ulceration can appear at site distant from injection site and can occur up to several months after treatment. Renal toxicity. Hemolytic uremic syndrome (uncommon). Interstitial pneumonitis/pulmonary fibrosis reported. Total cumulative dose should not exceed 50 mg/m^2 to avoid excessive toxicity. May potentiate cardiotoxicity of doxorubicin. Sensitivity to sunlight.
Mitotane (o, p′-DDD, Lysodren®)	2–10 gms in 3–4 divided doses PO qd continuous	Severe N/V, anorexia, diarrhea. Rash. Depression (lethargy and sedation), dizziness, vertigo.	Functional impairment and brain damage with prolonged use of high doses. Acute adrenal insufficiency—glucocorticoid and mineralcorticoid replacement may be needed.
Mitoxantrone (DHAD, Novantrone®)	10–12 mg/m^2 IV qd × 5d 12 mg/m^2 IV qd × 3d 12 mg/m^2 IV q 21–28d	BMD. Mild N/V, diarrhea, stomatitis. Alopecia.	Irritant. Cumulative cardiotoxicity; monitor left ventricular ejection fraction. Bluish discoloration in vein used for infusion, and of sclerae; blue-green discoloration of urine.
Paclitaxel (Taxol®)	135–250 mg/m^2 IV over 3–24 hrs q21–28d	BMD. Hypersensitivity reactions. Arrhythmias. Peripheral neuropathy. Complete alopecia. Fatigue, arthralgias, myalgias. Mild nausea, stomatitis, diarrhea are all rare.	Irritant. Premedication with steroid, antihistamine, and H$_2$ blocker may decrease or eliminate hypersensitivity reactions. Administer via polyethylene tubing and in-line filtration.
Pegaspargase (Oncaspar®, PEG asparaginase)	2500 u/m^2 IM or IV q14d	Fatigue. N/V, anorexia.	Polyethylene glycol (PEG) is combined with L-asparaginase to produce a drug that has reduced immunogenicity and prolonged half-life. Hypofibrinoginemia and other coagulation defects can occur.

Table 2C–3 (*Continued*)
Cancer Chemotherapy Agents

Drug (Synonym)	Dose, Route & Schedule When Used As Single Agent	Side Effects	Comments & Precautions for Safe Administration
Pentostatin (2'-deoxycoformycin, dCF, Nipent®)	4 mg/m^2 IV q2 wks	BMD. Moderate N/V, stomatitis, anorexia, diarrhea. Rash. Fever. Fatigue. Kerato-conjunctivitis, photophobia.	Hydration with 500–1000 ml of intravenous fluid before and after drug administration is recommended. Hepatotoxicity. Lethargy, seizures, and coma rare at conventional doses.
Plicamycin (Mithracin®, Mithramycin)	0.025–0.03 mg/kg IV qod × 3–8 doses or until toxicity Individual daily dose should not exceed .03 mg/kg	BMD. Moderate-severe N/V in 6 hrs lasting 12–14 hrs. Fever.	Irritant. Coagulation abnormalities and hemorrhage often preceded by flushing and epistaxis. Hepatotoxicity. Renal toxicity may be cumulative. Administer with caution to patients with hepatic or renal dysfunction. CNS toxicity with neuromuscular excitability, severe headache. Dermatitis. Proteinuria, azotemia, and electrolyte abnormalities (decreased levels of Phos, K, Mg, Ca).
Prednimustine (Leo 1031, stereocyte) [NSC 134087]	20–30 mg PO qd 100–160 mg/m^2 PO qd × 3–5d q2 wks Investigational	BMD. Mild N/V.	Gastritis can occur. N/V usually transient. Emotional lability. Rash, urticaria. Mild diarrhea. Edema.
Procarbazine (Matulane®)	50–200 mg PO qd × 14d or continuous	BMD. Moderate–severe N/V, anorexia. Skin rash, photosensitivity, urticaria. CNS abnormalities, including depression, nightmares, insomnia, mania, psychosis. Alopecia, stomatitis, diarrhea. Gonadal suppression.	Concurrent use of sympathomimetics, tricyclic antidepressants, other MAO inhibitors, foods rich in tyramine, benzodiazepams, opioid analgesics, barbiturates, phenothiazines, antihistamines may result in adverse effects. Postural hypotension. Interstitial pneumonitis/pulmonary fibrosis (rare).
Streptozotocin (STZ, Zanosar®)	500 mg/m^2 IV qd × 5d q6 wks 500–1500 mg/m^2 IV qwk	Mild BMD. Moderate-severe N/V in 1–4 hrs, anorexia, diarrhea. Reactive hypoglycemia due to insulin release. Vein irritation.	Irritant. Nephrotoxicity, glycosuria, proteinuria, hypophosphatemia, tubular necrosis, increased BUN. Mild to moderate hyperglycemia. Monitor BUN, serum creatinine, creatinine clearance, urinary protein. Severe hypoglycemia with insulinoma. Slow infusion to decrease local venous burning.

Continued

Table 2C–3 *(Continued)*
Cancer Chemotherapy Agents

Drug (Synonym)	Dose, Route & Schedule When Used As Single Agent	Side Effects	Comments & Precautions for Safe Administration
Teniposide (VM-26, Vumon®)	50 mg/m^2 IV 2× wk × 4 wks 100 mg/m^2 IV qwk × 6–8 wks	BMD. Mild N/V. Alopecia. Hypersensitivity reactions—hypotension, bronchospasm, tachycardia, urticaria (rare).	Irritant. Chemical thrombophlebitis common. Infuse over 30–60 mins to prevent hypotension.
Thioguanine (6TG)	2–3 mg/kg PO qd IV preparation investigational	BMD. Occasional N/V, stomatitis, diarrhea. Rash, dermatitis.	Reduce dose if stomatitis/diarrhea develops. Full dose can be given with allopurinol. Hepatotoxicity, cholestatic jaundice, veno-occlusive disease. Administer oral dose on an empty stomach to facilitate complete absorption. Administer IV dose over at least 30 min. Rapid IV administration may cause bronchospasm and cardiovascular collapse.
Thiotepa (Triethylene-thiophosphoramide, TSPA)	8 mg/m^2 IV qd × 5d q3–4 wks 30–60 mg IV, IM, or SC qwk; dose based on WBC	BMD. Occasional N/V, anorexia. Alopecia (rare), hives, rash, pruritis.	Well tolerated.
	1–10 mg/m^2 IT	Headache, dizziness, parasthesias.	
	30–60 mg q4 wks for intravesicular use	Local irritation. Hematuria, dysuria, urgency, frequency with bladder instillation.	Leukopenia can occur after bladder instillation.
	Higher doses (up to 900 mg/m^2) given in bone marrow transplantation	With high dose therapy: N/V, severe stomatitis, diarrhea. Alopecia, erythema and desquamation of skin. Stupor & coma.	
Topotecan (Hycamtin™)	1.5 mg/m^2 IV qd × 5 q3 wks	BMD. N/V, constipation, diarrhea, abd pain. Weakness, fatigue, lethargy. Alopecia.	Minimum of 4 cycles is recommended as median response time is 2.3 months.
Tretinoin (Vesanoid®, all-trans-retinoic acid)	45 mg/m^2 daily in 2 divided doses	Dry skin and mucous membranes. Skin rash. Xerostomia, cheilitis. Headache. N/V. Arthralgias.	Retinoic acid syndrome characterized by fever, weight gain, respiratory distress, interstitial pulmonary infiltrates, pleural/pericardial effusions and hypotension; can be fatal.

Table 2C-3 *(Continued)*
Cancer Chemotherapy Agents

Drug (Synonym)	Dose, Route & Schedule When Used As Single Agent	Side Effects	Comments & Precautions for Safe Administration
Vinblastine (Velban®, VLB)	6–10 mg/m^2 IV qwk 0.1–0.4 mg/kg IV qwk 1.5–2 mg/m^2 IV qd as CI × 5d q4 wks	Dose-related BMD. Jaw pain following injection. N/V (rare), constipation.	Tissue vesicant. Biliary excretion; decrease dose 50% for bilirubin >1.5; 75% for bilirubin >3.0 or for hepatic dysfunction. Peripheral neuropathy (rare at conventional doses). Sensitivity to sunlight; use of sunscreen is recommended. Syndrome of inappropriate ADH secretion. Ischemic cardiotoxicity.
Vincristine (Oncovin®, VCR, Vincasar PFS)	0.4–1.4 mg/m^2 IV q1–4 wks	Mild BMD (rare). N/V unusual. Jaw pain following injection. Alopecia. Peripheral neuropathy, paresthesias, and loss of DTRs. Abdominal pain, constipation, paralytic ileus, bladder atony, vocal cord paresis. Diplopia, ptosis, photophobia, cortical blindness, headache, seizures.	Tissue vesicant. Biliary excretion; decrease dose 50% for bilirubin >1.5; 75% for bilirubin >3.0 or for hepatic dysfunction. Increased neurotoxicity in elderly and immobile patients. Use of stool softeners recommended. Hyponatremia and a syndrome of inappropriate ADH secretion.
Vindesine (Eldisine) [NSC 245467]	3–4 mg/m^2 IV q7–14d 1–1.3 mg/m^2 IV qd × 5–7d q3 wks	BMD. Mild N/V. Alopecia. Peripheral neuropathy (common).	Tissue vesicant. Do not administer with other vinca alkaloids. Great potential for cumulative neurotoxicity if given with other vinca alkaloids.
Vinorelbine (Navelbine®)	30 mg/m^2 IV qwk	BMD. N/V. Peripheral neuropathies, constipation. Jaw pain following injection. Mild alopecia.	Venous pain upon injection which can be reduced by decreasing the infusion time to 6–10 min. and administering at least 75 ml. of IV fluid after the infusion is complete.

BMD—bone marrow depression; CHF—congestive heart failure; CI—continuous infusion; CNS—central nervous system; CSF—cerebrospinal fluid; CV—cardiovascular; D/C—discontinue; DSW—Dextrose 5%/water; DTR—deep tendon reflex; GI—gastrointestinal; HA—headache; IM—intramuscular; IP—intraperitoneal; IT—intrathecal; LFTs—liver function tests; MI—myocardial infarction; NS—normal saline; N/V—nausea, vomiting; RFTs—renal function tests.

Table 2C–4
Hormonal Agents

Drug (Synonym)	Dose, Route & Schedule When Used As Single Agent	Comments & Precautions for Safe Administration
Androgens Fluoxymesterone (Halotestin®)	10–40 mg/d PO	Hepatotoxicity—dose reductions required for hepatic dysfunction. Cholestatic jaundice. Increased appetite and weight gain. Hypercalcemia especially in immobile patients with bone metastases. Masculinization—hirsutism, acne, patchy alopecia, voice change, increased libido. Sodium and fluid retention—monitor weight; low-salt diet.
Testosterone	50–100 mg IM tiw	Aqueous suspension. Some injectable preparations are formulated using oil-based esters which result in slow release and prolonged biological activity. Patients may become sensitized to oil carrier.
Testolactone (Teslac®)	250 mg qid PO	
Testosterone proprionate (Oreton®)	50–100 mg IM tiw	Oil based.
Testosterone cypionate (Depo®-Testosterone)	200–400 mg IM q2–4 wks	Oil based.
Testosterone enanthate (Delatestryl®)	200–400 mg IM q2–4 wks	Oil based.

Table 2C–4 *(Continued)*
Hormonal Agents

Drug (Synonym)	Dose, Route & Schedule When Used As Single Agent	Comments & Precautions for Safe Administration
Estrogens		
Diethylstilbestrol (DES)	15 mg PO qd (breast) 1–3 mg PO qd (prostate)	Hypercalcemia in patients with bone metastases. Sodium and fluid retention with edema, hypertension, and CHF-monitor weight; low-salt diet. Thromboembolic complications. In men, feminization, loss of libido, gynecomastia, breast tenderness. In women: endometrial hypertrophy, uterine bleeding, areolar hyperpigmentation. N/V at high doses resembling morning sickness. N/V often subsides with continued treatment. Urinary frequency. Patients may become sensitized to oil carrier. Natural and synthetic compounds vary with regard to onset of activity, bioavailability, and duration of activity. Chlorotrianisene is extremely fat soluble and considerable fat storage occurs, accounting for delayed onset and prolonged duration of effect. Individual products should be chosen selectively based on such properties.
Diethylstilbestrol diphosphate (Stilphostrol®)	50–200 mg PO tid 500–1000 mg IV × 5 d then 250–1000 mg IV qwk	
Chlorotrianisene (Tace®)	12–25 mg PO qd (prostate)	
Conjugated estrogenic compound (Premarin®, Estracon)	10 mg PO tid (breast) 1.25–2.5 mg PO tid (prostate)	
Ethinyl estradiol (Estinyl)	1 mg PO tid (breast) 0.15–2 mg PO qd (prostate)	
Estrone	2–4 mg IM 2–3 times weekly (prostate)	
Antiestrogens		
Tamoxifen (Nolvadex®) Toremifene (Fareston®)	20 mg PO qd 60mg PO qd	Hot flashes. Disease "flare" with increase in symptoms such as bone pain. Hypercalcemia. N/V. Mild estrogenic activity seen; vaginal discharge, bleeding, and pruritus vulvae. Increased risk of endometrial cancer; therefore, any abnormal vaginal bleeding should be further evaluated. Thrombophlebitis, thromboembolism. Corneal opacity, cataracts and retinopathy.

Continued

Table 2C–4 *(Continued)*
Hormonal Agents

Drug (Synonym)	Dose, Route & Schedule When Used As Single Agent	Comments & Precautions for Safe Administration
Progestins		
Medroxyproges-terone (Provera® [PO], Depo-Provera® [IM])	20–200 mg PO qd 200–800 mg IM biw	Generally well tolerated. Minimal fluid retention with edema, hypertension and CHF. Occasional hypercalcemia in patients with bone metastases. Hot flashes. Thromboembolic complications.
Megestrol (Megace®)	40 mg PO qid (breast) 10–80 mg PO qid (endometrial)	Changes in menstrual pattern–spotting, breakthrough bleeding, amenorrhea. Increased appetite, weight gain. Natural progestins are rapidly inactivated.
Hydroxyproges-terone caproate (Delalutin)	1–2.5 gm IM biw	Some injectable preparations are formulated using oil-based esters which result in slow release and prolonged biological activity. Patients may become sensitized to oil carrier.
Corticosteroids		
Prednisone (Deltasone®)	40–60 mg/m² PO qd	Agents vary with respect to mineral corticoid potency (sodium and fluid retention); intermittent administration can decrease the risk of serious toxicity.
Prednisolone (Delta-Cortef)	40–60 mg/m² IM qd	Adrenalectomized patients must increase steroids in stress, infection, trauma. Oral preparations irritate GI mucosa—administer with antacids.
Methyl-prednisolone (Medrol) sodium succinate (Solu-Medrol®) acetate (Depo-Medrol®)	10–25 mg IV or IM	*Side effects associated with prolonged use:*
Hydrocortisone (Cortef) sodium succinate (Solu-Cortef®)	100–500 mg IV or IM qd	Immunosuppression—increased risk of infection. GI ulceration and hemorrhage. Hyperglycemia, diabetes, hyperlipidemia, weight gain. Thin fragile skin, impaired wound healing, petechiae, ecchymosis. Sodium and fluid retention, hypertension, edema, potassium wasting. Emotional lability, euphoria, psychosis. Muscle wasting, muscle weakness. Osteoporosis, aseptic necrosis of bones. Glaucoma, cataracts. Cushingoid appearance, acne, secondary amenorrhea, growth failure. Suppression of pituitary-adrenal axis requires slow withdrawal.
Dexamethasone (Decadron®)	0.5–20 mg PO, IV or IM qd	

Table 2C–4 *(Continued)*
Hormonal Agents

Drug (Synonym)	Dose, Route & Schedule When Used As Single Agent	Comments & Precautions for Safe Administration
Aromatase Inhibitors		
Amino-glutethimide (Cytadren®, Elipten)	250 mg PO qid	Usually given with hydrocortisone 40 mg/d. Skin rash which subsides with continued treatment. Lethargy, fatigue, vertigo, nystagmus, somnolence. Addisonian characteristics; secretion of aldosterone with postural hypotension and hyponatremia. Hypothyroidism. Virilization. Mild nausea, vomiting, loss of appetite. Adrenal insufficiency.
Anastrozole (Arimidex®)	1 mg PO qd	Thromboembolic complications. Mild fluid retention. Asthenia, headache. Hot flashes. N/V. Hepatotoxicity (increased SGOT and SGPT).
LHRH Analogues		
Leuprolide (Lupron®)	1 mg SC qd 7.5 mg IM depot q month	Disease "flare" with increased bone pain, urinary retention. In men, hot flashes, gynecomastia, breast tenderness, testicular atrophy, impotence, decreased libido. In women, hot flashes, amenorrhea, vaginitis, emotional lability, decreased libido, breast tenderness, acne. Anorexia, nausea.
Goserelin (Zoladex®)	3.6 mg SC depot pellet q month	Disease "flare" with increased bone pain, urinary retention. Hot flashes, decreased libido, impotence, gynecomastia in males; amenorrhea in females. Pain at injection site.
Antiandrogen		
Flutamide (Eulexin®, Anandron)	250 mg PO tid	Usually used with LHRH agonist or orchiectomy. Hot flashes, gynecomastia, breast tenderness, galactorrhea, impotence. Occasional N/V, diarrhea. Transient hepatotoxicity (increased SGOT and LDH).
Bicalutamide (Casodex)	50 mg PO qd	Side effects similar to flutamide. Major advantage is once a day dosage.

Table 2C-5
Adjunctive Drugs Used in Cancer Treatment

Drug (synonym)	Usual dose	Indication	Comments & Precautions for Safe Administration
Amifostine (Ethyol®, WR2721)	910 mg/m² IV over 15 min	Protectant against cisplatin-induced nephrotoxicity and peripheral neurotoxicity and cyclophosphamide-induced granulocytopenia. Enhanced efficacy of cisplatin in metastatic melanoma patients; protection against granulocytopenia secondary to radiation therapy also reported.	Administer 30 min prior to chemotherapy. Hypotension—monitor BP q 5 min during infusion. Infusion rates >15 min associated with higher incidence of adverse effects. Side effects include N/V, flushed feeling, drowsiness, hypocalcemia.
Dexrazone (Zinecard®, ADR529, ICRF-187)	Recommended dose ratio of dexrazone to doxorubicin is 10 to 1	Cardioprotective agent used in patients who have received a cumulative doxorubicin dose of >300 mg/m².	Administer doxorubicin within 30 min following dexrazone. Myelosuppression can be more severe.
Gallium nitrate	300 mg/m² daily × 7d by CI	Heavy metal, exact mechanism of action is unknown. Used in the treatment of symptomatic hypercalcemia of malignancy unresponsive to hydration.	Hypocalcemia occurs within 3–4 d of administration. Transient hypophosphatemia can occur. Elevation in BUN and serum creatinine can be dose-limiting; minimized with adequate hydration.
Leucovorin (citrovorum factor, Wellcovorin®)	As rescue for methotrexate: 10–25 mg/m² po or IV q6 hrs × 6–8 doses To potentiate 5FU: 20–500 mg/m² po or IV	Used as a rescue for methotrexate or to potentiate the cytotoxic effects of fluorouracil and floxuridine.	When used as rescue for methotrexate, it is critical that all doses be taken as prescribed. Leucovorin usually administered until the serum methotrexate level has decreased to $<5 \times 10^{-7}$.
Levamisole	150 mg po qd × 3d; given every 2 wks	Used in combination with fluorouracil in the treatment of Dukes C adenocarcinoma of the colon.	
Mesna	The usual dose is 20% of the ifosfamide dose, given immediately before, and 4 & 8 hrs after ifosfamide	Used to prevent ifosfamide-induced or cyclophosphamide-induced hemorrhagic cystitis.	
Pamidronate (Aredia®)	90 mg IV over 2–4 hrs q 4 wks	Bisphosphonate used in treatment of hypercalcemia and osteolytic bone metastases.	
Plicamycin (Mithracin®, Mithramycin)	0.025–0.030 mg/kg IV 1–3 times per wk	Used for the treatment of hypercalcemia of malignancy.	Administer over 30 min to 6 hrs. Can cause cellulitis or phlebitis if extravasated.

BP—blood pressure; CI—continuous infusion; N/V—nausea and vomiting.

Antimetabolites

An antimetabolite is a chemical analogue, a drug that resembles an essential metabolite so closely that it enters the essential metabolic pathways. An antimetabolite is a fraudulent substrate for essential biochemical reactions and interferes with or blocks normal biosynthesis of nucleic acids necessary for synthesis of DNA and RNA. Because their antitumor activity takes place when cells are in the synthetic phase of the cell cycle (S phase), antimetabolites are considered cell cycle specific. They are therefore most effective against rapidly growing tumors. Antimetabolites present minimal risk in terms of leukemogenesis or carcinogenesis and are not associated with prolonged or delayed myelosuppression.

Antimetabolites are subdivided into folic acid antagonists, and purine and pyrimidine analogues. The only folic acid antagonist in clinical use is methotrexate. Purine analogues include the guanine analogues mercaptopurine and thioguanine, and the adenosine analogues pentostatin, fludarabine and cladribine. Pyrimidine analogues include azacytidine, cytarabine, fluorouracil, and gemcitabine. Gemcitabine has been recently approved for the treatment of pancreatic cancer. Clinical trials are underway to evaluate its efficacy in other malignancies.

Antimicrotubule Agents

Vinca Alkaloids

Certain antitumor agents are derived from plants. Two of the most established compounds, vincristine and vinblastine, are derived from the pink periwinkle plant and, until 1994, were the only vinca alkaloids approved for use in the United States. Vindesine, a semi-synthetic form of vinblastine, has been in clinical trials since the 1970s. Vinorelbine, also a semi-synthetic form of vinblastine, was approved in 1994 for the treatment of non-small cell lung cancer. These agents bind to the protein *tubulin*, which normally polymerizes to form the microtubule apparatus during mitosis. The result of protein binding by the drug is metaphase arrest. The vinca alkaloids also inhibit DNA synthesis and RNA synthesis. Because their antitumor activity occurs during mitosis, they are considered cell cycle specific. Tubulin also serves as a conduit for the transport of neurotransmitters along nerve axons. This accounts for the neurotoxicity of some plant alkaloids.

Vincristine produces little bone marrow toxicity, but myelosuppression is the major side effect of vinblastine, vindesine, and vinorelbine. Neurotoxicity, the major toxicity with vincristine administration, is minimal with the use of vinblastine.

Taxanes

The taxanes are a new group of chemotherapeutic agents that include paclitaxel and docetaxel. Paclitaxel, derived from the bark of the western yew tree, was approved for the treatment of metastatic ovarian and breast cancer in 1993. Docetaxel, a semi-synthetic form of paclitaxel, was approved in 1996 for the treatment of metastatic breast cancer. The taxanes are novel antimicrotubule agents that promote the assembly of microtubules and stabilizes them against depolymerization. The dose-limiting toxicity of the taxanes is neutropenia. Neurotoxicity has also been reported and includes hyperesthesias, paresthesias, and decreased or absent deep-tendon reflexes. Administration of paclitaxel and docetaxel is associated with hypersensitivity reactions and requires medication prior to administration. Docetaxel is also associated with fluid retention which can be minimized with the administration of dexamethasone for 3 to 5 days beginning the day prior to treatment.

Topoisomerase I and II Inhibitors

Topoisomerases are enzymes that catalyze the coiling and uncoiling of the two strands of DNA. The uncoiling of DNA helix is essential for normal DNA function such as DNA replication or RNA transcription. There are two types of topoisomerases in humans, known as topoisomerase I and II. Topoisomerase inhibitors poison either the topoisomerase I or II enzyme by forming a stable complex of drug, enzyme, and DNA. The result is DNA damage that interferes with replication and transcription.

Two topoisomerase I inhibitors have recently been approved for use, irinotecan (Camptosar®) and topotecan (Hycamtin®). They are both derived from camptothecin, a naturally occurring alkaloid found in the bark and wood of a Chinese tree, *Camptotheca acuminata*. Irinotecan is approved for the treatment of advanced colorectal cancer in patients who have failed fluorouracil-based chemotherapy. Topotecan is approved for the treatment of relapsed or refractory ovarian cancer. Bone marrow suppression is the dose-limiting toxicity of both these agents. In addition, diarrhea can be dose limiting for irinotecan.

The antitumor topoisomerase II inhibitors currently in clinical use are etoposide (VP-16), teniposide (VM-26), and amsacrine (m-AMSA). Etoposide and teniposide are derived from the mayapple plant. The active substance in this plant is podophyllotoxin, and etoposide and tenopside are semisynthetic derivatives. A water soluble form of etoposide, known as etoposide phosphate or Etopophos®, has recently been approved for use, improving the ease of administration. Leukopenia is the dose-limiting toxicity. Mild neurotoxicity, such as decreased deep tendon reflexes and paresthesia, can also occur.

Antitumor Antibiotics

Antibiotics effective against cancer are a heterogeneous group of compounds produced by various bacterial and fungal organisms. Although they are too cytotoxic to treat bacterial infections, antitumor antibiotics are effective in treating a broad range of solid tumors as well as hematologic malignancies. Most antibiotics are cell cycle nonspecific. In general, antibiotics interfere with DNA synthesis by binding with DNA at various points and preventing dependent RNA synthesis.

The anthracycline antibiotics doxorubicin and daunorubicin are the most widely used antitumor antibiotics. Unfortunately these agents are associated with significant acute and late toxicities. The incidence of cardiotoxicity increases as the cumulative dose of each reaches 550 mg/m^2.

Anthracyclines and Anthracenediones

Mitoxantrone is an anthracenedione antibiotic, a new class of antitumor antibiotics. It intercalates with DNA and inhibits topoisomerase II. The cumulative lifetime dose of mitoxantrone is 140 mg/m^2. In patients who have received prior anthracycline therapy, the maximum dose is 120 mg/m^2. Cardiac toxicity is greater in patients with preexisting heart disease, prior anthracycline therapy, or radiation therapy to the mediastinum.

The development of analogues of commercially available antitumor antibiotics is currently being pursued. This effort is aimed at producing agents that have a greater therapeutic index or less toxicity than those now available. Idarubicin, an analogue of daunorubicin, has recently been approved for the treatment of acute nonlymphoblastic leukemia. Other analogues such as epirubicin and esorubicin continue in clinical trials.

Miscellaneous Agents

L-asparaginase is the only enzyme to be successfully used in cancer chemotherapy. It is prepared from various sources, including guinea pig serum, yeast, and *Escherichia coli* bacteria. The enzyme converts L-asparagine, an essential amino acid involved in protein synthesis, to L-aspartic acid. Many leukemic and some lymphoma cells require exogenous L-asparagine stored in body tissues, but normal tissues can independently synthesize this amino acid. Resistance to this drug could be related to an increased production of cellular L-asparagine synthetase, which converts L-aspartic acid to L-asparagine. L-asparaginase is effective in inducing remission of acute lymphoblastic leukemia. Its major life-threatening toxicity is anaphylaxis. Pretreatment skin testing and administration of a test dose is often used to predict hypersensitivity. Patients who exhibit hypersensitivity reactions must be desensitized before the therapeutic dose is administered. An investigational form of L-asparaginase that is prepared from *Erwinia* is available from the NCI for patients intolerant to *E. coli* preparation. Pegaspargase (Oncaspar®) is L-asparaginase combined with polyethylene glycol, and is also commercially available. It is less immunogenic than *Escherichia* or *Erwinia* asparaginase due to the polyethylene glycol coating. Myelosuppression is rare, but hemolytic anemia, liver dysfunction, severe nausea, and coagulation abnormalities are not uncommon. Acute pancreatitis and hypoglycemia (related to depressed serum-insulin levels) also can occur and are dose related.

Other drugs exist whose mechanism of action is unknown or which cannot be classified in any of the groups listed here. Although little is known about their mechanisms of action, the toxicity of many is well documented and should be understood by nurses administering them in cancer treatment.

New Formulations

Another recent advance in cancer chemotherapy has been the formulation of drugs in liposomes and/or with polyethylene glycol (PEG). Such formulations of chemotherapeutic agents were developed with the hope of reducing drug-related toxicities and selectively targeting drug to tumor. Liposomes are phospholipid layers surrounding an aqueous compartment. Chemotherapeutic agents can be inserted into this compartment. One difficulty associated with liposomal formulations of drugs has been the ability of macrophages to destroy these liposome-drug complexes. To circumvent this problem, polyethylene glycol has been used to coat the liposome. This prevents the liposome from being recognized and broken down by macrophages. This "stealth" liposome then enters the tumor and releases drug.

Liposomal doxorubicin (Doxil®) and daunomycin (DaunoXome®) are both approved and commercially available for the treatment of Kaposi's sarcoma. These formulations have significant distribution to cutaneous tissue, resulting in delivery of a sustained dose of drug to the tumor. Further clinical trials are underway to determine other tumors in which these formulations may be effective.

Pegaspargase is indicated and approved for the treatment of patients who are hypersensitive to native forms of L-asparaginase. The polyethylene glycol coating prevents the drug from being taken up by the reticuloendothelial system.

Hormones and Hormone Antagonists

Research into the mechanism of action of hormones has revealed that steroid-binding receptor glycoproteins exist in hormonally dependent or responsive tissue. When hormones bind to these receptor sites, these complexes interact with nuclear chromatin to alter the transcription of messenger RNA. This results in disturbance of cellular function and growth. Receptors for estrogens, progesterones, androgens, and corticosteroids have been identified and probably explain why these hormones are effective antitumor agents. Lack of responsiveness to hormonal manipulation is probably related to the absence of these receptors in the tumor. The major hormonal agents are described in Table 2C–4.

Tissues normally dependent on or responsive to endogenous physiologic hormones are often responsive to endocrine manipulation when the tissue develops a neoplasm. Such tissue includes that of the breast, endometrium, prostate, and thyroid. This hormonal dependency can often be exploited as therapy. For example, exogenous hormones can be administered that block the production of the hormone to which the tumor is sensitive. Progestins, which are compounds related to progesterone, have been used in the treatment of metastatic endometrial carcinoma. With the use of progestinal agents, remissions in endometrial cancer can last several years, especially in women who have experienced a long disease-free interval between primary resection and recurrent disease or who have well-differentiated tumors. Thyroid hormones have been used to control the growth of some papillary adenocarcinomas of the thyroid. These hormones act by inhibiting the secretion of thyroid-stimulating hormone (TSH) by the pituitary. Control with thyroxine is limited to tumors responding to the normal TSH feedback mechanism.

More recently, luteinizing hormone-releasing hormone (LHRH) analogues have been used in the treatment of carcinoma of the breast and prostate. This hormone is secreted by the hypothalamus and stimulates the pituitary to release luteinizing hormone (LH) and follicle-stimulating hormone (FSH). LH and FSH act on ovaries to secrete estrogen and progesterone or the testes to secrete androgens. When LHRH agonists are administered, the pituitary becomes desensitized to the effects of LHRH by decreasing the number of receptor sites. This results in a decrease in LH and FSH and, in consequence, a decrease in estrogen and androgen secretion.

The endogenous source of the hormone to which the tumor is sensitive can be ablated. Castration (oophorectomy and orchiectomy) has been used successfully to produce tumor regression in breast and prostate carcinoma. Diethylstilbestrol (DES) has been used to produce androgen ablation in prostate carcinoma. The antifungal agent ketoconazole has also been used in prostate carcinoma by inhibiting the conversion of 17 alpha-hydroxprogesterone to testosterone. Agents that compete with endogenous hormones for receptor sites can also be used to produce tumor regression. Tamoxifen, used in the treatment of breast cancer, competes with estradiol for binding to its receptor. When bound, tamoxifen causes the cell to resist estrogen stimulation. Similarly, flutamide, an antiandrogen used in the treatment of prostate cancer, competitively blocks the binding of androgens to the androgen receptor.

Adrenal corticosteroids can be administered in large nonphysiologic doses to alter the hormonal balance and to modify the growth of neoplasms. Prednisone is the most commonly used steroid hormone. The mechanism of action of corticosteroids is not clearly defined. It is thought that they might interfere at the cell membrane and inhibit RNA synthesis of protein. Corticosteroids are known to inhibit mitosis and have the capacity to destroy lymphocytic elements. Corticosteroids are active in a variety of neoplasms and are commonly used in combination chemotherapy because of their lack of bone marrow toxicity. However, corticosteroids are potent immunosuppressive agents, and their anti-inflammatory properties have the distinct disadvantage of disguising the cardinal signs and symptoms of infection.

Combination Chemotherapy

Treatment of advanced cancer, where the tumor burden is large, is frequently most successful with combination chemotherapy. Potentially curative dosages of a single agent could be so high that life-threatening or fatal toxicity precludes its use. Furthermore, repeated administration of tolerable dosages over prolonged periods can result in the development of resistant tumor cell lines. Various mechanisms for drug resistance have been proposed, including rapid repair of drug-induced DNA damage (alkylating agents), development of alternate metabolic pathways (antimetabolites), inadequate uptake of the drug by tumor cells (methotrexate), inadequate drug activation (antimetabolites), and increased inactivation of drugs (cytarabine). Tumors are also capable of spontaneous mutation to resistance with subsequent proliferation of the resistant clone.

Tumor resistance to single drugs stimulated the development of treatment programs that use drug combinations to circumvent the mechanisms of resistance and to reduce the tumor cell population. Effective drug combinations cause multiple lesions in cancer cells and produce a greater antitumor effect than would be achieved by giving each of the drugs in sequence. In addition, effective combinations decrease the cancer cell's ability to repair damage and delay or prevent the development of resistance. Drugs are selected for use in combination chemotherapy regimens using the principles outlined in Table 2C–6.

Unfortunately, the development of resistance to one agent often results in resistance to several agents. Although this phenomenon is not completely understood, it appears to be related to the presence of a cell membrane glycoprotein known as p170. This membrane glycoprotein acts as a drug efflux pump that reduces intracellular drug concentration. The gene responsible for encoding the p170 membrane glycoprotein is called mdr1. Currently under investigation are several agents that might be capable of blocking the p170 glycoprotein and thereby restoring, at least partially, a tumor's sensitivity to chemotherapy.

Adjuvant and Neoadjuvant Chemotherapy

Chemotherapy can also be combined with surgery and radiation to optimize the antineoplastic effects of each treatment modality and mini-

Table 2C–6
Rationale for Drugs Used in Combination Chemotherapy Programs

Active against tumor when used as single agent
Biochemical basis for suspected synergism
Different mechanisms of action
Different organ system toxicities
Different timing of toxicity

mize its toxic or disfiguring effects. Adjuvant and neoadjuvant chemotherapy programs are being successfully employed with several tumors. The preoperative or neoadjuvant use of chemotherapy reduces tumor size, thereby facilitating resection and/or preserving function (see Chapter 2A).

Adjuvant chemotherapy is now used to augment the curative potential of surgery or radiation in patients who have a high risk of recurrence. The use of prophylactic adjuvant therapy is an attempt to completely eradicate occult residual disease. Because measurable disease cannot be identified, only treatment programs with proven efficacy should be employed. Furthermore, the absence of measurable disease necessitates the use of randomized controlled trials to document improvement in disease-free survival. Because there are risks associated with chemotherapy administration, the potential benefits and risks of prophylactic adjuvant therapy must be carefully weighed. Adjuvant and neoadjuvant programs that effectively eradicate residual cancer cells have great potential for changing the primary surgical management of many tumors, permitting use of less extensive and less disfiguring surgical techniques.

DRUG DOSE CALCULATION

The dose of chemotherapeutic agent to be administered is usually determined based on the patient's body surface area. Body surface area (BSA), based on the patient's height and weight, allows for greater consistency in dosing agents than utilizing weight alone. Drug doses based on weight alone are expressed as mg/kg. BSA is expressed in meters squared (m^2); doses of agents to be administered based on BSA are expressed in mg/m^2. Special slide rules are available to calculate BSA easily, or a nomogram can be used (Figure 2C–1). An exception to dosing based on the patient's height and/or weight is that used for carboplatin, which is based on the patient's renal function, and may also take into consideration the platelet nadir. The majority of carboplatin excretion is renal, so dosages based on creatinine clearance prevent underdosing patients with above average renal function, or overdosing patients with impaired renal function. This type of dose calculation is referred to as the Area Under the

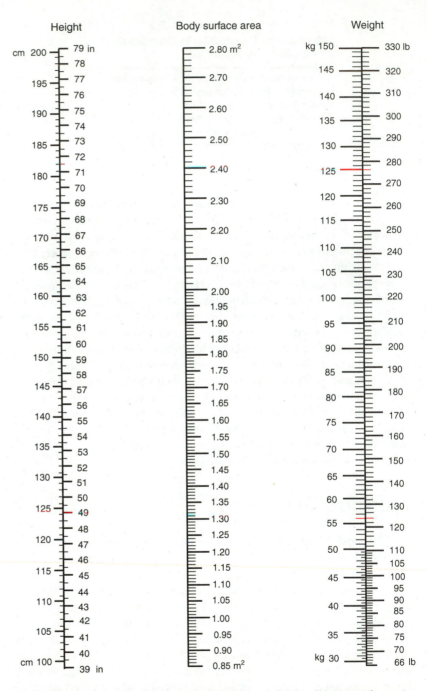

Figure 2C-1. Nomogram for the determination of body-surface area of adults from height and weight.

A straight edge connecting the individual's height and weight will intersect the center column at the individual's body-surface area.

Curve (AUC; the target area under the concentration versus time curve) method, and is expressed in mg. Dosages of chemotherapeutic agents might be modified for obese patients or those with ascites or amputation. Calculations of dosages of chemotherapeutic agents should be checked for accuracy prior to administration, as medication errors that result in over-dosage can have toxic effects, including treatment-related death.

NURSING CARE OF PATIENTS RECEIVING CHEMOTHERAPY

Acute and chronic side effects occur with most chemotherapeutic agents. Toxicities specific to individual drugs are summarized in Tables 2C–3 and 2C–4. Patients who are educated about potential toxicities can act to reduce or prevent complications related to treatment. The ability of patients to become involved in the management of their disease depends largely on their interactions with physicians and nurses. The development of a therapeutic relationship depends on professional competence and knowledge as well as the development of mutual trust. A good therapeutic relationship also facilitates effective education of the patient about treatment-related morbidity. Nurses should present information about specific neoplasms, available therapeutic options, and side effects associated with treatment, in terms of probabilities rather than absolutes. Although it is important to prepare patients for difficult realities that could lie ahead, it is also important to provide hope.

Gastrointestinal Side Effects

Nausea and vomiting are the most commonly encountered complications of antineoplastic agents (see Chapter 9). Symptoms might appear shortly after administration, be delayed by 8 to 12 hours, and persist for periods up to 48 hours with gradual resolution. Although they might occur separately, nausea and vomiting frequently appear as a clinical syndrome associated with physiologic changes such as dizziness, pallor, tachycardia, and diaphoresis. The incidence and severity of symptoms are dose-related with some, but not all, agents. Onset of symptoms might be related to any of the following: (1) direct irritation of the gastrointestinal tract (such as the mechanism of action of ipecac); (2) stimulation of a chemoreceptor trigger zone in the medulla oblongata that is sensitive to certain blood-borne compounds; (3) a central effect on the vomiting zone, a motor and reflex center in the floor of the fourth ventricle that regulates and coordinates the sequence of events during emesis; (4) anticipatory anxiety; or (5) a combination of factors. Symptoms can often be ameliorated with the prophylactic and regular use of antiemetic medications (see Table 2C–7).

These medications act in various ways, including depressing the vomiting center and blocking the effect of drugs on the chemoreceptor trigger zone. Patients should be encouraged to use antiemetics liberally and advised about their timing, scheduling, and side effects so that maximum relief can be achieved. Current research in the management of nausea and vomiting

Table 2C-7
Antiemetics in Current Use for Cancer Chemotherapy-Induced Nausea and Vomiting

Class	Example	Adult Usual Dose	Side Effects
Phenothiazine	Prochlorperazine	10 mg PO or IM, 25 mg PR q4–6hr 15 mg sustained release capsule PO q8–12hr	Sedation (mild) Orthostasis (IV) Anticholinergic Extrapyramidal
Butyrophenone	Droperidol	5–10 mg IV q2hr	Sedation (marked) Orthostasis Anticholinergic Extrapyramidal
Steroid	Dexamethasone	10–20 mg IV	Dysphoria, insomnia Perineal burning (rapid bolus)
Benzodiazepine	Lorazepam	1 mg PO/IV q4–6hr	Sedation Amnesia Confusion
Antihistamine	Diphenhydramine	50–100 mg PO/IM/IV q6–8hr	Sedation Anticholinergic Drowsiness
Cannabinoid	Dronabinol	5 mg/m^2 PO q2–4hr	Dysphoria Confusion Hallucination Tachycardia Orthostasis
Substituted Benzamide	Metoclopramide	up to 3 mg/kg IV/PO q2hr	Headache Restlessness Diarrhea Extrapyramidal
5-HT$_3$ (Serotonin) Antagonist	Ondansetron Granisetron	8 mg PO q 8–12hr 0.15 mg/kg IV q4 hr × 3 2 mg PO q24hr 10 mg/kg IV	Headache Constipation Dizziness Transaminase elevation

includes studies on diversion and relaxation techniques to reduce symptomatology as well as new antiemetic preparations. Delta-9- tetrahydrocannabinol (THC), the major active ingredient of marijuana, has been employed with some success in clinical settings where conventional antiemetics have failed. High-dose intravenous metoclopramide (2–3 mg/kg/dose), a substitute benzamide, has been successfully used in preventing and treating cisplatin-induced nausea and vomiting in many patients. Difficulties associated with its use include a relatively high incidence of extrapyramidal side effects and unsuitability for outpatient use. Selective 5-HT_3 serotonin receptor antagonists, ondansetron and granisetron, have significantly improved the management of nausea and vomiting associated with highly emetogenic chemotherapeutic agents. These drugs bind to serotonin receptors of the 5-HT_3 type located peripherally on vagal nerve terminals and centrally in the chemoreceptor trigger zone. This blocks serotonin stimulation and subsequent vomiting. They can be administered orally every 12 or 24 hours, making them easy to use in the outpatient setting. The addition of dexamethasone to ondansetron and granisetron enhances the efficacy.

Anorexia (see Chapter 9) can occur in conjunction with nausea and vomiting, or it might be related to physiologic changes (such as gastrointestinal obstruction and loss or distortion of taste) induced by tumor. Anorexia might also stem from emotional disturbances, especially depression and anxiety. A probable etiology should be identified and used to select appropriate therapeutic measures. Intervention can include nutritional counseling, dietary modification, nutritional supplements, and/or the use of intravenous parenteral nutrition to prevent severe nutritional deficiencies.

Diarrhea (see Chapter 9) can occur as a result of gastrointestinal mucosal irritation secondary to a direct toxic effect of the drug on the bowel. Antidiarrheal agents are often useful. When significant diarrhea occurs, hydration must be increased, especially when drugs that are nephrotoxic or eliminated in urine have been administered. Diarrhea associated with irinotecan can be a dose-limiting toxicity and must be treated early and aggressively. Diarrhea occurring during or within 24 hours of treatment is thought to be due to a cholinergic response. Recommended treatment is atropine 0.25 mg to 1 mg IV. Diarrhea occurring 2–12 days following treatment is due to direct cytotoxic effect. Loperamide 4 mg at the onset followed by 2 mg every 2 hours until the diarrhea has resolved for 12 hours is recommended.

Constipation (see Chapter 12B) is generally related to a direct effect on the nerve supply of the bowel, causing hypomotility. The vinca alkaloids are the group of drugs most often associated with this side effect. Constipation can also occur in patients taking selective 5-HT_3 receptor antagonists (ondansetron or granisetron) antiemetics. Prophylactic institution of a bowel program to prevent constipation is often warranted.

Cutaneous and Mucosal Toxicity

Mucositis or stomatitis (see Chapter 10B) is a serious, potentially life-threatening complication that is generally seen with antimetabolites and antitumor antibiotics. Toxicity manifests as erythema, pain, and ulceration of the oral mucosa. Dose reductions and/or interruptions in therapy are often necessary. Mucositis occurs when renewal of the epithelial cells lining the gastrointestinal tract is inhibited by chemotherapeutic agents. Bone marrow depression also influences mucositis, because lower granulocyte and platelet counts in conjunction with mucositis result in a higher incidence of infection and/or bleeding. Management of mucositis includes frequent cleansing of the oral cavity using sponge-tipped swabs and rinsing with saline. Topical anesthetics such as diclonine hydrochloride or viscous lidocaine are used as needed to control pain. Occasionally systemic analgesics are required. Topical antibacterial and antifungal therapy can prevent superinfection with opportunistic organisms.

Alopecia is a common complication of chemotherapy that, while not serious, has a profound psychological impact on clients. Patients receiving chemotherapeutic agents that can cause alopecia should be reassured that this side effect is temporary and that hair regrowth often occurs during therapy. The use of wigs, scarfs, and hats should be discussed.

Several techniques have been used to prevent or minimize alopecia, including scalp tourniquets and scalp hypothermia. These techniques reduce circulation to the scalp, thereby limiting contact of the chemotherapeutic agent with the hair follicle stem cell. These interventions have not been recommended for use in patients with hematologic malignancies or malignancies that metastasize to the scalp, because scalp cooling can prevent or limit tumor cell exposure to chemotherapy. Moreover, an FDA action calls into question the use of these techniques with any patient receiving chemotherapy. In 1990 the FDA halted the sale of commercially available scalp cooling devices on the grounds that their manufacturers had not provided adequate clinical data regarding their safety and efficacy. Patients who ask to use a scalp tourniquet or some form of scalp hypothermia should be made aware of the risks involved.

Macular or pustular rashes, desquamation, and epidermolysis can also occur as a direct effect of the drug on the skin or as an immunologically mediated allergic reaction. Areas of previous radiation are particularly susceptible to dermatologic toxicity. Severe toxicity might require dosage reductions, interruption, or cessation of therapy.

The cytotoxic action of chemotherapeutic agents can cause hyperpigmentation, banding, and retardation of nail growth. Patients should be reassured that these side effects of therapy are not related to disease progression. Photosensitivity can occur with administration of various agents. Patients should be instructed to limit sun exposure; to wear a wide-brimmed hat, long-sleeved shirts, and long pants; and to liberally apply sunscreen with an SPF of 15 or greater to exposed areas.

Hematologic Toxicity

Myelosuppression is the most common dose-limiting toxicity that is associated with chemotherapeutic drugs (see Chapter 10A). Bone marrow suppression is manifested as anemia, thrombocytopenia, and leukopenia and can sometimes be managed with blood component therapy. In the absence of concurrent cardiovascular disease, many patients will be asymptomatic if the hemoglobin level remains above 8 gm/dl. If symptoms such as excessive weakness, fatigue, and shortness of breath develop, packed red blood cell transfusions are used to prevent serious cardiovascular complications. In the thrombocytopenic patient, the risk of bleeding from all mucous membranes and skin and into the central nervous system or sites of trauma is increased. However, life-threatening hemorrhage is uncommon unless peripheral blood platelet counts fall below 20,000 cells/mm^3. Use of prophylactic platelet transfusions has reduced the incidence of fatal hemorrhage by more than 50 percent. If available, platelets obtained from histocompatible donors should be used when prolonged periods of thrombocytopenia are anticipated. Administration of certain drugs such as plicamycin and L-asparaginase can produce coagulation abnormalities that further increase the risk of serious bleeding when platelet counts are low. Important nursing interventions include assessment for evidence of increased bruising, petechiae, or oozing from mucous membranes, and counseling patients to avoid physical trauma and drugs, such as aspirin, that compromise platelet function.

Leukopenic, and more specifically granulocytopenic, patients are particularly susceptible to the development of infection. This increased risk of infection is often due to a combination of granulocytopenia and impaired immunocompetence. As patients become more granulocytopenic, the risk of sepsis increases dramatically. Classic signs and symptoms of infection are often absent because of the lack of granulocytes. Early recognition of infection is essential. Fever in the vast majority of leukopenic patients is due to infection. Febrile patients who are profoundly granulocytopenic should be hospitalized, with blood cultures performed promptly, and treated empirically with systemic, broad-spectrum antibiotics until the source of the fever is identified. Infection with gram-negative bacilli, fungi, parasites, and other opportunistic organisms is common. Granulocyte transfusions might be useful in the supportive care of patients who are expected to be leukopenic for prolonged periods. Hypersensitivity reactions to incompatible leukocytes can occur with granulocyte transfusions despite attempts to administer histocompatible cells.

Hematopoietic growth factors such as granulocyte macrophage colony-stimulating factor (GM-CSF) and granulocyte colony-stimulating factor (G-CSF) are used for 10 to 14 days following chemotherapy to reduce the degree and duration of neutropenia. These growth factors can allow higher doses of chemotherapy to be administered with fewer treatment delays, perhaps resulting in improved response rates.

Immunosuppression

In addition to having a direct effect on normal hematopoiesis, many commonly used chemotherapeutic agents are potent immunosuppressants. Impairment of the host's immune system increases the risk of infectious complications. Normal immune function might not return for as long as one to two years following the cessation of all therapy. Current chemotherapeutic programs are designed to provide intensive therapy that alternates with rest periods on a regular schedule to enhance immunologic recovery.

Hepatic, Pulmonary, and Renal Effects

Prolonged administration of chemotherapeutic agents could reversibly or permanently damage the liver, lung, and kidney. The incidence and severity of these effects are not fully appreciated at present. However, the potential for such toxicity must be considered when decisions about the duration of therapy are made, especially in patients receiving adjuvant therapy for undetectable residual cancer. Prolonged administration of both methotrexate and mercaptopurine is associated with chronic hepatotoxicity. Toxicity can include hepatic fibrosis, jaundice, and ascites. Prolonged treatment with busulfan, methotrexate, and carmustine have been linked to the development of diffuse interstitial and intra-alveolar pulmonary infiltrates. These infiltrates might gradually resolve when therapy is terminated and steroids are administered, or could result in progressive deterioration in pulmonary function despite discontinuation of the agent. Treatment with high doses of methotrexate, cisplatin, and the nitrosoureas is associated with renal toxicity. The incidence of permanent renal damage and renal failure following cessation of therapy with these agents is not yet appreciated.

Hyperuricemia can occur following the administration of chemotherapeutic agents when there is rapid lysis of tumor cells. High serum uric acid levels are due to breakdown of nucleoproteins in these cells. At high concentration, uric acid precipitates in the renal tubules and can cause serious or irreversible kidney failure. Allopurinol prevents the formation of uric acid and should be given prophylactically with hydration prior to the initiation of chemotherapy when rapid cell lysis is possible (see Chapter 16B). This is particularly important in patients with acute leukemia and lymphoma, where the use of chemotherapy can produce rapid and dramatic reductions in tumor volume. As noted in Table 2C–2, the dose of mercaptopurine should be decreased when allopurinol is given.

Long-Term Effects of Chemotherapy

Cancer chemotherapeutic agents, especially alkylating agents, can affect testicular and ovarian function. Therefore, a potential long-term complication of successful therapy is sterility. Although gonadal and reproductive capacity might return following the completion of treatment, patients who are in their reproductive years must be informed that irreversible sterility can occur. Chemotherapy can cause sublethal chromosomal damage to male or female gametes, so the risk of fetal abnormalities following therapy is real, although poorly defined to date. It is important to remember that although chemotherapy can cause infertility, methods of contraception should be discussed, because many agents are teratogenic and pregnancy should be avoided during therapy. Long-term storage of spermatozoa or eggs in special facilities might be considered for patients planning to have families.

Alkylating agents, antimetabolites, antitumor antibiotics, and procarbazine can produce cytogenetic aberrations, suggesting that these drugs have the potential for causing secondary malignancies in patients who have received them. A relationship between cancer and immunodeficiency has also been established in animals and in patients with congenital immunodeficiency syndromes (e.g., Wiskott Aldrich syndrome, ataxia telangiectasia), in patients with AIDS, and in renal transplant recipients who are being treated with highly potent immunosuppressive drugs to prevent organ rejection. The pathogenesis of second malignancies might also relate to the fact that drug-induced immunosuppression can permit cells damaged by drugs or radiation to proliferate and become clinically manifest as a second neoplasm. The risks of a second cancer must be balanced against the benefits to each patient in terms of quality of life and prolonged survival. Because the greater and more prolonged use of antitumor agents will place more patients at risk of developing drug-induced second neoplasms, it becomes even more important for nurses to understand the risk/benefit ratio thoroughly, to follow their patients carefully for any evidence of a second cancer, and to ensure that they are informed about this potential complication.

CONCLUSION

Although many advanced malignancies such as those listed in Table 2C–1 are now curable using drugs with or without radiation, the solid neoplasms of later life, particularly adenocarcinomas originating in the gastrointestinal tract and lung, remain a formidable therapeutic challenge. For these patients, the potential toxicities and risks of aggressive therapy must be carefully weighed and presented when discussing the potential benefits. The goal of cancer treatment should always be based on the potential for cure and a careful assessment of the side effects. At times, less intensive treatment or supportive care, consisting of control of pain and other symptoms, and psychological support, might be the wisest therapeutic choice. Although supportive care might not affect the ultimate outcome, it can often allow the patient extended periods of functional, pain-free life. It is essential, therefore, for nurses to be attuned to the psychological needs of patients as they care for their physical needs and to maintain a concerned and supportive attitude. There is no single, simple cure-all for cancer—and there probably never will be. Cancer is, in actuality, many different diseases, and each cancer must be approached as a unique entity. Many cancers can be cured now that systemic therapy with drugs can be used to eradicate undetected cancer cells left behind after surgery or radiation. There is great reason for continued optimism, given the research that is currently under way to improve effective therapies and to prevent and/or effectively manage untoward side effects.

BIBLIOGRAPHY

1. Burke, M. B., G. M. Wilkes, and K. Ingwersen. *Chemotherapy Care Plans: Designs for Nursing Care.* Jones and Bartlett Publishers, Inc., Boston. 1992.

   This pocket-size, spiral-bound reference book includes information about most chemotherapeutic agents in use today. It includes drug name, mechanism of action, metabolism, dosage range, preparation, administration, and special considerations. A unique feature is the inclusion of a nursing care plan for each drug. The care plan lists nursing diagnoses, defining characteristics, expected outcomes, and nursing interventions in a tabular format.

2. Chabner, B. A., and D. L. Longo, eds. *Cancer Chemotherapy and Biotherapy: Principles and Practice.* Lippincott-Raven Publishers, Philadelphia. 1996.

   This comprehensive resource on the preclinical and clinical pharmacology of chemotherapeutic agents includes information on chemical structure, cellular pharmacology, and pharmacokinetics not readily found in other resources. It is especially useful for oncology nurses involved in the clinical trials of investigational agents.

3. DeVita, V. T., S. Hellman, and S. A. Rosenberg, eds. *Cancer: Principles and Practice of Oncology,* 5th Ed. J. B. Lippincott Company, Philadelphia. 1997.

   This textbook presents the state of the art of basic scientific principles guiding the study, diagnosis, and treatment of cancer as well as the practice of treating the many forms of cancer and its complications.

4. Dorr, R. T., and D. D. Von Hoff. *Cancer Chemotherapy Handbook,* 2d Ed. Appleton & Lange, Norwalk, CT. 1993.

   This comprehensive resource includes data sheets for each conventional chemotherapeutic agent as well as selected agents under investigation. Information on complications and toxicities and administration of chemotherapy is provided.

5. Fischer, D. S., M. T. Knobf, and H. J. Durivage. *The Cancer Chemotherapy Handbook,* 5th Ed. Mosby, St. Louis. 1997.

   This easy-to-use resource includes information on conventional chemotherapeutic agents and some under investigation, including mechanism of action, indications, metabolism, dose, administration, toxicity, mixing, and storage. One chapter includes commonly prescribed chemotherapy combinations by disease site. An excellent section on the management of the patient and family includes chapters on topics such as ethics, infection, and pain.

6. Oncology Nursing Society. *Cancer Chemotherapy Guidelines and Recommendations for Practice.* Oncology Nursing Society, Pittsburgh. 1996.

   This series of modules was developed by the Clinical Practice Committee of the Oncology Nursing Society. It includes an outline for a basic chemotherapy course and associated practicum, policies, outcomes, and procedures related to chemotherapy administration. It is an excellent resource for nurses involved in establishing institutional policies, procedures, and course content related to the administration of chemotherapy.

7. Perry, M. C., ed. *The Chemotherapy Source Book.* Williams & Wilkins, Baltimore. 1992.

   This is a comprehensive and sophisticated textbook with 61 chapters. Topics covered include discussion of chemotherapeutic agents by class, management of drug toxicities, and chemotherapeutic treatment of major malignancies. It is excellent for oncology nurses who desire in-depth information.

8. Preston, F. A., and C. Wilfinger. *Memory Bank for Chemotherapy,* 2d Ed. Jones & Bartlett, Boston. 1993.

   This is a small, easily readable, spiral-bound reference book for the administration of chemotherapy, management of side effects, and related patient education. Chemotherapeutic agents are listed alphabetically with information on drug classification, indications, dosage, reconstitution, administration, stability, side effects, and a nurse alert that highlights important points. The chapter on nursing management/patient education includes information on side effects, highlighting patients at risk, assessment parameters, possible nursing diagnoses, nursing actions, and patient teaching.

2D

D. Biotherapy

S. Katharine Sandstrom

INTRODUCTION

Traditional cancer therapy consists of surgery, chemotherapy, and radiation therapy. These modalities have demonstrated therapeutic efficacy and safety in treating a broad range of neoplastic disorders, but there are still a vast number of cancers for which their efficacy has not been demonstrated. It has been shown that mammalian species have an innate mechanism for the control and/or destruction of cancer growth. This mechanism of immune surveillance suggests aberrant cells are constantly being produced within the host and destroyed by the immune system in response to tumor-specific antigens. This provides the foundation for biologic response modifier (BRM) therapy. Biologic response modifiers produce antitumor effects primarily through the action of the natural host defense mechanisms and/or by the administration of natural mammalian substances.

In the late 1800s Dr. William Coley and his associates observed a decrease in the incidence of cancer recurrence following postoperative opportunistic infections. These observations led to the discovery and use of Coley's toxin, in which active bacteria were injected into patients in order to elicit an immune response. Based on these observations, it has been hypothesized that a major role of the immune system is to prevent cell mutations. This concept became known as the *immune surveillance theory*. Although Coley's toxin failed to demonstrate a therapeutic value, it catalyzed the development of biologic-based therapies.

Scientists have been aware of the phenomenon of viral interference, the ability of infection by one virus to prevent the recurrence of a second, for more than 60 years. In the late 1950s, while studying viral interference *in vitro,* scientists reported the discovery of a substance released from virus-infected cells that would protect untreated cells from subsequent infection. They named the substance *interferon*. Subsequent studies revealed that interferon is a potent inducer of the immune response. In the 1960s, clinical trials evolved using immunomodulating agents, which were capable of initiating a host immune response. These agents included bacillus of Calmette-Guerin (BCG), methanol-extracted residue of BCG (MER-BCG), *corynebacterium parvum* (C. parvum), and levamisole. During the 1980s technical advances in molecular biology and recombinant DNA technology made it possible to produce large quantities of very pure proteins for clinical testing and treatment. Before these advances, these naturally occurring substances could not be isolated in sufficient quantities for clinical application. Recombinant proteins are created by excising the portion of human DNA that codes for the specific biologic response modifier that needs to be reproduced. This process involves placing the human portion of DNA and the DNA of a bacterial cell together into rapidly reproducing bacteria such as *Escherichia coli* or a yeast cell to produce the desired recombinant protein. BRMs produced this way are designated by an "r" (e.g., rIL-2).

AGENTS USED IN BIOTHERAPY

Cytokines are a general classification of cellular proteins that are produced and secreted in response to exogenous or endogenous stimuli. They encompass a large family of soluble polypeptide hormones that serve two essential functions: to regulate and differentiate cell growth and to augment cell activities. Cytokines can be further classified as either *monokines,* which are derived from mononuclear cells, or *lymphokines,* produced by sensitized lymphocytes (see Table 2D–1). Cytokines regulate the immune response of the host cell to activate and maintain the body's natural defenses; they are generally pleiotropic (producing many effects) in nature, possessing numerous functions that can be synergistic, overlapping or contradictory. Currently many clinical trials are underway to determine the effects of various cytokines on the immune system.

Interleukins represent a broad and expanding category of cytokines produced by activated lymphocytes. The biologic effects of the interleukins are pleiotropic and are part of a complex regulatory network of immunomodulatory and hematopoietic activities. The interleukins are designated with a numerical suffix that identifies each by its functional characteristics. The list of interleukins continues to grow; currently interleukins 1–17 have been identified and characterized.

Interleukin 2 (IL-2), also known as T-cell growth factor, is a glycoprotein, or lymphokine, that is produced primarily by T cells and is essential to the growth of T-lymphocytes. Interleukin 2 is by far the most extensively studied interleukin, as a single agent and in combination therapy with other BRMs. In addition to being a molecule with a potent effect on the immune system, it also mediates a wide spectrum of cytolytic activities. These include the activation of lymphocytes, generation of both natural killer (NK) cells and lymphokine-activated killer (LAK) activity, and the production of gamma-interferon and other cytokines. The enhancement of NK cell cytolytic activity appears to result from the ability of IL-2 to stimulate NK cells to produce gamma-interferon. In addition, IL-2 also stimulates its own growth by encouraging the formation of IL-2 receptors on T cells, monocytes, and macrophages. IL-2 therapy has substantial toxicities (see Table 2D–2). Used as a single agent in cancer treatment, IL-2 has been shown to be active in the treatment of metastatic renal cell cancer, melanoma, and non-Hodgkin's lymphoma.

Interferons constitute a family of naturally occurring glycoproteins that inhibit viral replication and exhibit antiviral, antiproliferative, and oncogene regulatory effects. To date, there are three species of interferon: alpha (α), beta (β), and gamma (γ). Structurally the interferons are similar, with 85 percent protein homology. The interferons are classified on the basis of their antigenic receptors. Alpha- and beta-interferons are located on the same chromosome and bind to the same receptor site on the cell surface. Gamma-interferon is located on a different chromosome and binds to a different receptor site from alpha- and beta-interferon. The biologic activity of alpha- and beta-interferon is predominantly antiviral and antiproliferative, whereas gamma-interferon functions more as an immunomodulatory agent, in addition to synergizing with other interferons and interleukins. Alpha-interferon has been approved by the Food and Drug Administration (FDA) for the treatment of hairy-cell leukemia, AIDS-related Kaposi's sarcoma, hepatitis non-A and non-B, and condyloma.

Tumor necrosis factor (TNF) was first discovered in mice immunized with BCG and subsequently treated with endotoxin. When the toxin was transferred into tumor-bearing animals, the result was hemorrhagic necrosis, giving this factor its name.

Table 2D–1
Types of Cytokines

Cytokine	Principal Cellular Origin	Biologic Activities
Interleukin 1 (IL-1)	Produced by monocytes and macrophages.	Stimulates proliferation of T-lymphocytes, interferon, and IL-2. Synergizes with growth factors and IL-2. Important mediator of inflammation. Chemoattractant for neutrophils and macrophages. Enhances NK activity.
Interleukin 2 (IL-2)	Produced by activated lymphocytes and helper T cells.	Promotes proliferation of T cells. Enhances killer T cell activities. Assists in synthesis of INFs and ILs 1, 2, 4, 5, and 6. Facilitates proliferation and activation of NK cells and LAK cell activity.
Interleukin 3 (IL-3)	Produced by T cells, NK cells, mast cells.	Hematopoietic growth factor. Stimulates histamine secretion.
Interleukin 4 (IL-4)	Produced by T cells, monocytes.	Enhances B cell growth and antibody production. Stimulates production of other cytokines.
Interleukin 5 (IL-5)	Activated T cells. Mast cells.	Induces proliferation and differentiation of B cells. Active in growth and differentiation of eosinophils. Co-regulator in stimulation of IgE production.
Interleukin 6 (IL-6)	Produced by various cell types— including fibroblasts, endothelial cells, monocytes/macrophages, T-cell lines, and mononuclear phagocytes—in response to immunologic and inflammatory processes.	Activates T-lymphocytes. Induces differentiation of cytotoxic T-lymphocytes and maturation of B lymphocytes. Involved in acute phase response. Hematopoietic growth factor.
Interleukin 7 (IL-7)	Bone marrow stromal cells.	Regulator of early lymphoid progenitors of T cell and B cell lineages. Potential role in platelet production.
Interleukin 8 (IL-8)	Chemotactic cytokine secreted during inflammatory response by a variety of cells.	Pro-inflammatory effects.
Interleukin 9 (IL-9)	T-cell-derived.	Potential for selectively stimulating erythroid development. Mast cell growth factor. Important in induction of T-helper cells.
Interleukin 10* (IL-10)	T-cell-derived. Produced by B cells.	Pleiotropic effects. Regulatory effects on immunologic and inflammatory responses.
Interleukin 11 (IL-11)	Fibroblasts, endothelial cells, adipocytes, & monocytes; bone marrow stromal cell line (oprelvekin).	Coregulator in proliferation of hemopoietic progenitor cells (specifically, megakaryocyte lineage). Involved in modulating antigen-specific antibody responses. Important in synthesis of hepatic proteins. Down regulates proinflammatory macrophage products.

Table 2D–1 *(Continued)*
Types of Cytokines

Cytokine	Principal Cellular Origin	Biologic Activities
Interleukin 12** (IL-12)	Heterodimeric cytokine produced by lymphocytes.	Growth factor for human T cells and NK cells. Synergistic with IL-2 in facilitating cytotoxic lymphocyte responses.
Interleukin 13 (IL-13)	Derived from Th$_2$-type lymphocytes. Similar to IL-4.	Inhibits monocyte & macrophage activation in chronic inflammation. Stimulates B cells. May contribute to replenishment of effector cells during a strong Th$_2$ response.
Interleukin 14 (IL-14)	Preliminary data available only.	
Interleukin 15 (IL-15)	Derived from peripheral blood monocytes dendritic cells.	Similar properties of IL-2; pleiotropic cytokine. Capable of activating NK cells. Cooperates with IL-2 during T cell mediated immune response.
Interleukin 16 (IL-16)	Produced by CD8+ lymphocytes.	Pro-inflammatory chemokine. Induces functional IL-2 receptors in T cells. Regulatory effects on lymphocyte activation. Chemotactic for CD4+ T cells.
Interleukin 17 (IL-17)	Preliminary data available only.	
Alpha (α) interferon (α-INF)	Produced by leukocytes, B cells, T cells, null cells, and macrophages.	Antiviral, antiproliferative, oncogene regulation, immunomodulation.
Beta (β) interferon (β-INF)	Produced by fibroblasts following exposure to viruses or foreign antigens.	Activation of NK cells, increased HLA antigen expression.
Gamma (γ) interferon (γ-INF)	Produced by T-lymphocytes and NK cells.	Immunoregulatory; enhances properties of other INFs, ILs, and TNFs.
TNF (tumor necrosis factor)	Produced by monocytes and macrophages.	Antiproliferative. Cytotoxic—may augment NK cytolytic activity. Stimulates IL-1 secretion.
M-CSF (monocyte colony stimulating factor)	Produced by monocytes and activated T cells.	Stimulates macrophage and monocyte function and cytotoxicity.

Continued

Table 2D–1 *(Continued)*
Types of Cytokines

Cytokine	Principal Cellular Origin	Biologic Activities
G-CSF (granulocyte colony stimulating factor)	Produced by monocytes, fibroblasts and endothelial cells.	Promotes proliferation, differentiation and maturation of granulocytes.
GM-CSF (granulocyte macrophage colony stimulating factor)	Produced by T cells.	Initiates differentiation of immature cells into granulocytes and monocytes.
EPO (erythropoietin)	Glycoprotein primarily produced and secreted by kidney.	Induces primitive erythroid progenitor cells to undergo differentiation; increases hemoglobin-synthesis-stimulated release of reticulocytes from bone marrow.
TPO/MGDF (thrombopoietin, also known as megakaryocyte growth and development factor)	Bone marrow, also produced in liver & kidney.	Promotes megakaryocyte progenitor cells. Promotes proliferation of megakaryocytes. Increases platelet production. Co-regulator in proliferation of hematopoietic progenitor cells.
SCF (stem cell factor)	Bone marrow stroma.	Stimulates pluriponent stem cell and progeniors for all cell lines.

*Previously called cytokine synthesis inhibitory factor (CSIF)
**Previously called cytotoxic lymphocyte maturation factor (CLMF)
INF—interferon; LAK cell—lymphocyte activated killer cell; NK cells—natural killer cells.

TNF is available in two recombinant forms: TNF-alpha (TNF-α) and TNF-beta (TNF-β). TNF-α is predominantly synthesized by monocytes and activated macrophages. It is often identified with the compound cachectin, which is associated with wasting syndrome in patients with cancer and chronic diseases. Structurally, TNF-α is very similar to lymphotoxin, another cytotoxic protein produced by lymphocytes. Because of its similarity to TNF-α, lymphotoxin is referred to as TNF-β. Both compounds appear to have cytotoxic and cytostatic effects and might cause vascular endothelial destruction in tumors, resulting in hemorrhage and tumor necrosis. As a single therapeutic agent, TNF has shown little antitumor activity. Studies have indicated that combination therapy with TNF and other cytokines (such as interferon and IL-2) could have synergistic effects in treating a variety of malignancies.

Human hematopoietic growth factors, also termed colony stimulating factors (CSFs), are a family of glycoprotein hormones that regulate the proliferation and maturation of hematopoietic precursor cells. In addition, the CSFs influence the functional activities of mature hematopoietic cells. Hematopoietic cell lines originate with the pluripotent stem cell, which is also known as a colony forming unit (CFU) blast, the most primitive of

Table 2D–2
Colony-Stimulating Factors

Growth Factor	Cell Lineage	Clinical Uses
IL-3	N, M, E, B. EO, Meg	Myelosuppression Bone marrow failure Combination therapy
IL-11	Meg	Chemotherapy induced thrombin cytopenia
G-CSF	N	Myelosuppression Bone marrow failure (e.g., MDS) Bone marrow transplant Leukopenia in HIV/AIDS and infectious diseases Aplastic anemia Peripheral stem cell mobilization
GM-CSF	N, M, E, EO, Meg	Myelosuppression Bone marrow failure (e.g., MDS) Bone marrow transplant Leukopenia in AIDS Aplastic anemia Leukemia in elderly
EPO	E	Anemia in cancer and chemotherapy treatment Bone marrow failure (e.g., MDS) Anemia in chronic renal disease

B—basophil; E—erythroid; EO—eosinophil; M—monocyte; MDS—myelodysplastic syndrome; Meg—megakaryocyte; N—neutrophil.

blood cells. The CFU blast is capable of self-renewal and further differentiation into CFUs for myeloid and lymphoid cell lineages. Hematopoietic growth factors are essential for the differentiation, proliferation, and maturation of early progenitor cells. When stimulated, these cells give rise to single or multiple cell lineages. Interleukin 3 (multi-CSF), for example, targets multiple cellular lineages, whereas granulocyte-CSF (G-CSF) affects granulocyte formation (see Table 2D–2). Many other cytokines (e.g. interleukin 11) have pleiotropic properties that also regulate hematopoesis. The potential uses of hematopoietic growth factors lie in their ability to enhance bone marrow function as a single agent or in combination with other treatment modalities such as chemotherapy and radiation therapy.

Activated lymphocyte therapy is a type of adoptive immunotherapy in which highly sensitized or activated biologic substances are administered to the patient. These substances are used for their direct cytotoxic effect and to augment other agents in mediating an antitumor response. The most extensively studied adoptive therapies are those with tumor-infiltrating lymphocytes (TILs) and LAK cells. LAK cells are produced after removing peripheral blood lymphocytes from the bloodstream by leukapheresis and incubating them with IL-2. The resulting LAK cells are then washed with normal saline solution, suspended in culture with albumin and IL-2, and then reinfused into the patient. TILs are derived from autologous (the patient's own) tumor samples or malignant body fluids and then expanded in culture with IL-2 or a mixture of IL-2 and IL-4. The resulting activated lymphocytes are prepared in the same fashion as LAK cells and reinfused into the patient. The chosen lymphocyte preparation (LAK or TIL) is then given concomitantly with systemic IL-2 infusion. Studies have indicated that TILs expand better in culture and have greater antitumor effects than LAK cells. In addition, TILs are tumor specific and display greater reactivity to autologous tumors than LAK cells. The therapeutic effects of these agents remain controversial and are being examined in clinical trials.

Monoclonal antibodies (MAbs) have specific antibodies produced by a single clone of B-lymphocytes, directed toward specific antigens located on the surface of cells. Single clones of B-lymphocyte cells derived from tumor cells are isolated and fused with rapidly reproducing mouse myeloma cells to form an antibody-producing hybridoma, which is then capable of producing large quantities of a specific antibody. These antibodies can be used alone or bound to radioisotopes, bacterial toxins, other BRMs, or chemotherapeutic agents. Because of their technical and biologic limitations for use in therapy, monoclonal antibodies have largely been used for diagnosis and screening. For this treatment to work, there must be enough tumor-specific antigen present to react with the antibody as well as minimal cross-reactivity with normal tissue. In addition, monoclonal antibodies derived from mouse antibodies can themselves trigger human anti-mouse antibody (HAMA) production. Various approaches to overcome antibody immunogenicity are currently being investigated, including the use of human MAbs, mouse-human chimeric MAbs, biochemical modification, and lymphoid radiation prior to administration.

Currently, MAbs are being tested in clinical trials with a variety of cancers, including lymphoma, leukemia, colorectal, breast, ovarian, renal, bladder, and prostate cancer.

Gene therapy involves obtaining metastatic tumor cells from the patient, altering the cells by laboratory methods to increase the presence of tumor necrosis factor, and then reintroducing these cells to the patient. The intended goal of the altered cells is to increase the presence of lymphocytes at the site of the diseased cancerous cells, ultimately causing the immune system to aggressively attack the cancer cells. As a new direction in therapy, this can be called immunization treatment for cancer. In other words, the altered cells are reintroduced to stimulate the immune system to attack the cancer cells, treating them as foreign bodies. If it proves successful, gene therapy, combined with other immunotherapy products, could be the forerunner of immunizations against cancer.

Vaccine therapy, also termed active specific immunotherapy (ASI) is another form of biotherapy that aims at inducing a specific immune response against the host tumor. Numerous studies have been conducted using various techniques to augment specific immunity against solid tumors. Attempts to enhance the immune response have involved the use of several different modifications, and the application of adjuvant treatments such as BCG, *C. parvum,* and GM-CSF. Although many of these preparations have been unsuccessful, the quality and purity of vaccines has improved greatly in the past few years.

Although there has been a diversity of approaches in the preparation of vaccines, two methods are primarily utilized: autologous and allogeneic. Autologous vaccine utilizes tumor obtained from the patient, which has been radiated. Surgery is required to obtain enough fresh tumor for vaccine preparation. One of the limitations is that the patient must have enough tumor obtainable in order to be a candidate and therefore often has advanced disease. Allogeneic vaccines are derived from radiated cell lines of more than one patient and have the advantage of being available to treat large groups of patients. Allogeneic vaccines might be of value as adjuvant therapy and in treating microscopic residual disease.

There are several problems in eliciting specific anti-tumor responses, including (1) the existence of numerous tumor antigens; (2) the frequent mutation of metastatic tumor cells, altering the nature of antigens; and (3) the immunodominance of specific antigens is unknown. Early clinical trials with many of these vaccines have failed to demonstrate significant responses. As new prospects for vaccine preparations develop and more is learned about the mechanisms of the immune system, vaccine therapy may be a reasonable approach with wider application in the treatment of solid tumors.

NURSING CARE OF PATIENTS RECEIVING BRMS

The side effects that may occur with biologic response modifiers (BRMs) therapy affect several systems: the neurologic, cardiac, pulmonary, gastrointestinal, hepatic, and cutaneous. In addition, flu-like symptoms are often present, indicating an alteration in the host's immune system. The side effect profile and the severity of toxicities are a function of dose, route of administration, schedule, and concurrent therapies. As with any cancer therapy, individual factors, such as age, functional performance status, concomitant medical problems, previous therapy history, and social-cultural expectations, can influence the side effects. Table 2D–3 presents the routes of administration and known side effects of BRMs and incorporates nursing considerations of the adverse reactions. Table 2D–4 describes nursing management of the commonly encountered toxicities in patients receiving BRMs.

Table 2D-3
BRMs: Routes of Administration and Known Side Effects

BRM	Routes of Administration	Side Effects	Nursing Considerations
Interleukin 2 (IL-2)	IV, SC	Flu-like syndrome,* malaise (cumulative) GI: N/V, diarrhea, anorexia (cumulative), GI bleeding Integumentary: Mucositis, xerostomia, dry skin, erythematous rash, pruritus, desquamation Neurological: Agitation, anxiety, confusion, impaired memory, sleep disturbances, depression, hallucinations, psychosis Cardiovascular: Capillary leak syndrome, edema, ascites, hypotension, arrhythmias, tachycardia, myocardial ischemia/infarction, cardiac onset, pericardial effusion Pulmonary: Respiratory compromise/failure, pulmonary edema, dyspnea, pulmonary congestion, tachypnea, nasal congestion Renal: Oliguria/anuria, elevated BUN/creatinine, proteinuria, hematuria Hepatic: Elevated LFTs Hematological: Anemia, thrombocytopenia, leukopenia, leukocytosis, coagulation disorders, eosinophilia	Patients should have normal cardiac, pulmonary, renal, hepatic, and neurologic function prior to starting therapy. Capillary leak syndrome may begin with 2–12 hrs. of initiation of therapy. Management may require the administration of IV fluids, colloids, or pressor agents. The hypotensive effects are dose- and route-related. Continuous-infusion administration produces less hypotension than bolus infusion. The side effects and toxicities resolve with the cessation of therapy. Some resolve quickly, while others, such as fatigue, anorexia, and skin desquamation, may persist for several weeks. Serum creatinine levels return to baseline within 1–2 weeks.
Interferons: alpha, beta, gamma	IM, SC, IV, Intraperitoneal, Intralesional	Flu-like syndrome Anorexia, taste alterations Fatigue General malaise N/V, diarrhea Neurologic: poor concentration, confusion, lethargy, drowsiness, mental slowing, psychosis, hallucinations Cardiovascular: arrhythmias, tachycardia Renal: increased BUN/creatinine Hepatic: elevation of liver enzymes Hematological: transient, non-dose-limiting leukopenia, thrombocytopenia	Many of the side effects and toxicities of INFs are dose-dependent and rapidly reversible. Cardiotoxic effects are seen mostly with elderly patients and those with cardiac history. Anorexia and fatigue are cumulative and may be dose-limiting. Fever/chills tend to occur 4–8 hrs post-injection, are most severe in the first 1–2 weeks, and diminish with continued therapy. PM dosing is often employed to improve management of side effects.

Agent	Route	Side effects	Comments
Tumor necrosis factor (TNF)	IV, IM, SC, bladder instillation	Flu-like syndrome Headache, back pain, tumor pain N/V, diarrhea, anorexia Orthostatic hypotension Dizziness, lethargy Elevated PFTs Transient hematologic changes	Headache is observed at all dose levels and may be severe. May be controlled at lower doses with acetaminophen. At higher dose levels of TNF, headaches may be less responsive or refractory to opioids and may be considered the dose-limiting toxicity. Fever and chills are mild and disappear with subsequent dosing.
M-CSF	SC, IV	Bone pain Flu-like syndrome	Phase I/II clinical trials ongoing.
G-CSF	IV, SC	Most common: Bone pain Less common: Fever Elevations in serum uric acid	Should be administered at least 24 hrs after last dose of chemotherapy and discontinued at least 24 hrs before next chemotherapy. Should be continued as directed until ANC is greater than or equal to 10,000/mm^3.
GM-CSF	IV, SC	Pain Arthralgia Myalgia Lethargy Skin rash	Many of the side effects are dose-related and more severe at higher doses. A "1st dose reaction" can occur (hypotension, tachycardia, flushing, dyspnea, N/V) in doses greater than 1 mcg/kg and more commonly with IV administration.
EPO	IV, SC	Hypertension (rare) Venous fistula clotting Functional iron deficiency Rare: Thrombocytosis, sweating, and bone pain	May decrease the need for maintenance transfusions in anemia and myclodysplastic syndrome.
Interleukin 11 (IL-11)	SC	Mild to moderate fluid retention Moderate decrease in Hgb/Hct due to increased plasma volume Transient atrial arrhythmias Transient visual blurring Fever, flu-like syndrome Conjunctival injection Dyspnea	Dosing should begin 6–24 hrs following completion of chemotherapy. Dosing should continue until post-nadir counts are >50,000/mm^3. Fluid balance should be carefully monitored during treatment; can require diuretics. Use with caution in patients with histroy of cardiac disease.

Continued

Table 2D-3 (Continued)
BRMs: Routes of Administration and Known Side Effects

BRM	Routes of Administration	Side Effects	Nursing Considerations
Activated lymphocytes (LAK cells and TILs)	Systemic or regionally: IV, IA, IC	Fever, chills/rigors Headache Respiratory compromise Hypotension Tachycardia N/V Pain/discomfort (with IC admin.)	A central venous access catheter with ≥20 gauge lumen is preferable for administration. There is not enough data on the potential damage from peripheral infiltration. Must be given by gravity (pumps may damage cells). Piggyback primary line with NS solution only. IL-2 is usually given concomitantly with activated lymphocytes and is not compatible. Give via separate line. Squeeze bag every 5 minutes during administration.
Monoclonal antibodies	Dose specific to murine or human antibody, IV	Anaphylaxis: generalized flushing, hives, bronchospasm, hypotension, loss of consciousness Flu-like syndrome Serum sickness N/V, diarrhea Urticaria, pruritus, erythema Dyspnea Renal failure related to HAMA resulting in obstruction of renal tubules Myelosuppression	Murine antibodies eventually recognized by human body as foreign antigen, triggering production of HAMA. Anaphylaxis possible during or shortly after drug administration. Appropriate medication should be available. Serum sickness may occur approximately 10 days after exposure, with possible renal dysfunction. Usually responds to steroid therapy. Radio-labeled isotopes should be handled appropriately according to state and federal regulations.
Vaccines	IM, ID, SC	Local reaction (swelling, erythema, induration, tenderness, possible ulceration) Mild flu-like symptoms	There is generally very minimal reaction to vaccine therapy and tends to be determined by the type of adjuvant used (virus or bacteria-based).

NOTE: The side effects listed in this table are known side effects identified from clinical trials. Some of the cytokines listed in this chapter are currently in laboratory or Phase I studies and the list of side effects is unknown or incomplete.

*Flu-like syndrome is defined as symptomatology including fatigue, fever, chills/rigors, arthralgias/myalgias, and headache.

ANC—absolute neutrophil count; BRMs—biological response modifiers; GI—gastrointestinal; HAMA—human anti-mouse antibodies; IA—intra-arterial; IC—intracavitary; INFs—interferons; LFTs—liver function tests; N/V—nausea/vomiting; PFTs—pulmonary function tests.

Table 2D-4
Nursing Management of Biotherapy-related Toxicities

Toxicities	Nursing Management/Intervention

I. Flu-like symptoms
  A. Fever
	A. Assessment
	   1. Body temperature every 4–12 hr. (Outpatient: every 6 hrs.)
	   2. Fluid intake and output. (Outpatient: ask the number of glasses of liquid taken in daily.)
	   3. Skin integrity
	   4. Neurological status
	B. Intervention
	   1. Hyperthermic resolution modalities
	     a. Tepid sponge baths
	     b. Ice packs
	     c. Cooling blanket
	     d. Outpatient
	       1. Instruction on self-management technique
	         a. Tepid showers
	         b. When to seek medical advice
	     e. Medicate as ordered
	       1. Acetaminophen—2 tabs every 4 hrs ATC
	       2. Indomethacin—25 mg TID
	         a. Contraindicated in renal insufficiency
	     f. Fluid replacement
	       1. 500 cc plus output in prior 24-hr period
	C. Documentation
	   1. Onset and duration—relationship to time dose administered
	   2. Accurate intake and output
	   3. Effective intervention

B. Chills/rigors	A. Assessment
	   1. Cardiovascular status
	   2. Respiratory status
	B. Intervention
	   1. Comfort measures
	     a. Blanket
	   2. Medicate as ordered
	     a. Diphenhydramine, 25–50 mg PO
	       1. Mild chills
	     b. Meperidine, 25–50 mg IV every 4–6 hr (with 1 repeated dose)
	     c. Hydromorphone, 2–4 mg SL every 30 minutes
	       1. Based on BSA
	       2. Outpatient therapy—written instruction on self-administration and total dose to be given
	     d. Morphine, 1–2 mg every 15 minutes up to 100 mg
	   3. Notify physician if unresolved
	   4. Standing order may help to facilitate care
	C. Documentation
	   1. Onset and duration—relationship to time dose administered
	   2. Effective intervention

Continued

Table 2D–4 *(Continued)*
Nursing Management of Biotherapy-related Toxicities

Toxicities	Nursing Management/Intervention

C. Arthralgia/myalgia	A. Assessment
	  1. Past medical history for arthritis (symptoms may be exacerbated)
	  2. Location of pain
	B. Intervention
	  1. Moist heat
	  2. Massage affected area
	  3. Administration of nonsteroidal anti-inflammatory drugs
	C. Documentation
	  1. Arthritic disease location
	  2. Onset and duration—relationship to time dose administered
	  3. Effective intervention

D. Headaches	A. Assessment
	  1. Location
	  2. Characteristics
	    a. Frequency
	    b. Duration
	    c. Alleviating factors
	    d. Aggravating factors
	B. Intervention
	  1. Comfort measure
	    a. Cool moist compresses
	    b. Darkening rooms
	    c. Relaxation techniques
	    d. Visual imagery
	  2. Medicate as ordered
	    a. Antihistamines (reduce prostaglandin release)
	    b. Prostaglandin inhibitors
	    c. Decongestants (e.g., pseudoephedrine)
	    d. Propranolol, 10–40 mg per day (vascular headaches)
	C. Documentation
	  1. Onset and duration—relationship to time dose administered
	  2. Effective intervention

E. Fatigue	A. Assessment
	  1. Performance status
	  2. Family support structure
	  3. Hematologic, cardiopulmonary fluid status, and nutritional status
	  4. Concurrent medications
	B. Intervention (see Chapter 8C)
	  1. Energy conservation technique
	    a. Prioritizing activities
	    b. Delegation of duties
	    c. Rest when fatigued
	  2. Optimize nutrition
	    a. Nutritional supplements
	    b. Small frequent meals
	    c. Diet rich in proteins, vitamins, and iron
	  3. Assist in correcting body systems malfunction that may exacerbate fatigue
	C. Documentation
	  1. Onset and duration—relationship to time dose administered
	  2. Effective interventions

Table 2D–4 *(Continued)*
Nursing Management of Biotherapy-related Toxicities

Toxicities	Nursing Management/Intervention

II. Neurologic and psychologic symptoms
  Confusion
  Irritability
  Impaired memory
  Expressive aphasia
  Sleep disturbances
  Depression
  Psychosis
  Hallucination
  Decreased level of consciousness
	A. Assessment
	  1. Neuropsychologic history
	  2. Level of consciousness
	  3. Cranial nerves
	  4. Cognitive abilities
	  5. Memory
	  6. Body system malfunctions
	  7. Concomitant medications
	B. Intervention
	  1. Reassure patient and caregiver this may be temporary if related to BRM therapy
	  2. Encourage caregiver to report cognitive and/or behavioral changes
	  3. Instruct patient to avoid hazardous activities
	  4. Encourage and promote environmental safety
	  5. Encourage patient's and caregiver's verbalization of concerns
	  6. Discontinue neurotoxic medication (e.g., sedative, opioid, alcohol, and H_2 blocker)
	  7. Patient may need to have dose reduced or therapy discontinued as indicated by protocol guidelines and/or by physician order
	  8. Notify physician of neurologic changes
	C. Documentation
	  1. Onset and duration—relationship to time dose administered
	  2. Body system malfunction that may exacerbate symptoms
	  3. Neurotoxic concurrent drugs

III. Cardiovascular
  Cyanosis
  Hypotension
  Neurological changes
  Dysrhythmias
  Peripheral edema
  Congestive heart failure
  Myocardia ischemia or infarction
	A. Assessment
	  1. Skin
	  2. Heart rhythm, regularity
	  3. Neck vein
	  4. Fluid output
	  5. Chest pain—may be confused with pulmonary congestion, which occurs with some growth factors
	  6. Vital signs every 4–24 hr
	    a. Inpatient every 4 hr
	    b. Outpatient daily
	  7. Neurologic changes
	B. Interventions
	  1. Decrease salt intake
	  2. Oral intake as prescribed
	    a. Fluid reduction with renal insufficiency
	    b. Fluid increase with some cases of vascular depletion
	  3. Elevation of lower extremities
	  4. Elevation of head of bed with respiratory insufficiency
	  5. Change position frequently when on bed rest
	  6. Maintain physical activity as much as possible
	  7. Ensure moisturizing lotions are placed on skin
	    a. Avoid those with perfume base or increased alcohol content
	    b. Moisturizers
	      1. Eucerin® cream
	      2. Lac-Hydrin® cream

Continued

Toxicities	Nursing Management/Intervention
	8. Instruct patient to change position slowly
	9. Reassure patient/caregiver of temporary nature if associated with BRM treatment
	10. Notify physician of cardiac abnormalities
	11. Administer medication as ordered
	a. Diuretic
	b. Oxygen therapy support
	c. Vasopressor may be indicated
	d. Discontinuation of BRM therapy
	C. Documentation
	1. Onset and duration—relationship to time dose administered
	2. Past medical history
	3. Effective interventions
	4. Diary card may be of assistance in monitoring toxicities in outpatient setting
	5. Standing orders may facilitate care

IV. Pulmonary
  Pleural effusions
  Pulmonary edema
  Shortness of breath
  Cyanosis
  Productive cough
  Chest congestion
	A. Assessment

	1. Respiratory status every 4 hrs
	a. Rate
	b. Rhythm
	c. Depth
	d. Breath sounds
	2. Other system malfunction that may exacerbate symptoms
	3. Arterial blood gases
	B. Intervention
	1. Comfort measure
	a. Elevation of the head
	2. Supplementary oxygen therapy
	3. Respiratory hygiene
	4. Energy conservation
	5. Administration of medication
	a. Diuretic
	b. Bronchodilation
	6. With some BRM therapies (TIL and LAK cells), slowing down the rate of infusion will ameliorate acute dyspnea
	7. Notify physician of pulmonary complications
	C. Documentation
	1. Onset and duration—relationship to time dose administered
	2. Diary card may be helpful
	3. Accurate intake and output
	4. Effects of interventions

V. Gastrointestinal
  Nausea
  Vomiting
  Diarrhea
  Anorexia
  Bowel perforations (rare case reported)
  Taste alterations
	A. Assessment

	1. Prior history of gastrointestinal disorders
	2. History of eating habits
	3. History of elimination patterns
	4. Increased abdominal pain may be associated with bowel perforation
	B. Interventions
	1. Educate patient and caregiver on potential side effects—give written material on:
	a. Side effects
	b. Self-care measures
	c. When to seek medical attention
	d. How to take prescribed medication

Toxicities	Nursing Management/Intervention
	2. Environmental intervention
	a. Remove body secretions and waste from care area as soon as possible
	b. Avoid strong-smelling food
	c. Encourage patient to have a companion at meal time
	d. Make meals attractive
	3. Oral hygiene prior to meals, at least 15–30 minutes
	a. Baking soda mouthwash
	4. Wine prior to meals, if not contraindicated, may stimulate the appetite
	5. Avoid gas-forming foods
	6. Avoid liquids with and prior to meal
	7. Try room temperature foods
	8. Clear liquid to reduce nausea
	9. Sour food to avoid nausea (e.g. lemon drops)
	10. Encourage small but frequent meals high in calories, protein, and carbohydrates
	11. Medicate as ordered
	a. Antiemetic—30 minutes prior to meals
	1. Lorazepam—1 mg PO or IV (has helped with anticipatory nausea)
	2. Prochlorperazine—5–10 mg PO or IV
	3. Ondansetron—8 mg PO or 0.15 mg/kg IV
	4. Granisetron—2 mg PO or 10 mg/kg IV
	b. Antidiarrheal—should be taken consistently
	1. Loperamide—2 tabs loading dose then 1 after each loose stool up to 8 per 24-hr interval
	2. Diphenoxylate with atropine
	c. Discontinuation or dose reduction of the BRM may be needed
	C. Documentation
	1. Number of stools/24-hr period (every shift inpatient)
	2. Number of episodes of vomiting/24-hr period (every shift inpatient)
	3. Taste alterations
	a. Salty
	b. Metallic
	c. Chemical taste
	d. Sweet
	4. Interventions that help relieve toxicity

VI. Hepatic
  Elevated SGOT
  Elevated SGPT
  Elevated LDH
  Elevated alkaline phosphatase
  Elevated total bilirubin
  Decreased albumin
  Decreased serum cholesterol
	A. Assessment

	1. Monitor liver function studies 2–3 times per week
	2. Performance status
	3. Nutritional status
	4. Elimination pattern
	5. Body characteristics
	a. Skin color
	b. Skin integrity
	6. Neurologic status
	7. Concurrent hepatotoxic medications
	B. Intervention
	1. Energy conservation
	a. Prioritize activities
	b. Delegate responsibilities
	c. Schedule strenuous activities when rest periods can follow

Continued

Table 2D–4 *(Continued)*
Nursing Management of Biotherapy-related Toxicities

Toxicities	Nursing Management/Intervention

	2. Skin care—especially with increased total bilirubin
	  a. Bathe with nondrying soap, rinse well
	  b. Keep skin moist
	3. Hepatotoxic or hepatic-metabolized medication may need close reduction
	4. Notify physician of:
	  a. Behavior changes
	  b. Elevated LFTs
	5. Discontinuation of BRM therapy or close reduction may be needed
	C. Documentation
	  1. Trend of liver function abnormalities
	  2. Acute changes in other systems

VII. Renal
  Decreased urine output
  Elevated creatinine
  Elevated serum BUN
  Protein uria
  Changes in acid base balances
  Alteration in calcium magnesium and phosphorus metabolism
  Third spacing
	A. Assessment
	  1. Urinary output
	  2. Laboratory value
	    a. Serum creatinine
	    b. BUN
	    c. Urinalysis
	    d. Serum CO_2
	    e. Arterial blood gases if indicated
	    f. Other body systems that may be involved
	B. Intervention
	  1. Educate patient and caregiver about potential side effects
	    a. Reassure of temporary nature if related to BRM therapy
	  2. Maintain strict I&O record
	  3. Daily weight
	  4. Notify physician if urinary output is less than 240 cc in 8-hr period
	  5. Medicate as ordered
	    a. Fluid challenge (250 cc normal saline bolus) used conservatively
	    b. Diuretics may be ordered if patient hemodynamically stable
	    c. Renal dose dopamine infusion may be initiated to increase renal perfusion
	    d. Discontinuation of BRM therapy or dose reduction may be needed
	C. Documentation
	  1. Strict I&O
	    a. Consider insensible loss with febrile status
	  2. Trends
	    a. Electrolyte
	    b. Metabolites
	  3. Other body system abnormalities

VIII. Skin integrity
  Transient generalized flushing
  Generalized and local erythema
  Generalized and local pruritus
  Dryness and exfoliative dermatitis
	A. Assessment
	  1. Past medical history of skin integrity abnormalities
	  2. Location, type, induration, size, breakage in integrity, or drainage every 4–8 hrs
	  3. Monitor lab values, especially liver function test
	  4. Monitor skin breakdown areas for potential infection
	B. Intervention
	  1. Encourage patient to verbalize concern regarding body image changes
	    a. Assist in referring patient to appropriate resources (e.g., cosmetologist, dermatologist)

Table 2D–4 *(Continued)*
Nursing Management of Biotherapy-related Toxicities

Toxicities	Nursing Management/Intervention

Alopecia
Ulcerations
Jaundice
Stomatitis
Psoriasis of the scalp
Infection via central
venous access
catheters
	2. Stomatitis (see Chapter 10B)
	  a. Oral care qid including 30 minutes prior to meals
	    1. Brush teeth with soft nylon tooth brush
	    2. Baking soda mouthwashes qid (1 tsp per 240 cc of water)
	    3. Moisten lips with lubricating jelly or lip balm prn
	  b. Avoid irritating substances (tobacco, alcohol, spicy food, too hot or too cold foods)
	3. Avoid frequent hot baths and/or showers
	4. Use a mild soap and rinse thoroughly
	5. Apply oil-based and/or mild acid-based moisturizers
	6. Avoid skin irritants
	7. Monitor lab values
	8. Avoid excessive shampooing, rinse thoroughly, pat hair dry, use low heat with electric dryers
	9. Satin pillows and scarves to decrease tangling
	10. Injection site should be rotated to decrease subcutaneous complications
	11. Observe invasive procedure sites; increased risk of infection associated with IL-2 based therapy
	12. Notify physician of complications
	C. Documentation
	  1. Onset and duration
	  2. Temperature, color, if skin intact, drainage, pain at site
	  3. Stomatitis—note the degree to which it interferes with oral intake

IX. Hematologic
  Anemia
  Leukopenia
  Neutropenia
  Thrombocytopenia
  Thrombocytosis
  Eosinophilia
  Leukocytosis
	A. Assessment
	  1. Sign and symptoms of anemia
	    a. Skin color (pale)
	    b. Neurologic symptoms (headache/vertigo)
	    c. Dyspnea with activity
	    d. Fatigue
	    e. Rapid pulse rate
	  2. Signs and symptoms of neutropenia
	    a. Fatigue
	    b. Chills/fever
	    c. Headache
	    d. General malaise
	  3. Signs and symptoms of thrombocytopenia
	    a. Petechiae
	    b. Increased bleeding tendency
	  4. Thrombocytosis
	    a. Deep vein thrombosis
	    b. Respiratory complications
	    c. Venous access device—increased risk of clotting
	  5. Signs and symptoms of infection
	B. Intervention
	  1. Supportive therapy—blood transfusion, platelet transfusion, growth factors
	  2. If neutropenic (as determined by institutional guidelines), instruct patient/caregiver to wash hands frequently, maintain nutritional status, and monitor temperature

Continued

Table 2D–4 *(Continued)*
Nursing Management of Biotherapy-related Toxicities

Toxicities	Nursing Management/Intervention
	3. Instruct patient to avoid hazardous activity that can increase skin breakage
	4. With low platelet counts, avoid valsalva maneuver, which increases intracranial pressure
	5. Notify physician of hematologic changes
	C. Documentation
	1. Signs and symptoms of anemia, neutropenia, thrombocytopenia, and thrombocytosis
	2. Interventions initiated and results
	3. Instructions given to patient and caregiver
X. Knowledge deficit	A. Assessment
	1. Patient understanding of treatment approach
	2. Patient knowledge of potential side effects
	B. Intervention
	1. Patient should be given written material that includes:
	a. Name of medication
	b. Dose
	c. Time
	d. Route
	e. Date to start
	f. Side effects (expected)
	1. Self-care measures
	2. When to seek medical attention
	g. Numbers to call in case of emergency
	1. Attending physician
	2. Primary nurse
	3. Contact person after working hours (include what information to tell person)
	a. Diagnosis
	b. Treatment receiving—start date, dose, how often given
	c. Present signs and/or symptoms
	4. If can not reach above, the patient should be informed go to local ER
	h. Supplies needed for self-care
	i. Diary card may facilitate toxicity assessment
	C. Documentation
	1. Instruction given to patient
	2. How well patient performed self-care instruction
	3. Printed material patient received

BRMs—biological response modifiers; LAK cell—lymphocyte activated killer cell; LFTs—liver function tests; TIL—tumor-infiltrating lymphocytes

SUMMARY

The integration of BRMs into the treatment of cancer and other diseases continues to progress rapidly. Advances in understanding the molecular biology of human tumors make possible more selective application of BRMs, but the therapeutic mechanisms of these agents remain poorly defined. The task of future studies will be to decipher the multifunctional nature of these agents and their complex interactions *in vivo*.

The use of many of these agents might be tempered only by their side effect profiles. In general, BRMs produce similar side effects that in most cases are related to changes in preexisting physiologic mechanisms. Many effects are dose related and increase in intensity at higher doses; however, nearly all of them disappear fairly rapidly when treatment is discontinued. As BRMs become a standard component of the medical armamentarium, the resolution and control of side effects will be of vital importance.

BIBLIOGRAPHY

1. Brogley, J. L., and E. J. Sharp. Nursing care of patients receiving activated lymphocytes. *Oncol Nurs Forum* 17(2): 187–193. 1990.

   This nursing journal article discusses the specifics of activated lymphocyte administration, common side effects, and nursing management strategies.

2. DeVita, V. T., S. Hellman, and S. A. Rosenberg, eds. *Biologic Therapy of Cancer*. J. B. Lippincott, Philadelphia. 1991.

   Detailed information presents the complexity of biologic cancer treatment from research principles to current treatments to new investigational modalities.

3. DeVita, V. T., S. Hellman, and S. A. Rosenberg, eds. *Cancer: Principles and Practice of Oncology,* 5th Ed. J. B. Lippincott, Philadelphia. 1997.

   This comprehensive explanation of cancer therapy includes scientific research into active cancer therapies with information about possible treatment-related complications.

4. Foon, K. A. Biological response modifiers: The new immunotherapy. *Cancer Res* 49(7): 1621–1639. 1989.

   This medical journal article discusses the role of immune therapy in cancer. It covers a broad range of BRMs and is technical in nature.

5. Groenwald, S. L., M. H. Frogge, M. Goodman, and C. H. Yarbro, eds. *Cancer Nursing Principles and Practice,* 4th Ed. Jones and Bartlett Publishers, Inc., Boston. 1997.

   This nursing-directed reference book is designed to address cancer nursing as a specialty associated with complex cancer treatments.

6. Haeuber, D. and J. E. DiJulio. Hemopoietic colony stimulating factors: An overview. *Oncol Nurs Forum* 16(2): 247–255. 1989.

   This nursing journal article describes the general nature of CSFs and therapeutic possibilities in patients with cancer.

7. Irwin, M. M. Patients receiving biological response modifiers: Overview of nursing care. *Oncol Nurs Forum* 14(6): Suppl. 32–37. 1987.

   This nursing journal article discusses the unique nursing care problems encountered with BRMs.

8. Kiegel, R. L. Interleukins, interferons, and tumor necrosis factor in cancer treatment. *AAOHN Journal* 35(4): 159–162. 1987.

   This journal article briefly discusses the general role of BRMs in cancer treatment.

9. Parkinson, D. R. The role of Interleukin-2 in the biotherapy of cancer. *Oncol Nurs Forum* 16(6): Suppl. 16–20. 1989.

   This nursing journal article describes the rationale, preclinical data, and clinical trial experience with IL-2 in cancer treatment.

10. Reiger, P. T., ed. *Biotherapy: A Comprehensive Overview.* Jones and Bartlett Publishers, Inc., Boston. 1995.

    This is a comprehensive overview of biotherapy written by oncology nurses. It is excellent source text for all levels of oncology nursing.

11. Roitt. I., Brossoff, J., Male, D., eds. *Immunology,* 3d Ed. Mosby-Year Book Europe Ltd., London. 1993.

    This is a comprehensive textbook on immunology and contains very technical and detailed information on the immune system.

12. Strauman, J. J. The nurse's role in the biotherapy of cancer: Nursing research of side effects. *Oncol Nurs Forum* 15(6): Suppl. 35–39. 1988.

    This nursing journal article outlines the unique toxicities of biologic response modifiers and symptom interventions.

Special Treatments

3

A. Marrow and Peripheral Stem Cell Transplantation

Patricia C. Buchsel

INTRODUCTION

Over the past 35 years, bone marrow transplantation (BMT) has become an established and effective treatment for selected patients with cancer or blood diseases. The use of peripheral blood stem cell transplantation (PBST) is developing rapidly; researchers predict that this therapy will eventually replace BMT. Research continues to evaluate the effectiveness of PBST compared with BMT (and other therapies) in achieving adequate bone marrow engraftment and improved patient survival. In 1995 alone, the International Bone Marrow Transplant Registry (IBMTR) reported 12,000 allogeneic (donor) BMTs and 18,000 autologous (self) BMTs performed in 330 centers in 47 countries (Figure 3A–1).

Improvements in supportive care and the development of recombinant colony stimulating factors have greatly decreased the morbidity and mortality rate of the transplant procedure. By generating earlier white blood cell recovery, the use of growth factors—such as granulocyte macrophage colony stimulating factors (GM-CSF) and granulocyte colony stimulating factors (G-CSF)—has significantly decreased the incidence of post-transplant infections (and therefore the use of antibiotics), length of hospitalizations, and number of hospital readmissions. Multilineage cytokines, including the interleukin-3, -6, and -11, are being studied to hasten both neutrophil and platelet engraftment. Single lineage cytokines such as thrombopoietin and erythropoietin are also under investigation as a means to reduce the need for blood product support after transplantation.

The frequency of autologous transplants now exceeds that of allogeneic transplants, and most centers use hematopoietic progenitor cells, or *stem cells*, collected from the peripheral blood. Fewer than 20 percent of autologous transplants are performed with bone marrow alone. BMT might be added to PBST if insufficient numbers of stem cells are available. In contrast, more than 90% of allogeneic transplants use bone marrow. Recently, interest in collecting allogenic cells from peripheral blood or umbilical cords has increased.

3A

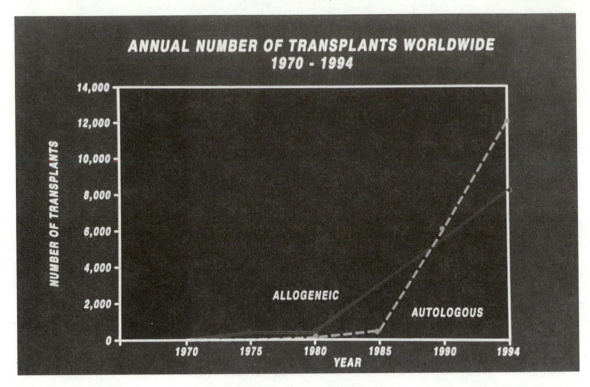

Figure 3A-1. Increasing use of blood and marrow transplantation.

Reprinted with permission from International Bone Marrow Transplant Registry.

Successful recruitment of more than 2 million unrelated donors from international and national donor banks has increased the availability of allogenic BMT. As peripheral blood stem cell transplantation becomes available in the allogeneic setting, the number of transplants will increase dramatically. Because of the shift from marrow to alternative stem cell sources, more patients will be treated in diverse care settings.

HISTORY

The earliest described BMTs in humans were administered by mouth, intramuscular injection, and intramedullary or intravenous routes, without success. After World War II, bone marrow failure following radiation exposure led to treatment with infusions of bone marrow. The first modern human marrow transplants were conducted without success in patients with end-stage disease. It was not until the 1960s that medical research focused on the importance of human tissue typing and applied these concepts to organ and marrow transplantation. By the late 1960s, following the institution of human leukocyte antigen (HLA) typing to identify suitable sibling donors, successful allogeneic transplants were performed in increasing numbers. Simultaneously, the technology of platelet transfusion and methods of prophylaxis against infection were developed.

In the past decade, improvements in Graft-versus-Host Disease (GVHD) management and prophylaxis and treatment of infection have decreased transplant-related morbidity and mortality. However, relapse after BMT remains a major problem and is a priority for research. The use of fractionated total body irradiation (TBI) rather than single-dose TBI has significantly reduced post-BMT complications. The increased use of busulfan and cyclophosphamide without TBI for pretransplant conditioning in the marrow transplant setting has also resulted in decreased acute complications and improved relapse-free survival; but long-term complications persist. Laminar airflow units (LAFs) and rooms with high-efficiency particulate (HEPA) filters are now rarely used because it is not clear that their use contributes to improved survival; simple protective isolation with scrupulous hand washing is commonly practiced.

Although PBST is thought of as a new approach to oncologic and hematologic diseases, the evolution of PBST from BMT began more than 100 years ago. As early as 1909, it was postulated that there were small cells circulating in the blood that had the capability to self-generate from a primitive stem cell. This discovery was debated until the mid 1950s as understanding of the nature and characterization of the stem cells improved. Studies in the 1950s and 1960s reported the existence of stem cells in the peripheral blood of rats, mice, guinea pigs, and dogs. Goodman and Hodgson, using the term "blood stem cell" were the first to record evidence that circulating stem cells are capable of restoring hematopoiesis after marrow ablation. Successful animal transplantation with peripheral stem cells soon led to the belief that human PBST was a possibility.

Subsequently, leukopheresis and cryopreservation techniques improved. The development of the continuous flow stem cell separator in 1965 gave birth to the first clinical PBSTs, but findings were not published until 1971. The first significant studies were reported in 1986 from four centers using PBST for patients with chronic myelogenous leukemia in accelerated phase. Although patients responded, treatment with PBST was not curative. In addition, the use of PBSTs was limited because multiple collections were needed to attain sufficient numbers of stem cells to repopulate the marrow successfully after cytotoxic therapy.

In the late 1980s, the use of cyclophosphamide and cytokines effectively mobilized larger numbers of stem cells, leading to earlier engraftment, fewer infections, less antibiotic use, and fewer hospital admissions.

MARROW TRANSPLANTATION VERSUS PERIPHERAL BLOOD STEM CELL TRANSPLANTATION

The rational for BMT and PBST is similar, but unique procedural differences exist. Generally speaking, BMT is a more lengthy procedure re-

Table 3A-1
**A Comparison of Peripheral Stem Cell Transplantation
and Marrow Transplantation**

Issue	PSCT	BMT
Care facility	May be performed in outpatient area	Hospital/acute care setting
	Available in community setting	Usually performed in major research settings
Granulocyte recovery	6–8 d	10–12 d
Platelet recovery	6–8 d	14–16 d
Long term engraftment	Long term survivors 6–7 years to date	Long term survivors to over 30 years
Tumor contamination	Yes, but extent not known	Yes
Overall morbidity and mortality	Less	More
Graft vs. leukemia effect	Rare	Predominantly allogeneic (30%–50%)
Average costs	$60,000–90,000	$90,000–250,000
Collection or harvest	No general anesthesia peripheral apherisis	Marrow harvest under general anesthesia
Types and sources available	Autologous	Autologous, allogeneic and unrelated BMTs
Patient and family time commitments	Approximately four to six weeks Caregiver burden may be more intense but of shorter duration	Approximately 6–12 months Caregiver burden intense over longer duration
Insurance coverage	Less available than BMT due to "experimental nature"	More available, but exceptions exist
Venous access	Large double bore catheter	Standard central lumen catheter
Hospitalization	Short or no length of stay	30–35 d hospitalization
Readmission Rate	Approximately 65%	Approximately 50%

Adapted from Buchsel PC, Kapustay P. Peripheral stem cell transplantation. *Oncology Nursing: Patient and Support.* 2(2): 1–14. 1995.

quiring extended hospitalization. Most marrow recipients receive TBI as part of the pretransplant conditioning regimen, whereas most peripheral blood recipients receive only combination chemotherapy. In addition, the methods for obtaining the cells to be transplanted differ. Marrow is "harvested" under general or spinal anesthesia, whereas peripheral blood stem cells are collected through apheresis methods in the outpatient setting. Recovery of blood cells (engraftment) following aggressive anti-tumor chemotherapy occurs more rapidly after PBST, because patients receive colony stimulating factors for stem cell mobilization. Table 3A–1 describes the advantages and disadvantages of each type of approach.

The rationale behind the use of either BMT or PBST is as follows:

- The dose of most chemotherapeutic agents administered to cure a patient of cancer is limited because of toxicity.
- The availability of marrow or stem cells for transplantation and subsequent engraftment makes it possible to administer chemotherapy and radiation therapy in higher potentially lethal doses to kill malignant cells (pretransplant conditioning regimens).
- The patient is rescued with marrow or stem cells to prevent death from profound pancytopenia (transplantation).
- The infused marrow or peripheral blood stem cells reconstitutes the patient's hematopoietic and immune system (engraftment).
- Acute and chronic complications that follow are the result of conditioning regimens, GVHD (allogeneic), and treatment failure (relapse).

TYPES OF TRANSPLANTS

Transplants are named according to the donor type—allogeneic (related or unrelated person), syngeneic (twin), or autologous (self)—and categorized by the hematologic stem cell source. The most common sources are marrow, blood, and umbilical or placenta stem cells. Other stem cell sources in preclinical studies are fetal liver cells and dendritic cells.

Allogeneic Transplantation

Allogeneic transplants are most commonly performed for leukemia or preleukemia (74 percent), including chronic myelogenous leukemia (22 percent), acute myelogenous leukemia (23 percent), acute lymphoblastic leukemia (19 percent), myelodysplastic syndromes (7 percent), and others (3 percent). Figure 3A–2 summarizes other diseases for which allogeneic transplant is used.

A successful allogeneic marrow or peripheral blood transplant depends on the availability of an HLA-matched donor. GVHD, a complica-

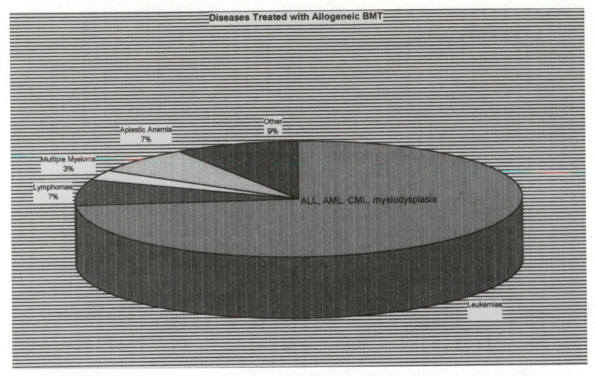

Figure 3A–2. Diseases treated with allogeneic bone marrow transplantation.

tion unique to allogeneic transplantation that occurs when the grafted marrow "rejects" the host, remains a major obstacle to successful transplantation. Intensive supportive care with protective environments, prophylactic and therapeutic antibiotics, and blood component therapy are required.

The National Marrow Donor Program (NMDP) contains data on more than 2.5 million unrelated bone marrow donors from more than 10 countries, most of whom are Caucasian. There is a special need for volunteer donors from other racial groups, including African Americans, Asian/Pacific Islanders, and the Hispanic and American Indian/Alaska Native communities.

Autologous Marrow and Peripheral Stem Cell Transplantation

In an autologous marrow or peripheral stem cell transplantation, a patient receives his or her own marrow or stem cells, which have been collected and cryopreserved during remission. This approach is used primarily for patients with breast cancer, lymphoma, or other solid tumors, or for selected patients with leukemia (Figure 3A–3). The major advantage of autologous tranplants is the fewer treatment-related toxicities, including GVHD. Research to induce mild GVHD in the autologous transplant re-

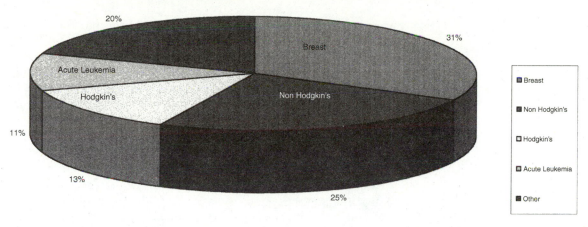

Lung, Brain, Bone, CML
Ovarian, Multiple Myeloma

20%

Breast

31%

Acute Leukemia

Non Hodgkin's

Hodgkin's

11%

13%

25%

Legend:
- Breast
- Non Hodgkin's
- Hodgkin's
- Acute Leukemia
- Other

Figure 3A-3. Diseases treated with autologous marrow and peripheral stem cell transplantation.

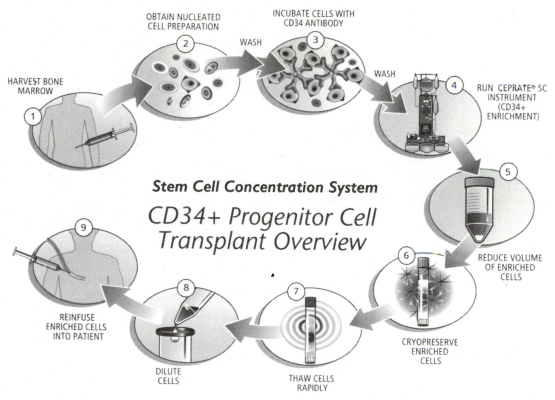

OBTAIN NUCLEATED
CELL PREPARATION

2

WASH

INCUBATE CELLS WITH
CD34 ANTIBODY

3

WASH

HARVEST BONE
MARROW

1

4

RUN CEPRATE® SC
INSTRUMENT
(CD34+
ENRICHMENT)

Stem Cell Concentration System

CD34+ Progenitor Cell Transplant Overview

5

REDUCE VOLUME
OF ENRICHED
CELLS

9

6

CRYOPRESERVE
ENRICHED
CELLS

REINFUSE
ENRICHED CELLS
INTO PATIENT

8

7

DILUTE
CELLS

THAW CELLS
RAPIDLY

Figure 3A-4. A schematic of a stem cell purging process.

Reprinted with permission from CellPro, Inc.

cipient to induce a "graft-versus-leukemia effect" holds promise in further reducing relapse rates in this patient population.

Autologous marrow is harvested from the patient in a manner similar to harvesting marrow from a donor for allogeneic transplant. More marrow might be needed if it is to be purged or otherwise manipulated. Autologous marrow is sometimes infused immediately after completion of the pretransplant high-dose conditioning regimen. More often, the marrow is cryopreserved to be used if the patient relapses. The length of time that marrow can be stored without compromising its viability is thought to range from one to eight years.

Relapse of the primary disease in the marrow is a concern following autologous transplantation. It can be caused by the failure of the conditioning therapy to eradicate malignant cells completely. For this reason, autologous marrow is purged to remove malignant cells before the marrow or peripheral blood is reinfused. Three methods can be used, alone or in combination: physical, immunologic, and pharmacologic. Physical purging requires separation of contaminated cells from marrow and blood using lectin separation, centrifugation in density gradients, and counterflow evaluations. Immunologic purging uses immunotoxins, or monoclonal antibodies alone or in combination with magnetic "immunobeads." Pharmacologic purging uses potent cytotoxic agents such as merocyanine 540, mafosfamide (ASTA-2-7557), 4-hydroperoxycyclophosphamide (4-HC), or alkyl-lysophospholipids. Figure 3A–4 illustrates a process for marrow purging using immunoadsorption beads.

THE TRANSPLANT PROCEDURE

Pretransplant Evaluation and Preparation

Transplant candidates require comprehensive evaluation to determine eligibility and ability to sustain the procedure. This evaluation, described in Table 3A–2, is usually performed in outpatient facilities. A family conference is scheduled to (1) obtain informed consent, (2) discuss the risk of transplant-related morbidity and mortality, and (3) discuss expected outcomes with the patient. Although the patient usually focuses on immediate concerns, it is equally important to familiarize him or her with possible long-term complications of transplantation. For example, the high-dose pretransplant conditioning regimens can cause gonadal failure. For male patients desiring children, sperm banking should be considered prior to hospitalization. In the future, ova storage might be an option for women.

Before the BMT patient is admitted or the PBST patient begins stem cell mobilization, the nurse might familiarize him or her with protective isolation and various treatment and research protocols to be used. Patients will have multi-lumen indwelling central catheters inserted. Large bore atrial catheters are essential to accommodate the blood volumes circulating

Table 3A–2
**Pretransplantation Evaluation for Peripheral Stem Cell
and Marrow Transplantation Candidates**

Patient	Donor
Complete medical history	X
Full discussion of marrow transplantation, including its rationale, risks and benefits with family and referring physician. Particular attention must be devoted to discussion of alternative therapies and long-term complications.	X
Complete medical history, including differential diagnosis	X
Previous treatment and results	X
Co-morbid medical problems that might complicate or preclude transplantation	
Allergies, especially to sulfa medications	X
Transfusion history	
Psychological assessment	
Bone marrow aspiration and biopsy	
Tumor staging studies for malignant diseases, central nervous system sanctuary sites	
Immunization history	
Organ toxicity screening:	X
CBC	X
Hepatic: liver function studies, hepatitis screen	X
Renal: urinalysis, serum creatinine, creatinine clearance	X
Pulmonary-arterial blood gases, pulmonary function tests	
Chest x-ray	X
Cardiac: Left ventricular function evaluation	
Endocrine: Fasting blood sugar, glucose tolerance test, thyroid function tests	

Continued

Table 3A-2 *(Continued)*
Pretransplantation Evaluation for Peripheral Stem Cell and Marrow Transplantation Candidates

Patient	Donor
Cholesterol and triglycerides	
Toxoplasma titers	X
Andrology for sperm banking	
Human chorionic gonadotropin	X
Follicle stimulating hormone levels	X
Histocompatibility testing for allogeneic and syngeneic marrow transplantation	X
Restrictive fragment length	
Serologic typing	X
Mixed leukocytes culture testing	X
Molecular studies	
Identification of marker of engraftment for allogeneic marrow transplantation	
Transfusion support planning evaluation of allosensitization status	X
ABO typing	X
Human Immunodeficiency Virus titer	X
Cytomegalovirus status	X
Nutritional evaluation	
	Iron supplements colony stimulating factors (PBST donor only)
Informed consent	X
Dental consultation, films	

through apheresis equipment during stem cell collection, and marrow transplant recipients require large volumes of parenteral fluids. Peripherally inserted catheters (PICs), placed by certified nurses, could be used, especially for patients receiving autologous marrow transplant.

Donor Selection

Selection of an appropriate marrow donor is based on blood tests for HLA and oligotyping techniques. Bone marrow cells have inherited surface antigens, called HLAs, that can recognize and reject foreign tissue. To date, four antigens have been identified: A, B, C, and D. Blood samples from donor and patient are compared, mixing small samples of white blood cells with blood sera negative for the HLAs; if cells are destroyed, incompatibility is indicated. The best possible donor would match all four antigen sites. Only about 25 percent of siblings have genetic HLA matching similar enough to be successful donors (Figure 3A–5). As the demand for transplantation increases, faster and more accurate methods will be needed to identify the most appropriate donor. Oligotyping allows the identification of HLA allelic polymorphism at the DNA level by hybridization with sequence-specific oligonucleotide probes after identification of DNA by polymerase chain reaction.

In addition to being HLA matched, selected allogeneic donors must be evaluated for general health, give informed consent, and be available for marrow or stem cell harvest. Donors who are minors present special legal and ethical considerations. Although risks are minimal, donors are carefully evaluated prior to marrow harvest for tolerance of general or spinal anesthesia. Donors weighing more than 50 kilograms donate units of whole blood prior to harvest, to be reinfused intraoperatively.

Marrow is harvested in the operating room under sterile conditions using general or spinal anesthesia. The marrow is obtained from the posterior iliac crests in 2–5 milliliter aspirates, to a total of 10–15 milliliters per

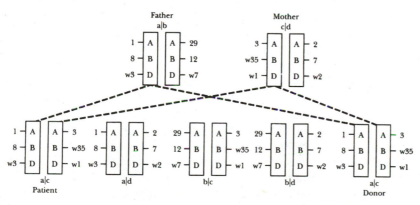

Figure 3A-5. Diagram of possible combinations of human leukocyte antigen (HLA) region of chromosome 6 inherited from parents to sibling. The recipient and donor have inherited the same two haplotypes and are genotypically HLA identical.

Reprinted with permission from Buchsel, P. C., and J. Kelleher. Bone marrow transplantation. Nursing Clinics of North America 24(4): 910.

kilogram of recipient's body weight. If necessary, the anterior iliac crests and sternum can be used. Although 150–200 aspirates are necessary to obtain sufficient marrow, only 6–10 skin punctures are made, because the aspiration needles are redirected to different sites under the skin. The heparinized marrow is passed through a series of progressively finer mesh screens to filter out bone particles and fat. Marrow is then placed in blood administration bags to be infused at a later time.

Allogeneic marrow donors are usually admitted to the hospital for harvest on the day of surgery and discharged 24 hours after surgery. Common side effects of marrow harvest are pain and bleeding at the puncture sites, low back pain, nausea, vomiting, sore throat, and fever. Follow-up care is essential for physical as well as psychologic support. Marrow from unrelated donors is typically harvested in a hospital other than the recipient's for reasons of confidentiality and convenience.

Stem Cell Harvest

The candidate for PBST receives chemotherapy and/or colony stimulating factors to stimulate stem cells from the marrow into the peripheral blood. This process is called *mobilization*. Under normal conditions, bone marrow has a concentration of stem cells 10 to 100 times higher than the peripheral blood. A chemotherapy-induced white blood cell nadir stimulates the bone marrow to undergo dramatic hematopoiesis, resulting in a 100-fold increase in the number of stem cells in the peripheral circulation. Stem cells are collected from the patient at this time to obtain the maximum yield of pluripotent stem cells, or CD34+ cells. (CD34+ cells are named for the antigen present on the cell surface; these cells are thought to be most capable of producing rapid regeneration of granulocytes and subsequent marrow engraftment.) An additional advantage to administering chemotherapy for mobilization is to further enhance tumor cell kill before transplantation. Alkylating agents are used because of their cell cycle non-specificity and subsequent cell recovery.

The most common alkylating agent used is cyclophosphamide at doses of 2 to 4 grams. Human recombinant growth factors (granulocyte-macrophage colony stimulating factor or granulocyte colony stimulating factor) are also used to stimulate regrowth of stem cells. (Care of the patient receiving colony stimulating factors is discussed in Chapters 2D and 10A.)

The stem cell collection process involves using apheresis technique. *Apheresis* uses commercial cell separators programmed to collect either lymphocytes or low-density leukocytes. Commonly used apheresis machines are the Cobe Spectra (COBE Laboratories, Lakewood, CO), Fenwal CS-3000 (Fenwal, Round Lake, IL), and Haemonetics V-50 (Haemonetics Corp., Brainier, MA). Apheresis is performed daily for approximately two to four hours, depending on the rate of blood flow (between 50 and 70cc/min) through the apheresis catheter to the machine and the total blood volume to be apheresed. Approximately 9–14 liters of blood are processed through a large bore central lumen catheter and returned to the patient. The number of apheresis procedures depends upon the viability of the collected stem cells and the number of CD34+ cells collected. Daily cell counts are performed to determine the number of CD34+ cells in the peripheral blood. Generally, several aphereses are required to collect sufficient stem cells, performed over several days. Optimal cell counts differ among institutions, but the number of cells needed for successful engraftment is approximately 2 to 5×10^6 mononuclear cells or 2×10^6 CD34+ cells per kilogram of body weight. Research is ongoing to develop a method for collecting sufficient cells for transplant in one collection.

The most common complications reported with apheresis are transient hypocalcemia secondary to the citrate infusion and catheter obstruction. These phenomena are directly related to anticoagulant citrate dextrose (ACD), which is mixed with the blood to prevent clotting during the apheresis process. Hypovolemia due to fluctuations in circulating blood volume during apheresis causes lightheadedness or dysrhythmias; this can be minimized by reducing the extra corporeal volume or slowing the flow rate. Hypocalcemia is manifested by paresthesia, muscle and/or abdominal cramps, chills, tremors, or chest pain. These symptoms can be managed with oral calcium supplements such as Tums®. If symptoms continue to increase despite administration of oral calcium, intravenous calcium gluconate can be administered every four hours until symptoms are controlled. Covering the patient with warm blankets might help. Obstructed catheters are managed by repositioning the patient or instillation of urokinase. A complete explanation of these adverse complications is necessary to reduce patient and family concern.

When collected, the stem cells are removed from the blood cell separator, and isolated using a density gradient or other apheresis procedure to reduce the number of potentially contaminating red cells and granulocytes. Further volume of the stem cell collection can be reduced or cells for tumor reduction manipulated through purging techniques similar to marrow purging. The stem cells collected are sometimes referred to as an *enriched stem cell product*.

Allogeneic peripheral blood cell donors are required to be healthy and willing to accept administration of colony stimulating factors for stem cell mobilization. Stem cells are collected through apheresis similar to the autologous recipient. As often as possible, central venous catheters are avoided in this population to minimize donor risk for infection and inconvenience. A major debate in transplant medicine is the possible acute or long-term adverse effects of colony stimulating factors on healthy donors. To date no adverse problems have been identified, but further research is needed, especially as the recruitment of volunteer peripheral blood cell donors is anticipated.

Cryopreservation

The average stem cell life span is three to seven days; consequently, stem cells are cryopreserved to prevent damage and ensure cell viability at the time of PBST. The cells are prepared for cryopreservation with one of two methods. The most recent technique involves the use of the cryoprotectant dimethylsulfoxide (DMSO) at a concentration of 10 percent by volume. The cells are cooled in a controlled-rate freezer and stored in the vapor or liquid phase of nitrogen. The second method uses DMSO at a concentration of 5 percent by volume combined with hydroxyethyl starch for cryoprotection. In the latter, but older method, the cells are placed in a $-80°$ C freezer for cooling and placed in the freezer for storage. The patient is then ready to proceed to high-dose therapy and/or TBI, often referred to as the preparative or pretransplant conditioning regimen.

ADMISSION TO THE BMT UNIT

Pre-transplant Conditioning Regimens

BMT/PBST recipients are usually admitted to the hospital one day prior to the start of their pretransplant conditioning, or preparative, regimen. Patients receive high doses of chemotherapy with or without lethal doses of radiation to eradicate residual malignant cells and, in the case of allogeneic transplant, to prevent rejection of the graft by the immune system. Table 3A–3 lists the most common conditioning regimens.

TBI is delivered in varying doses from cobalt or linear accelerator units and offers optimal tumor kill because of its capability to penetrate the central nervous system and other "privileged" sites. Lung shielding during TBI is often used to reduce life-threatening pulmonary complications. Although TBI can be delivered as a single dose, most centers employ fractionated doses to reduce toxicities. Pretransplant radiation therapy to sites of previous bulky disease has shown some success in preventing relapse.

The day of marrow or stem cell infusion is termed "day 0," with subsequent days numbered from this time (T+1, T+2, and so on). The infu-

Table 3A–3
Sample Marrow and Peripheral Stem Cell Transplantation Conditioning Regimens

Cyclophosphamide and Total Body Irradiation
Cytarabine and Total Body Irradiation
Busulfan and Cyclophosphamide
Antithymocyte Globulin
Carmustine
Etoposide/Teniposide
Melphalan

sion is a procedure similar to a blood transfusion. Marrow is infused through a central lumen catheter over several hours. Marrow cells pass through the lung to the marrow cavity. Possible complications include volume overload and pulmonary abnormalities secondary to fat emboli. Symptoms similar to blood transfusion reactions can occur—for example, chills, urticaria, and fever—and should be treated with antihistamines or antipyretics, or by decreasing the rate of infusion.

Peripheral stem cell reinfusion differs slightly from marrow infusion. With a PBST, the frozen stem cells are removed from the cryopreservation laboratory, thawed in a warm water bath in the patient's room; cross-referenced between the physician, nurse, or laboratory personnel; and infused by gravity drip. Needles are not used because of the possibility of stem cell destruction. Infusion-related complications, often due to the cryoperservative, DMSO, include nausea, vomiting, diarrhea, and facial flushing. Cellular debris from red cell lysis can cause allergic reactions as well. The patient usually experiences a garlic-like taste and smell. Table 3A–4 lists common complications associated with peripheral stem cell infusion and

Table 3A–4
Possible Complications of Peripheral Stem Cell Reinfusion

Potential Complication	Nursing Intervention
Pulmonary emboli, fluid overload	Monitor for cough, chest tightness, tachypnea, cardiac arrhythmias, hypo-hypertension
	Frequent vital signs, monitor I&O, administer oxygen, diuretics, if necessary
DMSO toxicity	Premedicate with diphenhydramine 50 mg, hydrocortisone 250 mg
Nausea, vomiting, chills, abdominal cramping, diarrhea, garlic-like taste, body odor, facial flushing	Administer antiemetics Offer cool cloths for facial flushing
Anaphylaxis	Premedicate with hydration beginning approximately four hours prior to stem cell infusion
	Administer hydrocortisone preinfusion, epinephrine if indicated
	Assess for shortness of breath, chest tightness, coughing
Renal dysfunction Hematuria from red cell lysis	Administer hydration

clinical support. Engraftment, with recovery of circulating red and white blood cells and platelets, usually occurs within two to four weeks.

ACUTE COMPLICATIONS OF BONE MARROW TRANSPLANTATION

Although transplantation holds promise for cure for several diseases, acute and chronic toxicities complicate the post-transplant course. Complications can result from the high doses of chemotherapy and radiation used for conditioning regimens, GVHD (with allogeneic transplants), and problems associated with recurrent disease. Complications of autologous marrow transplantation are similar to those seen with allogeneic transplantation, with the exception of GVHD. Acute complications occur several days after transplant and affect many organ systems. The toxicity of pretransplant conditioning regimens is most severe until engraftment occurs. Table 3A–5 offers a detailed summary of the cause, incidence, onset, manifestations, and interventions associated with acute complications of BMT.

Complications associated with PBST are largely dependent on the pretransplant conditioning regimen. In contrast to BMT, PBST recipients receive more diverse high-dose chemotherapeutic regimens, depending on their disease and prior treatment. It is imperative for oncology nurses caring for patients after transplantation to be familiar with the conditioning regimens and the acute and long-term side effects. Because these patients seldom receive TBI, the cataracts and growth and development problems that can result from TBI will not likely be observed in these patients.

Gastrointestinal Toxicity

Oral mucositis (stomatitis), or inflammation of the oral and pharyngeal tissues, begins two to three days after marrow infusion (seven to ten days after the conditioning regimen) and is a major clinical problem. Patients with stomatitis are at risk for herpes simplex lesions and other local or systemic secondary infections. Protracted oral pain is usually treated with intravenous morphine. Mucositis can be further complicated by severe thrombocytopenia, aspiration pneumonia, and nutritional depletion (see Chapter 10B). These problems resolve when engraftment occurs, and serious long-term problems are rare.

Nausea and vomiting following the conditioning regimen might be protracted if complicated by GVHD, cytomegalovirus esophagitis, or gastrointestinal infection. Differential diagnosis must be made and can include endoscopy with duodenal biopsy. The use of antibiotics and other concomitant medications can exacerbate nausea/vomiting (see Chapter 9).

In the first weeks after BMT, diarrhea occurs as a result of chemotherapy and radiation therapy, but seldom persists beyond day 15. Oral magne-

Table 3A–5
Acute Complications of Marrow and Peripheral Stem Cell Transplant

Complication	Inc. %	Onset	Signs/Symptoms	Nursing Intervention
GIT				
Mucositis due to high-dose prep regimen +/− coexistent infection	100	0–28d after BMT	Profuse watery to thick ropy mucous, severe pain, bleeding, ulceration, infection, potential airway obstruction, xerostomia	Assess nasal/oral cavity for integrity of mucous membrane; diligent mouth care, pain control
Esophageal mucositis	100	0–28d after BMT	Esophageal dysphagia, bleeding, infection	Pain control, frequent oral care
Gastric mucositis	100	0–28d after BMT	Anorexia, N/V, bleeding, infection	Monitor I&O, maintain fluid balance, pain control
Intestinal mucositis	100	0–28d after BMT	Watery diarrhea, cramping pain, ulceration, bleeding, infection	Monitor VS q 4 hr; I&O, pain control
Lower bowel mucositis due to high-dose prep regimen; GVHD	100	0–28d after BMT	N/V, diarrhea	Monitor I&O, electrolyte balance, effect of antiemetics, parenteral nutrition
Alopecia	100	7–10d after BMT	Loss of body hair	Assist with coping; provide psychological support
Infection				
Bacterial *E. coli, Staph epidermidis, Staph aureus, Streptococcus*	100	0–30d post-BMT	Neutropenia, oral fever >38°C, sepsis, cough, lethargy	Provide protective isolation, good handwashing, surveillance cultures, pan cultures; administer antibiotics, manage side effects of treatment; monitor and regulate BP; manage fluid & electrolyte balance; fever reduction measures
Viral *Herpes simplex*	70–80	70–80d post-BMT	Pain, ulceration, bleeding, fever, infection	Provide vigorous mouth care; pain control
CMV	10–70 (auto-allo)	60–70d post-BMT	Dyspnea, infiltrates on CXR, abnormal ABGs, PFTs	Administer medication
Fungal *Aspergillus*	80–90		Fever	Administer amphotercin B; monitor serum electrolytes, hydration, side effects

Continued

Table 3A–5 *(Continued)*
Acute Complications of Marrow and Peripheral Stem Cell Transplant

Complication	Inc. %	Onset	Signs/Symptoms	Nursing Intervention
Acute GVHD				
Skin	45	10–70d after BMT; median 25 d	Maculopapular rash on trunk, palms, soles, ears; generalized erythroderma with desquamation	Assess skin integrity; monitor for side effects of drug treatment; provide psychological support, pain control
Liver	45	same	Elevated LFTs, RUQ pain, hepatomegaly, jaundice	Monitor LFTs, skin care
GIT	45	same	Green watery diarrhea, abdominal cramping, anorexia, N/V	Monitor stool for blood; weigh patient, I&O, CVPs, CBC and electrolytes, provide antiemetics, pain control
Renal insufficiency	25	1–50d after BMT	Decreased urine output, azotemia, proteinuria, hypertension, renal failure, thrombocytopenia purpura, thirst, dizziness; flat or distended neck veins, peripheral edema; doubling of baseline serum creatinine	Monitor VS with postural BP; fluid management, I&O; monitor serum creatinine, BUN, electrolytes. Monitor urine electrolytes, specific gravity q 4 hr; measure daily abdomen girth, weight; assess for peripheral edema; monitor patient during dialysis
Veno-occlusive disease (VOD)	21 (6% fatal)	6–15d after BMT	Weight gain >12%; ascites, bilirubin >2.0 mg/dL, SGOT >40 mU/mL; RUQ pain; encephalopathy, hepatomegaly	Assess fluid balance, monitor weight BID, VS with postural BP, I&O; measure abdomen girth qd, fluid and sodium restriction; monitor narcotics and hemodynamics

RUQ—right upper quadrant; CMV—cytomegalovirus

sium and nonabsorbable antibiotics can cause mild diarrhea. Diarrhea associated with acute GVHD and infection is seen as early as day 7 (see Chapter 9).

Hematologic Complications

Transplant recipients are at high risk for hemorrhage and must be supported with radiated red blood cells and platelets until the donor marrow becomes fully engrafted and functional. Blood products are radiated to destroy T-lymphocytes that can cause GVHD in the allogeneic marrow recipient. Patients who become resistant to random platelet transfusions can receive HLA-matched platelets from family or community donors (see Chapter 10A).

Graft-versus-Host Disease

GVHD is an immunologic disease that is a direct consequence of allogeneic marrow transplantation. It occurs in both acute and chronic forms and can affect 30 percent to 50 percent of HLA-identical recipients. Marrow recipients receiving unrelated donor transplants experience significantly worse GVHD than those receiving HLA-identical sibling transplants. However, there appears to be no significant difference in the occurrence of GVHD with unrelated donors than with mismatched related donors. GVHD is thought to be a graft-host response in which the grafted donor T-lymphocytes recognize disparate non-HLA host cell antigens and initiate cytotoxic injury against host (patient) tissue. Acute GVHD targets the skin, liver, and gut. Risk factors for acute GVHD are increased patient age and mismatched BMT donors.

Acute GVHD of the skin typically begins with a maculopapular erythema that might be pruritic and covers 25 percent of the body. The disease can progress to a generalized erythroderma with frank desquamation and blistering similar to second degree burns. At the same time as or after the onset of GVHD of the skin, GVHD can involve the liver, causing increases in liver enzymes, right upper quadrant pain, and hepatomegaly. Gastrointestinal involvement of acute GVHD can result in nausea, vomiting, anorexia, abdominal cramping, and pain. A typical early symptom is green, watery diarrhea that can exceed two liters per day.

GVHD might be difficult to distinguish from symptoms secondary to infection or the side effects of high-dose conditioning regimens. Differential diagnosis is imperative and is usually made by skin and liver biopsy and by clinical, laboratory, and x-ray data.

One of the most important tasks in transplantation medicine is to prevent GVHD and its related symptoms. Immunosuppressive medications, such as cyclosporine and methotrexate, are used to remove or deactivate the T-lymphocytes that cause GVHD. They are more effective when used in combination than when used alone. Other medications used to prevent and modify GVHD are antithymocyte globulin (ATG) and monoclonal antibody therapy. Table 3A–5 describes nursing and medical interventions. Initial data report the incidence and severity of acute GVHD after allogeneic PBST to be not significantly different from that after marrow transplantation.

Renal Complications

Renal dysfunction occurs in more than 50 percent of marrow recipients and is defined as a doubling of the baseline serum creatinine level. Nephrotoxic drugs (amphotericin B, cyclosporine, methotrexate, aminoglycosides, acyclovir) used to prevent and treat transplant-related problems can exacerbate existing complications such as hypovolemia, impaired circulation of blood volume, or tumor lysis syndrome (see Chapter 16B). Early symptoms are anuria and oliguria. Renal dysfunction in marrow transplant patients is usually mild and can be managed by medication and careful fluid balance. However, 5 percent to 10 percent of allogeneic post-transplant patients require dialysis; mortality is 85 percent in this group.

Veno-Occlusive Disease

Veno-occlusive disease (VOD), which is almost exclusively related to BMT, is the most common liver problem that develops after BMT and is caused by the conditioning regimen. The incidence is 21 percent in adult patients; the mortality rate can be as high as 50 percent. Risk factors for developing VOD are (1) liver abnormalities prior to marrow transplant, (2) age greater than 15 years, (3) hematologic malignancies other than acute lymphocytic leukemia (ALL), and (4) allogeneic BMT.

Liver damage involves two histopathologic processes: (1) venule occlusion and/or veno-occlusive process involving terminal hepatic venules and sublobular veins and (2) hepatocyte necrosis. Clinical symptoms occur in the first weeks after transplant (Table 3A–5). Currently, there is no prevention method or treatment for VOD. Providing supportive measures to maintain the patient until the VOD has run its course is the mainstay of care.

Hemorrhagic Cystitis

More than 50% percent of marrow recipients develop some degree of hemorrhagic cystitis, most often as a result of the use of cyclophosphamide in the conditioning regimen. Recently, adenovirus has been implicated in this problem. Hemorrhagic cystitis can have a sudden onset, be delayed, or manifest itself months after BMT. Hemorrhagic cystitis can be prevented using continuous bladder irrigation and/or aggressive intravenous therapy.

Pulmonary Complications

Pulmonary complications are a major cause of morbidity and mortality, appearing as early (before day 100) or late sequelae of BMT (after day 100) (see Chapter 14). Pulmonary edema caused by sodium excess and cardiomyopathy, myocarditis, and volume overload from VOD can occur immediately after transplantation. Interstitial pneumonia causes symptoms similar to those of adult respiratory distress syndrome (ARDS) and occurs early or late post-transplant (Figure 3A–6).

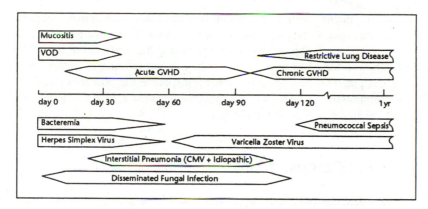

Figure 3A–6. Temporal sequence of major complications after allogeneic bone marrow transplantation from day 0 to one year after BMT.

Interstitial pneumonia is a nonbacterial, nonfungal process that occurs in the interstitial spaces of the lungs. It develops in approximately 35 percent of allogeneic marrow recipients and is the most frequent cause of death during the first 100 days after transplant. The overall mortality rate from interstitial pneumonia is approximately 20 percent in allogeneic recipients transplanted for advanced hematologic malignancy.

Cytomegaloviral (CMV) pneumonia is a leading cause of infectious pneumonia that occurs in 20 percent of allogeneic BMT recipients and 2 percent to 3 percent of autologous marrow recipients. The fatality rate is as high as 85 percent. The median time of onset for early CMV is between five and thirteen weeks after transplantation. Risk factors include (1) age greater than 30 years, (2) severe GVHD, (3) TBI conditioning regimen, (4) CMV-seropositivity, and (5) advanced hematologic malignancy. The use of CMV-negative blood products for the 100 days following BMT is the most effective prophylaxis. Patients who are initially CMV-seropositive or who have donors who are seropositive might benefit from the use of antiviral agents such as acyclovir or passive antibody prophylaxis with immunoglobulin.

Idiopathic pneumonia accounts for 30 percent of all interstitial pneumonia in marrow recipients and is thought to be a result of high-dose radiation. Idiopathic pneumonia is diagnosed when no specific organism is recovered in bronchial lavage washing or biopsy of lung tissue.

Other pneumonias can occur in marrow transplant patients, caused by viruses (e.g., adenovirus, herpes simplex, varicella zoster), bacteria, or fungi. These account for 15 percent of pneumonia in marrow recipients and can be successfully treated.

Neurologic Complications

Neurologic complications occur in 60–70 percent of marrow recipients with a resulting 6 percent fatality rate. Underlying causes are conditioning regimens, central nervous system infection, and immunosuppressive agents such as cyclosporine, steroids, and intrathecal methotrexate.

Leukoencephalopathy has been reported in the 7 percent of transplant patients who have had prior cranial radiation and intrathecal methotrexate (see Chapter 11). Patients receiving cyclosporine for post-transplant immunosuppression have developed hypomagnesemia, which can have neurological sequelae such as seizure activity.

Cardiac Complications

Cardiac complications can develop within several days after the administration of high-dose cyclophosphamide. Patients can develop cardiomegaly, congestive heart failure, and fluid retention, which can be managed with fluid balance to avoid pulmonary edema.

Infection

Infection as a result of profound immunosuppression following the conditioning regimen is a major cause of morbidity and mortality in the BMT recipient. The most common sites of infections are the gastrointestinal tract, oropharynx, lung, skin, and indwelling catheter sites. During the first month following BMT, gram-negative and gram-positive bacteria infections, together with fungus (e.g., aspergillus, candida) and/or herpes simplex virus, prevail. During the second and third months, patients are at risk for infection from cytomegalovirus, fungi, gram-positive bacteria, and pneumocystis carinii. After engraftment is established, recipients remain at risk for infection from encapsulated bacteria, varicella zoster, and pneumocystis carinii (Table 3A–6).

DISCHARGE FROM THE HOSPITAL

The average discharge for allogeneic BMT recipients is approximately 30–35 days after BMT. Patients receiving autologous BMT and PBST typically have shorter hospitalizations, decreased BMT-related toxicities, and earlier engraftment.

Ideally, preparation for discharge begins when the patient arrives at the BMT center. Technical preparations usually start when engraftment is established and BMT-related problems are stabilized. Patient and family must be taught clearly and consistently what they should know to prevent and promptly recognize transplant-related problems. They are taught to prevent infections by avoiding crowds, school, and work for one year after BMT.

Table 3A-6
Late Effects of Bone Marrow Transplantation

Late Effect	Incidence[a]	Causes	Typical Onset Post-Transplant	Signs and Symptoms	Medical Management
Pulmonary Complications	50% with chronic GVHD 21% without chronic GVHD 2% autologous BMT	Cytotoxic agents Radiation Structural and functional damage Impaired immunity from chronic GVHD Infectious pathogens	100 days or until immune reconstitution	Fever, shaking chills, malaise, cough, dyspnea, wheezing, bronchospasm, bilateral interstitial infiltrates, and abnormal PFTs	Chest x-ray PFTs and ABGs Open lung biopsy Antibiotic therapy
Interstitial pneumonitis	10%–15% allogeneic BMT	Radiation Cytotoxic agents Impaired immunity Infectious pathogens	80–150 d	Nonproductive cough, fever, wheezing, dyspnea, bronchospasm, hypoxia, and reduced expiratory flow	Chest x-ray ABGs BAL Steroid and antibiotic therapy
Restrictive disease	20%	Radiation Cytotoxic agents Chronic GVHD	365 d	Cough, dyspnea upon exertion, abnormal PFTs, mean loss in total lung capacity, reduced vital capacity, and impaired diffusion capacity May be asymptomatic	Respiratory therapy Bronchodilators
Obstructive disease	10%–15%	Radiation Cytotoxic agents Chronic GVHD	100–400 d	Dyspnea, cough, hypoxia, shortness of breath, reduced forced expiratory volume, and reduced IgG and IgA levels	Chest x-ray ABGs, pulse oximetry, and PFTs Lung biopsy Oxygen therapy and mechanical ventilation Immunosuppressive therapy

Continued

Table 3A–6 (Continued)
Late Effects of Bone Marrow Transplantation

Infectious Complications

Late Effect	Incidence[a]	Causes	Typical Onset Post-Transplant	Signs and Symptoms	Medical Management
Bacterial organisms: Blood and sinopulmonary sites • Encapsulated bacteria • Streptococcus pneumonia • Hemophilus influenzae	38% MUD BMT 22% HLA-matched BMT Rare with autologous BMT	Immunodeficiency caused by chronic GVHD, HLA disparity, and hypogamma-globulinemia	100–365 d	*General:* Fever, sepsis, shaking chills, malaise, hypotension, changes in mental status, and headache. *Site specific:* Ear pain, sore throat, sensation of pressure/pain in frontal or maxillary sinuses, postnasal drip, cough, shortness of breath, abdominal pain/cramping, diarrhea, nausea, and vomiting	Appropriate cultures (e.g., blood, nasal, sputum, urine) Chest and sinus x-rays CBC with differential and immunoglobulin levels PFTs Antibiotics and IVIG
Fungal organisms: Oral, esophageal, and sinopulmonary sites • Aspergillus • Mucomycosis	50%	Immunodeficiency GVHD HLA disparity	100–365 d	Positive blood culture, sore throat, difficulty swallowing, mucositis, and pulmonary infiltrates	Appropriate cultures (e.g., blood, nasal, sputum, urine); x-rays; CBC with differential and IgG levels; PFTs; and antifungal prophylaxis or IVIG therapy
Viral organisms • CMV pneumonia	10%–15% allogeneic BMT 2%–3% autologous BMT	Immunodeficiency CMV seropositive patient and donor GVHD	100–365 d	Rapid onset with fulminant respiratory failure in days or slow onset with nonproductive cough, prolonged fever, dyspnea, or lethargy May be asymptomatic	Rule out bacterial infection Shell viral cultures Chest x-rays ABGs, PFTs, bronchoscopy, and BAL IgG and IgA levels Prophylaxis with ganciclovir, foscarnet, and acyclovir Surveillance cultures of blood, urine, and pharyngeal secretions Leukocyte-depleted blood products, CMV-negative blood products, and IVIG or CMV IVIG with ganciclovir

Complication	Incidence	Risk Factors	Onset	Clinical Manifestations	Management
• VZV integument	>50% with chronic GVHD 33%–50% without chronic GVHD	Immunodeficiency GVHD CMV seropositive patient and donor Immunosuppression	180–365 d	Prodromal symptoms: Headache, irritability, malaise, pain, itching, burning along affected nerve tract, fever, chills, and vesicular lesions localized or disseminated along dermatomes Neurologic manifestations: Facial palsy and hearing loss	VZV cultures Acyclovir IV 500 mg/m² q8hr × 10 d Strict isolation until lesions are crusted Calamine lotion and antihistamines for pruritus Pain management as needed
• Visceral VZV dissemination	16%	Immunodeficiency GVHD CMV seropositive donor and recipient Immunosuppression	180–365 d	Midepigastric or peri-umbilical pain, with or without nausea, vomiting, or fever	Monitor for possible complications: Pancreatitis, hepatitis, GI hemorrhage, and disseminated intravascular coagulation Acyclovir IV 500 mg/m² q8hr × 10 d
Protozoal organisms • Pneumocystis carinii pneumonia	8% with chronic GVHD	Immunosuppression Chronic GVHD	100–200 d	Fever, nonproductive cough, dyspnea, tachypnea, hypoxia, reduced midexpiratory airflow, and progressive airflow obstruction	Chest x-ray Lung biopsy Oxygen therapy and mechanical ventilation Pulse oximeter and ABGs Prophylactic TMP-SMX
Central Nervous System Complications Neurologic sequelae	59%–70%	CNS radiation Intrathecal methotrexate Immunosuppressive agents (e.g., steroids, cyclosporine) Drug withdrawal	Variable	Tremors, seizures, musculoskeletal changes, visual disturbances, peripheral neuropathy, and encephalopathy Depression, mood swings, nervousness, sleep disturbances, agitation Myopathy	Head CT and MRI scan to rule out organic disease Drug dose adjustment Psychiatric, neurologic, and neuropsychiatric consultation

Continued

Table 3A–6 (Continued)
Late Effects of Bone Marrow Transplantation

Late Effect	Incidence[a]	Causes	Typical Onset Post-Transplant	Signs and Symptoms	Medical Management
Central Nervous System Complications					
Leuko-encephalopathy	7%	Prior CNS radiation Intrathecal methotrexate Conditioning regimens	30–150 d	Lethargy, confusion, somnolence, coma, and irritability Ataxia, tremors, and seizures Personality changes, impaired memory, and shortened attention span Ventricular dilation, calcification of brain tissue, and white-matter hypodensity	Head CT and MRI scan Neurologic and psychiatric consultations: Psychometric evaluation, symptom management, and periodic screening Occupational counseling Vocational rehabilitation Special education
Cognitive disabilities	Preliminary anecdotal reports	Prior CNS radiation Intrathecal methotrexate Systemic treatment	90 d to years	Short-term memory loss and shortened attention span Visual-motor coordination, abstract thinking, spatial processing, and behavioral and language processing deficits	(See Leukoencephalopathy above)
Ocular Complications					
Cataracts	>50% with single dose TBI <50% with fractionated dose TBI	TBI Steroids	1.5–5 years	Poor (cloudy) vision	Ophthalmology consultation and slit lamp microscopy Surgical removal and intraocular lens replacement
Endocrine Complications					
Thyroid dysfunction	15%–25% with fractionated dose TBI 30%–50% with single dose TBI	TBI	Immediate to years	Increased TSH and reduced thyroxine levels Lethargy, sluggishness, depression, sleep disturbances, weight gain, sparse/thinning hair, and dry skin	Endocrine consultation: Thyroid scan and thyroid replacement therapy

Complication	Incidence (%)	Cause	Onset	Signs and Symptoms	Management
Growth and Development Alterations	100% Not yet known in children age nine or younger 100% in children older than age nine	Cranial radiation, TBI Glucocorticosteroids GVHD Busulfan and cyclophosphamide together (cyclophosphamide alone will not cause these problems)	At puberty	Delayed development/absence of secondary sexual characteristics, primary gonadal failure, reduced growth velocity curves, abnormal bone age, reduced growth hormone level, increased gonadotropin levels, reduced estradiol levels (females), azoospermia, reduced testicular volume (males), and reduced T4 levels	Pediatric endocrine consultation Health history, physical examination, and monitoring of growth Tanner staging Menstrual history Semen analysis Growth hormone replacement (testosterone/estrogen) Sexual and reproductive counseling
Gonadal Complications Ovarian and testicular dysfunction	100% but varies with age and treatment; with TBI or combination chemotherapy (busulfan plus cyclophosphamide) or in women older than age 26, effects generally are permanent and irreversible With cyclophosphamide alone or in women younger than age 26, effects usually are transient	TBI Chemotherapy	Immediate Transient effects last 3–24 months	*Females:* Menstrual irregularities (scanty flow/amenorrhea), sterility, night sweats, hot flashes, vaginal atrophy, vaginal adhesions, osteoporosis, decreased libido, palpitations, dyspareunia, depression, altered self-esteem, elevated luteinizing and follicle-stimulating hormones, and decreased estradiol *Males:* Sterility, azoospermia, elevated luteinizing and follicle-stimulating hormones, premature ejaculation, and altered self-esteem	*Females:* Care by gynecologist familiar with BMT Monitor gonadotropin and hormone levels Cyclic hormone therapy, water-soluble vaginal lubricants, and topical estrogen creams Vaginal stents and dilation Sexual counseling *Males:* Urology consultation Monitor gonadotropin and hormone levels Semen analysis and sperm banking prior to transplantation Sexual counseling

Continued

Table 3A–6 *(Continued)*
Late Effects of Bone Marrow Transplantation

Late Effect	Incidence[a]	Causes	Typical Onset Post-Transplant	Signs and Symptoms	Medical Management
Dental/Oral Complications					
Retarded dental and facial bone development in children	Unknown Preliminary/ anecdotal reports	Cranial radiation and TBI	Months to years	Asymmetrical face (e.g., reduced lengths of mandible and maxilla, reduced vertical growth of upper face) Abnormal tooth/root development, delayed tooth eruption, and disproportion between tooth and jaw size Pain and difficulty chewing	Cephalometric measurements and facial bone x-rays Annual orthodontia consultation and interventions
Dental caries	Common	TBI GVHD Immunosuppression Reduced IgA and IgG levels in saliva	90 d to 1 year	Tooth decay, pain, and sensitivity	Regular dental examinations: Panorex films, fluoride gels and rinses, and oral hygiene instruction
Temporomandibular joint dysfunction	Not known Anecdotal reports	Not known	Not known	Toothache and facial pain Dizziness, ringing in the ears, and headache	Rule out CNS disease, infection, and dental or periodontal disease Dental consultation Treat underlying pathology Occlusal splints, physical therapy, tricyclic antidepressants, and muscle relaxants
Skeletal Complications					
Avascular Necrosis	10%	Glucocorticoid therapy GVHD	90 d to 1 year	Pain, discomfort, inflammation in femoral or humeral heads, limited range of motion in leg/ hip or shoulder joints, and contractures	Pain management Antimicrobial therapy Femoral head replacement and physical therapy

Genitourinary Complications					
Chronic renal failure	Not known Anecdotal reports	Radiation injury to renal system/ kidneys Chemotherapy regimens Antimicrobial and cyclosporine toxicity	4.5–26 months	Hematuria, proteinuria, increased serum creatinine levels, decreased glomerular filtration rate, fluid and electrolyte imbalances, anemia, and hypertension	Nephrology consultation, urinalysis, 24-hr creatinine clearance, and intravenous pyelogram Monitor BUN, serum creatinine, and electrolytes. Antihypertensive medications, erythropoetin, dialysis, and renal transplantation
Late hemorrhagic cystitis	Not known	Cyclophosphamide Ifosfamide Adenovirus	>100 d	Microscopic or gross hematuria, dysuria, vague abdominal pain, anemia, bladder wall scarring, urinary musculature atrophy, and infection	Nephrology consultation, urinalysis, cystoscopy, and hydration Analgesics and antimicrobial therapy Urinary diversion CBC and viral cultures
Hemolytic uremic syndrome	Usually associated with renal failure	Possibly high-dose chemotherapy regimens Infection Cyclosporine	30–875 d	Microangiopathic hemolytic anemia, renal insufficiency, thrombocytopenia, hematuria, increased creatinine levels, reduced creatinine clearance, fluid retention, and fatigue	Nephrology consultation, urinalysis, 24-hr creatinine clearance, BUN, serum creatinine, electrolytes, and radiated packed red blood cell and platelet transfusions Hemodialysis
Graft Failure/ Marrow Dysfunction	1% HLA-matched sibling donors 2% HLA 1-antigen- mismatched related donors 5%–40% T-cell- depleted marrow 20% autologous transplant	HLA disparity, chronic GVHD, T-cell-depleted marrow, disease status at time of transplant, insufficient stem cells the donor graft, disease reoccurrence, infection, drug-related marrow suppression (e.g., TMP-SMX, ganciclovir), and damaged or insufficient stem cells	Weeks to months	Pancytopenia, hypocellular bone marrow, infection, bleeding, and anemia	CBC, bone marrow aspiration and bone biopsy, and cytogenetic studies Identification of underlying cause Interferon and hematopoietic growth factors Second BMT Supportive care interventions and hospice care

Continued

Table 3A–6 (Continued)
Late Effects of Bone Marrow Transplantation

Late Effect	Incidence[a]	Causes	Typical Onset Post-Transplant	Signs and Symptoms	Medical Management
Secondary Malignancy Lymphoproliferative disorders (e.g., Hodgkin's and non-Hodgkin's lymphomas, acute or chronic leukemia) Basal cell and squamous cell carcinoma	2%–22%	Associated with TBI, Epstein-Barr virus, antithymocyte globulin, anti-CD-3 monoclonal antibody, immunosuppression, chronic immune stimulation, T-cell-depleted grafts, and HLA disparity	1–14 years	Fever, fatigue, swollen glands, abnormal CBC, night sweats, and pain	Periodic follow-up examination and screening Health history CBC, bone marrow aspiration, and bone biopsy CT scans Biopsy suspicious lesions Health teaching
Psychosocial Complications	5%–10%	Neuropsychological deficits, body image changes, malaise, sexual dysfunction, altered functional status, ineffective coping skills, and post-traumatic stress disorder	Months to years	Depression; feelings of loss, sadness, and helplessness; disruptive anxiety; inability to concentrate or make decisions; social isolation; altered interpersonal relationships; suicidal ideation; pathologic regression; and delirium	Rule out organic disease with psychometric tests (e.g., Beck's Depression Scale, Haberman's Demands of BMT Recovery) Head CT and MRI scans Psychiatric evaluation and psychotherapy Antidepressants and antianxiety medications

| *Quality of Life Disruption* | Probably 100% | Immediate to years | *Physical:* Decreased strength and stamina, altered level of function, visual disturbances/cataracts, recurrent infections, infertility, effects of chronic GVHD, and inadequate nutritional intake. *Psychological:* Increased anxiety, fear of recurrence, depression, cognitive deficits, and altered role function. *Social:* Difficulty in resuming intimate or sexual relationships, inability to return to former vocation or employment, increased anxiety regarding caregiver, and financial burden | Per patient and family self-report | Symptom management according to physical findings. Appropriate referrals (e.g., social worker, psychologist, financial counselor, vocational counselor). Physical therapy. BMT support groups. Antidepressants and antianxiety medication |

[a]Figures are intended as general guidelines. Incidence will vary/be uncertain depending on the number of patients, diseases, and transplant variables.

Abbreviations: BAL—broncho alveolar lavage; BMT—bone marrow transplant; CMV—cytomegalovirus; GVHD—graft-versus-host disease; HLA—human lymphocyte antigens; IgA—immunoglobulin alpha; IgG—immunoglobulin gamma; IVIG—intravenous immunoglobulin; MUD—multiple unmatched donors; TBI—total body irradiation; TMP-SMX—trimethoprim-sulfamethoxazole; TSH—thyroid-stimulating hormone; VZV—varicella zoster virus.

Reprinted with permission from Buchsel, P. C., E.W. Leum, and S. R. Randolph. Delayed Complications of Bone Marrow Transplantation: An Update. Oncology Nursing Forum. 23: 1267–1291. 1996.

Table 3A–7
Discharge Criteria for Bone Marrow Transplant Patients

Oral intake @ 30% baseline requirements
<2000 ml parenteral fluid within 24 hrs required
Nausea and vomiting controlled
Diarrhea controlled @ <500 ml/d
Afebrile (may be on IV antibiotics)
Platelet count >15,000 mm^3
Granulocytes >500 mm^3 for 48 hrs
Hematocrit >25%
Responsible caregiver in home
In close proximity to multidisciplinary BMT team

Discharge criteria for marrow recipients differ among institutions and depend on (1) the stability of the patient, (2) the presence of skilled outpatient teams, and (3) the caregiver support in the home. Established discharge criteria are outlined in Table 3A–7.

If possible, allogeneic recipients should remain near the transplant center until approximately 50 days after BMT. This time period has been established as necessary to allow sufficient immune system recovery to prevent immediate life-threatening complications. Comprehensive outpatient care consists of daily to weekly clinic visits to assess the BMT patient's stability. Blood component therapy, parenteral nutrition, intravenous medications, research medications, and procedures can be delivered effectively in ambulatory care and home settings.

Community Practice

Community-based physicians and nurses can expect to see a patient at least weekly during the first month home. If no new medical problems develop and the patient is stable, these intervals can be lengthened to two weeks for the next two months, and eventually to three weeks or monthly intervals depending on the patient's clinical status. Typically, patients return to the BMT center for annual evaluations for up to three years after BMT.

LATE COMPLICATIONS OF BMT

Late complications of BMT are those that develop 100 days or more after transplant. Nursing management is discussed in Table 3A–8. The complications, incidence, manifestations, and medical management and diagnostic measures are outlined in Table 3A–9.

Table 3A–8
Nursing Care of the Late Effects of Bone Marrow Transplantation

Nursing Diagnosis	Nursing Interventions
Knowledge deficit regarding late effects of bone marrow transplant (BMT)	Instruct patient/caregiver about potential late complications. Teach reportable signs and symptoms. Emphasize the importance of follow-up and medication compliance. Set mutual, realistic goals for return to school or work. Provide written instructions regarding medication schedule, central lumen catheter care, diet, activities of daily living (ADL), and personal hygiene measures. Identify activity restrictions necessary until immune reconstitution. • Avoid crowds, infectious people, and construction areas. • Refrain from gardening. • Refrain from changing animal litter boxes. Monitor compliance with instructions. Communicate with primary physician and homecare and interdisciplinary team members about patient status and treatment plan. Provide 24-hr emergency number. Refer patient to community support services such as support groups, the American Cancer Society, and the National Coalition of Cancer Survivors.
Knowledge deficit regarding clinical manifestations of chronic graft-versus-host disease (GVHD)	Assess patient's and caregiver's understanding of chronic GVHD. Provide information about chronic GVHD and symptom management. Teach adverse effects of immunosuppressive medications. • Cyclosporine: Hypertension, seizures, magnesium wasting, and hirsutism • Steroids: Hypertension, fluid retention, aseptic necrosis of bone, and mood swings • Thalidomide: Drowsiness and constipation Document teaching plan and patient and family level of understanding. Monitor medication compliance.
Impaired skin integrity related to chronic GVHD and infection	Assess skin for signs and symptoms of altered integrity. • Texture: Scaling and dermatosclerosis • Color: Hypo/hyperpigmentation and erythema • Ulceration: Desquamation • Infection: Redness, drainage, and tenderness Clean skin with nonirritating soap. Apply creams such as Eucerin® (Beiersdorph Inc., Norwalk, CT) and Aquaphor® (Beiersdorph Inc.) moisturizing lotion. Avoid direct sunlight, and apply sunscreen. Administer medications (e.g., immunosuppressive therapy, antibiotics, topical steroids, antihistamines), and monitor for desired effects. Promote range-of-motion exercises to prevent contractures. Provide consultation with a dermatologist familiar with BMT recipients.
Altered body image related to chronic GVHD and side effects of medication	Instruct patient about alterations in skin color and texture and other skin-related side effects of medications such as weight gain, hirsutism, alopecia, muscle wasting, and gingival hyperplasia. Reassure patient that appearance will improve with effective treatment. Offer counseling regarding cosmetic aids, make-up, wigs, hats, and scarves. Provide emotional support. Refer patient to a support group.

Continued

Table 3A–8 *(Continued)*
Nursing Care of the Late Effects of Bone Marrow Transplantation

Nursing Diagnosis	Nursing Interventions
Altered oral mucous membranes related to chronic GVHD, sicca syndrome, and infection	Assess oral cavity for pain; xerostomia; striae on mucous membranes lining cheeks, lips, and palate; erythema progressing to ulceration; burning; loss of taste; and dental caries. Monitor immunosuppressive therapies. Culture suspicious lesions for bacteria, virus, and fungus. Instruct patient in oral hygiene regimen. • Use a soft toothbrush, and floss daily. • Rinse regularly with saline or water. • Avoid commercial mouthwashes. • Use artificial saliva. Provide salivary gland stimulants, such as sugarless mints, gum, and hard candy. Encourage patient to eat a soft, bland diet. Avoid spices, acidic foods, and foods served at extreme temperatures. Refer patient to a nutritionist. Monitor response to topical anesthetics and parenteral analgesics.
Altered nutrition (less than body requirements) related to chronic GVHD, infection, and medications	Assess signs and symptoms of esophageal dysfunction, such as difficulty swallowing, retrosternal pain, and esophageal stricture. Assess nutritional status, including monitoring weight, calorie count, and tissue turgor. Provide a low-bacterial diet. Administer antibiotic therapy as ordered. Record anthropometric measurements. Refer patient to a nutritionist, if necessary. Assess signs and symptoms, including anorexia, nausea, vomiting, diarrhea, malabsorption, and weight loss. Provide nutritional supplements, enteral feeding, and total parenteral nutrition as ordered. Culture suspicious sites. Determine whether esophageal dilation is necessary. Monitor serum albumin, ferritin, and electrolytes. Administer analgesics, antiemetics, antidiarrheal agents, fluid, and electrolyte replacements as ordered; monitor for desired effects.
Altered metabolic processes (impaired hepatic function) related to chronic GVHD, infection, and medications	Assess and monitor hepatic function, including liver function tests (SGOT, SGPT, gamma glutamyl transferase, bilirubin, alkaline phosphatase), impaired hepatic function, hepatitis antigen and antibody levels, right-upper quadrant pain, hepatomegaly, and ascites. Obtain medication and transfusion history. Assess current medication profile. Monitor abdominal girth. Monitor for signs and symptoms of infection. Observe for changes in level of consciousness. Assess coagulation profile (e.g., prothrombin time, partial thromboplastin time, fibrin split products). Observe sclera and skin for jaundice.

Table 3A–8 *(Continued)*

Nursing Care of the Late Effects of Bone Marrow Transplantation

Nursing Diagnosis	Nursing Interventions
Altered metabolic processes (thyroid dysfunction) related to total body irradiation	Instruct patient about signs and symptoms of hypothyroidism such as sluggishness, depression, lethargy, sleep disturbances, weight gain, sparse or thinning hair, and dry skin. Assess thyroid stimulating hormone and thyroxine levels. Monitor and instruct patient regarding thyroid replacement therapy compliance. Provide symptom management interventions. Discuss changes in functional capacity and ability to perform ADL. Reassure patient that thyroid replacement therapy will restore adequate thyroid function. Refer patient to an endocrinologist.
Altered growth and development related to cranial or total body irradiation, GVHD, and glucocorticosteroids	Discuss growth and developmental effects with patient and family prior to BMT. • Delayed development of or difficulty in performing cognitive skills • Delayed development or absence of secondary sexual characteristics • Delayed or altered growth velocity Assess and monitor growth and development, including physical assessment: Tanner staging; neuropsychological evaluation; luteinizing and follicle stimulating hormone levels; semen analysis (males); and menstrual history (females). Refer patient to a pediatric endocrinologist. Monitor compliance with sex and growth hormone replacement. Monitor school performance history. Collaborate with school officials regarding development of social and cognitive skills. Refer for appropriate counseling (e.g., reproductive, educational, vocational).
Altered growth and development (retarded dental and facial bone development) related to cranial or total body irradiation	Assess cephalometric measurements and dental development, including abnormal tooth/root development, delayed tooth eruption, disproportion between tooth and jaw dimensions, pain, and difficulty chewing. Refer for orthodontic consultation.
Altered ovarian function (in women over age 26) related to total body irradiation and cyclophosphamide	Assess signs and symptoms of ovarian failure such as sterility, premature menopause, amenorrhea, hot flashes, vaginal atrophy and dryness, heart palpitations, and osteoporosis. Monitor luteinizing and follicle stimulating hormone and estradiol levels. Assess for alterations in sexual response including painful intercourse and decreased libido. Assess psychological status, including depression, poor self-esteem, and performance anxiety. Refer patient to a gynecologist who is familiar with BMT recipients. Recommend water-soluble vaginal creams and topical estrogen creams. Discuss/explain vaginal stents and dilation. Monitor patient response to hormone replacement therapy. Refer for sexual counseling as appropriate.

Continued

Table 3A–8 *(Continued)*
Nursing Care of the Late Effects of Bone Marrow Transplantation

Nursing Diagnosis	Nursing Interventions
Impaired testicular function related to total body irradiation	Discuss sperm banking prior to transplant. Assess for signs and symptoms of testicular dysfunction such as sterility, azoospermia, increased luteinizing and follicle stimulating hormone, and premature ejaculation. Refer patient to a urologist.
Sexual dysfunction related to testicular/ovarian failure, chronic GVHD, fatigue, and impaired self-esteem	Establish a therapeutic relationship. Implement PLISSIT model interventions (i.e., P = permission, LI = limited information, SS = specific instructions, and IT = intensive treatment). Encourage communication between patient and partner. Assess etiology of sexual dysfunction, including altered body structure or function (e.g., vaginal dryness, stenosis, impotence, premature ejaculation), low self-esteem, altered body image, and anxiety/depression. Provide information about sexual aids, lubricants, vaginal dilator, and relaxation techniques. Refer for sexual counseling as appropriate.
Altered visual sensory perception related to chronic GVHD, ocular sicca, infection, and plugged lacrimal ducts	Assess ability to perform ADL and changes in functional capacity. Assess/monitor for signs and symptoms of ocular alterations such as dry eyes/itching, corneal ulceration, photophobia, and pain/discomfort. Recommend artificial tears. Instruct patient about wearing sunglasses. Monitor for signs and symptoms of infection.
Altered visual sensory perception related to cataracts	Assess risk for cataract development including transplant conditioning regimen, corticosteroids, and chronic GVHD. Assess for visual changes such as cloudy or blurred vision and opaque cornea. Refer patient to an ophthalmologist. Help explain surgical options. Reassure patient that vision will return with cataract removal or lens replacement.
Activity intolerance related to chronic GVHD, anemia, and infection; musculoskeletal, peripheral nervous system, or psychological late effects; and aseptic bone necrosis	Assess functional capacity (e.g., Karnofsky performance status. World Health Organization performance scale). Monitor signs and symptoms of physiologic and psychological peripheral dysfunction including reports of weakness and fatigue, abnormal heart rate or blood pressure; dyspnea; pain; muscle weakness and wasting; limited range of motion; neuropathy; depression; social isolation; stress; and inability to complete ADL. Identify underlying etiology and contributing factors, and collaborate with interdisciplinary team to treat underlying causes. Promote balanced activity rest patterns. Teach stress management. Establish mutual and realistic goals.

Table 3A–8 *(Continued)*
Nursing Care of the Late Effects of Bone Marrow Transplantation

Nursing Diagnosis	Nursing Interventions
Impaired gas exchange, ineffective breathing pattern related to chronic GVHD, infection, restrictive/obstructive airway disease, and bronchiolitis obliterans	Assess for decreased activity tolerance and fatigue. Monitor for altered respiratory function including abnormal or absent breath sounds; quality and rate of respiration; dusky or cyanotic color; dyspnea, shortness of breath on exertion, or wheezing; bronchospasm; and productive or nonproductive cough. Perform chest auscultation and percussion with each clinic or home visit. Assess vital signs and pulse oximeter regularly. Monitor pulmonary function tests, arterial blood gases, complete blood count, immunoglobulin gamma levels, and blood and sputum cultures. Prepare patient for bronchial lavage procedure and lung biopsy. Discuss potential for hospitalization with respiratory support, including mechanical ventilation. Administer supportive therapies, as ordered, such as ganciclovir, trimethoprimsulfamethoxazole (TMP-SMX), pentamidine, amphotericin B, and broad-spectrum antibiotics; bronchodilators; immunosuppressive therapy; and immunoglobulins.
Risk for infection related to chronic GVHD, immunosuppression, and graft failure	Assess and monitor for signs and symptoms of infection, such as fever, chills, and hypotension; cough and dyspnea; painful urination, difficult urination, and foul-smelling urine; diarrhea, vomiting, and abdominal pain; redness, swelling, tenderness, and drainage; and malaise/arthralgia. Monitor complete blood count, immunoglobulin gamma, and IgA levels. Instruct patient regarding infection precautions. • Wash hands meticulously. • Avoid crowds and infectious individuals. • Avoid live vaccines. • Avoid trauma and invasive procedures. • Eat a low bacterial diet. Monitor compliance with prophylactic medications such as TMP-SMX, ciprofloxin, nystatin/fluconozole, and acyclovir.
Risk of second malignancy related to chronic immune suppression, T-cell-depleted graft, total body irradiation, alkylating chemotherapy, antithymocyte globulin, CD-3 monoclonal antibodies, and Epstein-Barr virus	Assess risk factors for development of a secondary malignancy. Discuss possibilities with patient and family. Instruct patient to report possible warning signs such as fever, fatigue/malaise, abnormal bleeding, night sweats, pain, and appearance of a painless lump. Emphasize the need for health screening and periodic check-ups.

Reprinted with permission from Buchsel, P. C., E. W. Leum and S. R. Randolph. Delayed Complications of Bone Marrow Transplantation: An Update. Oncology Nursing Forum 23: 1267–1291. 1996.

Table 3A-9
Complications of Chronic Graft-Versus-Host Disease

Site and Incidence	Signs and Symptoms	Medical Management
Skin, 70%	Dyspigmentation, erythema, hyperkeratosis, desquamation, facial butterfly rash, patchy hyperpigmentation, reticular mottling, perifollicular papules, and pruritus Hidebound skin texture, joint contracture, and guttate lesions (stretch marks) Ulcerations with serous drainage and concomitant infection Alopecia, nail ridging, and premature graying Loss of sweat gland function	Clinical examination and 3 mm skin biopsy Immunosuppressive therapy: Cyclosporine, corticosteroids, thalidomide, rapamycin, tacrolimus, psoralen, and ultraviolet irradiation Diphenhydramine and topical steroids for itching Burn treatment measures with silver sulfadiazine ointment, whirlpool debridement, and skin allografts
Mouth, 70%	Erythema, tissue atrophy, and lichenoid changes Hyperkeratotic striae, plaques, papules, and patches Pseudomembranous ulcerations of buccal mucosa and lateral tongue Infection Pain, burning, xerostomia, and loss of taste Sensitivity to spices, acidic foods, and temperature Difficulty opening mouth Dental caries	Immunosuppressive therapy Lip biopsy Salivary analysis for proteins and antibodies Culture and sensitivity for bacteria, fungus, and virus Pilocarpine and anetholetrithione for xerostomia Analgesics as needed Fluoride gels and mouthwashes
Esophagus, 10%	Difficulty swallowing Retrosternal pain Weight loss Esophageal web formation and stricture	Endoscopy and x-rays for diagnosis Esophageal dilation
Gastrointestinal tract, rare	Anorexia, nausea, and vomiting Diarrhea and malabsorption Weight loss	X-rays for diagnosis Stool culture and sensitivity Total parenteral nutrition Immunosuppressive therapy
Liver, 30%	Jaundice Elevated bilirubin, SGOT, and alkaline phosphatase Increased prothrombin time and partial thromboplastin time Abdominal pain in the right quadrant	Immunosuppressive therapy Rule out viral and fungal infection, hepatotoxic drug reactions, gallstones, and neoplastic disease Biopsy for diagnosis Liver function tests Prothrombin time, partial thromboplastin time, and fibrin split products Ursodeoxycholic acid
Eyes, 80%	Sicca syndrome Pain, burning, and itching Photophobia Corneal ulceration or scarring Cataracts Infection Positive Schirmer's tear test (less than 10 mm wetness)	Immunosuppressive therapy Ophthalmology consult Slit lamp microscopy examination Lacriset plugs and punctural ligation Keratoplasty and tarsorrhaphies Ocular lens replacement

Table 3A–9 *(Continued)*
Complications of Chronic Graft-Versus-Host Disease

Site and Incidence	Signs and Symptoms	Medical Management
Lungs/bronchiolitis obliterans, 10%	Persistent cough, dyspnea, and wheezing Decreased forced expiratory volume and vital capacity Decreased serum immunoglobulin gamma and IgA levels	Immunosuppressive therapy Chest x-ray Pulmonary function tests Arterial blood gases and pulse oximetry
Vagina, incidence unknown	Vaginal stenosis and atrophy Decreased libido Fatigue Painful intercourse Obstruction of menstrual flow (swollen abdomen, pain, bloating)	Immunosuppressive therapy Gynecology consult Vaginal biopsy and Pap test Vaginal dilation and vaginal lubricants Sexual counseling
Myofascial, 10%	Muscle pain, aches, and cramping Arthralgia Synovial effusion Tendonitis and arthritis Limited range of motion	Immunosuppressive therapy Muscle biopsy and x-rays for diagnosis Analgesics as needed Physical therapy consult
Peripheral nervous system, extremely rare	Myasthenia gravis: Eyelid ptosis, extraocular weakness, and proximal limb and facial muscle weakness Polymyositis: Proximal muscle weakness and tenderness, dysphagia, and cardiac muscle involvement Demyelinating polyneuropathy: Difficulty chewing, swallowing, and speaking; progressive quadriplegia	Neurology consult Electromyography and nerve conduction studies Sural nerve biopsy Cholinesterase inhibitors (e.g., diphenhydramine prochlorperazine) Immunosuppressive therapy Plasmapheresis Immunoglobulins Physical therapy consult
Immune system, 20%–40%	Leukopenia, lymphopenia, and granulocytopenia Eosinophilia and thrombocytopenia Infection Anemia and bleeding Fatigue and malaise	Physical examination and health history Bone marrow aspiration and bone biopsy Complete blood count and immunoglobulin levels Prophylactic antibiotics Immunoglobulins Granulocyte and granulocyte-macrophage colony-stimulating factors and epoetin alfa Irradiated packed red blood cell and platelet transfusions Surveillance cultures of urine and central venous catheter sites Sepsis work-up: Blood, urine, stool, sputum, catheter exit site culture and sensitivity Chest x-rays Antibiotics

Reprinted with permission from Buchsel, P. C., E. W. Leum and S. R. Randolph. Delayed Complications of Bone Marrow Transplantation: An Update. Oncology Nursing Forum 23: 1267–1291. 1996.

Chronic Graft-versus-Host Disease

Chronic GVHD, a major cause of late transplant-related morbidity, occurs in 33 percent of HLA-identical transplants, 49 percent of HLA-non-identical-related transplants, and 65 percent of unrelated donor BMTs. It is life-threatening in about 5 percent of patients if left untreated. Chronic GVHD typically develops more than three months post-transplant and differs from acute GVHD in its target organs and clinical presentation (see Table 3A–6). Clinical and pathologic findings resemble several naturally occurring autoimmune diseases, such as scleroderma, lupus erythematosus, lichen planus, rheumatoid arthritis, and Sjogren's or sicca syndrome.

The onset of chronic GVHD can be progressive, quiescent, or de novo. Progressive onset follows as a direct extension of acute GVHD and carries the poorest prognosis. Quiescent onset develops in patients who have had a clinical resolution of acute GVHD; these patients have a fair prognosis. Patients with de novo onset have the best prognosis, because they have had no prior acute disease.

Medical treatment of chronic GVHD involves the use of immunosuppressive therapy with one or more medical regimens that include cyclosporine, corticosteroids, and imuran. New treatment strategies currently being explored are psoralen ultraviolet (PUVA) therapy, thalidomide, cytokine antagonists, oxypentifylline, and photopheresis monitoring. Table 3A–9 describes the organ systems affected by chronic GVHD, signs and symptoms, and medical management.

Gonadal Dysfunction

Conditioning regimens of high-dose chemotherapy and TBI affect gonadal function in men, women, and children. Table 3A–6 describes possible gonadal dysfunction and related management in BMT recipients.

Patients who receive only single-agent chemotherapy often demonstrate recovery of fertility and can successfully bear children. The adverse effects of high-dose chemotherapy on gonadal function depend on the age of the patient at the time of BMT. Girls and boys who are prepubertal at the time of BMT develop normally. Women under 26 years of age can expect return of menstrual periods, but only a few have borne children. Women over the age of 26 develop early menopause. Men usually have return of normal gonadotropin levels and low to normal sperm counts, and can father children. The effects of newer conditioning regimens, such as high-dose busulfan and cyclophosphamide without TBI, on gonadal function are as yet unknown.

Almost all female recipients conditioned with TBI have gonadal dysfunction, including sterility and early menopause. Except for women who have received transplants for breast cancer, cyclic oral or transdermal hormone replacement therapy can be administered post-BMT to reduce symptoms of premature menopause and to prevent long-term disorders such as osteoporosis or vulvar and vaginal atrophic changes. Vasomotor symptoms such as hot flashes, sweating, palpitation, irritability, headache, sleep disturbances, and genitourinary tract symptoms are common and might be the primary cause of sexual dysfunction. Most men conditioned with TBI preserve Leydig cell function and testosterone and luteinizing hormone production, but spermatogenesis is usually absent. Sensitive counseling by gynecologists, nurse practitioners, or staff nurses working in ambulatory and home care settings can support affected women in their intimate relationships (see Chapter 13).

Most prepubertal girls who receive TBI have primary ovarian failure, do not achieve menarche, and do not develop secondary sexual characteristics. Prepubertal boys conditioned with TBI develop secondary sexual characteristics, but most have delayed onset of puberty. The most profoundly affected children are prepubertal boys who received testicular radiation prior to marrow conditioning. Testosterone therapy could be effective, but longer follow-up is needed.

Growth and Development

Children who are conditioned with high-dose cyclophosphamide have normal growth and development. However, all children have decreased growth rates following TBI; children who have chronic GVHD in addition are the most significantly affected. Deficits in adrenocortical function, growth hormone levels, and thyroid function occur, especially in children with prior cranial radiation. Nurses should make parents aware of the potential late effects of radiation; this issue should be addressed prior to and at regular intervals after transplant. Growth patterns should be evaluated annually, and patients who demonstrate a decreased growth rate should be referred to a pediatric endocrinologist. Growth hormone replacement therapy could be indicated. Careful long-term follow up care through puberty will be necessary.

Relapse

Relapse is a significant problem after transplant and can be attributed to the reinfusion of malignant cells contained in the marrow or stem cells or residual cancer cells not eradicated by the high-dose conditioning regimen. Several approaches aimed at reducing disease relapse or recurrence are under investigation, such as post-transplant active immunization, salvage chemotherapy, second transplant, withdrawal of immunosuppressive medications (allogeneic), cytokine therapy, donor leukocyte infusions, and monoclonal antibody therapy.

Graft Failure

Graft failure rarely occurs in HLA-matched marrow transplants. HLA-mismatched or T-cell-depleted marrow grafts can fail early or several months following BMT. Graft failure is defined as (1) primary graft failure, that is, the absence of hematologic recovery in patients surviving more than 21 days after BMT, or (2) transient engraftment, or complete or partial recovery of hematopoiesis, in the absence of moderate to severe GVHD, followed by recurrent pancytopenia.

Aseptic Necrosis

Aseptic necrosis of the bone, particularly of the humerus or femur head, is commonly due to the use of glucocorticosteroids. Patients complain of pain and limited range of motion. Antibiotic treatment and orthopedic surgery for joint replacement is usually indicated.

Dental Effects

Dental effects related to conditioning and GVHD can lead to oral hygiene and dental decay. Oral sicca, or dry mouth syndrome, is a common late effect and results in oral caries and infection. TBI can directly affect dental and facial bone development, resulting in poor calcification and root blunting, which can cause facial disfigurement in children.

Neurological Complications

Following conditioning regimens using radiation and chemotherapy, impaired memory, shortened attention span, and impaired verbal skills can occur. Pediatric BMT recipients, when tested against controls, performed less well intellectually.

Signs and symptoms of chronic leukoencephalopathy might not appear for months or years after transplant. Learning disabilities in children have been reported, with abnormal motor, perceptual, behavioral, and language performance. Clinical signs and symptoms can be subtle and require careful observation of behavior.

Second Malignancies

Second malignancies after BMT are reported with increasing frequency and occur at a rate of up to seven times normal. This phenomenon is similar to second malignancies experienced by solid organ transplant recipients and could be the result of lengthy immunosuppressive periods, the use of corticosteroids, TBI, viral infection, chronic immune stimulation, or genetic predisposition. The presentation of a second malignancy occurs from two to fourteen years after BMT. Common second malignancies after BMT include the lymphoproliferative disorders as well as solid tumors, such as acute lymphocytic leukemia, acute nonlymphocytic leukemia, granulocytic sarcomas, non-Hodgkin's lymphoma, carcinomas, malignant melanomas, glioblastoma multiforme, and invasive vulvar carcinoma. An analysis of 1,926 combined allogeneic and autologous marrow recipients transplanted for hematologic malignancies in Seattle reported an incidence of 35 BMT recipients with a second malignancy. Data from the International Bone Marrow Transplant Registry reflect similar statistics.

Quality of Life

Early quality of life (QOL) studies focused mainly on morbidity as measured by the Karnofsky Performance Scale. More recently, researchers have attempted to measure QOL in four domains: physical, social, psychological, and spiritual. Prospective studies show physical and psychosocial status improved following BMT for women and younger recipients, while men and older recipients did less well. Other results demonstrate that severe chronic GVHD, coupled with pretransplant family conflict, predicts subsequent impaired physical and emotional recovery. Most studies show that patients report QOL to be good or excellent. Consistent themes are that patients perceive lack of social support, dissatisfaction with their body images, lack of stamina, and inability to attain sexual satisfaction. According to Sjralya and others, patients with previous GVHD were most adversely affected.

Few studies address pediatric QOL issues, but anecdotal evidence from parents shows improved family life among disease-free survivors. Recent encouraging studies demonstrate stable cognitive and psychological function of children following BMT. More prospective studies that follow pediatric recipients over longer periods of time are needed. Patient/family referral to local community support groups will facilitate their reintegration into the community following the BMT/PBST experience.

BIBLIOGRAPHY

1. Buchsel, P. and P. Kapustay. *Blood Cell Transplantation.* Mosby Year Book, St. Louis. In press.

   This is the first nursing text exclusively devoted to the peripheral blood transplantation and includes chapters on umbilical stem cell transplantation, gene therapy, cell therapy, and the new Standards of the Foundation for Accreditation of Hematopoietic Cell Therapy.

2. Buchsel, P. C, E. W. Leum, and S. R. Randolph. Delayed complications of bone marrow transplantation: An update. *Oncol Nurs Forum* 23: 1267–1291. 1996.

   This article serves as an update of a classic review of the known chronic or long-term complications of BMT. The signs, symptoms, time of onset, nursing and medical interventions, and diagnostic tools are described, with helpful tables.

3. Buchsel, P., and M. B. Whedon. *Bone Marrow Transplantation: Administrative Strategies and Clinical Concerns.* Jones and Bartlett, Boston. 1995.

   Marrow and stem cell transplantation is increasingly moving out of the research center to community settings. Oncology teams wishing to implement a transplant program will find this a helpful book to structure both inpatient and ambulatory care units.

4. Burt, R. K., H. J. Deeg, and S. T. Lothian. *Bone Marrow Transplantation.* R. G. Landes Company, Austin. 1996.

   Written as a therapeutic manual designed as a quick practical guide and reference for the entire transplant team, this book provides one of the most comprehensive overviews of current practice in hematopoietic transplantation. Indications for transplantation, complications, drug doses, and approaches to clinical management problems are emphasized. Requirements for a bone marrow transplant unit are described. Chapters with procedures on patient evaluation, unrelated donors, marrow processing, engraftment/relapse, and general patient care are included.

5. Ezzone, S. *Blood Cell Transplantation: Recommendations for Nursing Practice and Education.* Oncology Nursing Press, Pittsburgh. 1997.

   This manual is a comprehensive description of peripheral stem cell transplantation and the nursing management of persons undergoing PBST throughout the treatment course.

6. Ferrell, B., M. Grant, and G. M. Schmidt. The meaning of quality of life for bone marrow transplant survivors, Part 2: Improving quality of life for bone marrow transplant survivors. *Cancer Nurs* 15(4): 247–253. 1992.

   This article offers answers to the question "What makes quality of life better?" The researchers make a solid contribution to the nursing literature and to the care of the BMT recipient.

7. Kurtzberg, J., M. Lauglin, M. L. Graham, et al. Placental blood as a source of hematopoietic stem cells for transplantation into unrelated recipients. *N Engl J Med* 335(3): 157–166. 1996.

   This is the seminal article describing the value of using placental blood for unrelated transplantation. The important finding of this study is that in placental-blood transplants that differed by as many as three HLA, antigen or alleles engrafted and produced all major lines of blood cells without causing clinically significant GVHD.

8. Shapiro T. W., D. B. Davison, and D. Rust. *A Clinical Guide to Stem Cell and Bone Marrow Transplantation.* Jones and Bartlett, Boston. 1997.

   This book is compact in size and provides tools and information for day-to-day management of the marrow and stem cell recipient. The information is presented in a succinct format for ease in obtaining information in a rapid fashion. The book can easily be placed in a laboratory coat pocket.

9. Weaver C., L. S. Schwartzberg, J. Hainsworth, et al. Treatment-related mortality of 1000 consecutive patients receiving high-dose chemotherapy and peripheral blood progenitor cell transplantation in community cancer centers. *Bone Marrow Transplantation* 19(7): 671–678. 1997.

This definitive article demonstrates the feasibility of performing peripheral stem cell transplants in the community setting. The data support the vision that marrow and stem cell transplants can be given by an oncologist in the patient's community setting, rather than a distant research center.

10. Whedon, W. B., and D. Wujcik. *Blood and Marrow Transplantation: Principles, Practice, and Nursing Insights, 2d Ed.* Jones and Bartlett, Boston. 1997.

This book is the second edition of one of the mainstays of bone marrow transplantation for oncology nurses. The recent edition updates history, procedures of transplantation, and immunologic interventions, and provides new information about hematologic concepts, pharmacologic and biologic agents, radiation therapy, and gene therapy. Particular attention is given to peripheral blood transplantation.

B. Parenteral Therapy: Access and Delivery

Myra Woolery-Antill

3B

INTRODUCTION

Administration of chemotherapeutic and/or biological agents is one of the major methods of treating cancer. There are many classes of chemotherapy and types of biologics that have proven effective in causing toxicity to cancer cells. Unfortunately, many are also toxic to normal cells, producing potentially serious problems, such as local tissue necrosis caused by extravasation of drug from the vein. Venous access devices, such as tunneled (Hickman) or nontunneled central catheters, can be used to administer therapies and thereby decrease the risk of local irritation to veins. The toxicities associated with systemic therapy have led scientists and physicians to develop better ways to administer agents. Delivering large concentrations of therapy directly to the site of disease while sparing normal tissue is the rationale behind several of the access devices and routes discussed in this chapter. Nurses need information about how to assess, prevent, and manage problems that might be encountered while caring for patients receiving parenteral therapy. The following guidelines address these issues for a variety of access routes.

IRRITANT AND VESICANT DRUGS

Despite precautions taken by physicians, nurses, and other health care professionals, local reaction to antineoplastic drugs is always possible. Reactions can be caused by the properties of the agent, volume or characteristics of the diluent, site of therapy injection, or technique of administration. Agents that commonly produce local necrosis or irritation are dactinomycin, daunorubicin, doxorubicin, epirubicin, estramustine, mechlorethamine, mitomycin, vinblastine, vincristine, and vindesine.

Vesicants cause tissue inflammation and pain when extravasated or when they leak out of the vein into the tissue. Skin discoloration and loss of venous patency can follow erythema. Vesicants (e.g., doxorubicin, mechlorethamine) can cause ulcers that require surgery, debridement, or skin grafting to repair extensive tissue damage. Irreversible changes in tendons and underlying tissue can result in loss of limb function. Agents classified as irritants (e.g., carmustine, dacarbazine, etoposide, streptozotocin, and teniposide) can cause severe burning and pain but do not result in blisters, ulceration, or skin burns. Other agents can create phlebitis of the vein, resulting in discomfort and loss of venous patency (Table 3B–1).

As new agents are clinically investigated, it is important for the nurse to assess each therapy's potential effects on veins or other access sites. Animal studies that precede human testing might indicate potential effects, but human studies will validate if the agent is a vesicant or irritant, or has other

Table 3B–1
Potential Damage from Chemotherapy

Local Necrosis	Irritation
Amsacrine	Carmustine
Bisantrene	Dacarbazine
Dactinomycin	Etoposide
Daunorubicin	Fluorouracil
Doxorubicin	Mitoxantrone
Epirubicin	Paclitaxel
Idarubicin	Plicamycin
Mechlorethamine	Streptozotocin
Mitomycin	Teniposide
Vinblastine	
Vincristine	
Vindesine	
Vinorelbine	
At very high concentrations:	
Cisplatin	
Mitoxantrone	
Paclitaxel	

serious effects. It is unknown whether biotherapy will have similar toxicities to chemotherapy, so these agents require careful assessment as well.

Management

Nursing management consists of preventive and supportive measures. Knowing which agents are vesicants or irritants allows the nurse to prepare and evaluate the patient. Completion of a chemotherapy competency program is recommended for nurses who administer antineoplastic agents. Similar competency programs in biotherapy will continue to develop as this treatment option expands. To assume this important job responsibility, the nurse must know about the potential for serious toxicities, the basic skills necessary to administer these agents as recommended, and management of treatment effects. This information can then be shared with the patient. The patient should be educated about the therapy's side effects, including information on signs and symptoms to be reported during administration. Complaints of pain, burning, swelling, or redness at the injection site might be a sign of extravasation. Hypersensitivity or flare reaction is often hard to distinguish from actual tissue seepage. Suggestions for monitoring therapy instillation are given subsequently.

The treatment should be administered in a quiet, unhurried environment. In anticipation of possible extravasation and/or hypersensitivity, the appropriate antidote, emergency medications, and equipment should be available. Review the patient's history and experiences with cancer therapy. Review the orders for therapy. Double-check agent, dose, and route of administration with another nurse. Ensure that hydration, diuresis, or other pretreatment requirements have been administered. Assist the patient into a comfortable position and proceed to establish peripheral venous access. Evaluate both arms for best vein selection. Proceed from the hand to forearm. Avoid the side of a mastectomy. Lower extremities should not be used because they are more susceptible to emboli formation. Do not use antecubital fossa, sites distal to recent venipuncture, or bruised, sore areas; avoid joints. Impaired venous circulation is also a reason to avoid a site and might indicate the need for other access routes, such as a central venous access device. Use heat to distend veins to aid in finding a site.

Therapy via Peripheral Venous Access

Procedure
1. Explain procedure to patient.
2. Wash hands. Don gloves.
3. Inserting a new intravenous (IV) prior to administration of a vesicant is strongly recommended.
4. Apply the tourniquet. When necessary, ask the patient to pump a fist to distend veins.
5. Cleanse the site with an alcohol or povidone-iodine (Betadine®) swab.

6. Insert the butterfly needle or over the needle catheter (e.g., angio-cath®), observe for blood backflow, remove the tourniquet, and connect the flush intravenous solution. Infuse enough fluid to ensure venous patency.

7. Tape the needle to make the insertion site easy to see and to stabilize the needle.

8. Administer agent using the side arm technique. The side arm technique involves administering an agent through a free flowing IV at the closest y-site or injection port to the patient.

9. While administering the agent, observe for signs of infiltration such as redness or swelling at the injection site, change in quality or decrease in IV flow rate, inability to obtain a blood backflow, or burning, stinging or pain experienced by the patient. Check vein patency every 1–2 milliliters and at end of administration by verifying blood backflow.

10. Irrigate the line with flush solution in between and after all drugs.

11. When treatment is complete, remove the needle and apply pressure and dressing as needed. Discard used equipment using safe handling methods to avoid needle sticks and hazardous waste exposure.

12. Document all actions, site, gauge, type of needle, agent administered, observations made during administration, patient response, and outcomes of the process.

Itching, inflammation, and rash can appear at the point of entry but usually disappear within seconds. Allow flush solution to run for a few seconds. Diphenhydramine (Benadryl®) might be needed in the case of a hypersensitive flare reaction. If there is any doubt as to the patency of an existing IV line, the treatment should be interrupted and the line removed. A new IV site should be started either proximal to the previous site or in the other arm.

Management of vesicant extravasation is controversial. Several antidotes have been proposed in the literature, but little experimental information has been published. Further research is needed to evaluate the effectiveness of the agents listed in Table 3B–2. Until definitive research is available, each institution needs to formalize standard orders for treatment of vesicant seepage into the tissue. Supportive nursing management requires knowledge of possible treatments for therapy infiltration. Use of isoproterenol (Isuprel®), dimethylsulfoxide (DMSO), corticosteroids, isotonic sodium thiosulfate, hyaluronidase, and sodium bicarbonate have been reported. Heat or ice might be indicated. The following management plan is one that can be used for suspected drug extravasation (courtesy of the National Institutes of Health, Nursing Department).

Extravasation Treatment

Procedure

1. If extravasation occurs, immediately stop the administration of the agent.

2. Explain procedure to patient.

Table 3B–2
Extravasation Treatments

Antidote	Agent
Hyaluronidase (Wydase)*	Vinblastine
	Vincristine
	Vindesine
	Vinorelbine
	Etoposide
	Teniposide
Sodium thiosulfate*	Cisplatin (high concentrations)
	Mechlorethamine
Topical cooling	Dactinomycin
	Doxorubicin
	Epirubicin
	Idarubicin
	Mitoxantrone
	Mitomycin
Topical warming	Paclitaxel
Dimethylsulfoxide (DMSO)	Doxorubicin
	Daunomycin
	Mitomycin
	Mechlorethamine
General antidotes:	
Cold	
Corticosteriods	
Lidocaine	
Isoproterenol (Isuprel®)	
EDTA	

*Can be injected through existing intravenous line and subcutaneously at extravasation site. See Oncology Nursing Society Guidelines for more information.

3. Leave the needle in place and aspirate any residual agent and blood from the intravenous tubing, needle, and suspected infiltration site. If unable to aspirate residual agent from the IV tubing, *do not* instill the antidote through the needle.
4. Inform the patient's prescriber (e.g., physician, nurse practitioner, physician assistant) and initiate appropriate treatment measures.
5. Administer antidote if appropriate.
6. Inject the antidote through the IV needle if appropriate.
7. Remove the IV needle. Inject the antidote subcutaneously clockwise into the infiltrated area using a 25 gauge needle. Change the needle with each new injection. Avoid applying pressure to the suspected area of infiltration.

8. Mark skin around IV site and note any area of induration, swelling, or erythema.
9. Determine the size of the suspected extravasation by measuring a perpendicular length and width at the widest points.
10. Cover lightly with an occlusive sterile dressing. Instruct the patient in care of the site and follow-up.

Observation and care depend on agent, dose, amount of drug suspected to have infiltrated, extent of suspected injury, and patient's needs and concerns. Discuss with the physician the need to consult with a surgeon if pain, erythema, induration, and/or tissue breakdown occurs.

The patient might receive restitution for injury resulting from extravasation. Thus, the therapy administration process must be well documented whether or not complications occur. A photograph of the site can serve to document a suspected extravasation. Documentation in the patient's medical record should include date and time of extravasation, needle size and type, insertion location site, therapy sequence, method of drug administration, how venous patency was verified, the patient's comments prior to extravasation, approximate amount of agent infiltrated, dimensions of extravasation site, nursing management of the extravasation, date of follow-up evaluation, and any consultations. Additional notes should include instructions to the patient regarding follow-up care, resources to call, and emotional care provided. On the patient's next visit, the area of extravasation should be assessed and observations noted in the patient's record. Plan to follow up by telephone in the interim. Damage might not occur immediately but might become apparent in several days.

VENOUS ACCESS DEVICES

Many patients with cancer have poor venous access because of their disease (e.g., leukemia) and treatment. Deterioration of peripheral veins can result from repeated venipunctures. A variety of venous access devices (VADs) have been developed to assist clinicians in providing and managing cancer therapy (see Figures 3B–1 and 3B–2). VADs ensure reliable access. They help decrease the trauma associated with multiple venipunctures while allowing easy access for drug delivery and blood sampling. For cancer clinicians, VADs offer the advantage of minimizing the risk of drug extravasation associated with chemotherapy administration.

VADs are primarily used for long-term therapies. They are used to administer intravenous fluids, blood products, continuous drug infusions, medications (e.g., antineoplastics, antibiotics, biologics, opioids); parenteral nutrition; and for venous blood sampling.

After a VAD is inserted, correct placement should be verified by obtaining an x-ray. Complications associated with VAD placement include

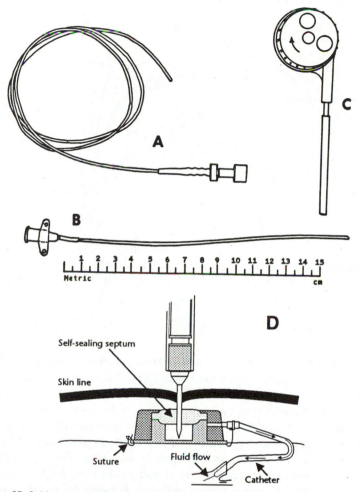

Figure 3B-1. Venous access devices: (A) Hickman-type catheter;
(B) percutaneous central venous catheter; (C) PICC line; (D) Port-a-Cath.

Reprinted with permission of Pharmacia: Port-a-Cath Drug Delivery System, professional manual.

(1) pneumothorax; (2) thrombus formation; (3) catheter damage, kinks, migration, malposition, and occlusion (blood or precipitate); (4) fibrin sheath formation; (5) pulmonary embolus; (6) infection: exit, tunnel, port pocket; (7) extravasation (needle dislodgment is the most common cause); and (8) phlebitis in peripherally inserted catheters. When the VAD is not in use, its patency should be ensured by irrigation with heparin or saline. Forceful irrigation is contraindicated. When entering the VAD (except Groshongs), the catheter or tubing should be clamped to avoid air embolus or bleedback into the catheter IV tubing. In addition, only luer-lock devices (e.g., infusion caps, tubing) should be used with VADs.

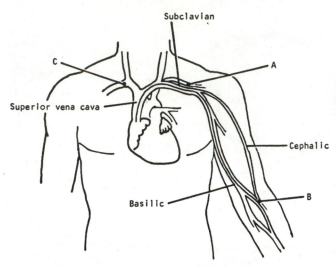

Figure 3B-2. Sites of catheter placement: (A) percutaneous central venous catheters; (B) PICC lines; (C) Hickman-type catheters, Groshongs.

Nontunneled Catheters

Nontunneled catheters are available in a variety of materials; however, most are made of polyurethane. These catheters are generally inserted using local anesthesia. Percutaneous central venous catheters (CVCs) are placed through a large vein (e.g., subclavian, internal jugular, external jugular). The tip of the catheter is threaded into the superior vena cava just outside the right atrium of the heart. In general, the CVC is placed to deliver short duration therapies (weeks or less) or to provide venous access until a tunneled catheter or port can be placed. CVCs can also be used to monitor central venous pressure. Peripherally inserted central venous catheters or PICC lines provide an additional venous access option and are generally utilized for therapies lasting weeks to months. They are placed by physicians or by nurses who have been certified in placement techniques. PICC lines are placed in the anterior area of the nondominant forearm into one of the brachial veins (basilic or cephalic). The catheter is threaded into the subclavian vein. Nontunneled catheters are less expensive than surgically implanted devices; delays waiting for surgical placement can be avoided.

Tunneled Catheters

There are several types of tunneled catheters, such as Hickman-type catheters and Groshongs. Tunneled catheters are made of silicone rubber and are surgically placed using local or general anesthesia. First, an entrance incision is made to isolate the subclavian vein. Then a subcutaneous tunnel is created from the point of entry to the exit site. The most common exit site is located at approximately the fourth or fifth intercostal space. Less common exit sites include the abdomen, back, chest wall, or arm. The catheter is then passed through this tunnel into the subclavian vein, and finally, the tip of the catheter is threaded into the superior vena cava. Tunneled catheters have a dacron cuff that anchors the catheter subcutaneously and provides a barrier to infection. Hickman-type catheters are open ended, whereas Groshongs are closed ended and have a two-way slit valve at the distal end. Tunneled catheters are available in single, double, and triple lumens. A variation of the Hickman-type catheter is utilized for apheresis and hemodialysis. These tunneled catheters are shorter in length, have a larger diameter, and are usually placed into the subclavian vein. When tunneled catheters are not in use, irrigation with heparin or saline is needed to maintain patency. Hickman-type catheters require the instillation of heparin once a day to maintain patency; Groshongs require the instillation of saline once a week. Dressings are required on these catheters. Complications associated with tunneled catheters include infection, malposition, catheter occlusion, difficulty aspirating blood, kinks, and catheter breakage or leakage.

Tunneled catheters are fragile and susceptible to breaks and leaks that require repair. Patients should be instructed in securing the catheter to minimize the risk of damage and in interventions to be taken if the catheter is damaged. Breakage of Hickman-type catheters can be minimized by the use of only smooth-edged cannula clamps. A cannula clamp should be with the patient at all times. Most Hickman-type catheters are now made with a clamp attached. Should the catheter leak or break, it should be clamped immediately above the leak. A permanent repair should be done as soon as possible. A temporary repair can be done if there is a delay in obtaining a permanent catheter repair kit. The patient can be taught how to do a temporary repair and/or to call for assistance. Groshongs should never be clamped. If the catheter develops a leak or breaks, it should be folded over and taped. The patient should be instructed to call so that arrangements can be made for a permanent repair.

Subcutaneous Venous Access Devices

Subcutaneous venous access devices (SVADs) also referred to as ports (e.g., Port-a-Cath™, Infus-a-Port™, Mediport™, Groshong™) are used primarily for venous access. In addition, SVADs are available for arterial, intraperitoneal, and epidural administration. A port has a silicone domed reservoir with a self-sealing membrane and is attached to a catheter. The distal end of the catheter can be open ended like Hickmans or closed ended with a slit valve like Groshongs. The port is implanted in the subcutaneous tissue in an area where access is easiest. The catheter is threaded into a large vein, artery, organ, or cavity where therapy is desired.

The central venous port is implanted under local or general anesthesia, generally in the upper chest area. The peripheral access system PAS-port™ is implanted via cutdown or percutaneous approach using local anesthesia in the outpatient setting, in the anterior area of the nondominant forearm into one of the brachial veins (basilic or cephalic) and threaded into the subclavian vein. The CathFinder™ Catheter Tracking System is used to locate the catheter and to ensure proper placement. CathLink™ is a new implantable port that can be placed either through peripheral access, like the PAS-port™ or centrally like other ports. In addition, unlike the other SVADs, which are accessed using a noncoring needle, the CathLink™ is accessed using an over-the-needle catheter that is at least $1\frac{3}{4}$ inches long. When accessed, the needle is removed, creating a needleless access.

Complications associated with SVADs include infection, malposition, flipping of port, and catheter occlusion. In addition, port pocket cellulitis, vein phlebitis, and difficulty aspirating blood have been noted with the PAS-port™. When SVADs are not in use, irrigation is needed at least once a month to maintain patency. Heparin is used for most SVADs; however, saline is used for Groshong-type SVADs.

After the surgical site is healed, no dressing is necessary when the SVAD is not being used. Accessing the SVAD requires attention to detail. The disadvantage of a SVAD is that access requires a needle stick. A topical anesthetic agent such as EMLA® cream (lidocaine 2.5 percent and prilocaine 2.5 percent) can be applied to the SVAD site one hour prior to access to decrease the discomfort associated with the needle stick. A sterile field is established, and povidone-iodine is used to prepare the site for needle entry. Only noncoring right angle needles are used to access ports with sealing membranes. Over the needle catheters (e.g., angiocath®, jelco™) are used to access the CathLink™ device. The needle should be inserted straight into the septum. If done at an angle or with a twisting motion, the septum might be cut, resulting in leakage of fluid. During continuous infusions or drug administration lasting many days, the needle should be changed at least every seven days. Establishing blood return prior to drug administration, especially with vesicants and irritants, is essential. A procedure for accessing an implanted port follows.

Implanted Port Access Procedure

Supplies
Sterile gloves
Sterile barrier
3 alcohol swabsticks
3 povidone-iodine swabsticks
20 or 22 gauge noncoring right angle needle, with attached tubing and clamp, or use extension tubing with clamp
Syringe with 5 ml 0.9% saline
Dressing supplies

Procedure for accessing self sealing ports

1. Explain procedure to the patient.
2. Wash hands.
3. Open sterile barrier and place SVAD access supplies on the sterile field.
4. Palpate site to locate SVAD septum.
5. Administer local anesthetic if necessary.
6. Don sterile gloves.
7. Cleanse SVAD site and surrounding tissue with alcohol swabs. Using a spiral motion, begin at the SVAD septum and work outward approximately 2 inches. Repeat twice.
8. Repeat step 7 using povidone-iodine swabsticks. Allow povidone-iodine to dry.
9. Connect syringe of 0.9% saline to tubing of noncoring right angle needle or to extension set.
10. Flush tubing and needle with 0.9% saline to expel air and clamp tubing.
11. Locate the SVAD by palpation and stabilize the SVAD between the thumb and index finger of the nondominant hand.
12. Insert the needle through the skin and SVAD septum at a 90-degree angle. Insert the needle until it meets the bottom of the port chamber.
13. Unclamp the tubing, and flush the SVAD with 0.9% saline. Draw back on syringe to obtain a blood return.
14. Infuse medication, obtain blood samples, or flush system as appropriate. If needle is to be left in place, excess povidone-iodine should be removed from the skin and the needle secured with a transparent or other appropriate dressing.

Assessment

The nurse should know about the advantages and disadvantages of the various types of venous access devices available. The factors that should be considered when selecting the appropriate VAD are listed in Table 3B–3.

Management

Nursing management of a patient with a VAD consists of (1) monitoring for complications, (2) developing procedures for care of the VAD, and (3) patient education concerning the device. Nursing assessment is discussed in Table 3B-4. Certain complications associated with VADs, such as infection or occlusion, might require the removal and replacement of the

Table 3B-3
Factors Guiding the Selection of Venous Access Devices

Patient age
Patient/family intellectual skills
Psychomotor skills
Psychosocial factors
Medical history
Lifestyle
Duration of therapy
Treatment regimen/complications
Catheter maintenance requirements
Frequency of access
Condition of peripheral veins
Patient preference
Risks of anesthesia
Cost

device. Occlusion is a common complication when VADs are used. The only symptom of occlusion is encountering resistance when trying to inject or infuse fluid through the device. To restore the patency of the device a thrombolytic agent such as urokinase might be needed to dissolve a clot in the catheter; 70 percent ethyl alcohol might be needed to dissolve a lipid precipitate or sodium bicarbonate ($NaHCO_3$) 0.1N hydrochloric acid (HCL) or ammonia chloride might be needed to dissolve a drug precipitate.

Each institution should establish standards of care for the various devices utilized. The following are examples of procedures for changing dressings, flushing, and drawing blood with VADs.

Sterile technique is used when changing the exit site dressing of percutaneous CVCs, PICCs, and tunneled catheters in the hospital. However, prior to discharge, patients with tunneled catheters are instructed to use clean technique at home. There are a variety of dressing materials available. An occlusive dressing is used on tunneled catheters until the site is healed.

Sterile Technique
Dressing Change

Supplies (available in a preassembled kit)
Sterile gloves (2 pairs)
Sterile barrier
3 alcohol swabsticks
3 povidone-iodine swabsticks
Skin prep swab
Dressing material of choice:
 Transparent dressing (e.g., Bioclusive®, Tegaderm®)
 Occlusive gauze dressing (e.g., sterile 2x2 gauze and tape,
 CoverLet® O.R. 4x4 dressing that incorporates 2x2 gauze and
 paper tape)

Table 3B–4
Nursing Protocol for Assessment of Patients with Venous Access Devices

Problem	Intervention
Preplacement	
Decision	Evaluate patient's mental status
	Share information with health care provider
	Factors to consider in identifying the best VAD:
	• Patient's ability to care for the VAD
	• Availability of family members to assist with care
	• Resources
	• Activity level
	• Anticipated length of therapy
Patient's need for information	Discuss procedure with patient: Why, how, expectations after insertion, care responsibilities, and potential complications
Insertion	
Complications of VAD placement	Assess the patient for the following potential complications:
	Pneumothorax: cyanosis, dyspnea, chest pain, tachycardia, respiratory embarrassment, absent breath sounds in affected area
	Pulmonary embolism: dyspnea, tachypnea, pleuritic pain, cyanosis, unexplained deterioration of patient's condition, engorgement of neck veins
	Pleural effusion: increasing dyspnea, minimal or absent breath sounds
	Notify physician if these symptoms occur
	Obtain x-ray to verify findings
Post-placement	
Potential complications	
Local	Evaluate for pain, bleeding, leakage of fluid, or hematoma
	Assess for signs of infection such as redness, irritation, fever, or discharge from catheter exit site (if applicable)
	Periodically check patient's dressing
Mechanical (catheter function)	
Aspiration difficulties	Fluid infuses freely, but blood return is sluggish or absent. Causes include catheter occlusion, catheter malposition, fibrin sheath formation, kinked catheter, "pinch off" syndrome, blood vessel obstruction. Solutions include checking for kinks or tight sutures, changing patient position, alternately flushing and aspirating, x-ray to verify position, dye study, instilling urokinase
Occlusion	Signs and symptoms include inability to infuse or sluggish infusion of fluids; resistance during flushing; absent blood return. Assess cause of occlusion (blood clot, drug precipitate, lipid precipitate, kinked catheter, "pinch off" syndrome, catheter malposition). Instillation of urokinase to dissolve blood clot; $NaHCO_3$, 0.1N HCL or ammonia chloride to dissolve drug precipitates; 70% ethyl alcohol to dissolve lipid precipitates might be necessary. If unable to remove occlusion, catheter might have to be replaced
Displacement	An x-ray or scan might be required to evaluate catheter position
Damage	Depending on type of device, catheter could be damaged by use or trauma. Tunneled catheters and some PICCs can be repaired. The nurse will need to review individual VAD information to determine necessary precautions

Alcohol swab (tunneled catheters)
Steri-strips™ (PICCs and SVADs)
Adhesive tape remover (optional)
$\frac{1}{2}$ strength hydrogen peroxide solution (optional)

Procedure
1. Explain procedure to patient.
2. Wash hands.
3. Open sterile barrier and place dressing change supplies on the sterile field.
4. Don sterile gloves and remove old dressing. Discard gloves and old dressing. Wash hands.
5. Observe site for erythema, irritation, bleeding, drainage, tenderness, swelling, or signs of skin breakdown and document. Culture any drainage.
6. Don second pair of sterile gloves.
7. If crusting is present, cleanse exit site with $\frac{1}{2}$ strength hydrogen peroxide using cotton tip applicators.
8. Cleanse exit site and surrounding tissue with alcohol swabsticks. Using a spiral motion, begin at the exit site and work outward approximately 2 inches. Repeat twice. Allow alcohol to dry.
9. Cleanse exit site and surrounding tissue with povidone-iodine swabsticks. Using a spiral motion, begin at the exit site and work outward approximately 2 inches. Repeat twice. Allow povidone-iodine to dry.
10. *For tunneled catheters:* Cleanse catheter using an alcohol swab. Anchoring catheter at the exit site, gently wipe swab from proximal to distal end of the catheter.
11. Sterile steri-strips® can be placed on PICC to provide stability and prevent catheter migration. They can be placed on noncoring right angle needle to increase stability.
12. Apply skin-prep to area where dressing will be applied.
13. Apply dressing of choice. Recommended dressing change frequency is as follows: transparent every 72 hours, and gauze, transparent with gauze under it, or CoverLet® every 24 hours. In addition, change whenever dressing becomes wet, soiled, or loose.
14. Loop catheter and secure with tape. A catheter holder device can be used to secure the catheter.
15. Remove gloves. Label dressing with date, time, and initials. Document.

Clean Technique Dressing Change

Supplies
3 alcohol swabsticks
3 povidone-iodine swabsticks

Skin prep swab
Dressing material of choice:
   Transparent dressing (e.g., Bioclusive®, Tegaderm®)
   Occlusive gauze dressing (e.g., sterile 2x2 gauze and tape,
   CoverLet® O.R. 4x4 dressing that incorporates 2x2 gauze and
   paper tape)
Alcohol swab (tunneled catheters)
Adhesive tape remover (optional)
$\frac{1}{2}$ strength hydrogen peroxide solution (optional)
Sterile cotton tip swabsticks (optional)

Procedure
1. Prepare clean work area and gather supplies.
2. Wash hands with soap.
3. Remove old dressing, being careful not to tug on catheter or touch the exit site.
4. Look at the site for redness, irritation, bleeding, drainage, tenderness, swelling or signs of skin breakdown.
5. Rewash hands with soap.
6. If crusting is present, cleanse exit site with $\frac{1}{2}$ strength hydrogen peroxide. Dip cotton tip swabstick in $\frac{1}{2}$ strength hydrogen peroxide solution. Then take swabstick and gently attempt to remove crusting from around the exit site of the catheter.
7. Open and holding only the end of the alcohol swabstick remove one from package. Clean catheter exit site and surrounding tissue. Using a spiral motion, begin at the exit site and work outward approximately 2 inches. Never return to the exit site with the same swabstick. Repeat twice using the remaining swabsticks. Allow alcohol to dry.
8. Open and holding only the end of the povidone-iodine swabstick remove one from package. Clean catheter exit site and surrounding tissue. Using a spiral motion, begin at the exit site and work outward approximately 2 inches. Never return to the exit site with the same swabstick. Repeat twice using the remaining swabsticks. Allow povidone-iodine to dry.
9. *For tunneled catheters:* Clean catheter using an alcohol swab. Using nondominant hand lift the catheter. Using dominant hand place alcohol swab around catheter and grip. Gently run alcohol swab down catheter from exit site toward the cap.
10. Apply skin-prep to cover the area where the tape part of the dressing will be placed (optional).
11. Apply dressing of choice. Be careful not to touch the part which will be covering the exit site.
12. Loop catheter to decrease pulling and secure with tape. A catheter holder device may be used to secure the catheter.

Routine Flushing

Supplies

Syringe with needle or needleless cannula containing appropriate flush solution

VAD	Flush Solution	Amount
Nontunneled Catheters		
Percutaneous CVC	Heparin (100u/ml)	1 ml
PICC	Heparin (100u/ml)	2 ml
Groshong PICC	0.9% saline	10 ml
Tunneled Catheters		
Apheresis	Heparin (1000u/ml)	1.5 ml
Hickman	Heparin (100u/ml)	2.5 ml
Groshong	0.9% saline	10 ml
Venous SVADs (ports)		
Hickman	Heparin (100u/ml)	3 ml
Groshong	0.9% saline	10 ml
PAS-port™	Heparin (100u/ml)	5 ml
CathLink™	Heparin (100u/ml)	5 ml

Syringe containing 5 mls of 0.9% saline (use 10 ml syringe or larger for CathLinks™ and PICCs)

Empty 3 cc syringe (apheresis catheters)

Alcohol swab

Intermittent infusion cap

Nonsterile gloves

Procedure

1. Explain procedure to patient.
2. Wash hands.
3. Don nonsterile gloves.
4. Cleanse intermittent infusion cap with alcohol pad and allow to dry.
5. Clamp catheter (except Groshongs). For apheresis catheters withdraw 2 mls of blood using empty 3 cc syringe and discard prior to flush.
6. Insert syringe containing appropriate flush solution into the infusion cap.
7. Unclamp the catheter and flush gently. For PICCs flush using the push-pause technique.
8. Clamp catheter (except Groshongs). Remove and discard syringe in appropriate container.

A benefit of a VAD is that it can be used for blood drawing; however, in general, SVADs are not accessed only for blood sampling. One method for blood drawing utilizes a vacutainer and stopcock system to minimize exposure to needles and blood. In addition, this method of blood drawing maintains a closed system and decreases manipulation of the catheter (see Figure 3B–3). Many institutions reinfuse the discarded blood, especially with pediatric and critically ill patients (see Figure 3B–4). Refer to your institutional policies.

Blood Drawing

Supplies
4 way double stopcock
Vacutainer® holder and needle
1 syringe containing heparin (100 u/ml)
   CVC: 1 ml
   Hickman: 2.5 ml
   SVAD: 3 ml
   PAS-port™/CathLink™: 5 ml
   PICC: 5 ml
1 syringe containing heparin (1000 u/ml)
   Apheresis catheters: 1.5 ml
1 syringe containing 0.9% saline
   CVC, Hickman, or SVAD: 5 ml
   Groshong: 10 ml
Needle or needleless cannula
Labeled collection tubes for blood specimens
For discard:
   extra blood collection tube
   1–10 ml syringe (optional)

Figure 3B–3. Blood drawing procedure using double stopcock setup (Vacutainer® can be substituted for syringe to draw blood samples).

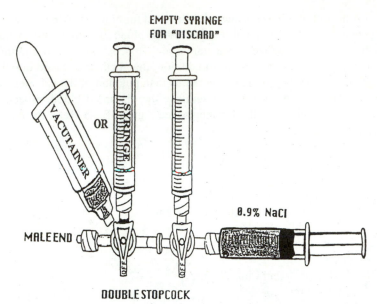

Figure 3B-4. Blood drawing procedure: Double stopcock setup for reinfusion of discard blood. (Vacutainer® can be substituted for syringe to draw blood samples.)

Nonsterile gloves
19 gauge 1-inch needle (optional)
Intermittent infusion cap

Procedure
1. Explain procedure to patient.
2. Assemble equipment for obtaining blood specimens as follows:
   a. Attach needle or needleless cannula to luer lock end of double stopcock.
   b. Attach vacutainer holder in first stopcock closest to luer lock of double stopcock system.
   c. Attach syringe containing 0.9% saline to second stopcock.
   d. Attach syringe containing heparin to distal end of double stopcock system.

Capped line procedure
3. Wash hands and don gloves.
4. Cleanse intermittent injection cap with alcohol pad and allow to dry.
5. If patient has a multi-lumen device, turn off infusion to the other catheter lumens and clamp.
6. Insert the double stopcock system through infusion cap or remove intermittent infusion cap and attach double stopcock system directly.

7. Turn stopcock open to vacutainer, unclamp catheter, and insert vacutainer tube for discard. Fill tube with blood, remove, and set aside.
8. Insert remainder of specimen tubes and fill to appropriate level.
9. Turn stopcock "off" in direction of vacutainer and "on" to 0.9% saline. Slowly inject.
10. Turn stopcock "on" in direction of syringe containing heparin and slowly inject.
11. Clamp catheter; remove and discard double stopcock system. Change or replace intermittent infusion cap.
12. Remove gloves and wash hands.

Continuous infusion procedure
1. Wash hands.
2. Stop all intravenous infusions.
3. Don gloves.
4. Cleanse connection with alcohol pad and clamp catheter.
5. Detach infusion, placing a capped sterile needle on the end of the detached tubing.
6. Attach double stopcock system directly to the catheter.
7. Continue according to blood drawing procedure above (steps 7–9 of capped line procedure).
8. Clamp catheter; remove and discard double system. Reconnect infusion.
9. Resume infusion(s).

Patient Teaching

The patient and/or significant other should be taught the appropriate care of the venous access device (Table 3B–5). It is important to provide emotional support while the patient learns the detailed procedures so that the patient becomes comfortable with them. A written booklet is very helpful to patients and their families. Patient education should include type of device, maintenance requirements (e.g., heparinization, dressing change, flushing procedure), special precautions, whom to notify should they experience a problem, and available resources. Booklets are available that (1) describe the various venous access devices along with their advantages, and (2) review maintenance care.

Because venous access devices are important in easing the administration of therapy, patients often become dependent on them. Patients worry that problems, when they occur, will not be correctable and that their venous access device will need to be removed. Nurses can alert patients to potential causes and symptoms of complications and the interventions to correct them, thus prolonging the life of the VAD and increas-

Table 3B-5
Guidelines for the Care of Venous Access Devices

Venous Access Device	Dressing		Flushing			Cap/Needle change
	Gauze	Transparent	Solution	Amount	Frequency	
Nontunneled Catheters						
Percutaneous CVCs	Daily	Every 72 hrs or whenever dressing is wet, loose or soiled	Heparin (100 u/ml)	1 ml	Daily and after each use	Cap change every 48 hrs and after each use. Once a week at home
PICC		Initial dressing changed within 48 hrs and then weekly or whenever dressing is wet, loose, or soiled	Heparin (100 u/ml)	2 ml	Daily and after each use using the push-pause technique	Cap change every 48 hrs and after each use. Once a week at home
Groshong PICC		Initial dressing changed within 48 hrs and then weekly or whenever dressing is wet, loose, or soiled	0.9% saline	10 ml	Weekly and after each use	Cap change every 48 hrs and after each use. Once a week at home
Tunneled Catheters						
Hickman/ Broviac	Daily in hospital / Twice a week at home	Every 72 hrs or whenever dressing is wet, loose, or soiled	Heparin (100 u/ml)	2.5 ml	Daily and after each use	Cap change every 48 hrs and after each use. Once a week at home
Groshong	Daily in hospital / Twice a week at home	Every 72 hrs or whenever dressing is wet, loose, or soiled	0.9% saline	10 ml (adults) 5 ml (peds)	Weekly and after each use	Cap change every 48 hrs and after each use. Once a week at home

SVADs (ports)

Hickman SVAD (ports)	Every 72 hrs or whenever dressing is wet, loose, or soiled	Heparin (100 u/ml)	3 ml	At least monthly and after each use	Needle change every 7 days
Groshong SVAD (ports)	Every 72 hrs or whenever dressing is wet, loose, or soiled	0.9% saline	10 ml	At least monthly and after each use	Needle change every 7 days
PAS port™	Every 72 hrs or whenever dressing is wet, loose, or soiled	Heparin (100 u/ml)	5 ml	At least monthly and after each use	Needle change every 7 days
CathLink™	Every 72 hrs or whenever dressing is wet, loose, or soiled	Heparin (100 u/ml) 0.9% saline	5 ml 10 ml 20 ml	At least monthly and after each use After infusions After blood draws	Over the needle change every 7 days

ing the chances patients will have them for the duration of therapy. Patients should be encouraged to wear a Medic-alert necklace or bracelet and carry an identification card to alert medical personnel to the presence of the VAD.

INTRA-ARTERIAL THERAPY

Arterial catheter or arterial SVAD placement is another method used to obtain access to administer cancer therapy. These VADs can be used for continuous arterial blood sampling without frequent punctures. Cancer patients might require an intra-arterial access for an infusion of antineoplastic agents or monitoring for complications of disease or treatment. Arterial drug administration allows a high concentration of therapy to be delivered to tumor sites with a theoretical decrease in systemic toxicity. Tumors treated in this way are colorectal, liver, head, neck, brain, pancreatic, bladder, cervical, and breast cancers; melanoma; and sarcomas. The major artery chosen for catheter placement depends on the disease site; possible choices are the celiac, femoral, brachial, radial, hepatic, axillary, and external or internal carotid arteries. Agents tested by arterial administration are fluorouracil, FUDR, IUDR, BUDR, carmustine, cisplatin, doxorubicin, methotrexate, etoposide, mitoxantrone, mitomycin, and biotherapies such as IL-2 and monoclonal antibodies.

Experimental interventions that enhance drug levels within the artery are being evaluated because their effectiveness seems to be related to dosage. These interventions include (1) embolization of drug carrier albumin microspheres that facilitate tumor entry; (2) administration of angiotensin II to cause vasoconstriction and increase the tumor-to-liver blood flow ratio; (3) balloon occlusion of the artery; and (4) isolated regional perfusion.

Regional perfusion is most commonly performed in the limbs. Regional perfusion isolates both arterial and venous blood supply to and from the region so that high concentrations of the therapeutic agent can perfuse the tumor site and the agent can be removed before it is spread systemically. Any of these therapies alone, or in combination with other treatments such as surgery, other agents, or radiation, are often locally effective, but systemic disease can occur. Because arterial access has disadvantages, current clinical trials are evaluating what role this alternative route of administration will ultimately play.

An arterial catheter can be placed percutaneously by a radiologist or surgically. An arterial SVAD is placed surgically. Preplacement angiography can be done to determine the anatomy of the arterial blood supply. Surgical placement allows a more stable and permanent placement of the catheter, because it is sutured in place, but this procedure requires general anesthesia. The catheter can be hooked to a port that is implanted subcutaneously. Intermittent flushing of the surgically placed catheter is necessary because it stays in place for longer periods of time.

When a radiologist performs the procedure, the catheter is placed percutaneously using local anesthetic, and—because the catheter is radiopaque—its placement is checked by x-ray. The percutaneous catheter might or might not be sutured in place; it is used for short-term therapy and usually needs continuous IV heparinization. Steri-strips™ are used to anchor the catheter if it is not sutured. Totally implanted pumps have also been tested for arterial therapy administration (Infusaid®, Medtronics®). Arterial SVADs are flushed with 5,000 u/ml of heparin. Angiography is used to check proper placement and patency.

Assessment

The nurse should be familiar with the percutaneous arterial catheter, arterial SVAD, and the surgical methods of arterial catheterization so that the patient can be prepared for insertion. Baseline information—such as color, temperature, pulses, nerve sensation, Allen test, and blanching time of the area around the proposed site—should be observed and documented. Table 3B–6 discusses in detail problems that require assessment before and after placement, together with appropriate nursing interventions.

Management

Medical decisions to be made include anticipated length of therapy, appropriate device selection, and site of catheter placement. Care continues with follow-up for problems encountered during therapy (e.g., a clotted catheter). If the intra-arterial device becomes occluded with a blood clot, the medical team must decide whether to remove the catheter or attempt to declot it with urokinase.

Nursing management focuses on preparing the patient for insertion and care of the catheter. The patient must be educated about what to expect, potential problems, and preventive care of the exit site. Care will depend on routines of each individual institution; the following are general guidelines.

The nurse or patient should note the color and temperature of the exit site extremity every four hours. The site should be checked for bleeding. Pressure should be applied to the site and maintained while the dressing is removed to observe for any disconnections. Strict sterile technique must be maintained any time the external catheter is manipulated. This includes insertion, blood drawing, changing the line components, and therapy preparation. If an implantable port or pump is used, less stringent care is required, but sterile technique must be used whenever the implantable device is accessed. Care of the site should be performed daily.

Table 3B–6
Nursing Protocol for Management of Patients with Intra-arterial VADs

Problem	Intervention
Preplacement	
Decision about best type of arterial VAD for the patient	Evaluate the patient's needs. Can patient care for the catheter and recognize complications, precautions, and reasons to call for help? Share this information with the physician. Assess availability of family members to assist in catheter care. Items to consider:
	Resources: Percutaneous catheter must be placed by a radiologist, anesthesiologist, or physician. A surgically placed arterial catheter requires use of an operating room.
	Need for device: The surgically placed catheter is sutured in place and is more permanent. The percutaneous catheter is more appropriate for short-term use. A port can be attached to the catheter to allow long-term access with less maintenance care.
	Activity level: The surgically placed catheter can be capped and flushed intermittently with heparin, allowing greater mobility than the percutaneous catheter, which often requires continuous IV irrigation to prevent clotting.
	Safety: Both types of intra-arterial VADs present a tremendous danger from hemorrhage. If the patient or family members are unable to demonstrate safety measures necessary to stop bleeding, then this type of therapy should not be considered.
Patient's need for information	Discuss procedure with the patient: why, how, preparation for catheter placement, post-insertion expectations, care responsibilities, and potential problems.
Postplacement	
Potential complications: Local	Assess for bleeding at insertion site, hematoma development, or swelling. If present, apply direct pressure to the site. Whenever an arterial catheter is removed, pressure must be applied to the site for at least 5 minutes to prevent a hematoma.
Dislodgement of catheter Patient's need for information	Teach patient to report excessive side effects of treatment. These might include nausea and vomiting, diarrhea, dyspepsia, stomach pain, twitching, paresthesia, motor weakness, or problems with vision.
Mechanical (catheter function)	Assess for decreased or absent pulse distal to the insertion site. This might be caused by an occluded catheter. Preventive treatment involves heparin flushing either every 4–6 hr and then every 24 hr for a surgically placed catheter, continuously for a percutaneous catheter, and weekly for arterial SVADs. Intermittent flushes can occasionally be used, and if so, careful monitoring for backflow of blood between flushes is necessary. Pain or numbness in the extemity might signal a problem.
	An arterial catheter can be broken by wear and tear or trauma. The patient needs to have a clamp available and be taught what to do if breakage should occur. Luer lock connectors need to be used with arterial infusions to prevent hemorrhage, such as blood backup caused by loose connections, leakage of fluid from site, or frank bleeding. Safety measures include evaluation of all connection sites frequently, use of luer lock connectors, and use of a built-in alarm system to monitor pressure changes within arterial line. If patient is to go home, it is essential to teach the patient and his or her family to immediately apply pressure to the site and elevate the affected part should bleeding occur.

Table 3B–6 *(Continued)*
Nursing Protocol for Management of Patients with Intra-arterial VADs

Problem	Intervention
Postplacement	
Therapy effects	Toxicities that occur are site and drug specific. Nurse and patient need to know what is expected, and to report the unexpected or severe. Potential effects include the following:
	Brain arterial infusions: eye pain, decreased vision, seizures, hemiparesis, decreased hearing, confusion, dermatitis on forehead.
	Head and neck: visual changes, hemiparesis, seventh nerve palsy, mucositis, dermatitis, ulceration.
	Extremity infusions: edema, nerve and muscle damage, thrombophlebitis, tissue necrosis, decreased joint mobility, dermatitis.
	Pelvis: cellulitis, fistula, leg pain and nerve damage, cystitis, mucositis, myelosuppression.
	Colon: stomatitis, nausea, vomiting, diarrhea, myelosuppression, chemical hepatitis, biliary sclerosis, ulcers, cholecystitis, pancreatitis.

Guidelines for Intra-arterial Exit Site Care

Supplies
sterile gloves
alcohol swabs
povidone-iodine swabs
povidone-iodine ointment
2-by-2 inch sterile gauze
cotton applicators
tape

Procedure
1. Explain procedure to patient.
2. Wash hands.
3. Remove old dressing. Check the site for signs of infection such as redness, swelling, or discharge. If signs of infection are present, blood cultures should be drawn. Culture any drainage.
4. Don sterile gloves.
5. Clean the exit site with alcohol and then povidone-iodine.
6. With an applicator, apply ointment to the exit site.
7. Place 2-by-2 inch gauze over the catheter and secure the dressing.

Drawing Blood from an Arterial Line

Supplies
sterile gloves
one 3 ml syringe for discard
alcohol swabs

syringes for blood specimens
labeled collection tubes for blood specimens
saline and heparin per physician's order

Procedure
1. Explain procedure to patient.
2. Wash hands.
3. Don sterile gloves.
4. Remove the cap from the in-line stopcock and cleanse the stopcock with alcohol. Insert the 3 ml syringe. Turn stopcock to open, and blood will flow freely into the syringe. Withdraw 3 ml for discard. Discard may be reinfused for pediatric and critically ill patients at the discretion of the institution.
5. Close the stopcock halfway to stop blood flow and quickly remove discard syringe. Insert specimen syringe, turn stopcock to full open, and obtain blood specimens.
6. Turn stopcock to off position and remove the specimen syringe.
7. Transfer the blood to collection tubes.
8. Immediately flush the line with saline or heparin solution until the catheter is clear.
9. Clean the outside of the stopcock with the alcohol swab and replace the cap.

Management of intra-arterial therapy infusions requires a high level of responsibility as well as technical skill. The nurse needs to know as much as possible about this method to ensure that patients are adequately prepared. Many patients who receive intra-arterial therapy via an infusion pump will be at home. The nurse generally initiates the therapy, but the patient monitors the administration.

A checklist provided by the nurse might be helpful to the patient. Good teaching, including frequent supervision and practice opportunities, will ensure that the patient is confident and comfortable about (1) performing maintenance care, (2) maintaining the infusion, and (3) identifying signs and symptoms of problems or abnormal effects. Greater patient awareness will encourage prompt communication with the staff, so that problems can be recognized early. Should problems occur, nurses are valuable resources for patients.

Because this method of therapy has become more popular, new implantable devices have been designed that decrease the incidence of complications, including thrombosis and infection, and reduce the patient's responsibilities. However, either kind of catheter can be dislodged. Home care places demands on the patient and family. The nurse is the source of support both during hospitalization and after discharge. Therapy evaluation will continue to address whether this mode of treatment offers an improvement in both quantity and quality of life to the patient.

AMBULATORY PUMPS

Several drugs used in the treatment of cancer work best when the drug is infused continuously into the bloodstream. This method of administration avoids the peak-and-valley effects of bolus injections while maintaining therapeutic drug levels. Over the past decade, many ambulatory pumps have been developed that facilitate the administration of cancer treatments in the outpatient and/or home setting. A variety of ambulatory pumps are available; they can be classified as implantable pumps, portable external pumps, and syringe pumps. This section focuses on implantable pumps.

Implantable pumps are designed for long-term therapy in the ambulatory patient. They are placed subcutaneously. One of their advantages is the capability of delivering medications to a specific target area. In cancers such as hepatoma or colon carcinoma, this is particularly important because the blood supply is almost exclusively arterial. The implantable pump can be inserted so that it delivers chemotherapy by infusion directly into the hepatic artery. Because most of the drug passes through the liver, where it is metabolized, and not out into the systemic circulation, systemic side effects are decreased.

Safe and effective use of implantable pumps requires knowledge of the pump, its function, its problems or limitations, and the need for follow-up care. An example of an implantable pump is the Infusaid (Figure 3B–5), which is composed of a lightweight metal that encloses two chambers separated by a flexible metal bellows. The interior chamber holds the drug; the surrounding outer chamber holds a two-phase charging fluid, which is the power supply. The charging fluid is in either a vapor or liquid state, depending on a number of variables. Pressure differences between the two chambers activate the pump. The vapor pressure of the charging fluid exerts a constant pressure on the bellows, causing the drug to flow from the pump into the catheter and to the selected body site. When the

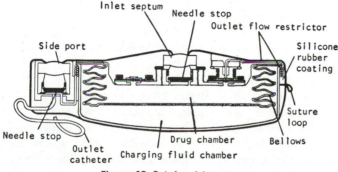

Figure 3B–5. Infusaid pump.

pump is refilled, the increasing volume causes pressure on the charging fluid, which condenses from the vapor to the liquid state. The liquid once again vaporizes, which provides the energy to move the bellows and deliver the desired drug flow. The flow rate is calibrated at the factory, but variations can be caused by changes in body temperature or altitude, which can alter the rate at which the charging fluid is converted from liquid to vapor. Each pump is delivered with specific calibration curves defining the flow characteristics for the planned catheter placement site, hometown elevation, and the drug to be used.

Attached to the pump is a silicone rubber catheter, which is placed in the vein, artery, or other site. The pump is refilled by percutaneous injection. The refill septum, which is in the center of the pump, can be easily palpated. The pump also has a side port, which can be used to bypass the reservoir and inject boluses of medication through the catheter. The technique for using this side port is the same as that described above for other similar implantable access ports.

Refilling the Infusaid pump on schedule is important. The dose and volume should be calculated by the physician, considering the factory-set flow rate of the pump, drug concentration, and individual factors, such as hometown elevation. The Infusaid Corporation holds classes to teach the pump refill procedure, which is as follows:

Infusaid Pump Refill

Supplies
Sterile gloves
22 gauge special Infusaid needle
Povidone-iodine swabsticks
Anesthetizing agent
Stopcock
Sterile syringe
Medication syringe

Procedure
1. Explain procedure to patient.
2. Wash hands.
3. Scrub the pump site with povidone-iodine swabsticks.
4. Anesthetize the injection site.
5. Don sterile gloves.
6. Attach 22 gauge needle to sterile stopcock.
7. Attach syringe to stopcock.
8. Using sterile technique, feel the outer edges of the pump to locate the refill septum located in the pump center.
9. Puncture the skin and septum and allow the pump's pressure to expel the infusate from the reservoir into the empty syringe. Precaution: The needle must be held securely against the needle stop. Do not put the needle at an angle within the septum.
10. When fluid has stopped returning, close the stopcock and remove the syringe barrel and stopcock from the needle. Air does not

enter into the needle because of the pressurized system. Record the volume. Precaution: If no fluid returns into the syringe, the possibilities are that the septum was not penetrated, the pump is empty, or there is a malfunction. Inject 5 ml of bacteriostatic water into the pump and then release the plunger. If fluid still does not return, repeat the procedure, beginning with reinsertion of the needle. If you think that you have penetrated the septum but have been unable to get return flow to the syringe, a pump failure may have occurred; notify the Infusaid Corporation.

11. Connect a warmed syringe of medication to the needle in the septum and slowly inject the contents. Remove syringe and needle when completed. Precaution: Make sure the needle point remains against the needle stop throughout the injection cycle.

12. The refill schedule should be planned several days before the end of the cycle to avoid an empty drug chamber.

Assessment

Nursing assessment of the patient's suitability for a totally implantable system involves the factors discussed in Table 3B–7. Interventions presented must be individualized.

Table 3B–7
Nursing Protocol for Management of Patients with Implantable Pumps

Problem	Intervention
Preimplantation	
Examine any contraindications to having an implantable pump	Assess the patient for severe emotional or psychologic disturbances that might indicate unreliability; a small thin body size that could not accommodate the weight of the pump; frequent travel, because altitude affects drug flow; or involvement in vigorous or rough occupations or activities, such as sports. Share this information with the physician.
Patient need for information	Use the teaching booklet supplied by pump manufacturer to supplement discussion of why, where, how, and patient responsibilities. Review instructions for contraindications, what to report, and use of an identification card, especially in the airport, where the pump will set off the metal detector.
Postimplantation	Tailor wound care to patient's needs. Review preimplantation instructions regarding what needs to be reported to doctor or nurse. Emphasize the necessity of returning on time for pump refills.

Management

Surgical site care depends on the location of pump implantation, but it usually consists of keeping the area clean and dry. The wound should be allowed to heal for three to seven days after implantation before beginning chemotherapy.

Nursing focus is primarily on the education of the patient. Each type of implantable pump has specific precautions. Patients need to know and understand the precautions relevant to their pump. The nurse plays an important role in sharing this information with the patient and family. Also helpful are the booklets that have been developed for the patients by many pump manufacturers. Instructions include avoiding rough physical activities, changes of altitudes (such as long airplane flights or scuba diving), and long hot baths or saunas, which elevate pump temperature. In addition, patients are advised to consult their physician during febrile illnesses and to report unusual signs and symptoms, and to notify hospital personnel about the pump if other medical procedures are planned. Most booklets encourage patients to return at the prescribed time for pump refill.

An identification card should be provided to the patient with an implantable pump. This might be needed during emergencies or if the patient is passing through an airport metal detector. The pump might be detected by the weapon surveillance machine, but performance of the pump will not be affected.

INTRAVENTRICULAR SUBCUTANEOUS RESERVOIRS

Other implantable devices are available without a pump attached. Some examples of intraventricular access devices are the Ommaya and Rickham reservoirs. These allow repeated administration of medications (e.g., cytotoxic drugs) and sampling of cerebrospinal fluid (CSF) without the need for repeated lumbar punctures. The Ommaya reservoir (Figure 3B–6) is the most common intraventricular subcutaneous device used in cancer treatment. It is a mushroom-shaped, silicone domed device with a catheter attached. The dome provides easy external access while the catheter allows communication with CSF in the lateral ventricle.

The Ommaya is surgically inserted by the neurosurgeon in the operating room under general anesthesia and is usually placed in the nondominant frontal lobe over the coronal sutures. The reservoir is placed subcutaneously, and the catheter is positioned through a burr hole into the lateral ventricle. The dome of the reservoir rests between the scalp and the skull, creating a quarter-size bulge on the scalp. Skin sutures or staples are closely spaced. They are removed seven to ten days after placement. Correct placement is verified by a CT scan or magnetic resonance imaging (MRI). Flow studies are also often done.

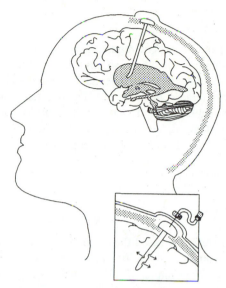

Figure 3B–6. Ommaya reservoir.

The Ommaya reservoir is used primarily in the treatment of meningeal carcinomatosis, the infiltration of the leptomeninges of the brain by cancer. Although these devices have been used for the administration of chemotherapy for brain tumors, lymphoma, cystic tumor drainage, ventricular drainage, special diagnostic studies, treatment of cancer pain, recurrent or chronic central nervous system (CNS) infections, and measuring CSF pressure, the reservoir is particularly useful for the management of recurrent CNS leukemia.

The reservoir has a self-sealing membrane that allows repeated punctures, thus facilitating the frequent administration of intraventricular chemotherapy and sampling of CSF. The most commonly reported chemotherapeutic agents administered by this route are methotrexate, cytarabine, and hydrocortisone. Investigational agents include diaziquone, mercaptopurine, thiotepa, topotecan, and mafosfamide. These drugs (except high-dose methotrexate) given systemically would not effectively cross the blood brain barrier to provide optimal therapy for the disease. In contrast to the administration of intrathecal chemotherapy, the use of the Ommaya for drug administration produces optimal consistent CSF levels, allows a decrease in dosage to achieve the same CSF level, enhances drug distribution, and facilitates the exploration of alternative administration schedules. An example of an alternative schedule is "concentration $\times$ time" (C $\times$ T). In this approach, multiple low doses of an agent are administered in order to achieve constant CSF levels and decrease the peak concentrations observed when larger doses are given. C $\times$ T increases the duration of exposure of malignant cells to the agent.

Assessment

Assessment of the patient requiring an Ommaya reservoir consists primarily of evaluating the patient's/family's understanding of the procedure, purpose, potential complications, and activities to avoid that may result in head injury (e.g., contact sports). Factors that should be addressed are presented in Table 3B–8. The patient's neurological status, level of consciousness, history of headaches, seizures, and any other problems; knowledge about drugs being administered; and need for teaching should be assessed first.

Management

After the operation to insert the Ommaya, the nurse must monitor the patient for any changes in neurological status and signs of increasing intracranial pressure (see Chapter 15A). The patient will return from the operating room with a pressure dressing in place. The dressing is monitored for integrity and signs of bleeding. If excessive drainage or bleeding is

Table 3B–8
Nursing Protocol for Management of Patient with Ommaya Reservoir

Problem	Intervention
Preoperative	
Patient's need for information	Evaluate ability to comprehend instructions. Discuss rationale, preparations needed. Teach care of surgical site. Instruct to report any signs of infection or changes in neurological status. Advise to prevent head trauma.
Postoperative	
Potential complications: Catheter malfunction	Assess patient for pain; assess ability to aspirate fluid from catheter, and for inflow obstruction. May necessitate catheter removal. A CT scan, x-ray, or flow study may be needed to verify placement.
Infection	Assess site for redness, irritation, swelling, or drainage. Assess for fever or neck stiffness. Culture may be needed if any symptoms are present.
Neurologic deficits	Assess for changes in mental alertness or behavior, seizures, headaches, or dizziness. Report any changes to the physician.
Side effects of drugs	These vary according to drug, dose, and schedule. Provide patient with information about side effects.

noted, notify the physician. After 24 hours, a 4x4 gauze dressing with paper tape is sufficient until the sutures or staples are removed.

The risk of infection, the primary complication of the Ommaya reservoir, remains relatively small. Antibiotics are often given prophylactically and for 72 hours following placement. The skin over the reservoir should remain intact. Notify the physician if skin integrity is compromised by breakdown or erythema. Strict adherence to the practice of sterile technique while accessing (or tapping) this device is essential and helps decrease the incidence of infection. Most infections can be successfully treated with antibiotics and do not require removal of the reservoir. Patient education should include preventive measures, such as care and observation of the surgical site.

Additional potential complications associated with Ommaya placement include malfunction, catheter migration, and displacement. These complications, though rare, do occur. The Ommaya is pumped by gently rolling an index finger over the reservoir. The reservoir should refill with CSF as the depressed area is released. If the reservoir is difficult to pump, does not refill, or is sluggish in refilling, it might be malfunctioning or displaced; notify the physician. Complications associated with unresolvable infection, catheter malfunction (e.g., migration, plugging), and malposition could necessitate removal and replacement of the device.

The reservoir can be used as early as 48–72 hours after the operation; however, the neurosurgeon should be consulted prior to accessing the reservoir for the first time after its insertion. In many institutions it is the physician who accesses the Ommaya. In some institutions, nurses who are certified can do it. The following is a suggested procedure for accessing intraventricular reservoirs.

Scalp Preparation

(If scalp over reservoir does not need to be shaved, proceed to "Accessing the Reservoir.")

Supplies
Sterile barrier
Sterile basin
Four 4x4 sterile gauze sponges
Sterile razor
Sterile water
Chlorhexidine (Hibiclens®)
Sterile gloves

Procedure
1. Explain procedure to patient.
2. Wash hands.
3. Guide patient into supine position; moisten or tape hair down away from reservoir to minimize area to be shaved.
4. Prepare work area by placing a sterile barrier on table. Place sterile basin, 4x4 gauze sponges, and razor on barrier. Pour sterile water

into basin. Pour small amount of chlorhexidine on three of the 4x4 gauzes. (The fourth will be used for drying.)

5. Don sterile gloves.
6. Dip gauzes with chlorhexidine into water and scrub scalp area and reservoir.
7. Carefully shave scalp over reservoir. Shave the smallest area necessary to provide sterile exposure.
8. Wipe off area with dry gauze.
9. Remove gloves.

Accessing the Reservoir

Supplies
Mask
2 pairs of sterile gloves
Lumbar puncture tray (pediatric or adult); adult tray contains manometer
Povidone-iodine
Chlorhexidine
Four 2x2 sterile gauze sponges
25 gauge butterfly needle
adhesive bandage
5 ml or 10 ml syringe for removal of CSF
Appropriate size syringe for medication
3 ml syringe for CSF flush
19 gauge needle (for drawing up medication)
Alcohol prep pad
Medication (make sure it is room temperature)
Paper tape (optional)

Procedure
1. Explain procedure to patient.
2. Wash hands.
3. Position patient. If patient has hair, expose reservoir by moistening or taping it down away from reservoir.
4. Pump reservoir 8 times to allow reservoir to fill.
5. Prepare lumbar puncture tray with povidone-iodine, chlorhexidine, syringes, butterfly needle, and sterile 2x2 gauze sponges.
6. Don mask and one sterile glove.
7. Cleanse medication vial with alcohol prep pad. Using sterile technique, draw up medication in appropriate size syringe based on volume of the drug. Remove all air bubbles from syringe and place on sterile field.
8. Don second glove. Remove needle from syringe with medication and cover syringe with a sterile 2x2.
9. Cleanse area over reservoir with chlorhexidine proceeding in a circular pattern from the center outward; repeat twice. Cleanse

area with povidone-iodine in similar manner; repeat twice. Allow to dry.

10. Change gloves and drape area.
11. Insert butterfly needle into reservoir.
    a. Measurement of CSF Pressure
       1. Allow butterfly tubing to fill with CSF. When filled, pinch tubing and connect manometer with stopcock.
       2. Position manometer at external auditory meatus.
       3. Allow manometer to fill. Once the flow has stabilized, measure ventricular pressure by reading the bottom of the meniscus.
       4. If specimens are needed, attach a syringe to the stopcock and collect samples.
       5. Turn stopcock to off position. Pinch tubing and remove manometer with stopcock.
       6. Proceed to medication instillation if needed or to step 12.
    b. Ventricular CSF Sampling (only)
       1. Pinch butterfly tubing and connect 5 ml syringe.
       2. Obtain specimens as ordered.
       3. Proceed to step 12. Reservoir does not need to be pumped.
    c. Medication Instillation
       1. Pinch off butterfly tubing and connect 5 ml or 10 ml syringe to tubing. Remove the volume of CSF equivalent to amount of medication volume instillation (withdraw at rate not exceeding 2 ml/min) and place on sterile field.
       2. Pinch off butterfly tubing, connect 3 ml syringe, and remove 1 ml of CSF to be used as a flush after medication. Cap syringe or cover with a 2x2 gauze sponge and place on sterile field.
       3. Pinch tubing and connect medication syringe. Slowly instill medication at a rate not exceeding 2 ml/min. Make sure there is no air in the tubing.
       4. Connect 3 ml syringe with CSF flush and instill slowly.
12. Remove needle from reservoir, cover area with sterile 2x2 gauze, and pump 8 times to distribute the medication in the ventricular CSF.
13. Cover with adhesive bandage.
14. Distribute CSF into specimen tubes. Label and send specimens as ordered.
15. Instruct the patient and family regarding indicated care.

After accessing the Ommaya, document the procedure in the patient's medical record. Include the patient's reaction to the procedure, patient's neurological status, medication(s) administered, specimens obtained, patient teaching, and any untoward reactions and interventions implemented.

EPIDURAL THERAPY

The use of the epidural route for administration of pain management in the cancer patient has increased dramatically over the past several years. Epidural access devices are placed primarily postoperatively in patients having thoracic surgery, limb salvage, or amputations and for patients who do not achieve effective pain relief with less invasive methods of administration. They are contraindicated in the management of patients with coagulopathy or increased intracranial pressure or patients receiving anticoagulation therapy.

Epidural access devices are placed between the vertebral column and the dura mater into the epidural space. The insertion site into the epidural space will determine the dermatomes affected and location of anticipated pain control. Medical decisions regarding epidural access include determining anticipated length of therapy, type of device, and site of catheter placement to achieve the desired outcome. Devices available for epidural administration include catheters or ports. Epidural catheters are very long and thin. They are used for short duration therapy and are removed no later than 72 hours after placement. In most cases the catheter has a filter in place. In many institutions epidural catheters are placed by the anesthesiologist or nurse anesthetist. Epidural ports are placed under general anesthesia. Currently there is no standard placement site for these ports; however, they are usually located on the lower rib cage or abdomen with the catheter threaded into the epidural space.

Advantages of this route of drug administration include the following: lower doses (approximately one-tenth usual opioid dose) with longer duration of action are needed to achieve effective relief of pain, steady drug levels can be achieved, local anesthetics can be utilized, and patients report less drowsiness. Disadvantages of this route of administration include increased cost due to placement, earlier development of tolerance, migration of catheter, and potential infection of exit site or epidural space leading to meningitis or epidural abscess. Pruritus and urinary retention might be more common in patients receiving analgesia via the epidural route than any other route of administration.

Agents administered through this route affect the opiate receptors of the spinal canal. Analgesics administered through this route are generally preservative free and include fentanyl, morphine, and/or long-acting anesthestics such as bupivacaine. Analgesics are administered either by continuous infusion or by intermittent dosing. The use of patient-controlled analgesic (PCA) adminstration is often employed. This gives the patient the ability to control the level of analgesic needed to effectively control his or her pain within the limits specified by the prescriber.

Assessment

The nurse should be familiar with the management of percutaneously placed epidural catheters and epidural ports. If the patient has more than one port, it is imperative to label the ports so as to minimize confusion between the one used for venous access and the one for epidural access.

During administration of analgesics through the epidural route it is important for patients to be assessed and monitored closely. Assessment parameters include determining location and level of insertion site, monitoring motor strength of all four extremeties, monitoring touch sensation (presence, absence, tingling, numbness) of the affected dermatome(s) including one dermatome above and below the insertion site, assessing pain control, assessing level of sedation, observing the exit site, and ensuring the catheter connections are secured.

Management

Nursing management includes preparing the patient for placement and care of the device. The patient must be educated about the type of device that will be placed, the anticipated length of therapy, potential problems associated with the device, and symptoms to report. Care depends on routines of each individual institution. Site care depends on the type of device placed. In general, patients with epidural catheters usually have large occlusive transparent dressing across the spinal column over the exit site to secure the catheter. This dressing is generally left in place until the catheter is removed because it is easy to dislodge the catheter when removing the dressing. Most catheters are then brought up over the shoulder and secured to facilitate easier access. All connections should be luer locked and checked. The exit site should be inspected for signs of infection or leakage. Epidural ports are accessed like venous SVADs using noncoring right angle needles. Epidural analgesics are generally administered through an ambulatory pump. The pump and tubing should be well marked to avoid confusion. Many companies manufacture tubing specifically for epidural administration that is color coded to decrease the potential for infusion errors.

INTRAPERITONEAL THERAPY

As a result of the successful use of implantable intraventricular and venous access devices for administration of cancer therapy, a similar need was noted for treating peritoneal tumors. An intraperitoneal catheter for therapy infusions with implanted or external access theoretically presents an advantage over IV therapy because higher concentrations of the agent can be delivered directly into the abdominal cavity. Only the cells in close contact (less than 2 cm) with the peritoneal fluid will be subject to the effects of this therapy. Clinical trials have focused on this method of drug administration in patients with minimal residual disease or who might benefit from adjuvant therapy.

Because most agents administered by this method are cleared directly by the liver, only low levels of the agent enter the systemic circulation. As a result, side effects are fewer.

The Tenckhoff catheter is an access device used by several treatment centers for peritoneal dialysis. Peritoneal SVADs that have a Tenckhoff type catheter attached have also been utilized for this type of therapy. Previously used for renal dialysis, the technique was adapted for intraperitoneal delivery of therapeutic agents in ovarian cancer, where the abdominal cavity is often a site of tumor involvement. It has also been used in colon cancer and gastric cancer, where the liver and peritoneal surfaces are often a major site of recurrence. Agents tested intraperitoneally (see Table 3B–9) include chemotherapeutic, biologic (i.e., IL-2, TNF), and radioactive agents. These devices are also used to drain fluid that accumulates and to obtain cytologic specimens.

Assessment

Assessment of the patient receiving intraperitoneal therapy includes evaluation of the need for information and for catheter monitoring. Assess the peritoneal VAD frequently to monitor patency and identify signs of infection. Variables to be evaluated are presented in Table 3B–10.

Management

Medical management includes placement of the Tenckhoff catheter or SVAD with a Tenckhoff catheter attached to the port, and close follow-up in case problems occur. Implantation customarily takes place under local anesthesia in an operating room because bowel perforation is a potential complication. When the catheter is properly placed in the peritoneal cavity, it is threaded subcutaneously to exit through a small incision about 5 to 7 cm from the initial incision. During healing, the cuff on the catheter causes proliferation of fibroblasts in the subcutaneous tunnel, creating a seal around the catheter and decreasing the possibility that infection will travel into the abdomen. Peritoneal SVADs do not exit the abdomen at an external site but are anchored subcutaneously with the attached catheter entering the abdominal cavity. They are generally placed in a subcutaneous pocket and secured to an area at the bottom of the rib cage. It is accessed like the venous SVADs using a noncoring right angle needle.

Nursing management consists of preventive measures against infection. Infection can occur around the exit site of a Tenckhoff catheter or within the peritoneal cavity. Patient education is essential because catheter function is directly related to how well the patient maintains it. The advantage of the implanted port device is that less external care is necessary. Sterile technique is observed in caring for the external Tenckhoff catheter

Table 3B–9
Agents Used for Intraperitoneal Therapy

	Agent	Dose Range (mg/m^2)
Ovarian cancer	Fluorouracil	845–2080
	Methotrexate	13.5–45
	Doxorubicin	10–50
	Melphalan	12–90
	Cytarabine	10–1000 umol
	Mitoxantrone	10–40
	Cisplatin	50–270
	Carboplatin	150–650
	Combinations:	
	Cisplatin + cytarabine + doxorubicin	
	Cisplatin + cytarabine + bleomycin	
	Cisplatin + bleomycin	
	Cisplatin + etoposide	
	Cisplatin + etoposide +thiosulfate	
	Cisplatin + doxorubicin + cyclophosphamide	
	Carboplatin + etoposide + GM-CSF	
	IP-32	
	Monoclonal antibodies, radiolabeled antibodies	
	Gamma interferon, alpha 2-b interferon	
	Autologous monocytes activated ex vivo	
Colon cancer	Fluorouracil	1 gm
	Fluorouracil + mitomycin	
Gastric cancer	Fluorouracil	1,040–1,539
	Melphalan	30–90
	Mitoxantrone	10–40
	Recombinant beta interferon	
	Combinations	
	Fluorouracil + cisplatin	
	FUDR + leucovorin	
	Mitomycin + cisplatin	
	Mitomycin + OK432	
Malignant Ascites	Recombinant IL-2	
	Recombinant TNF-alpha	
	LAK cells + IL-2	
	Streptozotocin	
	Liposomal MTP-PE activated autologous monocytes	

until the exit site is completely healed. The site should be completely healed about two to four weeks after insertion, and no redness or tenderness should be present. After the exit site has healed, the patient will perform a daily "clean" dressing change. The prescribed procedure for care follows; the patient must be able to demonstrate proficiency in this procedure.

Table 3B–10
Nursing Protocol for Management of Patients
with Intraperitoneal Catheters

Problem	Intervention
Preplacement	
Patient's ability to care for catheter	Evaluate patient's mental status and ability to comprehend instructions and report complications. Share this information with physician. Assess availability of family members to assist in catheter care.
Patient need for information	Discuss the procedure with the patient—why, how, expectations after insertion, care responsibilities, and potential problems. Teach patient to report signs of infection. These include fever, chills, pain, or discharge around the catheter.
Postplacement	
Potential complications	
Leakage of fluid	Leakage around the catheter is normal postoperatively because the seal is not tight until after 10–14 days. If leakage occurs during first 2 weeks, catheter dressing must be changed frequently to prevent infection.
Catheter malfunction	Assess the patient for pain with dialysis or problem with drainage. May need to irrigate catheter forcefully with 50 ml normal saline using sterile technique to remove blockage.
Infection	Evaluate the characteristics of the dialysis fluid: It will be bloody initially but should become clear. If the fluid becomes cloudy, or pain, redness, irritation, or drainage occurs around the exit site, peritoneal fluid and exit site should be cultured.
Respiratory distress	If the patient has problems taking deep breaths when the dialysate is in the abdomen, the volume might need to be decreased.
Pain	Pain postoperatively is to be expected, and analgesics should be administered for relief. Pain caused by cold dialysate can be relieved by warming the fluid prior to administration. Pain caused by intraperitoneal infection is also accompanied by fever. Cultures should be obtained to determine the presence of an infectious organism. Pain related to the therapeutic agents is hard to distinguish from pain caused by infection. It is related to agent, dose, and schedule. Analgesics should be administered for relief once a bacterial source has been ruled out. Several agents cause abdominal adhesions that can also be painful.

Special points: Aseptic technique is to be maintained when caring for the Tenckhoff catheter. Any entry into the catheter requires a thorough cleansing of the port with povidone-iodine in order to minimize the risk of infection.

Supplies (often available as a kit)
one sterile barrier disposable towel
10 packages sterile 4x4 in. gauze pads (2/package)
one package sterile applicators (2/package)
povidone-iodine solution
one package povidone-iodine ointment
hydrogen peroxide
roll of 2-inch paper tape
sterile gloves

Procedure
1. Explain procedure to patient.
2. Wash hands.
3. Open sterile barrier towel and place sterile 4x4 gauze pads on sterile field, in three separate piles: one pile with eight 4x4s, two piles with six 4x4s each.
4. Pour povidone-iodine solution on the eight 4x4s and hydrogen peroxide on six 4x4s. Open and place applicators on barrier. Squeeze povidone-iodine ointment on barrier.
5. Remove old dressings and then put on sterile gloves.
6. Hold distal end of Tenckhoff catheter in nondominant hand with one 4x4 gauze saturated with povidone-iodine (continue to hold catheter while cleansing suture line and exit site).
7. Wash area directly surrounding catheter exit site with hydrogen peroxide saturated 4x4s (until sutures are removed and area is healed). Repeat twice. Note any signs of infection, erythema, exudate, or tenderness.
8. Scrub abdominal area with povidone-iodine saturated 4x4s. Use a circular motion, working from the catheter exit site outwards. Repeat twice.
9. Hold catheter by cap with povidone-iodine saturated 4x4 pad. Clean cap using rotating motion. Cleanse entire length of the exposed catheter with povidone-iodine-saturated 4x4s. Work from the catheter exit site to the catheter cap using a gentle rotating motion. Repeat twice.
10. Apply povidone-iodine ointment around catheter exit site with applicator.
11. Redress with sterile 4x4 pads. Place one on abdomen under the catheter. Two additional 4x4s are applied, overlapping, to completely cover catheter and exit site. Secure with paper tape.
12. Secure the catheter to the abdomen to prevent dislodgement.

Tenckhoff Catheter Care

Any time the dressing is opened to permit catheter connection or disconnection from the dialysis set, sterile technique is used; that is, sterile gloves are worn and the connector site is cleaned with povidone-iodine. This procedure is essential because it is very easy to introduce bacteria through the lumen of the catheter if precautions are not taken.

When the site is healed, the patient can do the daily dressing changes using clean, instead of sterile, technique. This requires good handwashing because gloves are not needed. Povidone-iodine swabsticks should be used to clean the site and catheter. This decreases the special attention the patient must devote to the catheter, without increasing the risk of infection.

If an implantable SVAD is used for peritoneal access, less care is required because no external catheter is present. However, access still requires careful cleansing of the needle insertion site to prevent peritonitis. Risk of infection appears to be lower with an implantable port, but other disadvantages might exist.

Nurses play a critical role in managing the care of patients receiving intraperitoneal therapy. They are responsible for managing catheter sterility, administering and managing the dialysis treatments, and teaching patients to manage catheters independently.

INTRACAVITARY MANAGEMENT OF PLEURAL EFFUSIONS

Like the intraperitoneal administration of drugs, intracavitary injection of agents can be used to prevent the reaccumulation of a pleural effusion. A *pleural effusion* is an accumulation of fluid in the pleural space that can interfere with pulmonary and cardiovascular function. Causes include congestive heart failure, pneumonia, malignancy, late complication of progressive cancer, or other pathologic conditions. Cancers most frequently associated with malignant effusions are breast, lung, gastrointestinal, and ovarian cancers; lymphoma; and leukemia. Malignant effusions can result from primary disease infiltration or metastasis.

A thoracentesis can help establish the diagnosis of malignant effusion (Table 3B–11), if pleural fluid removed during the procedure is analyzed. Thoracentesis alone, either by needle or by placement of a chest tube, cannot prevent reaccumulation of fluid. It does, however, help achieve the primary treatment goal, relief of respiratory symptoms, by permitting greater lung expansion and making breathing easier. Reaccumulation of fluid is generally the result of metastatic infiltration and can directly compromise the patient's quality of life. Management of metastatic pleural effusions is primarily supportive, with little chance of cure.

Systemic chemotherapy can be effective in controlling malignant effusions if the primary disease is responsive to these treatments. Like the intraperitoneal administration of drugs, intracavitary injection of agents can be used to prevent reaccumulation of fluid caused by metastatic effusions.

Table 3B-11
Findings of Thoracentesis Fluid

Test	Findings
Gross appearance	Exudate or transudate could signal malignancy but is also associated with other causes such as TB, pneumonia, and congestive heart failure.
RBC count	Grossly bloody fluid is suggestive of malignancy ($>$100,000 RBC/mm^3).
Total WBC count	Usually 4,000 cells/mm^3, but malignant pleural effusions have relatively low numbers of WBCs.
Differential WBC count	Lymphocytes predominate in a malignant pleural effusion. Predominance of neutrophils may be indicative of an inflammatory reaction.
Cytology	Positive in 60% of the effusions caused by malignancy.
Glucose	In 15% of malignant effusions, this is $<$60 mg/100 ml.
Amylase	Can be elevated with malignancy, pancreatitis, and esophageal rupture.
Fluid culture	Can indicate infection.
CEA	$>$12 ng/ml suggestive of malignancy.
Absolute cell count	A cellular pleural fluid indicates obstruction. 50–1,000 cells/mm^3 indicates serosal surface tumor. 1,000–4,000 cells/mm^3 indicates free-growing tumor.

CEA—carcinoembryonic antigen; TB—tuberculosis; RBC—red blood cell; WBC—white blood cell.

This is achieved through thoracentesis. The effectiveness of the treatment depends primarily on the agent's ability to sclerose (cause irritation and adhesions to) the pleural tissue, rather than on its antineoplastic activity. Agents commonly used are shown in Table 3B–12. In general, dosage is the same as for drugs administered systemically; however, the toxicities are less. Other treatment options for pleural effusions include radiation and pleurectomy. Radiation might be helpful for some pleural effusions, but pneumonitis is a risk. Because pleurectomy is a surgical procedure, it is associated with greater risks of morbidity and mortality.

Assessment

The nurse's assessment of the changes in the patient's clinical condition alerts the physician to the potential need for a thoracentesis to relieve

Table 3B–12
Sclerosing Agents for the Pleural Cavity

Class	Agent
Antineoplastic agents	Bleomycin
	Dactinomycin
	Doxorubicin
	Fluorouracil
	Mitomycin
Antimicrobial agents	Doxycycline
	Minocycline
Colloidal radioisotopes	Radiogold colloid
	Radioactive phosphorus
Other	Talc

symptoms. Factors to be considered in the care of patients undergoing thoracentesis are presented in Table 3B–13.

Management

Nursing management of a patient undergoing a thoracentesis is primarily supportive. During the procedure, which lasts approximately 15 to 30 minutes, a needle is inserted into the pleural space under a local anesthetic. Fluid is removed, and a sclerosing agent is injected if necessary. Evaluation of pre- and post-treatment respiratory symptoms is essential to measuring effectiveness of the drug injection as well as potential complications associated with thoracentesis (e.g., pneumothorax). A chest x-ray is taken after the thoracentesis is completed. The nurse should monitor the patient's pulse, respirations, and blood pressure. The patient might feel some soreness at the puncture site but should not experience any difficulty in breathing. Frequent thoracentesis might be necessary, depending on the cause of the effusion, effectiveness of the drug in sclerosing the cavity, and patient tolerance to fluid buildup.

If the drug is to be instilled via chest tube, hospitalization is necessary. The chest tube is inserted under water seal and the effusion evacuated. Pain medication might be necessary before the sclerosing agent is instilled. The chest tube is then clamped and the patient instructed to rotate through several positions to ensure maximum contact between the pleural surfaces and the sclerosing agent. The tube is then unclamped and drainage from the pleural space maintained for several days before the tube is removed. Instillation of the sclerosing agent can be repeated. Effectiveness of the treatment can be monitored by assessment of symptom relief, as well as by chest x-ray.

Table 3B–13
Nursing Protocol for Patients Undergoing Thoracentesis

Problem	Intervention
Pretreatment Symptoms indicating a pleural effusion	Evaluate patient for symptoms of pleural effusion: increasing dyspnea, minimal or absent breath sounds, fatigue with exercise or minimal exertion, dull aching or pleuritic chest pain. Report these findings to the physician.
Patient's need for information	Discuss throracentesis with the patient. Instruct patient regarding need to remain still during procedure. Children might need to be sedated. Explain post-treatment expectations: A small pressure dressing will be applied; a chest x-ray will be done and vital signs monitored. Explain to the patient that soreness at the puncture site can occur. Instruct patient to report any breathing difficulty to the nurse. If sclerosing agent is to be used, explain that a drug injection will be administered through the needle. If drug is to be instilled via chest tube, explain nature and purpose of the procedure: that a tube will be inserted into the chest cavity and will remain in place for several days. Explain that body position needs to be changed frequently to ensure maximum contact of sclerosing agent with pleural surfaces. Explain that eventually the tube will be unclamped and drainage will be maintained for several days. Pain medication might be required.
Post-Treatment Potential complications	Assess the patient for symptoms of pneumothorax: cyanosis, dyspnea, chest pain, tachycardia, tachypnea, respiratory compromise.
Response to Treatment	Pain secondary to thoracentesis or presence of chest tube may require medication for relief. Evaluate patient for decrease or recurrence of symptoms of a pleural effusion. Frequency of thoracentesis depends on cause of effusion, effectiveness of the drug in sclerosing the cavity, and patient tolerance of fluid accumulation.

CONCLUSION

Numerous advances have been made in the delivery of cancer therapy. It is imperative that nurses keep abreast of the changes in the care and management of the variety of venous and other access devices available. Continued research is needed to determine the optimal flushing techniques, dressing materials, and frequency for dressing changes. The nurse plays a critical role in educating patients and families about access devices and management.

BIBLIOGRAPHY

1. Baird, S., R. McCorkle, and M. Grant. *Cancer Nursing: A Comprehensive Textbook.* W. B. Saunders Co., Philadelphia. 1996.

   This is an excellent comprehensive reference book for the oncology nurse. Delivery of cancer chemotherapy chapter addresses preparation, handling, and administration of therapy. Types of drug delivery methods are described.

2. Blaney, S., F. Balis, and D. Poplack. Pharmacologic approaches to the treatment of meningeal malignancy. *Oncology* 5(5): 107–115. 1991.

   Meningeal disease and progress of treatment approaches (intralumbar, intraventricular, and systemic administration of medications) are briefly discussed. Current medications being utilized and/or studied for the treatment of meningeal disease are reviewed.

3. Brown, J. Peripherally inserted central catheters—use in home care. *Journal of Intravenous Nursing* 12(3, May/June): 144–148. 1989.

   This reviews the historical development of intravenous catheters, components of a training program for placement, catheter selection, and clinical experience. An insertion procedure and quality assurance data collection tool are included.

4. Camp-Sorrell, D. (ed). Advances in access devices for chemotherapy and pain management. *Seminars in Oncology Nursing* 11(3): 153–227. 1995.

   This entire issue provides a comprehensive review of VADs. Topics include comparison of VADs, selection of VADs and nursing care, management of infection and occlusion associated with VADs, rare complications of VADS, arterial, peritoneal, and intraventricular access devices, the use of access devices in cancer pain control, ambulatory infusion pumps: application to oncology, and patient education and compliance issues.

5. Dorr, R. Antidotes to vesicant chemotherapy extravasations. *Blood Rev* 4(March): 41–60. 1990.

   This summary article covers potentially dangerous vesicants, clinical case reports, and discussion of antidote testing results.

6. Huk, I., P. Entsheff, M. Prager, F. Schulz, L. Polterauer, and J. Furovics. Patency rates of implantable devices during long term intra-arterial chemotherapy. *Angiology—The Journal of Vascular Diseases* 41(November): 936–941. 1990.

   In this review, 64 intra-arterial catheter systems are compared to evaluate function and complication rate. Complications and infection rates were better for the implanted device when compared with an external catheter.

7. Kemeny, M. Continuous hepatic artery infusion (CHAI) as treatment of liver metastases. Are the complications worth it? *Drug Safety* 6(May/June): 159–165. 1991.

   This article discusses complications of this mode of therapy administration. Comparisons are made of the complications, toxicity, and effects of intra-arterial and systemic therapy for colorectal cancers.

8. Markman, M. *Regional Antineoplastic Drug Delivery in the Management of Malignant Diagnosis*. The Johns Hopkins University Press, Baltimore. 1991.

   A brief synopsis is given of types of regional antineoplastic drug delivery technique, including intra-arterial, intraperitoneal, intravesical, intrathecal, and other methods to treat malignancy.

9. Oncology Nursing Society. *Access Device Guidelines: Recommendations for Nursing Practice and Education*. Oncology Nursing Press, Pittsburgh, 1996.

   These guidelines present information on the use and care of various access devices. Developed by oncology nurse experts, they also provide standards for nursing education.

10. Oncology Nursing Society. *Cancer Chemotherapy Guidelines and Recommendations for Practice*. Oncology Nursing Press, Pittsburgh, 1996.

    Also developed by oncology nurse experts, these guidelines contain information regarding content for basic chemotherapy courses as well as information related to administration of cancer chemotherapy.

11. Schlag, P. Regional chemotherapy: Different operative techniques and clinical results. *Cancer Treatment Reviews* 17(November): 177–182. 1990.

    This summarizes principal considerations for regional chemotherapy and how to access specific treatment sites. It describes potential techniques and methods.

12. Sundaresan, N., and N. Suite. Optimal use of the Ommaya reservoir in clinical oncology. *Oncology* 3(12): 15–20. 1989.

    This article reviews concepts related to Ommaya reservoir and administration.

13. VanGroeningen, C. J. New technical developments in antineoplastic drug delivery and their role in cancer treatment. In Domellof, L., ed. *Drug Delivery in Cancer Treatment*. Springer-Verlag, New York. 1987.

    This presents external and implantable devices for infusion of cancer therapy.

14. Wickham, R. Advances in venous access devices and nursing management strategies. *Nurs Clin North Am* 25(June): 345–364. 1990.

    Information concerning nontunneled catheters, tunneled catheters, and venous access ports is reviewed. It provides a review of various catheter-related complications (infection, catheter occlusion, catheter thrombosis, extravasation, and catheter damage).

4

Principles of Clinical Research

Susan A. DiStasio
Susan Molloy Hubbard

INTRODUCTION

Oncology has emerged as an important area of clinical specialization over the past three decades, largely because of the success of clinical research in identifying effective cancer treatments. Whereas cancer clinical research investigates the use of radiation therapy, biological agents, surgical intervention, and mechanical devices, this chapter focuses on chemotherapy clinical research. Other trials not discussed here include cancer prevention and control, detection, and diagnosis, as well as the psychological impact of the disease and quality of life perspectives. Included is a discussion of the history of cancer clinical trials, the role of the nurse in study implementation, ethical considerations, and available resources.

CANCER TREATMENT STUDIES

Drug Development

The drug development process begins with the identification of a compound with observed or potential antitumor activity. When identified, the compound is subjected to careful scrutiny for antitumor activity in experimental tumor systems. This screening process permits scientists to narrow the number of compounds to be tested. At the conclusion of the screening, the compound's potential ability to retard the growth of cancer cells is assessed. If the drug demonstrates activity, it is considered a potential candidate for clinical trials.

When its biologic activity is established, the test compound must undergo the second preclinical step in development: purification and formulation. During this process, the compound is refined, its chemical structure is identified, and it is formulated so that it can be administered. The refined material is tested in rodents and large animals in an attempt to identify a starting dose that is not likely to produce toxicity to normal tissue in humans. After a starting dose for humans is estimated and acute and chronic side effects in animals established, an application for approval for use in patients with cancer is made to the U.S. Food and Drug Administration (FDA). The compound can then be used in clinical trials.

Clinical Trials

A clinical trial is a research study designed to answer a question that has therapeutic implications for patients. It is an experiment performed in a clinical setting rather than in a research laboratory. Although a clinical trial does not always produce a definitive answer, it should always yield data that are biologically valid and ethically sound. A sound clinical trial depends on a clear definition of the research question, a clear description of the data that support the hypothesis, and a research protocol that incorporates clinical and laboratory data on all of the biologic variables known to be important. Unlike laboratory research, in which experimental variables can often be precisely manipulated, conditions in clinical research are not so easily controlled. Patients, families, scheduling, transportation, finances, and various psychosocial factors complicate clinical research, requiring cooperation by many members of the health care team.

There are a variety of clinical trial designs. An *open-label study* is one in which both study participant and study personnel know what is being administered. Generally, data collected from this type of design are compared with that collected from a control group in which a conventional form of therapy has been used. A blinded study is one in which the participants are unaware of whether they are in the treatment group or the control group, and care must be taken to be sure that conditions for the two groups are as similar as possible. A *double-blinded study* is one in which neither the participants or study personnel know who is in the treatment or control group. The majority of trials include some form of *randomization,* which means that participants are randomly assigned to treatment groups, which allows for differences to be spread across treatment groups. The goal of randomization is to prevent systematic bias that can lead to one treatment group receiving more favorable or significantly different conditions during the treatment, which confounds the data and makes interpretation of results difficult.

Phase I Trials

Clinical trials are classified according to phases determined by their major objectives (Table 4–1). The Phase I trial, the initial phase of clinical investigation, represents the first time that a new treatment is evaluated in cancer patients. The goals of the Phase I study are to establish a maximum tolerated dose, to define toxicity to normal tissues, and to determine an optimal dosage and schedule for future clinical trials. Phase I studies are also

Table 4–1
Phases of Clinical Trials

Study Phase	Goals
I	a. Establish maximum tolerated dose b. Define toxicity to normal tissue c. Determine optimal dosage and schedule for future trials d. Obtain pharmacokinetic data on human absorption, bioavailability, metabolism, and excretion
II	a. Determine antitumor activity in specific cancers b. Evaluate toxicity further c. Estimate response rates
III	a. Compare to standard treatment b. Determine response rate and duration c. Continue toxicity evaluation
IV	a. Evaluate value of regimen as adjuvant therapy

designed to obtain pharmacokinetic data on human absorption, bioavailability, metabolism, and excretion.

Most cancer patients considered eligible for Phase I trials have little or no chance of deriving significant benefit from other established forms of treatment. These patients generally have cancers that are known to be unresponsive to current therapeutic modalities or that have progressed while receiving conventional therapy. The probability of obtaining a beneficial response to a new treatment during a Phase I clinical trial is difficult to estimate. The primary objective of the Phase I trial is the establishment of a safe dose of the new agent, not the identification of antitumor activity. Often the optimal dosage and schedule for administration of the new therapy are unknown, and in the interest of patient safety, the initial dosages are often well below the therapeutic dose range. This issue is an ethical concern for research nurses because patients who participate in this phase of research often do so on the assumption that they will derive some therapeutic benefit, though in reality the probability that this will occur is small.

The identification of any evidence of antitumor activity in a Phase I trial represents an important observation. It is important to emphasize that the lack of observable objective responses during Phase I trials does not necessarily mean that the treatment will not demonstrate antitumor activity in subsequent clinical trials, when an optimal dose and schedule are established. The absence of objective responses in this phase is not a sufficient reason to disqualify the agent under investigation from further trials. The only reason for not advancing a new antitumor agent or therapeutic approach to Phase II is the presence of unacceptable toxicity to normal tissues.

Phase II Trials

Phase II clinical trials are designed to evaluate the new drug or treatment program, employing a dosage and schedule established as safe during Phase I studies. The goals of Phase II trials are to determine a response rate in a statistically measurable number of patients with specific types of cancer or stage of disease and to determine the spectrum of antitumor activity by evaluating the new agent in a broad range of common cancers (Table 4–1). Several Phase II drugs or treatments can also be studied concurrently, so that results can be compared, thus allowing identification of more effective treatments.

For results to be scientifically and ethically sound, the number of patients with a specific tumor type fully evaluable at the end of Phase II studies must be sufficient to establish a response rate (or lack of response) with statistical confidence. Therefore, patients being considered for Phase II protocols must be carefully evaluated for eligibility. If the criteria are not carefully observed and treatment or follow-up is not properly performed, the clinical trial will fail to generate meaningful data about therapeutic efficacy. An important responsibility of the nurse is to inform the principal investigator of any concerns about patient eligibility and/or protocol violations.

Phase III Trials

In Phase III clinical trials, the major focus is on the attainment of complete responses. In these studies, a new agent or treatment approach that has demonstrated significant antitumor activity in Phase II studies is compared with standard or conventional form of treatment (see Table 4–1). Phase III trials are designed to determine response rate in a specific cancer as well as the duration of complete and partial responses that can be achieved with the new treatment. Patients are randomly allocated to one of the treatment groups to prevent the investigators from introducing bias into the selection of therapy. To ensure comparability between treatments, only newly diagnosed; previously untreated patients are generally considered eligible. For such clinical trials to be ethical, the investigational treatment must be promising enough to justify administering it to some patients instead of a treatment of known efficacy, and the protocol design must be adequate to compare the two therapies definitively. Therefore, the clinical protocol must be carefully constructed to ensure that patient eligibility is clearly defined, that there are enough patients in each treatment group, and that there is *stratification* of patients by all known important prognostic variables. Stratification is a means of assigning patients to treatment groups. It yields groups that are comparable because the characteristics of the individuals in each group are similar. Objective criteria to determine complete and partial responses and disease progression must be clearly established. In addition, the period of treatment and follow-up must be adequate to allow meaningful comparisons of overall therapeutic efficacy and toxicity.

Phase IV Trials

In Phase IV, the final phase of clinical investigation, new treatments that have proven effective in producing complete remissions in patients with advanced cancers are integrated into multimodal therapies for patients with cancers that appear to be localized at the time of diagnosis but are known to have a significant incidence of recurrence after apparently curative surgery or radiation therapy. These clinical trials are commonly known as *studies of adjuvant therapy*. Because all patients are clinically free of disease when adjuvant therapy is instituted and a certain, albeit unknown, fraction are already cured and do not need the adjuvant treatment, the prevention of treatment-related morbidity and documentation of all long-term complications are especially important, so that a complete assessment of the risk of potential morbidity can be made.

NURSING IN CLINICAL RESEARCH

Overview

The role of the nurse in oncology clinical research was one of the first that emphasized active collaboration in research. This expanded role developed at research centers in the beginning of the 1970s during early clinical trials to evaluate the therapeutic potential of drugs in the treatment of advanced cancer. It has grown as the curative potential of modern cancer treatments has become widely appreciated and applied in the medical community, stimulating the need for skilled nurses who share responsibility for the safe administration of investigational cancer treatments. For the first time, the nurse is considered an integral member of the primary research team, rather than a member of the ancillary support staff. In this capacity, nurses participate in patient-care rounds and conferences that enable them to learn about the biology of cancer, the natural history of the cancers under investigation, the special needs of the cancer research patient, and the fundamentals of clinical research. This allows the nurse to participate actively in clinical research and incorporates nursing considerations into research protocols. By assuming major responsibilities for the collection, analysis, and publication of research data, oncology nurses have become coinvestigators in clinical trials.

The role of the clinical research nurse has provided many nurses with the skills to design, perform, and evaluate clinical research and to perform independent studies. Nurses conduct clinical research to evaluate the efficacy of nursing interventions in dealing with the special needs demanded by new treatment approaches, and they have initiated clinical studies to assess the impact of innovative nursing care on the incidence and severity of disease and treatment-related morbidity. Areas of research include quality of life, long-term sequelae, psychosocial aspects, and decision-making skills. Many of these nursing studies have been conducted in conjunction with protocols of medical treatment regimens.

Nursing Roles

The roles enacted by nurses in clinical research can be divided into two major categories: those that emphasize the provision of direct patient care and those that emphasize improving care through research and conducting safe, effective clinical trials. The responsibilities and concerns of each role are complementary and should be combined to serve the care needs of the research patient. Because research is conducted in a variety of settings—including community hospital, comprehensive cancer centers, inpatient units, outpatient clinics, and physician offices—the role of the nurse can vary. In some settings, the staff nurse provides direct patient care, the research nurse is responsible for eligibility and protocol adherence, and a data manager provides data collection services. In other settings, such as the physician office, the staff nurse might be responsible for all of these activities. The role of the nurse throughout study implementation is summarized in the following sections.

Study Initiation and Eligibility

Before the clinical study is started, the research team—consisting of principal investigator, research nurse, data manager, primary nurse, advanced practice nurse, and anyone else involved in the study—should meet to review specific details of the protocol. Responsibilities are clearly delineated at this meeting. Impact on nursing resources should be evaluated prior to study initiation. For example, staffing changes might be necessary for a protocol that requires hourly vital signs in the outpatient setting. The principal investigator and research nurse might present an inservice education program to the appropriate staff involved in patient care. This presentation includes discussion of the scientific background, purpose, treatment plan, potential toxicities, study endpoints, and patient care implications. Research nurses often design a protocol summary (Table 4–2), which provides a quick, one-page description of the study. Documentation sheets (Figure 4–1) could be designed to assist nursing staff in collecting clinical information or scheduling and implementing

Table 4-2
Elements of a Protocol Summary Sheet

Protocol Title and Number
Study Phase and Objectives
Eligibility Requirements
Treatment Plan
Dose Modifications/ Retreatment Criteria
Expected Toxicities
Patient Care Considerations
Name and contact numbers for study personnel

Phase 1 Study of Drugs Z and Q in Patients with Advanced Malignancies: IRB # 7341
DAY 1   DOSE LEVEL: _____

Patient Name: _____   Actual Dose: _____

Unit Number: _____   Date: _____

Drug Z given at _____ (time)

COLLECTION TIME	ACTUAL TIME	BLOOD SAMPLE RED TOP TUBE	R.N. INITIALS
Before Drug Z **BASELINE**		5 cc	
Before Drug Q time = 30 min post Drug Z		5 cc	
End Drug Q infusion time = 1 hr & 30 min post Drug Z		5 cc	
2 hrs post Drug Z		5 cc	
4 hrs post Drug Z		5 cc	
6 hrs post Drug Z		5 cc	
12 hrs post Drug Z		5 cc	
24 hrs post Drug Z		5 cc	

RN initials and signature _____

RN initials and signature _____

Figure 4-1. Example of pharmacokinetic documentation sheet designed by clinical trials nurse and staff nurse.

protocol specific activities such as frequent vital signs or collection of specimens for pharmacokinetic studies.

When a potential study participant is identified, the physician initiates a discussion of the study background, risks and benefits, and alternatives available for the patient. A consent form is given to the patient for further details and review by other family members. The research nurse meets with the patient to discuss details of the protocol further and initiate determination of eligibility for the study. The research nurse coordinates prestudy testing with the patient/family. Final eligibility is reviewed by the physician prior to the registration of the patient on study. Many centers require central office registration to ensure that eligibility is met prior to study initiation.

Treatment

Following the exact specifications of the protocol cannot be emphasized enough. Violations can result in removal of the patient from the study or determination that the patient is unevaluable and that the data collected cannot be used in the final study analysis. Even worse, patients are exposed to unnecessary or life-threatening results. Although the principal investigator and research nurse are responsible for assuring protocol compliance, everyone involved in the patient's care should review the prescribed regimen before administering treatment. Unlike known chemotherapeutic agents, staff might not be familiar with doses for investigational drugs. All prescribed doses should be compared directly with the written research protocol. Many institutions utilize standard printed order sheets or computerized orders to decrease the likelihood of error. Retreatment criteria and dose modifications must be checked for each new cycle.

Documentation in research studies is essential. All disease- and treatment-related effects should be recorded in the patient's medical record as they occur and summarized on what is commonly called a *flow sheet* (Figure 4–2). Flow sheets concisely summarize the data on drugs administered and on therapeutic response and toxicity. Entries requiring a more detailed description or comment can be numbered and explained in the designated area. A human figure might be included so that clinical data, such as location of malignant lesions, can be illustrated if appropriate. Fluctuations in hematological and biochemical parameters, diagnostic studies, specific tumor markers, and performance status are easily assessed, as are the rate of response, remission duration, and time to maximal response. Important data can be extracted readily from the flow sheet and computerized to permit rapid analysis, thus facilitating the early recognition of important trends. Clinical research nurses together with staff nurses and advanced practice nurses play a major role in the development and enhancement of these flow sheets.

Toxicities

A major concern of the clinical research nurse is the early recognition and management of expected and unexpected side effects, representing acute, delayed, or cumulative toxicity. Accurate and detailed documentation of observations by the nurse are critical to the patient's welfare and constitute a major contribution to the quality of the clinical trial.

Nursing responsibilities include physical assessment of patients, documentation of objective and subjective changes in clinical parameters of response and/or progression, and documentation of normal tissue tolerance and drug toxicity. Documentation of toxicities should include the start and stop dates, severity, treatment, and response and should be complete and quantified. For example, "experienced four to six loose stools and mild abdominal cramping on 2/13 and 2/14; denies blood in stool; did not wake him at night; resolved on its own without treatment." Every symptom should be documented in this manner, even if it is felt to be unrelated to the investigational agent. Toxicities are graded on a 0- to 4-point scale. Examples of the National Cancer Institute's Common Toxicity Criteria are described in Table 4–3.

Serious adverse events that are life-threatening, initiate or prolong a hospitalization, or are unexpected require reporting to the principal investigator for notification to the responsible sponsoring agency, FDA, and institutional review board. Consent form revisions might be necessary for the addition of newly discovered toxicities. The nurse can help to maximize the impact of a therapeutic response by teaching the patient how to minimize or prevent treatment complications. Reduction of avoidable toxicity can ensure that therapeutic benefit will not be lost because of unnecessary treatment delays.

Response

Response to treatment is established as being either evaluable or measurable as defined in the individual protocol. Disease is measured at baseline, prior to initiating protocol treatment and at designated time periods throughout the treatment. Standardized criteria for therapeutic responses are described in Table 4–4.

Follow-Up

During this period of post-treatment observation, the nurse's concerns shift from the management of acute nursing care problems to health care

Patient's Name _____

Coordinating Group Protocol No. _____

Hospital Number _____

Protocol No. _____

Coordinating Group Patient Seq. No. _____

Institution/Affiliate _____

Patient Sequence No. _____

Page _____

Ht _____ cm   BSA _____

(REMARKS: R_1, R_2, R_3, etc. and date)

PROTOCOL TREATMENT	Date 19__ (mo./day)								
	Cycle/day								
	RECORD ACTUAL DOSE; IF MODIFIED OR NOT GIVEN, EXPLAIN								
OTHER THERAPY	Radiation (cGy/cum to date)								
	Transfusions								
	Analgesics								
	Antiemetics								
	Antibiotics								
PATIENT STATUS	Performance Status/Weight (kg)								
	Temperature								
	Blood Pressure								
	CIRCLE REACTIONS DUE TO PROTOCOL TREATMENT								
(Grade 0–5 CTC)**	Hemorrhage (clinical)								
	Infection								
	Fever in Absence of Infection								
	GU, SPECIFY								
	Nausea/Vomiting								
	Diarrhea								
	Stomatitis								
	Other GI, SPECIFY								

NORMAL LB VALUES
THESE VALUES MUST BE COMPLETED

Plt (x 1000)	(nl	to)
HGB (gms%)	(nl	to)
HCT (%)	(nl	to)
BUN (mg%)	(nl	to)
Creat. (mg%)	(nl	to)
Biliburbin (mg%)	(nl	to)
SGOT (units)	(nl	to)
SGPT (units)	(nl	to)
Alk. Ptase. (units)	(nl	to)
LDH (units)	(nl	to)

Investigator Signature _____ Date _____

TOXICITIES
- Liver (clinical)
- Pulmonary
- Cardiac, SPECIFY
- Skin
- Allergy
- Phlebitis
- Local (other than Phlebitis)
- Alopecia
- Neuro Sensory, SPECIFY
- Neuro Motor, SPECIFY
- Neuro Psychiatric, SPECIFY
- Neuro Clinical, SPECIFY
- Metabolic, SPECIFY

LABORATORY VALUES

REFER TO PROTOCOL PARAMETERS—
PROVIDE NORMALS IN THE ADJACENT TABLE

- WBC (x 1000)
- Granulocytes (%)/Bands (%)
- Lymphocytes (%)
- Platelets (x 1000)
- HBG (gms%)/HCT (%)
- BUN/Creatinine (mg%)
- Proteinuria/Hemturia
- Bilirubin (mg%)
- SGOT/SGPT (units)
- ALK. Ptase. (units)
- LDH (units)
- Ca/PO_4
- Uric Acid

OTHER
- Chest X-ray
- Bone Scan
- CT Scan, SPECIFY

*ECOG—Eastern Cooperative Oncology Group
**CTC—common toxicity criteria

Figure 4-2. ECOG* common toxicity criteria flow sheet.

Table 4–3
NCI Common Toxicity Criteria

			Grade		
Toxicity	0	1	2	3	4
Blood/Bone Marrow					
WBC	≥4.0	3.0–3.9	2.0–2.9	1.0–1.9	<1.0
PLT	WNL	75.0–Normal	50.0–74.9	25.0–49.9	<25.0
Hgb	WNL	10.0–Normal	8.0–10.0	6.5–7.9	<6.5
Granulocytes/Bands	≥2.0	1.5–1.9	1.0–1.4	0.5–0.9	<0.5
Lymphocytes	≥2.0	1.5–1.9	1.0–1.4	0.5–0.9	<0.5
Hemorrhage (clinical)	None	Mild, no transfusion	Gross, 1–2 units transfusion/episode	Gross, 3–4 units transfusion/episode	Massive, >4 units transfusion/episode
Infection	None	Mild Fever during leukopenia No organism recovered	Moderate Localized infection (e.g., cystitis pneumonia)	Severe Bacteremia	Life-threatening Septic shock
Gastrointestinal					
Nausea	None	Able to eat reasonable intake	Intake significantly ↓ but can eat	No significant intake	—
Vomiting	None	1 episode in 24 hrs	2–5 episodes in 24 hrs	6–10 episodes in 24 hrs	>10 episodes in 24 hrs or requiring parenteral support
Diarrhea	None	↑ of 2–3 stools/d over pre-Rx	↑ of 4–6 stools/d or nocturnal stools or moderate cramping	↑ of 7–9 stools/d incontinence or severe cramping	↑ of ≥10 stools/d or grossly bloody diarrhea or need of parenteral support
Stomatitis	None	Painless ulcers erythema or mild soreness	Painful erythema, edema, or ulcers but can eat	Painful erythema, edema, or ulcers & cannot eat	Requires parenteral or enteral support
Liver					
Bilirubin	WNL	—	<1.5 × N	1.5–3.0 × N	>3.0 × N
Transaminase (SGOT, SGPT)	WNL	≤2.5 × N	2.6–5.0 × N	5.1 × 20.0 × N	>20.0 × N

Table 4-3 (Continued)
NCI Common Toxicity Criteria

	Toxicity	0	1	2	3	4
				Grade		
Liver	Alk. Phos. or 5′ nucleotidase	WNL	$\leq 2.5 \times N$	$2.6–5.0 \times N$	$5.1–20.0 \times N$	$>20.0 \times N$
	Liver Clinical	No changes from baseline	—	—	Precoma	Hepatic Coma
	Local	None	Pain	Pain & swelling with inflammation or phlebitis	Ulceration	Plastic surgery indicated
	Weight gain/loss	<5.0%	5.0–9.9%	10.0–19.9%	$\geq 20.0\%$	—
	Fatigue/malaise (non-treatment days)	None	Occasional naps or early to bed, able carry on usual ADL or work full-time	Requires planned rest periods, bedrest 3–6 hrs. of waking hrs., unable to work full-time	Bedrest >6 hrs. of waking hrs. dyspnea on exertion, difficulty concentrating, disinterest in ADL, unable to work, maintains only basic care needs	Withdrawn, Unable to care for self
	Flu-like Symptoms in absence of infection	None	Mild, low back pain, myalgias or chills, no treatment required	Transient shaking chills (rigors), backpain, myalgias, tolerable with acetometaphen	Severe rigors, myalgias or arthralgias requiring narcotic analgesics or bedrest >4 hrs. on treatment days	Intractable discomfort
	Pain	None	Mild pain controlled by non-narcotics	Moderate pain, occasional po narcotics as needed	Severe pain requiring daily narcotics	Intractable pain, IV narcotics required
Metabolic	Hyperglycemia	<116	116–160	161–250	251–500	>500 or ketoacidosis
	Hypoglycemia	>64	55–64	40–54	30–39	<30
	Amylase	WNL	$<1.5 \times N$	$1.5–2.0 \times N$	$2.1–5.0 \times N$	$>5.1 \times N$
	Hypercalcemia	<10.6	10.6–11.5	11.6–12.5	12.6–13.5	≥ 13.5
	Hypocalcemia	>8.4	8.4–7.8	7.7–7.0	6.9–6.1	≤ 6.0
	Hypomagnesemia	>1.4	1.4–1.2	1.1–0.9	0.8–0.6	≤ 0.5

Continued

Table 4-3 *(Continued)*
NCI Common Toxicity Criteria

Toxicity	0	Grade			
		1	2	3	4
Fibrinogen	WNL	0.99–0.75 × N	0.74–0.50 × N	0.49–0.25 × N	≤0.21 × N
Prothrombin time	WNL	1.01–1.25 × N	1.26–1.50 × N	1.51–2.00 × N	>2.00 × N
Partial thrombo-plastin time	WNL	1.01–1.66 × N	1.67–2.33 × N	2.34–3.00 × N	>3.00 × N

(left margin label: Coagulation)

Table 4-4
Standardized Criteria For Therapeutic Responses

Response	Description
Complete remission (CR)	a. Complete regression of all evidence of cancer by every criterion (physical, radiological, biochemical) b. Return to normal performance status c. All residual symptomatic abnormalities must be related to side effects of therapy d. Duration of complete remission must exceed one month
Partial remission (PR)	a. Objective regression of 50 percent of all measurable tumor b. Subjective improvement c. Duration of partial remission is expressed in months d. Appearance of any new lesion or increase in size of residual lesions terminates the remission
Minor response (MR)	a. Objective tumor regression of 25 percent to 50 percent b. Subjective improvement
No response (NR)	a. No objective change in the tumor mass is seen or the response represents less than 25 percent regression b. No significant subjective improvement is seen
Progression (P)	a. Documented growth of measurable disease b. Appearance of any new disease

maintenance and from delineation of acute toxicity to the identification of chronic or long-term complications of treatment.

Apprehension and anxiety about treatment failure can become a major psychological problem for patients in prolonged adjuvant treatment programs. Compliance with an extended course of adjuvant chemotherapy when there is no evidence of disease can often be difficult. If nurses recognize this as a potential problem, they can assist patients in dealing with any ambivalence about treatment and making necessary adaptations in their lifestyle. In these situations, education must be reinforced with reassurance, encouragement, and support to help patients reestablish a sense of control.

Data Management

Data management responsibilities include accurate collection and submission of research data. The clinical research nurse or a trained clinical research associate can do this. In many instances, this includes the coordination of data for patients treated in several institutions, by different teams of physicians and nurses. Data are collected from such source documentation as hospital medical records, clinic and physician office records, and home care charts. These data are then entered onto a case report form, which can be abstracted for the development of research abstracts, publications, or presentations. Audits are performed by sponsoring agencies for the purpose of verification of the case report form data in comparison with source documentation. It is helpful for all members of the research team to participate in the audit summary.

ETHICAL CONSIDERATIONS FOR NURSES IN CLINICAL RESEARCH

Overview

Because ethical considerations are the foundation of every clinical trial, certain general issues must be considered by all nurses and physicians involved in research. Balancing the need for better cancer treatment and the requirements of a specific individual is crucial to a sound clinical trial. Furthermore, it is essential to differentiate between an individual's human rights and his or her personal needs. Protection of rights is essential, even when the needs of each individual cannot be completely met. Nurses in the research setting can provide invaluable assistance in ensuring that these rights are protected in clinical trials.

Components of a Protocol

To be ethical, every clinical trial must ask a question of significant scientific and humanitarian value. Moreover, the need for the therapeutic experiment must justify the risk of discomfort or harm to study subjects. To ensure that this need exists, each research protocol must clearly articulate the scientific rationale, the ratio of potential benefits to risks, the safeguards to be used to protect subjects from injury, and specific information about the proper execution of the study. The components of a research protocol are as follows:

1. Clear statement of the research question and the study objectives;
2. Clear description of scientific data supporting the specific research question to be tested;
3. Explicit criteria for eligibility and exclusion of patients;
4. Information regarding the activity and administration of the study agent;
5. The treatment plan, including randomization scheme and stratification variables;
6. Dose and schedule information: specific details about the dose, schedule, route, timing, and duration of each drug or treatment modality that is to be administered; dose-modification schedules specified by type of tissue toxicity (e.g., bone marrow depression, gastrointestinal toxicity, neurotoxicity);
7. Evaluation criteria: description of all parameters to be evaluated for response and/or disease progression; definition of criteria for complete and partial response, stabilization, disease progression, and treatment failure; criteria for evaluation of performance status (Karnofsky rating or other scale);
8. Research parameters to be evaluated, with intervals clearly specified; clinical parameters; laboratory studies; diagnostic examinations (e.g., x-rays, radionuclide scans, CAT);
9. Statistical methods utilized to evaluate study objectives;
10. Criteria for study termination;
11. Data collection requirements;
12. Informed consent document;
13. Proof of review and approval by an institutional review board established for the protection of human subjects participating in research. The qualifications and membership of this review board are established by federal regulation.

Nurses involved in clinical research assume major responsibilities for ensuring that these requirements are met and that any special requirements for nursing care and patient education are incorporated into the protocol during the design of the clinical trial.

Informed Consent and Patient Education

Another ethical concern is informed consent. In the United States, informed consent, obtained without coercion, is a legal prerequisite for participation of human subjects in clinical trials. Although legal responsibility for obtaining the informed consent rests with the primary physician, it is a moral responsibility shared by all members of the research team (see Chapter 6A). Moreover, each research patient must be adequately informed about the investigational nature of the clinical trial, because personal benefit cannot be guaranteed.

Because informed consent must continue in order to be valid, it is an ongoing process. Therefore, the nurse's ethical responsibilities in clinical research must be considered within the framework of patient education. At the outset of any educational program, the nurse should assess the nature of the patient's previous health care experiences, identify exactly what the patient knows, what the patient thinks that he or she needs to know or learn, and his or her level of anxiety. Only by identifying the patient's perceived needs can the nurse plan an educational program that will involve the patient in the learning process.

Education about any therapy should include information about immediate and long-term benefits as well as the adverse effects. By developing materials that explain why certain procedures and treatments will be used, the nurse can assist patients to become informed, active participants in the treatment process. Staff nurses have devised booklets, each of which describes a diagnostic test, its discomforts and/or side effects, and why it is needed to plan or evaluate therapy. When procedures are proposed, patients receive the appropriate booklets in time to review them, formulate questions, and discuss the procedure with the nurse prior to giving written consent. Information cards on cytotoxic chemotherapy and booklets on the indications for and care of vascular access devices are also frequently provided to patients. Use of these tools permits nurses to clarify information as needed and to ensure that the patient's consent is informed and voluntary.

RESOURCES

Clinical trial information is available to the public and health professional community through a variety of sources. Chapter 6B of this book describes several resource groups available to the patient and oncology nurses. Many of these groups offer specific clinical trial information. In addition, organizations such as the Oncology Nursing Society and cooperative groups provide an opportunity for networking among clinical trial nurses through special interest groups. These groups offer national and international networking and collaboration on important projects such as a development of a standards manual, newsletter publications, and the development of presentations specific to clinical trials.

The National Cancer Institute (NCI) sponsors a Cancer Information Service accessible by calling (800) 4-CANCER. Information provided includes general cancer information and specific clinical trial descriptions. More than 1,500 protocols are described in detail in the Physician's Data Query (PDQ). Health professionals can request a specific search by calling (800) 345-3300. Information can be mailed or faxed upon request.

The Internet offers an enormous amount of information about health care, including cancer clinical trials. The NCI is collaborating with advocacy groups as well as cooperative groups to provide lay-oriented information about cancer clinical trials to patients and the public on the World Wide Web. To view the CancerNet™ and the Clinical Trials home page, use the URL http//cancernet.nih.gov. Select "patient and public" to access clinical trial information. Selecting "Health Professionals" provides a direct link to the full PDQ protocol descriptions. Many cancer centers, advocacy groups, and cooperative groups provide clinical trial information on their own Web site. With the availability of computers at local libraries, work, schools, and in homes, the Internet offers another way for patients to search for information about their specific cancer and available studies.

BIBLIOGRAPHY

1. Benoliel, J. Q. The historical development of cancer nursing research in the United States. *Cancer Nurs* (August): 261–268. 1983.

   This article traces the development of cancer nursing research from the start of the 20th century to the publication date. It describes the growth of nursing research in general and specifically as a function of the development of oncology nursing as a specialty.

2. Cassidy, J., and D. Macfarlane. The role of the nurse in clinical cancer research. *Cancer Nursing* 14(3): 124–131. 1991.

   This is an overview of the role of the nurse in clinical trials expanding in detail the administrative aspects, adherence to protocol guidelines, research records, and audits.

3. Cassidy, J. The role of the data manager in clinical cancer research. *Cancer Nursing* 16(2): 131–138. 1993.

   This article discusses the qualifications, duties and responsibilities, data collection, audits, and maintenance of records for data managers.

4. Cox, K., and M. Avis. Psychosocial aspects of participation in early anticancer drug trials. *Cancer Nursing*. 19(3): 177–186. 1996.

   This is a pilot study of seven patients as they progressed through an anticancer drug trial. Informed consent process, decision making, and impact of participation on the lives of the patients are explored. Provides valuable insights into the process of informed consent and experience of trial participation.

5. DiGiulio, P., C. Arrigo, H. Gall, C. Molin, R. Nieweg, and B. Strohbuker. Expanding the role of the nurse in clinical trials: The nursing summaries. *Cancer Nursing* 19(5): 343–347. 1996.

Description of a nursing summary of the medical protocol that provides short and easy-to-read selection of protocol-relevant information highlight this selection. It enables nurses to safely and more easily implement the research protocol and improve the care of patients in clinical trials.

6. Fall-Dickson, J. M. Clinical trials and research in the community. *Semin Oncol Nurs* 9(1) (February): 38–43. 1993.

This article reviews requirements for the establishment of a successful community-based clinical research program and discusses the role and responsibilities of the nurse serving as protocol coordinator.

7. Fischer, D., S. Alfano, T. Knobf, C. Donovan, and N. Beaulieu. Improving cancer chemotherapy use process. *Journal of Clinical Oncology* (December) 14(12): 3148–3155. 1996.

This includes review of the practices/policies of chemotherapy use and recommendations for changes in policy/practice to prevent errors. Includes a section on special considerations for investigational drug use.

8. Fischer, D. S., M. T. Knobf, and H. J. Durivage. *The Cancer Chemotherapy Handbook, 5th Ed.* Mosby, St. Louis. 1997.

This practical handbook includes brief descriptions of currently used chemotherapeutic agents in tabular form. Each drug is explained according to its mechanism of action, indications, metabolism, dose and route of administration, toxicity, preparation, and storage. Also provided are sections on management of common side effects.

9. Frank-Stromborg, M. *Instruments for Clinical Nursing Research.* Appleton & Lange, Norwalk, CT. 1988.

This book provides a review of instruments used in clinical nursing research. It presents evaluations by subject, such as cancer attitudes, pain, skin integrity, quality of life, and coping. The material is useful to nurse researchers who are developing their own tools to measure clinical phenomena or who wish to utilize already tested instruments.

10. Gross, J. Clinical research in cancer chemotherapy. *Oncol Nurs Forum* 13(1): 59–65. 1986.

This review article describes drug development from preclinical screening and testing to clinical studies in humans. It includes a brief overview of the statistical considerations for each phase of clinical investigation, as well as the responsibilities of the nurse in this type of research.

11. Hill, M. and E. Schron. Opportunities for nurse researchers in clinical trials. *Nursing Research.* (March/April) 41(2): 114–115. 1992.

This article describes ancillary, data-based substudies that can be conducted within clinical trials.

12. McCabe, M. S., C. G. Varricchio, and R. M. Padberg. Efforts to recruit the economically disadvantaged to national clinical trials. *Semin Oncol Nurs* (May) 10(2): 123–129. 1994.

This describes the efforts of the National Cancer Institute to identify barriers to patient participation in clinical trials, and recruitment efforts targeted toward minority and impoverished patients are discussed.

13. McCabe, M. S., J. A. Piemme, eds. Cancer clinical trials. *Semin Oncol Nurs* (November) 7(4). 1991.

This entire issue is devoted to a review of cancer clinical research, both medical and nursing. Articles by nursing leaders in oncology include a historical review of clinical trials, programs sponsored by the National Cancer Institute and others, issues of concern in planning and implementing clinical trials, a review of nursing companion studies, and reviews of the various roles and responsibilities of nurses involved in clinical research.

14. Oncology Nursing Society. *Standards of Oncology Nursing Practice, 1996; Standards of Oncology Education: Patient/Family and Public, 1995; Standards of Advanced Practice in Oncology Nursing, 1997; Cancer Chemotherapy Guidelines, 1996.* Oncology Nursing Press, Pittsburgh, PA.

These publications include professional practice and performance standards for oncology nurses at various skill levels, guidelines for patient and family education, and guidelines and recommendations for chemotherapy administration. All of these publications were developed and reviewed by nursing experts in cancer care.

15. Tabak, Nili. Decision making in consenting to experimental cancer therapy. *Cancer Nursing* 18(2): 89–96. 1995.

Review of the decision-making process, criteria for valid decision making, and decision-making patterns are explored. Studied the decision making process of 23 end-stage cancer patients, 23 patients suffering peripheral arterial occlusion disease (requiring leg amputation versus experimental therapy), and 23 patients receiving conventional treatment for immunological disorders as well as implications for practice are discussed.

16. White-Hershey, D., and B. Nevidjon. Fundamentals for oncology nurse/data managers: Preparing for a new role. *Oncol Nurs Forum* 17(3): 371–377. 1992.

This article describes the role of the oncology nurse as data manager, which includes activities such as data collection, patient education, and communication. It provides information for both the nurse acting as data manager and the nurse caring for patients participating in clinical trials.

UNIT

II

COMMON CLINICAL PROBLEMS

Chapter 5 Prevention and Early Detection		**5**
Chapter 6 Information and Resources		**6**
A. Information		**6A**
B. Resources		**6B**
Chapter 7 Coping		**7**
Chapter 8 Comfort		**8**
A. Pain		**8A**
B. Sleep		**8B**
C. Fatigue		**8C**
Chapter 9 Nutrition		**9**
Chapter 10 Protective Mechanisms		**10**
A. Bone Marrow		**10A**
B. Mucous Membranes		**10B**
C. Skin		**10C**
Chapter 11 Neurologic Complications		**11**
Chapter 12 Elimination		**12**
A. Anatomical Alterations		**12A**
B. Functional Alterations: Bowel		**12B**
C. Functional Alterations: Bladder		**12C**
Chapter 13 Sexuality		**13**
Chapter 14 Pulmonary Function		**14**

5

Prevention and Early Detection

Bonny Libbey Johnson

INTRODUCTION

Prevention and early detection are two distinct but related approaches to reducing the morbidity and mortality of cancer. Whether any disease can be *prevented* depends upon the degree of knowledge about and control over the cause, as well as upon adequate access to the population at risk. *Early detection* is of paramount importance when the cause is not known or cannot be controlled and when the course of disease can be altered by early treatment, during an asymptomatic state. Therefore, programs for prevention and early detection are designed for populations or persons at risk for the disease or those who have it but do not yet show symptoms.

CONCEPTUAL CONSIDERATIONS

The principal role of the nurse as a provider of information in the prevention and early detection of cancer requires a basic understanding of the etiology and epidemiology of the disease. In addition, an understanding of the motivations for individual health-seeking behaviors and of the appropriate and available health care services will ensure effective management.

The concept of disease prevention has been classified according to three levels, focusing on the maintenance of health rather than the cure of disease. These levels are described as follows:

- *Primary prevention.* In primary prevention, risk of cancer is reduced or eliminated by avoidance of causative agents (e.g., cigarettes) or by removal of target organ (e.g., rectal polyps).
- *Secondary prevention.* In secondary prevention, the natural course of disease is favorably altered by early detection and effective and prompt treatment (e.g., breast self-examination).
- *Tertiary prevention.* In tertiary prevention, the morbidity of cancer is reduced by prompt and effective antitumor treatment, symptom control, and rehabilitation.

The focus of this chapter is on primary and secondary prevention. The remaining chapters of this handbook describe the nursing component of tertiary prevention.

EPIDEMIOLOGIC CONSIDERATIONS

Current American Cancer Society (ACS) statistics for the incidence of cancer by site are shown in Table 5–1. These data come from the Surveillance, Epidemiology, and End Results (SEER) Program of the National Cancer Institute (NCI), and the National Cancer Data Base. The National Cancer Data Base was organized by the American College of Surgeons Commission on Cancer and is funded by the American Cancer Society. Such statistics are important for determining the prevailing tumor types to target for public education and screening programs and also show changes in incidence, which could reflect alterations in lifestyles or changes in environmental factors related to cancer causation.

On the basis of what is currently known or suspected to cause cancer in the United States and the overall incidence of specific tumor types, it is estimated that up to 80 percent of the cancers are associated with environmental factors. The influence of these factors on the incidence of cancer is reflected in Figure 5–1. The death rate from cancer continues to rise each

Table 5–1
Estimated New Cases and Deaths for Major Sites of Cancer—1998

Site	Number of Cases	Deaths
Lung	171,500	160,100
Colon/rectum	107,000	58,200
Breast	180,300	43,900
Prostate	184,500	39,200
Urinary	86,300	24,700
Uterus	49,800	11,200
Skin (melanoma)	41,600	7,300
Oral	30,300	8,000
Pancreas	29,000	28,900
Leukemia	28,700	21,600
Ovary	25,400	14,500

Adapted with permission from Landis, S. H., T. Murray, S. Bolden, and P. A. Wingo. Cancer Statistics: 1998. *CA: A Cancer Journal for Clinicians*. 48(1): 10–11. 1998.

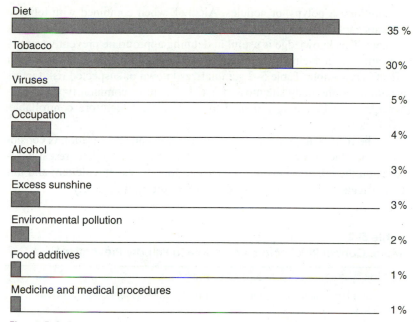

Figure 5-1. Percentage* of cancer cases attributable to various risk factors.

*Average of varying estimates available from the literature. Adapted from Office of Cancer Communications. Cancer Prevention: A Program to Inform the Public About Cancer Risk and Risk Reduction. National Cancer Institute, Bethesda, MD. January 1984.

year, primarily because of the impact of lung cancer; it is estimated that if lung cancer deaths were excluded, males would show no increase in cancer mortality, and the rate for women would decrease.

Recent SEER data demonstrate a high variability in cancer incidence and mortality rates among different racial and ethnic groups in the United States. African American men have the highest incidence of cancer (most frequently prostate, lung, and colon/rectum), and the highest mortality rates for these cancers. Among women, African American, Alaska natives, and Caucasians have approximately equal death rates for all cancers. The contributions of specific risk factors, such as smoking, obesity, diet, and poverty (inadequate or inaccessible medical care) require further research, as these health problems are correlated with specific racial and ethnic groups.

PREVENTION CONSIDERATIONS

Certain of these factors are defined as either initiators or promoters (see Chapter 1). An *initiator*, such as cigarette smoke or radiation, causes irreversible cellular damage and potential malignant change. A *promotor* is believed to stimulate initiated cells to proliferate in focal collections such as papillomas, polyps, or nodules. Alcohol, when combined with tobacco use, appears to be such a promoting factor in the causation of head/neck cancers. This knowledge is useful in defining appropriate preventive strategies aimed at reducing or eliminating exposure to promoters, because their effect is reversible. Table 5–2 summarizes known or suspected risk factors according to the body site most affected. The most common types of cancer appear to be strongly related to external, and therefore controllable, risk factors.

The role of *dietary deficiency or excess* in cancer causation is considered a risk factor for about 35 percent of all cancers. To date, research focuses on the relationship among high-fat, low-fiber diet; calcium; and micronutrients such as vitamins A, C, and E in preventing cancer.

Table 5–2
Major Cancer Risk Factors Amenable to Primary Prevention*

Factor	Site of Cancer
Diet: fat; fiber; vitamins A and C	Oral cavity, pharynx, esophagus, colon/rectum
Tobacco	Lung, oral cavity, pharynx, larynx, esophagus, kidney, bladder
Viruses	
Hepatitis B	Liver
Epstein-Barr	Nose/throat, Burkitt's lymphoma
Herpes simplex II	Cervix
Occupational hazards	
Asbestos	Lung
Chromate	Lung
Nickel, uranium	Lung
Alcohol	Oral cavity, pharynx, larynx, esophagus, liver, pancreas, colon/rectum, stomach, breast (suspected), melanoma (suspected)
Radiation	
↑ dose	Leukemia, thyroid, lung, breast, stomach, bone, liver
↓ dose (ultraviolet light, x-rays)	Skin, site exposed to x-rays (dental, chest x-rays)
Estrogens	Uterine (especially endometrium), cervix
Premalignant conditions	
Cervical dysplasia	Cervix
Rectal polyps	Colon/rectum
Leukoplakia	Skin, oropharynx, bladder

*In order of suspected or known degree of risk.

The excessive use of *alcohol* is associated with an increased risk for cancers of the head and neck, esophagus, and liver, and possibly breast and rectal cancers. Alcohol is believed to act as a promotor in causing cancer, enhancing, in particular, the carcinogenic effect of smoking.

According to the U.S. Public Health Service, the use of *tobacco* in our society is responsible for 85 percent of lung cancer cases and is implicated in cancers of the head and neck, esophagus, pancreas, bladder, and kidney, as well. Cigarettes account for 30 percent of all cancer deaths, or approximately 170,000 people per year. Although a slight decline in the number of adult smokers is evident, 25 percent to 30 percent of the U.S. adult population smokes and, according to the U.S. Office on Smoking and Health, smokes heavily. The risk for smoking-related cancer increases with number of years smoking, number of cigarettes, and depth of inhalation. Changing to low-tar/nicotine cigarettes appears to reduce the risk for cancer only slightly. The synergistic carcinogenic effect of cigarettes and alcohol, radiation, or occupational agents (e.g., asbestos) compounds the risk.

Study of the potential positive effect of *physical activity* in preventing cancer is currently underway. Of interest are studies that show that the incidence of colon cancer is lower among people who are occupationally active, and that physical inactivity might increase the risk for breast cancer.

Viruses are associated with several types of cancer: primary hepatocellular carcinoma, Burkitt's lymphoma, nasopharyngeal carcinoma, Hodgkin's disease, Kaposi's sarcoma, cancers of the cervix and genital organs, leukemia, and lymphoma. The strength of the association between the virus and the cancer varies among tumor types. The presence of certain cofactors (e.g., aflatoxin, alcohol, infection) might be necessary for cancer to result. For example, the hepatitis B virus in human serum is believed to precede and lead to a high incidence of hepatocellular carcinoma; this association becomes even stronger when aflatoxin or chronic alcohol intake is a factor.

The Epstein-Barr virus (EBV), a DNA virus of the herpes group, infects B lymphocytes and, perhaps due to a genetic defect, can progress to Burkitt's lymphoma, Hodgkin's disease, or nasopharyngeal carcinoma. EBV is endemic in Africa, where the incidence of related tumors is high.

The infectious etiology for cervical cancer is believed to involve more than one viral agent. Herpes simplex virus II and cytomegalovirus are two agents that show a strong association with cervical cancer. Both can be transmitted by sexual contact.

Estrogens have been reported to induce neoplasms when used (1) as replacement therapy after menopause (endometrial cancer); (2) for oral contraception (rare benign liver tumors); and (3) to prevent threatened abortion (clear cell adenocarcinoma of the vagina and cervix in daughters of women who took estrogen during pregnancy). Of particular note is the synthetic estrogen, diethylstilbestrol (DES), which was used for both (1) and (3). The benefit derived from the therapeutic use of estrogens must be weighed against each person's risk for developing cancer. Because the risk appears to be directly related to the dose of drug and duration of therapy, shorter courses with low doses of estrogen might be recommended. (A detailed discussion of *chemical* and *radiation* carcinogenesis is provided in Chapter 1. Table 5–8 incorporates these risk factors into a program of prevention.)

Genetic predisposition to cancer is a growing field. The ongoing Human Genome Project is an effort to completely map the human DNA molecule and, in its course, will aid in the discovery of new genes associated with cancer. Two new genes, the BRCA1 and BRCA2 genes, have demonstrated an association with breast cancer, though they account for only 5 percent of cases. Familial aggregations of cancer suggest the role of inherited susceptibility but might also point to shared environmental exposure.

CHEMOPREVENTION

Chemoprevention refers to the use of chemical agents to prevent, reverse, or delay the carcinogenesis process. Because the vast majority of cancers arise from external causes (e.g., diet, environment, tobacco) in the initiator/promotor model of carcinogenesis, it is theorized that chemicals might be useful in disabling the initiated cells from progressing to a malignant form when exposed to a promotor or in preventing the promotor from acting on the initiated cell(s). Chemopreventive agents such as the carotenoids appear to act as inhibitors of both initiation and promotion in the laboratory. Other agents under investigation include selenium, vitamin E (alpha-tocopherol), vitamin C (ascorbic acid), and molybdenum. Because the target population for chemoprevention trials is composed of persons deemed to be at risk for cancer but with no sign of disease, agents to be used in clinical trials must demonstrate little or no toxicity, be acceptable for continuous administration, and be feasible for a group requiring follow-up for a long period of time. Table 5–3 describes chemopreventive agents currently under investigation.

CONSIDERATIONS IN EARLY DETECTION

The concept of early detection can be applied in two ways: on an individual basis for a person at risk for specific reasons or as the basis for mass screening of a population at risk. In either case, the underlying assumption is that the smaller the tumor is when diagnosed, the better the chance for effective treatment.

The early detection of cancers relies on two conditions: The existence of a premalignant, or detectable preclinical phase (DPCP), and the availability of appropriate tests that can detect the tumor during the preclinical phase.

Table 5–3
Agents Currently Used in Chemoprevention Trials

Agent	Site(s)	Rationale
The retinoids 13-cis-retinoic acid Isotretinoin All-trans-retinoic acid Retinamide	Head/neck Leukoplakia (head/neck cancer); lung Acute promyelocytic leukemia Myelodysplastic syndrome	Vitamin A deficiency has been associated with the formation of precancerous lesions; retinoids influence cell differentiation and proliferation.
Tamoxifen	Breast	Tamoxifen is known to be effective in reducing new breast cancer primaries and prolonging survival of women with breast cancer; it is well tolerated and has added estrogen-like benefits on bone density and lipids.
Finasteride	Prostate	Finasteride might decrease androgen stimulation of the prostate gland; it decreases prostate volume and urinary flow; it is well tolerated.
Aspirin	Colon, rectum	Aspirin interferes with prostaglandin activity and cell proliferation and boosts immune system; it is well tolerated, inexpensive, and has added benefits.

In theory, cancers progress from a low to a high degree of anaplasia with metastatic potential (see Chapter 1). If a specific cancer demonstrates a defined, prolonged premalignant state, the chance for early detection and cure is maximized. The time during which a premalignant or malignant tumor exists prior to the onset of symptoms, or the DPCP, must be sufficient to allow purposeful diagnostic intervention. In addition to available tests, there must be treatments that will alter the course of disease even before symptoms occur.

Tests for early detection of cancer are judged according to their sensitivity and specificity for a particular tumor type. Briefly stated, test *sensitivity* is reflected by the percentage of people who test positive for the disease in question; test *specificity* refers to the percentage of people who are without the disease and test negative. Sensitivity and specificity are closely interrelated concepts. For example, a test that has a 100 percent sensitivity is capable of detecting everyone who has the disease in question with no false positives. A test that is 100 percent specific will be negative for

Table 5–4
Major Cancer Risk Factors Amenable to Secondary Prevention

Factor	Cancer
Endocrinopathies	
Infertility	Endometrium
Obesity	Breast, endometrium
Diabetes	Breast, endometrium
Family history of cancer	Lung, breast, thyroid
Nulliparity or late first pregnancy	Breast
Preexisting disease	
Xeroderma pigmentosum	Skin
Breast fibrocystic disease	Breast
Ulcerative colitis	Colon
Bloom's syndrome	Leukemia
Fanconi's syndrome	Leukemia
Mongolism	Leukemia

everyone without the disease (no false negatives). In tests that are neither 100 percent sensitive nor 100 percent specific, the results are affected by (1) the test itself and (2) the way it is applied and interpreted. In addition to a high degree of sensitivity and specificity, the optimal screening test for early detection is convenient for most people, comfortable, low-cost, and without side effects. For any program to be well received, a system must be established for immediate reporting of results and for follow-up.

Whereas preventive programs are based on controllable risk factors, individual programs for early detection target those who are at risk because of both controllable and uncontrollable factors. Examples of uncontrollable risk factors and associated tumors are listed in Table 5–4.

ASSESSMENT

Prevention

An understanding of risk factors for cancer allows the nurse to focus a preventive approach on those factors that a person can decrease exposure to or avoid. This knowledge is combined with an assessment of the psychologic and environmental factors that guide each person's health-related behaviors. Rosenstock's Health Belief Model provides a useful framework to assess a person's risk for cancer and his or her ability to alter that risk by changing behavior. Briefly, the model states that a person's health behaviors are governed by (1) knowledge of personal susceptibility to an illness (e.g., knowledge of risk factors), (2) perception that the risk is severe, and (3) belief that any behavior will positively alter that risk.

These personal factors are acted upon by such external or environmental factors as (1) accessibility/availability of health care service, (2) family/peer support, (3) cost of service, and (4) logistical concerns (time, transportation, work schedule).

Despite the knowledge that lifestyle changes could result in a significant decrease in cancer incidence and mortality, the majority of Americans continue to use tobacco, eat a high-fat diet, and shun regular exercise. It is reasonable to surmise that lack of knowledge about specific risk factors and a sense that "there is not much a person can do to prevent cancer" contribute to an inability or unwillingness of people to adopt a healthier lifestyle. Experience of tobacco control in the United States demonstrates the importance of combining strategies from the community, media, and public policy to affect societal norms and values and change behaviors. Similar approaches are underway to target dietary and exercise behaviors. In 1990, a consortium led by the Department of Health and Human Services established national health goals titled *Healthy People 2000: National Health Promotion and Disease Prevention Objectives*. Its objectives relate to (1) reducing the incidence of specific cancers believed to be amenable to lifestyle behaviors; (2) changing specific behaviors, such as smoking, dietary fat intake, and sun exposure; and (3) increasing health care availability and accessibility.

In summary, assessment of the person's ability to benefit from a primary prevention or risk-reduction program must include the following:

1. Knowledge base of risk factors;
2. Attitude toward cancer;
3. Knowledge of risk reduction techniques;
4. Motivation for change.

Early Detection

Assessment is an integral part of any program of secondary prevention. Only when an adequate baseline assessment reveals specific risk factors can an appropriate plan be made for ongoing diagnostic examination.

On an individual basis, the standard history and physical examination provides a comprehensive format for early detection of cancer. Emphasis is placed on the following areas:

1. History
   A. Family: family history of cancer;
   B. Social: cigarettes, alcohol use, sexual history;
   C. Occupational: exposure to chemicals, radiation, inhalants;
   D. Medical: previous malignancy;
   E. Medications: hormone replacement (DES), cytotoxic agents.

2. Review of systems
  A. Pulmonary: cough, pain, dyspnea, hemoptysis;
  B. Gastrointestinal: change in bowel habits, bleeding;
  C. Breast: nipple discharge, masses;
  D. Gynecological: vaginal discharge, dyspareunia, unusual bleeding;
  E. Skin: slow-healing sore, changing mole;
  F. Oropharynx: hoarseness for more than one week, abnormal bleeding, pain.
3. Physical examination
  A. Lymphadenopathy;
  B. Suspicious moles;
  C. Breast mass;
  D. Prostatic enlargement;
  E. Thyroid mass;
  F. Oral leukoplakia.

Of note is an increased risk for second tumors recognized in persons with cancer (Table 5–5). Awareness of this risk can assist those who conduct the physical examination. Table 5–6 presents a summary of data de-

Table 5–5
Summary of Second Cancers Following Initial Cancer

Sex	Initial Cancer	Second Cancer
Female	Breast	Buccal cavity
		Pharynx
		Breast
		Lung
		Ovary
		Corpus uteri
		Leukemia
	Cervix	Buccal cavity
		Pharynx
		Lung
		Bladder
Male	Lip and mouth	Buccal cavity
		Skin
		Lung
		Pharynx
	Pharynx	Esophagus
		Lung
		Prostate
	Salivary	Lung
		Prostate

Reprinted with permission from Newell, G. R. Cancer: Etiology and prevention. In Nixon, D. W., ed. *Diagnosis and Management of Cancer*. Addison-Wesley Publishing Co., Menlo Park, CA. p. 37. 1982.

Table 5–6
Major Risk Factors and Common Signs and Symptoms
for Common Cancers

Type of Cancer	Risk Factors, Signs, and Symptoms
Colon/rectum	History of rectal polyps Family history of rectal polyps History of ulcerative colitis Age 40+ Blood in stool Human papilloma virus
Lung	Heavy cigarette smoker > age 50 Started cigarette smoking at age 15 or before Smoker working with or near asbestos Exposure to uranium, radium
Uterine/endometrial	Late menopause (> age 55) Diabetes, high BP, and overweight Age 50+ Unusual bleeding or discharge
Uterine/cervical	Frequent sex in early teens or with many partners Poor socioeconomic background Poor care during or following pregnancy Unusual bleeding or discharge Tobacco use Human papillomavirus
Breast	History of breast cancer Close relatives with history of breast cancer Never had children; first child after age 30 Age 35+; especially > age 50 Lump in breast or nipple discharge
Skin	Excessive exposure to sun Fair complexion Work with coal tar, pitch, or creosote
Oral	Heavy smoker and drinker Poor oral hygiene
Ovarian	History of ovarian cancer among close relatives Never had children Age 50+
Prostate	Age 60+ Difficulty in urinating
Stomach	History of stomach cancer among close relatives Diet heavy in smoked, pickled, or salted foods History of *H. pylori* bacterial infection

Table 5–7
Special Diagnostic Tests

Test	Purpose	Comments
Tumor markers		
CEA	Cancers of the pancreas, colon, breast, lung, stomach, ovary	High levels correlate with high tumor burden.
AFP	Hepatocellular carcinoma Germ cell tumors	Used to monitor treatment response.
HCG/AFP	Malignant trophoblastic disease, cancer of the testes	Return to normal indicates cure.
Acid phosphatase	Cancer of the prostate	May be used to monitor response to treatment or recurrence.
Estrogen/ progesterone receptors	Cancer of the breast	Defines certain tumors that may be more responsive to hormonal therapy.
Calcitonin	Medullary cancer of the thyroid	Occurs as a manifestation of Multiple Endocrine Neoplasia (MEN) Type 2
Catecholamines	Pheochromocytoma	Dopamine, epinephrine, and/or norepinephrine may be produced by tumor.
PSA	Cancer of the prostate	Used particularly to monitor response to treatment.
Monoclonal immunoglobulins	Multiple myeloma	Malignant clone can be IgG, IgM, or IgA.
CA 125	Epithelial ovarian cancer	A tumor associated antigen that might be used in conjunction with vaginal ultrasound for screening.
CA 19-9	Cancers of the pancreas, colon, cervix and ovary	A relatively specific tumor associated antigen.
X-rays		
Mammography	Breast cancer	Average radiation exposure = 0.1–0.7 cgy.
Lymphangiography	Lymph node involvement, especially Hodgkin's disease, lymphoma, cancer of the testes	Blue dye, injected into lymphatic channel at great toe, visualizes abdominal lymph nodes.
Radionuclide scan	Shows function and size of specific organ (brain, bone, liver, spleen, kidney)	Used for staging because of specificity; radioisotope injected peripherally.
Ultrasound	Visualizes structural changes, mass (stomach, pancreas, kidney, uterus, ovary)	Uses high-frequency sound waves.
Computed axial tomography (CAT, CT, ACTA)	Cross-section images of internal structures	X-ray ± contrast dye; high specificity, especially brain tumors.
Microscopic examination		
Pap smear	Cancer of the cervix or uterus	Cytological examination of cells obtained by swab of vagina, endocervical canal, and exocervix.

Table 5-7 (Continued)
Special Diagnostic Tests

Test	Purpose	Comments
Bone-marrow aspirate	Tumor involvement, especially by leukemia or lymphoma	Needle aspirate of marrow from iliac crest or sternum.
Sputum cytology	Bronchogenic cancer	
Stool guaiac	Cancer of the colon/rectum	Patient must eat meat-free, vitamin-C free, high-fiber diet for 2 days, then submit 2 samples on each of 3 consecutive days.

AFP—α-fetoprotein; CEA—carcinoembryonic antigen; HCG—human chorionic gonadotropin; PSA—prostate specific antigen.

rived from the history and physical examination as they relate to different sites of cancer.

Secondary prevention, or early detection, is facilitated by the accuracy of laboratory or radiologic tests. Tests most commonly used in the detection of cancer are presented in Table 5–7.

Tumor markers are substances (antigens, enzymes, proteins, hormones) that are secreted in response to or by tumors and can be detected in the bloodstream or urine. For the most part, tumor marker tests are extremely sensitive, because tumor marker activity occurs prior to signs and symptoms. Although they are not sufficiently sensitive to use as screening tools, they can be useful in making a diagnosis and in following response to treatment.

The most sensitive and specific of the markers is the beta subunit of *human chorionic gonadotropin* (HCG), which is secreted by malignant trophoblastic disease (choriocarcinoma) and some germ-cell testicular tumors. *Carcinoembryonic antigen* (CEA) is less specific, occurring with some tumors of the colon, breast, and lung, and usually signifies a tumor burden of more than 10^8 cells. *Acid phosphatase* and *prostate specific antigen* (PSA) elevations demonstrate more advanced cancer of the prostate, and are therefore more useful as indicators of response to antitumor therapy than in diagnosis. Likewise, radioimmunoassay of *alpha-fetoprotein* (AFP) can be useful in the diagnosis of hepatoma, embryonal carcinoma, or liver metastases.

In most instances, the diagnosis of cancer is made as a result of a combination of tests and physical findings. The tests listed in Table 5–7 are specific but not limited to the diagnosis of cancer. Definitive diagnosis is made only by pathological examination of malignant cells *(cytology)* or tissue *(biopsy)* (see Chapter 2A).

MANAGEMENT

Prevention

A protocol for the preventive management of persons at risk for cancer is provided in Table 5–8. The primary role of health care providers must be to educate the public at large (e.g., the NCI Cancer Prevention Awareness Program) as well as individual consumers of health care. Coordination with existing organizations, such as the ACS, the American Lung Association, and the NCI Office of Communications, will result in maximum audience participation. Collaboration with various professionals is necessary to provide effective psychological support and counseling, nutritional guidance, surgical intervention, and/or medical follow-up.

Early Detection

Early detection programs are established with the goal of finding cancer as early as possible. Two different approaches are used to meet this goal: (1) *case-finding*, in which a person at risk is closely assessed and monitored (e.g., a person with a family history of colorectal cancer), and (2) *screening*, whereby an asymptomatic population is tested to define who might have disease and who probably does not. Both programs require (1) knowledge of high-risk patients and (2) available tests that are safe, effective, and affordable.

Case-Finding

Early detection programs prescribed for specific persons at risk usually occur in outpatient settings, where a one-to-one relationship between caregiver and patient allows greater communication, better patient adherence, and close follow-up. Therefore, the tests used can be more complex and the benefits/risks more carefully explained than is possible in mass screening programs.

Procedures that involve active patient participation require teaching and follow-up evaluation. Two examples are breast self-examination (BSE) and testicular self-examination (TSE).

Figure 5–2 demonstrates the three-step process of BSE recommended by the ACS. Position changes facilitate complete assessment of the breast by displacing normal breast tissue around any possible masses. Gentle palpation while showering eliminates extra movement by friction. Patients are instructed to perform BSE monthly one week after menses, or if postmenopausal, at the same time each month.

Testicular self-examination is especially indicated for men aged 20 to 35 years, for men whose testes never descended or descended into the scrotal sac after age 6 years, and for men with a family history of testicular cancer. Young men should be taught to examine each testicle with both

Table 5–8
Nursing Protocol for the Preventive Management of Persons at Risk for Cancer

Factor*	Intervention
Diet	Provide nutritional consultation of balanced diet; vitamins A and C, low fat, high fiber. Individualize diet according to general health status. Assist in maintenance of ideal body weight. Avoid salted, pickled or smoked foods. Increase calcium intake.
Exercise	Encourage regular exercise, active recreation, increase in total activity.
Tobacco	Educate: prevent youths from starting; motivate smokers to take active role in quitting. Counsel: multicomponent plan under professional guidance; achieve intolerance by smoking to excess, low tar/nicotine cigarettes; nicotine chewing gum; cold turkey. Provide follow-up support; maintain attitude of experimentation; individualize plans as needed; enlist support of family/friends. Decrease cues to smoke: encourage nonsmoking areas in public places or workplace; run a media campaign; act as a role model by not smoking. Use outside resources: NCI Office of Cancer Communications (physician's kit; "Helping Smokers Quit"); ACS, ALA, self-help groups.
Viruses	Immunize against infecting agent, such as hepatitis B vaccine. Educate: avoid exposure to venereal disease: avoid promiscuity, use barrier contraceptive; improve general hygiene.
Occupational hazards	Provide public education to inform persons at risk about chemicals, dusts, radiation. Use masks or respirators when appropriate. Maintain close monitoring of persons at risk.
Alcohol	Educate: encourage moderate consumption; promote cessation if exposed to (1) upper respiratory tract carcinogens, (2) hepatitis B surface antigen. Counsel: obtain psychologic consultation for behavioral modifications; use self-help groups (AA).
Radiation	Educate: avoid unnecessary x-ray tests; avoid excess sun exposure: minimize time exposed to midday sun; use sunscreens as needed (fair-skinned need sun protection factor of 8–15); take extra caution with sun exposure while on sensitizing drugs (e.g., tetracycline).
Estrogens	Educate: discuss risks/benefits of prolonged use of exogenous estrogens. Maintain close monitoring of persons exposed to DES.
Premalignant condition Large-bowel polyps	Suggest surgical consultation for possible removal. Provide follow-up: annual stool guaiac; sigmoidoscopy every 2–3 yr.
Cervical dysplasia	Repeat Pap smears to confirm. Advise colposcopy with biopsy if necessary. Refer for surgical treatment depending on extent of lesion: cryosurgery; conization; hysterectomy.

*Ordered according to degree of risk.

AA—Alcoholics Anonymous; ACS—American Cancer Society; ALA—American Lung Association; DES—diethylstilbestrol; NCI—National Cancer Institute.

1: IN THE SHOWER

Examine breasts during bath or shower; hands glide easier over wet skin. Fingers flat, move gently over every part of each breast. Use right hand to examine left breast, left hand for right breast. Check for any lump, hard knot or thickening.

2: BEFORE A MIRROR

Inspect breasts with arms at sides. Next, raise arms high overhead. Look for any changes in contour of each breast, a swelling, dimpling of skin or changes in the nipple.

Then, rest palms on hips and press down firmly to flex chest muscles. Left and right breast will not exactly match - few women's breasts do.

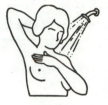
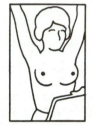
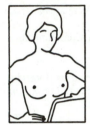

3: LYING DOWN

To examine right breast, put a pillow or folded towel under right shoulder. Place right hand behind head - this distributes breast tissue more evenly on the chest. With left hand, fingers flat, press gently in small circular motions around an imaginary clock face. Begin at outermost top of right breast for 12 o'clock, then move to 1 o'clock, and so on around the circle back to 12. A ridge of firm tissue in the lower curve of each breast is normal. Then move in an inch, toward the nipple, keep circling to examine every part of breast, including nipple. This requires at least three more circles. Now slowly repeat procedure on left breast with a pillow under left shoulder and left hand behind head. Notice how breast structure feels.

Finally, squeeze the nipple of each breast gently between thumb and index finger. Any discharge, clear or bloody, should be reported to physician immediately.

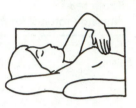
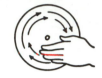

Figure 5–2. Breast self-examination.

Reprinted with permission from American Cancer Society, Inc., New York. 1977.

hands, gently rolling the sac between the thumb and fingers, feeling for a small lump.

Important to any self-examination procedure is instructing the person to call the appropriate health care provider if an abnormality is suspected or detected.

The ACS has recommended guidelines for early detection of cancer in asymptomatic persons (Table 5–9). The Society emphasizes that these are not appropriate as a mass-screening program, because the risk/benefit ratio is not yet established. The guidelines are based on (1) research demonstrating the effectiveness of each procedure for smaller samples of patients and (2) the known natural history of the most common tumor types. An attempt is made to make the cost incurred commensurate with the benefit expected.

Screening

Cancers amenable to cost-effective public screening programs are those that (1) cause significant morbidity and mortality, (2) have a prolonged DPCP, and (3) can be detected by tests that are safe and low cost. The higher the yield of positive results from any one screening test, the more effective the program is considered to be.

To date, cancers of the cervix, breast, and colon/rectum have proved to be amenable to screening programs. Studies have been undertaken to

Table 5–9
Protocol for the Early Detection of Cancer in Asymptomatic Persons

Test or Procedure	Sex	Age in Years	Frequency
Sigmoidoscopy	M & F	≥50	every 3–5 years based on physician's advice
Stool guaiac slide test	M & F	≥50	every year
Digital rectal exam	M & F	≥40	every year
Prostate exam (Digital rectal exam & PSA)	M	≥50	every year
Pap test	F	18–65; <18 if sexually active	every year; less frequently at physician's discretion following 3 consecutive normal annual exams
Pelvic examination	F	18–40 >40	every 3 years every year
Endometrial tissue sample	F	at menopause women at high risk[†]	at menopause and thereafter at physician's discretion
BSE	F	≥20	monthly
Breast physical exam	F	20–40 >40	every 3 years every year
Mammography	F	40–49 ≥50	every 1–2 years beginning at 40 years every year
Chest x-ray			not recommended
Sputum cytology			not recommended
Health counseling and cancer checkup[‡]	M & F	>20 >40	every 3 years every year

PSA—prostate specific antigen; BSE—breast self exam.

[†]History of infertility, obesity, failure of ovulation, abnormal uterine bleeding, or estrogen therapy.

[‡]To include examination for cancers of the thyroid, testicles, prostate, ovaries, lymph nodes, oral region, and skin.
Adapted with permission from American Cancer Society. Guidelines for the cancer-related checkup: Recommendations and rationale. *CA—A Cancer Journal for Clinicians* (Jan/Feb): p. 45. 1993.

demonstrate the role of screening for cancers of the lung, prostate, head/neck, testis, bladder, and stomach, and for melanoma.

The following major tumor types are described in order to further explain specific screening programs and reasons for their success or failure.

Cervical Cancer

There is a subtle but important distinction between prevention and early detection of this disease with the use of the Papanicolaou (Pap) smear. The Pap smear allows *prevention* of invasive disease by detecting cervical dysplasia (mild, moderate, or severe) or cervical intraepithelial neoplasia (CIN) (grades 1, 2, or 3), a premalignant condition. These lesions are usually asymptomatic and would not be detected on a routine pelvic examination. The Pap smear is also critically important in the *early detection* of carcinoma in situ (CIS), which, though invasive and malignant, has a 100 percent five-year survival rate when treated surgically. Progression of CIS to invasive carcinoma of the cervix (ICC) with involvement of local or regional tissues has 79 percent and 45 percent average rates of five-year survival respectively. Because CIS can last for years before progressing to ICC and because spontaneous regression can occur, close monitoring with repeated Pap smears will assist the physician in understanding the natural course of each patient's disease.

Breast Cancer

One out of nine American women will develop breast cancer during her lifetime, accounting for 180,300 estimated new cases in 1998. The principle tests available for the early detection of breast cancer are BSE, physical examination, and mammography. A survey of American women by the ACS revealed that 35 percent perform BSE monthly, though the impact of this statistic on early diagnosis is not known. The role of screening remains unclear, because the risk factors for developing breast cancer are not fully understood. In a large prospective study of American women carried out by the ACS to determine the significance of several suspected risk factors, only age, country of birth, and either a mother or sister with a history of breast cancer were found to constitute significant risk; two-thirds of the breast cancer cases could not be explained on the basis of these factors.

Therefore, the ACS recommends that all women over 35 years of age be considered at substantial risk, with a focus on specific women at *especially* high risk. Although the incidence of breast cancer is rising, the mortality remains somewhat constant, perhaps reflecting the influence of earlier diagnosis and more effective treatment.

Prostate Cancer

Prostate cancer has recently surpassed lung cancer as the most commonly diagnosed cancer in men, excluding skin cancer, with an estimated annual incidence of 184,500 cases. Currently 1 out of every 11 men will develop prostate cancer during his lifetime. For African American men in the United States, the risk is 50 percent higher than for Caucasian men, and African American men tend to be diagnosed at a more advanced stage of disease. Risk factors include a high-fat diet, family history of prostate cancer, and prolonged occupational exposure to cadmium.

Currently, 40 percent of cases of prostate cancer are diagnosed after the cancer has spread beyond the prostate. However, for men over age 40 years, the diagnosis of early prostate cancer might be possible by combining transrectal ultrasound and the blood test, prostate specific antigen (PSA), with the traditional digital rectal exam.

Lung Cancer

The incidence of lung cancer in the United States continues to rise (171,500 estimated cases in 1998), and the overall five-year survival rate remains less than 10 percent. Early detection succeeds in identifying only one-third of the entire group with local disease, which carries a 27 percent five-year survival rate. At present, studies have been undertaken to determine whether periodic screening of asymptomatic male smokers—using questionnaires, sputum tests for cytology, and chest x-rays—will detect lung cancer early enough to alter the natural course of disease by effective treatment. Because the DPCP appears short and available treatment inadequate, early detection programs to date appear not to affect mortality. Therefore, prevention, by decreasing the use of tobacco, remains the focus of large-scale programs.

Malignant Melanoma

Although the incidence of malignant melanoma is low (41,600 estimated new cases in 1998) compared with other cancers, it is growing at a faster rate than any other cancer in the United States. Early detection and effective treatment have resulted in a five-year survival rate for this cancer of 80 percent, because melanoma can be detected while confined to the dermis (less than 0.76 mm thickness). Health professionals must be aware of the early signs of malignant melanoma and teach patients to perform self-examination of both new and preexisting nevi using the ABCDs:

A = Assymmetry
B = Border irregularity
C = Color variegation (blue, red, brown, black)
D = Diameter generally greater than 6 mm

Any changes in preexisting nevi or the development of any new lesion after age 40 should raise suspicion of malignant melanoma and warrants professional examination.

Colorectal Cancer

Cancer of the colon/rectum can be detected early by means of a digital examination, occult blood test of the stool (stool guaiac), and barium enema or proctoscopy. The incidence of colorectal cancer is high (139,400 cases per year) and the five-year survival rate for asymptomatic patients is 90 percent (compared with 40 percent overall), underscoring the importance of early detection. Screening programs using the digital examination and stool blood tests have not been cost-effective, however, for the following reasons: (1) The 1 percent to 2 percent incidence of false-positive tests necessitates a diagnostic workup, which is expensive and time-consuming; (2) digital examinations and sigmoidoscopy cannot detect tumors that originate proximal to the sigmoid colon (half of all cases); and (3) negative public attitude toward cancer of the colon/rectum makes voluntary screening difficult. Current recommendations according to age are described in Table 5–9 for asymptomatic persons at normal risk. Table 5–6 defines asymptomatic persons at high risk for colorectal cancer; from age 40, these persons should undergo annual digital rectal examination, annual fecal occult blood testing, and either air-contrast barium enema with proctosigmoidoscopy, or colonoscopy every three to five years.

Any discussion of public education programs for the early detection of cancer would be incomplete without inclusion of the ACS "7 Warning Signals that can Save Your Life":

1. Change in bowel or bladder habits;
2. A sore that does not heal;
3. Unusual bleeding or discharge;
4. Thickening or lumps in breast or elsewhere;
5. Indigestion or difficulty in swallowing;
6. Obvious change in wart or mole;
7. Nagging cough or hoarseness.

Although these warning signals indicate that the disease has progressed to the point of symptomatology, the overall goal of early detection is facilitated by this approach, because it increases public awareness and decreases public fear.

BIBLIOGRAPHY

1. American Cancer Society. Guidelines for the cancer-related checkup: Recommendations and rationale. *CA—A Cancer Journal for Clinicians* (September/October). 279–282. 1993.

   This article presents rationale for recommendations made concerning both individual early detection and mass screening programs. It organizes discussion by specific tumor types: lung, breast, colon/rectum, and cervix.

2. American Society of Clinical Oncology. Statement of the American Society of Clinical Oncology: Genetic testing for cancer susceptibility. *Journal of Clinical Oncology*. 14: 1730–1736. 1996.

This important position statement is intended to inform the community about issues related to genetic testing of cancer risk.

3. Bernstein, L., B. E. Henderson, R. Hanisch, et al. Physical exercise and reduced risk of breast cancer in young women. *Journal of the National Cancer Institute* 86: 1403–1408. 1994.

A correlation is made in this article between active exercise and late menarche, a factor known to be associated with low risk for breast cancer.

4. Calzone, K.A. Genetic predisposition testing: Clinical implications for oncology nurses. *Oncology Nursing Forum* 24(4): 712–718. 1997.

This article presents implications for nursing practice of genetic testing. Issues such as cancer risk management, psychosocial sequelae, and legal and professional liability are addressed.

5. Cartmel, B., and M. Reid. Cancer control and epidemiology. In *Cancer Nursing: Principles and Practice*. S. L. Groenwald, M. H. Frogge, M. Goodman, and C. H. Yarbro, eds. Jones & Bartlett Publishers, Sudbury, MA. 50–74. 1997.

This is an excellent and comprehensive presentation of the suspected or known causes of cancer and the design of screening programs.

6. Frank-Stromberg, M., and R. F. Cohen. Assessment and interventions for cancer detection. In *Cancer Nursing: Principles and Practice*. S. L. Groenwald, M. H. Frogge, M. Goodman, and C. H. Yarbro, eds. 133–174. Jones & Bartlett Publishers, Sudbury, MA. 1997.

This is a comprehensive discussion about the methods for early detection of several common tumor types. For each tumor type, elements of the history, physical examination, and patient education are included.

7. Fraser, M. C., K. A. Calzone, and A. M. Goldstein. Familial cancers: Evolving challenges for nursing practice. *Oncology Nursing Updates: Patient Treatment and Support* 4(3):1–18. 1997.

This article describes patterns of familial cancers, identification of families at risk, and management strategies, with a focus on counseling. Social and ethical issues are discussed.

8. Hirschman, R. S., and H. Leventhal. The behavioral science of cancer prevention. In Kahn, S. B., R. R. Love, C. Sherman, and R. Chakrovorty, eds. *Concepts in Cancer Medicine*. 229–240. Grune & Stratton, Inc., New York. 1983.

This chapter provides a model for understanding and changing health behaviors using principles of behavioral science and biomedical science.

9. Landis, S. H., T. Murray, S. Bolden, and P. A. Wingo. Cancer Statistics: 1998. *Ca: A Cancer Journal for Clinicians*. 48(1): 6–30. 1998.

This is an annual report offered by the American Cancer Society showing statistics for cancer incidence and mortality, and compares them to other causes of death in the United States.

10. Loescher, L. J., Guest Editor. Cancer prevention and detection. *Seminars in Oncology Nursing* 9(3): 133–209. 1993.

This entire issue presents topics ranging from the Human Genome Project to early detection programs for specific tumors and assessment of cancer risk in ethnically diverse populations.

11. Lovejoy, N. C., M. L. Thomas, P. Halliburton, and L. Mimnaugh. Tumor markers: Relevance to clinical practice. *Oncology Nursing Forum* (September/October): 75–82. 1987.

    This article presents a comprehensive discussion of tumor markers used for early diagnosis, monitoring effects of treatment and assessing tumor prognosis or recurrence.

12. Murphy, G. P., W. Lawrence, and R. E. Lenhard. *American Cancer Society Textbook of Clinical Oncology.* American Cancer Society, Atlanta. 1995.

    This easily readable text provides overviews of cancer prevention and early detection and includes the scientific bases behind individual and public preventive health care strategies.

13. Parker, S. P., K. J. Davis, P. A. Wingo, L. A. G. Ries, and C. W. Heath. Cancer Statistics by Race and Ethnicity. *Ca: A Cancer Journal for Clinicians.* 48(1): 31–48. 1998.

    This is a special additional report that shows cancer incidence and mortality by racial or ethnic group within the United States.

14. Rosenstock, I. M. Why people use health services. *Millbank Memorial Fund Quarterly* (July): 94–127. 1966.

    This classic article describes the Health Belief Model as a means of understanding a person's health-related behaviors.

15. Swan, D.K., and B. Ford. Chemoprevention of cancer: Review of the literature. *Oncology Nursing Forum* 12(4): 719–727. 1997.

    This article provides an overview of current chemoprevention research and rationale.

16. Willson, P. Testicular, prostate and penile cancers in primary care settings: The importance of early detection. *Nurse Practitioner* (November): 19–25. 1991.

    This is a summary of risk factors, screening, early presentation, and professional examination for cancers of the male reproductive tract.

Information and Resources

A. Information

Deborah K. Mayer

INTRODUCTION

Trends in society and health care are affecting patient needs for information and resources. The U.S. population is becoming older, ethnically more diverse, and better educated. Access to a wider range of information is growing through the use of technology. Overall, patients are becoming more assertive and knowledgeable health care consumers, and at the same time, health care providers are learning the value of sharing responsibility for health care decisions. Our health care system continues to evolve, with projections that 80 percent of the U.S. population will have some form of managed care by the year 2000. A transition from an emphasis on acute care to chronic care is shifting the focus of care toward self-care and family-delivered home care. Community health care and empowered consumers will provide the cornerstone for many of these health care changes. This chapter reviews what the cancer patient and family need to know and ways to facilitate the sharing of cancer-related information.

Information Needs of the Cancer Patient

Like everyone else, the cancer patient is continually required to acquire information and make decisions, in order to prepare for and participate in health care and reduce anxiety. Over the course of the illness, there are both specific and general information needs. According to Mullan (1985), the "acute survival" phase begins with the diagnosis of cancer; the "extended phase" is when the initial treatment is completed when a period of recovering and watchful waiting ensues; followed by "permanent survival," when long term effects of living with the disease and treatment are confronted. Interpreting and integrating information about the diagnosis and disease process into one's life is a major activity during these phases of survival.

Today, most cancer patients prefer, in varying degrees, to receive information and to participate in decision making regarding their health care;

however, many are dissatisfied with their ability to obtain desired information (see Table 6A–1). Times that require special attention to treatment options and potential lifestyle changes include (1) the time of diagnosis, (2) the completion of therapy, (3) the first recurrence, and (4) the terminal phase of illness. Information needs can also be influenced by other factors such as age (e.g., the special needs of children and the elderly), gender, cultural influences, personal information styles, and literacy levels. The Cancer Information Service (CIS), sponsored by the National Cancer Institute, receives many patient calls just after diagnosis or during treatment. Exploring treatment options in order to discuss treatment plans with physicians was cited as the main reason for the CIS call. Most of these individuals seek information from at least three sources, including books, medical journals, friends and relatives, the American Cancer Society, or other organizations in addition to their health care provider.

A variety of studies have evaluated the information needs and preferences of cancer patients and their families and have similar findings (see Table 6A–2). Some of these studies are reviewed subsequently.

Frequently, after receiving a diagnosis of cancer, the patient has overwhelming feelings of loss of control, which can lead to feelings of helplessness and hopelessness. Cassileth et al. (1980a) found that the most hopeful patients were those who were actively involved in their own care. Brockopp et al. (1989) evaluated cancer patients' perceptions of five psychosocial needs and found hope and the desire for honest information to be the most important. Derdiarian (1986) studied recently

Table 6A-1
Patient Information Needs and Preferences

A substantial percentage of cancer patients want to be informed of their diagnosis.

Cancer patients are dissatisfied with the kind and/or amount of medical information they receive from their physicians and nurses.

Physicians and, to some extent, nurses underestimate the amount and misperceive the type of information that patients desire.

The physician is the preferred source of medical information.

Younger (less than 60 years), well educated patients desire more information than older, less educated patients.

Some patients prefer, and benefit from, ambiguous information because the uncertainty allows them to maintain hope for a positive health outcome.

Reprinted with permission from Degner, L., J. Farber, and T. Hack. *Communication between cancer patients and health professionals: an annotated bibliography.* p. 5. Joint Medical Affairs Committee of the Canadian Cancer Society and the National Cancer Institute of Canada, Toronto, Canada. 1989.

Table 6A–2
Type of Information Desired by Patient

Diagnosis

Stage of disease

Prognosis (probable outcome, chance for cure)

Treatment options/purpose of treatment

Side effects

Self-care needs/minimizing side effects

Effects on work, relationships

diagnosed cancer patients and describes a hierarchy of desired information, which she hypothesized to be based on the amount, imminence, and likelihood of anticipated harm. Her subjects ranked highest disease-related information, information about treatment; personal information about physical well-being; and effect on family and social relationships, particularly employment. In a randomized study of the effects of providing information, referral, and counseling for cancer patients and their spouses, Derdiarian (1989) found that members of the group that received more information were more satisfied with their care than members of a control group.

Lauer, Murphy, and Powers (1982) compared nurses' and patients' perceptions of learning needs and found significant differences between the two groups. Patients identified as most important knowing about their diagnosis, the plan of care, how to care for themselves at home and work, what they would experience during diagnostic procedures, and how to choose foods to help maintain weight. Patients noted the most important treatment-related information was the purpose, schedule, and side effects of treatment, and especially ways to minimize side effects during chemotherapy or radiation therapy. Campbell-Forsyth (1990) studied 80 patients receiving radiation therapy and did not find that information needs differed significantly based on age. Dodd (1982) evaluated patients' knowledge of the chemotherapy they were receiving and its potential side effects, particularly bleeding and infection as possibly lethal problems. She found that patients were not absorbing and retaining this information but that comprehension and understanding could be improved with education. In another study evaluating radiation therapy patients, Dodd and Ahmed (1987) found that their subjects preferred cognitive information describing the how, when, why, who, and where of the radiation treatments to behavioral information about actions that the individual could perform.

Frequently patients and families feel overwhelmed about what questions to ask or information to seek out. When 256 oncology patients were

surveyed about what type of information they desired, for 7 of the 12 topics included, more than 50 percent of the patients polled felt they ab-
solutely needed this information (Cassileth et al. 1980b; Table 6A–3).
These questions can be used by the nurse to assess the patient's comprehension of the situation.

Knowledge of these and other studies can help the nurse anticipate
some of the information needs of the individual cancer patient and family
or in addressing group needs. Baseline and periodic assessment of the patient's need for information should be conducted.

Table 6A–3
Type of Information Desired by Patient

	Patient Response		
	I absolutely need this information %	I would like to have this inforXmation %	I do not want this information %
What are all the possible side effects?	62.9	35.2	2.0
What will the treatment accomplish?	62.1	36.3	1.2
Is it cancer?	60.5	37.1	2.0
What is the likelihood of cure?	58.6	37.5	3.9
Are all parts of the body involved?	58.2	36.3	5.1
Exactly what will the treatment do inside my body?	57.4	37.9	4.7
What is the day-to-day (week-to-week) progress?	51.2	41.4	6.6
What is the specific medical name of illness?	48.4	44.5	6.3
Is it inherited, or contagious?	46.1	44.5	9.0
How effective has the treatment been for other patients?	44.5	48.4	7.0
Are there examples of cases where the treatment has been effective?	42.2	48.4	9.0
Are there examples of cases where the treatment has not been effective?	32.2	44.9	21.9

Adapted with permission from Cassileth, B., R. Zupkis, K. Sutton-Smith and V. March. Information and participation preferences
among cancer patients. *Ann Int Med* (June): 834. 1980.

Information Seeking Behaviors

Each patient brings an individual style and preference for seeking information to the cancer experience. Miller (1987) has described two styles, which can account for some of the differences seen in practice. Monitors are individuals who seek both general and specific information and might gather it from time of diagnosis. Blunters may want to avoid or distract themselves from specific information and want it only at a general level or on an "as needed" basis.

Degner and colleagues (1988, 1992, 1993, 1996) have studied the decision-making role cancer patients desire for information (see Table 6A–4). Statements reflecting role preferences range from passive to active and include "I prefer to leave all decisions regarding my treatment to my doctor" (passive), "I prefer that my doctor makes the final decision about which treatment will be used, but seriously considers my opinion" (passive), "I prefer that my doctor and I share responsibility for deciding which treatment is best for me" (collaborative), "I prefer to make the final selection of my treatment after seriously considering my doctor's opinion" (active), "I prefer to make the final selection about which treatment I will receive" (active). Most patients prefer some form of shared or collaborative decision making with the physician rather than with a family member. There were differences based on age (older patients tend to prefer a more passive role), gender (women preferring a more active role), and education (higher education more strongly correlates with an active role preference). Therefore, assessing individual preferences and helping patients to develop questions and comprehend information is an important nursing intervention.

Table 6A–4
Patient Participation in Treatment Decision Making

The majority of patients prefer to share treatment control with their physicians.

Younger patients prefer more active involvement than older patients.

Patients who want to play an active role are female, single, and well-educated.

More active participation by patients may increase treatment compliance and hope for a favorable health outcome.

Physicians may overestimate the degree to which patients want to participate in decision making.

Reprinted with permission from Degner, L., J. Farber, and T. Hack. *Communication between cancer patients and health professionals: an annotated bibliography.* p. 56. Joint Medical Affairs Committee of the Canadian Cancer Society and the National Cancer Institute of Canada, Toronto, Canada. 1989.

Table 6A–5
Suggestions for Effective and Meaningful Communication

Speak frankly with your doctor.

Bring a family member or friend.

Jot down your questions in a notebook.

Tape important conversations.

Insist on privacy during important interviews.

Give your doctor "cues" as to how much information you want and need to know.

Ask for interpretations of long, puzzling medical words or terms.

Do not forget that doctors are people, too.

Do not present yourself to your doctor as a disease, but as a person living with a disease.

Be sure that you understand your treatment plan before you leave the doctor.

If you find yourself unable to communicate with your doctor, try to find another one.

Reprinted with permission from Hoffman, J. *A cancer survivor's almanac: Charting your journey.* 40–43. Chronimed, Minneapolis. 1996.

Communication is the process of sharing information with another person so that the message sent is actually understood. Approximately 65 percent of a message is nonverbal (e.g. body language, vocal tone, facial expression). It has been documented that there is poor retention of health-related communication; in one study there was a 50 percent memory loss five minutes after visiting the physician. Effective communication improves participation in and satisfaction with care. Various strategies have been proposed to improve communication between patients and families and health professionals (see Table 6A–5).

Patient Education

Patients and their families have a right to information that will aid them in participation in therapy and self-management. Patients prefer initial verbal communication from their physicians, followed by printed materials, at least during the pretreatment period (Hinds 1995). Audiovisual materials are also available to augment learning. Having information available in a timely manner appropriate to each patient and situation, whether by individual teaching, group classes, or the use of printed or audiovisual materials regardless of setting of care will facilitate these goals. It is projected that in the future "telecomputers" integrating telephone, computer, and fax machines will link the home to health care providers for continuous health information and monitoring, possibly making printed materials obsolete.

Cancer patient education consists of structured or unstructured interventions designed to affect the knowledge, attitudes, skills, or other behaviors of persons with cancer. Thus, education is an important component of total patient care, helps increase patients' participation in their care, and contributes to improving quality of life. It will help patients adapt to their disease and ease their rehabilitation. Care that includes structured teaching, independent study, and counseling is effective in improving patient outcomes as measured by both psychological and physical quality of life indicators (e.g., anxiety, nausea, pain) (Devine and Westlake 1995). In a representative study on the effects of patient education by Jacobs, Walker, and Stockdale (1983), conducted with patients who had Hodgkin's disease, those who received educational materials experienced a decrease in anxiety, treatment problems, depression, and life disruption, compared with a control group of patients in a peer support group. The first group also showed improvement in psychologic and social behaviors. Ensuring adequate patient education is the nurse's professional role and responsibility.

Factors that can influence patient comprehension include information-seeking preferences, anxiety level, literacy level, and cultural background; nurses need to be sensitive to and adapt planned interventions based on these factors. In addition, the following basic steps will facilitate understanding and the retention of information during educational interactions:

1. Tell the patient what information will be presented during that session.
2. Present the material using short words and sentences and common words. What is the one idea that is important to convey and have comprehended?
3. Organize the information from the patients' viewpoint and into related clusters or categories, with the most important information first.
4. Have the patient restate or demonstrate the information.
5. Summarize and review the material presented.

The Oncology Nursing Society has established patient education standards that delineate the educational process (1995). These apply to teaching situations both structured and unstructured, formal and informal. They include an assessment of learning needs and establishment of mutually agreed-upon goals and objectives with patients and family, the selection of appropriate educational methods, and implementation and evaluation of the educational program. The educational process is completed by documentation in the patient's medical record, a requirement of the Joint Commission on Accreditation of Healthcare Organizations.

Available Resources

Many resources available both for cancer patients and their families and for the nurses involved in their care are listed at the end of this chapter. One must be particularly aware of issues related to literacy. Approximately 20 percent of adults read below the fifth grade level; however, most patient education material is developed at the tenth grade level (Morra and Varricchio 1993). It is important, therefore, to match the appropriate materials to the patient's literacy level. At the other extreme, the Internet has become a rich resource of information, advice and support. Information on the Internet can be overwhelming or unreliable. Careful appraisal is necessary as to how credible, reasonable and useful the information is.

Garrison et al. (1983), found that only 37 percent of patients received educational information at the time of diagnosis, though 72 percent expressed a desire for it. These patients were also not able to identify commonly available resources such as the American Cancer Society. Of 78 patients surveyed, 68 stated they would read material if it were available to them in the physician's office or clinics. The nurse should help patients and families become aware of available materials and how to obtain pertinent publications. Patients usually want and will use any information about cancer in general, their specific disease, and their treatments.

Many patients undergoing chemotherapy demonstrate inadequate knowledge of the drug they are taking and/or its side effects. There is no lack of written or audiovisual information available on chemotherapy, many common types of cancers, or other treatments. Many group and individual interventions, such as the American Cancer Society's "I Can Cope" course, are also well established. Other resources or programs might also be available within a specific practice setting or community. Support groups, many of which are disease oriented, have become a major arena for information sharing among cancer patients and families. Some of these resources are listed in Chapter 6B.

Patients are now being taught to assume a greater role in their own care. Self-care management includes providing relevant information about disease and treatment; skills and support to perform such technical aspects as monitoring blood counts, caring for venous access devices, administering therapy, and managing symptoms at home. Generally, compliance has been high, and patients benefit with greater self-esteem, stronger relationships with health care providers, and more control over their care. In addition, an increase in self-care reduces costs and improves the quality and efficiency of care (Dodd 1997).

Informed Consent

Informed consent is another important example of patient participation in decision making. There are many ethical, legal, and regulatory interactions involved, but the primary goal of informed consent is that patients have a full understanding of the relevant details of their proposed care. There are, however, problems related to the consent process (see Table 6A–6).

According to the U.S. Department of Health and Human Services, informed consent is "the knowing consent of an individual or his legally authorized representative so situated as to be able to exercise free power of choice without inducement or any element of force, fraud, deceit, distress, or any other form of constraint or coercion." The process of obtaining informed consent is followed for any invasive procedure, but it is usually observed in greater detail and monitored more closely for higher-risk and investigational procedures or treatments. Although it is the physician's legal obligation to obtain informed consent, it is the nurse's ethical obligation to make sure that this consent has been obtained.

The actual consent process consists of two parts: the oral and the written explanations. The consent form is not intended to replace verbal interaction, but to supplement and document it. The content of the standard consent form is required by law and enforced by institutional review boards (Table 6A–7). Unfortunately, much attention has been focused by all parties involved on obtaining a signed consent form, rather than on the process it was meant to facilitate. In one survey conducted by Cassileth, Zubkis, and Sutton-Smith (1980b), approximately 80 percent of patients viewed consent forms as a way to protect physicians' rights, although they also felt the forms were necessary and helpful in decision making.

In another study, conducted by the Psychosocial Collaborative Oncology Group (Penman et al. 1980), patients and their physicians were interviewed within three weeks of signing a consent form; 50 percent of patients stated that they had not asked questions that they had, and 75 percent of these patients also had lingering unspoken doubts and concerns about their treatment. The nurse, acting as patient advocate, can help avoid this kind of situation. Patients and families should be encouraged to write

Table 6A–6
Informed Consent Procedures

Informed consent forms are poorly understood by the majority of cancer patients who sign them.

Consent forms and procedures could be made more effective by making simple changes in wording and presentation.

Many physicians feel that using informed consent procedures has a negative impact on their relationship with patients and their patient's health.

Reprinted with permission from Degner, L., J. Farber, and T. Hack. *Communication between Cancer Patients and Health Professionals: An Annotated Bibliography.* p. 93. Joint Medical Affairs Committee of the Canadian Cancer Society and the National Cancer Institute of Canada, Toronto, Canada. 1989.

Table 6A–7
Standard for Consent Form Content

Section	Content
Purpose	A statement that the study involves research, an explanation of the purposes of the research, and the expected duration of the subject's participation.
Procedure	A description of the procedures to be followed and identification of any procedures that are experimental.
Benefits	A description of any benefits to the subject or to others that may reasonably be expected from the research.
Risks	A description of any reasonable foreseeable risks or discomforts to the subject.
Alternatives	A disclosure of appropriate alternative procedures or courses of treatment, if any, that might be advantageous to the subject.
Guarantees of right to confidentiality; financial remuneration; questioning; withdrawal from study	A statement describing the extent, if any, to which confidentiality of records identifying the subject will be maintained; explanation of any compensation and/or medical treatments that are available if injury occurs; the name of the person to contact for answers to questions about the study, the subject's rights, or research-related injury; acknowledgment that participation is voluntary and that participants will not be penalized for withdrawal.

Based on Food and Drug Administration regulations regarding the protection of human subjects. *Federal Register* (January 27): 8951. 1981.

down any questions they have. The nurse can help the patient raise questions for the physician that the patient may have forgotten or not thought of. The nurse should also ascertain how well the patient and family understand the information brought up in such a discussion. The nurse can then restate, reinforce, or expand on the information shared.

The usefulness of the consent form is much enhanced by its readability. Most consent forms are too technical and difficult for the average patient to comprehend. Four out of five surgical consent forms are written at the scientific journal level, whereas most newspapers are geared to the seventh to ninth grade level. Readability can be easily improved by using shorter sentences and fewer polysyllabic words.

The following recommendations, instituted to improve the consent process, might be helpful in other patient education as well:

1. Give the patient and family a copy of the consent form *at least* a day before it should be signed.

2. Encourage them to read it carefully.
3. Encourage them to write down any questions or concerns they wish to have addressed.
4. Set up an appointment for the patient and a family member (or significant other) to discuss treatment options with the physician and nurse.
5. Have the meeting in a private area where all participants can sit around a table or in comfortable chairs.
6. Tape-record discussions if possible, to enable the patient to refer to them later.
7. Ascertain how well the patient understands afterward by asking the patient questions about the subjects discussed.
8. Document the consent process in the patient's record.

By following these guidelines, the nurse can help patient and physician fulfill the intent of the consent process.

What and how health professionals communicate to the patient and family will play an important part in shaping the illness experience. The time spent providing information and promoting the patient's participation is worthwhile because the patient and family are more likely to be involved and satisfied with their care.

BIBLIOGRAPHY

1. Bilodeau, B. and L. Degner. Information needs, sources of information, and decisional roles in women with breast cancer. *Oncol Nurs Forum* 23(4): 691–696. 1996.

   Seventy-four women recently diagnosed with breast cancer were evaluated for personal preferences in decision making regarding their treatment. Most preferred and assumed a more passive role and preferred obtaining information from personal versus written sources.

2. Brockopp, D., D. Hayko, W. Davenport, and C. Winscott. Personal control and the needs for hope and information among adults diagnosed with cancer. *Cancer Nurs* 13(2): 112–116. 1990.

   Fifty-six cancer patients participated in a study to examine the relationship between perceived personal control and the need for hope and information. Significant correlations were found between hoping that pleasurable experiences were still possible and the desire to share with others what had been learned during the illness; other important needs are also noted.

3. Campbell-Forsyth, L. Patients' perceived knowledge and learning needs concerning radiation therapy. *Cancer Nurs* 13(2): 81–89. 1990.

   Eighty subjects shared their perceived knowledge and perceived learning needs about radiation therapy. No significant differences were noted between patients less than or more than 60 years of age.

4. Cassileth, B., R. Zupkis, K. Sutton-Smith and V. March. Information and participation preferences among cancer patients. *Ann Intern Med* 92(June): 832–836. 1980a.

   This study evaluated the response of 256 oncology patients to the Information Styles Questionnaire and the Beck Hopelessness Scale. Trends were identified in the areas of age, education, and race.

5. ———. Informed consent—Why are its goals imperfectly realized? *N Engl J Med* 302(April): 896–900. 1980b.

   This study evaluated the immediate recall of 200 cancer patients after signing a consent form. Education, medical status, and the care with which patients read the consent form were related to recall.

6. Chamorro, T., and J. Appelbaum. Informed consent: Nursing issues and ethical dilemmas. *Oncol Nurs Forum* 15(6): 803–807. 1988.

   Controversies related to ethics, advocacy, regulations, and scientific progress are reviewed. Issues discussed include patient protection, witnessing a consent document, legal accountability, disclosure, and comprehension related to informed consent.

7. Cooley, M., H. Moriarty, M. Berger, D. Selm-Orr, B. Coyle, & T. Short. Patient literacy and the readability of written cancer educational materials. *Oncol Nurs Forum* 22(9): 1345–1351. 1995.

   Reading ability of a sample of patients was tested and compared with the written materials used in their education. Forty-four percent of the patients had reading levels below that used in the 30 booklets. The majority of patients preferred more than one method of learning.

8. Degner, L., J. Farber, and T. Hack. Communication between cancer patients and health care professionals: An annotated bibliography. *National Cancer Institute of Canada* (August): 1–143. 1989.

   Ninety-five studies published since 1975 are critically reviewed in a variety of categories. These categories include patient information needs and preferences, disclosure of information by physicians, patient participation in treatment decision making, and informed consent procedures.

9. Degner, L., and C. Russell. Preferences for treatment control among adults with cancer. *Research in Nursing & Health* 11: 367–374. 1988.

   The preferences of adults with cancer about roles in decision making—about treatment were evaluated. The authors report that most patients prefer to share control in this process with the physician.

10. Degner, L. & Sloan, J. Decision making during serious illness: What role do patients really want to play? *J Clin Epidem* 45(9): 941–950. 1992.

    Two surveys were used to determine the roles people assume in selecting cancer treatment. Variables were assessed in relation to choosing more or less active roles.

11. Derdiarian, A. Information needs of recently diagnosed cancer patients. *Nurs Res* 35(5): 276–281. 1986.

    Sixty recently diagnosed cancer patients were assessed in relation to their disease and their personal, family, and social concerns. Few differences were found based on gender, age, or stage of cancer, implying that the need for information is universal.

12. ———. Effects of information on recently diagnosed cancer patients' and spouses' satisfaction with care. *Cancer Nurs* 12(5): 285–292. 1989.

    A randomized study of 30 recently diagnosed male cancer patients and their spouses received information, referrals, counseling, and follow-up care. They gained more information and were more satisfied with their care than a control group.

13. Devine, E., and S. Westlake. The effects of psychoeducational care provided to adults with cancer: meta-analysis of 116 studies. *Oncol Nurs Forum* 22(9): 1369–1381. 1995.

    An analysis of 116 psychoeducational studies demonstrating psychologic and physiologic benefits to cancer patients is reviewed.

14. Doak, L., C. Doak, and C. Meade. Strategies to improve cancer education materials. *Oncol Nurs Forum* 23(8): 1305–1312. 1996.

    This is an article outlining practical ways to develop effective cancer education materials, including those with limited literacy.

15. Dodd, M. Self-Care: Ready or not! *Oncol Nurs Forum* 24(6): 981–990. 1997.

    This is a review of almost twenty years of studies working with cancer patients and families regarding self-care.

16. ———. Cancer patients' knowledge of chemotherapy: Assessment and informational interventions. *Oncol Nurs Forum* 9(3): 39–44. 1982.

    Forty-eight cancer patients were studied about their knowledge of their chemotherapy. Patients were found to lack critical information such as potential side effects and drug names.

17. Dodd, M., and N. Ahmed. Preferences for type of information in cancer patients receiving radiation therapy. *Cancer Nurs* 10(5): 244–251. 1987.

    Sixty patients receiving radiation therapy were studied and found to prefer cognitive information about the treatment of its side effects.

18. Garrison, J., J. Abner, M. Oakley, and P. Hagen. Accessibility and utilization of educational materials for cancer patients. *Oncol Nurs Forum* 10(2): 60–62. 1983.

    Seventy-eight cancer patients were surveyed to determine the accessibility and utilization of education materials.

19. Hinds, C., A. Streater, and D. Mood. Functions and preferred methods of receiving information related to radiotherapy: Perceptions of patients with cancer. *Cancer Nurs* 18(5): 374–384. 1995.

    Patients were interviewed before and after receiving radiation therapy, identifying the usefulness of information in promoting active participation, anxiety reduction, and preparation. Verbal communication, especially from the physician, was the most preferred method with written material the next highest rated source.

20. Hoffman, B. *National Coalition for Cancer Survivorship's A Cancer Survivor's Almanac: Charting Your Journey.* Chronimed, Minneapolis. 1996.

    This is a consumer book addressing medical, emotional, spiritual, and social needs; insurance; employment; and legal and financial matters for the cancer survivor.

21. Jacobs, C., R. Ross, I. Walker, and F. Stockdale. Behavior of cancer patients: A randomized study of the effects of education and peer support groups. *Am J Clin Oncol* 10(June): 347–350. 1983.

Eighty-one Hodgkin's disease patients were evaluated with the Cancer Behavior Scale before and after entering either a support group, an educational group, or a control group.

22. Lauer, P., S. Murphy, and M. Powers. Learning needs of cancer patients: A comparison of nurse and patient perceptions. *Nurs Res* 31(1): 11–16. 1982.

The learning needs of cancer patients as perceived by 33 nurses and 27 patients were identified and compared. Significant differences existed; patients ranked "minimizing side effects of therapy" as most important, whereas nurses ranked "dealing with feelings" as most important.

23. Lenz, E. Information seeking: A component of client decisions and health behavior. *Adv Nurs Sci* 6(April): 59–72. 1984.

Information seeking is explored from a theoretical perspective. Factors such as sociodemographics, willingness to experiment, and personality are reviewed for their possible effect on information behaviors. Research implications are delineated.

24. Lewandowski, W., and S. Jones. The family with cancer: Nursing interventions throughout the course of living with cancer. *Cancer Nurs* 11(6): 313–321. 1988.

Sixty-two patients evaluated helpful nursing interventions during three phases of living with cancer: initial, adaptation, and terminal. Giving information was rated highly throughout the three phases.

25. Meade, C., J. Kiekmann, D. Thornhill. Readability of American Cancer Society patient education literature. *Oncol Nurs Forum* 19(1): 51–55. 1992.

American Cancer Society literature was evaluated for readability. The mean grade level of materials samples was twelfth grade; more recent materials are written at lower reading levels.

26. Miller, S. M. Monitoring and blunting: Validation of a questionnaire to assess styles of information seeking under threat. *J Personal Soc Psychol* 52(2): 345–353. 1987.

This article describes and validates a tool for predicting behavioral strategies, such as seeking information, in response to physical and psychological stress.

27. Morra, M. and C. Varricchio. Teaching patients with limited reading skills. *Cancer Practice* 154–156. 1993.

This is a step-by-step guide for developing written and audiovisual materials for those with limited reading skills.

28. Morra, M., and M. Grant, guest eds. Cancer patient education. *Semin Oncol Nurs* 7(2): 77–148. 1991.

This issue contains nine articles that address a wide range of patient education issues. Learning theories, styles, education systems, and programs are among the topics covered.

29. Mullan, F. Seasons of survival: Reflections of a physician with cancer. *N Engl J Med* 313(4): 270–273. 1985.

A physician describes his experience with cancer within the framework of surviving. This work led to the current survivorship movement, including the formation of the National Coalition of Cancer Survivors.

30. Neufeld, K. A nursing intervention strategy to foster patient involvement in treatment decisions. *Oncol Nurs Forum* 20(4): 631–635. 1993.

This article describes an intervention for supporting patients in decision-making, with a focus on assessing the degree to which they want to participate in medical treatment decisions.

31. Penman, D., G. Bahna, J. Holland, G. Morrow, et al. Patients' perception of giving informed consent for investigational chemotherapy. Proceedings of *ASCO/AACR* 21: 188. 1980.

Fifty-one patients and their physicians were interviewed after giving consent to participate in an investigational chemotherapy protocol. Most patients relied heavily on their physician's advice and had limited recall about the details of the study and treatment they were participating in.

6B

B. Resources

Marion E. Morra

This section lists some of the major national organizations that provide informational, social, financial, or psychological support for patients, their families, and health professionals. It also contains information on Internet government resources, along with Web site addresses for the major agencies.

GENERAL INFORMATION AND EDUCATION

Major Cancer Agencies

American Cancer Society, Inc.
1599 Clifton Road
Atlanta, GA 30329-4251
(404) 320-3333
Cancer Response System: (800) ACS-2345
http://www.cancer.org

The American Cancer Society (ACS) is a national voluntary organization that offers a wide range of services to cancer patients and their families and carries out programs of research and education. It also provides printed materials, films, and reprints for patients and professionals. The ACS has divisions and units throughout the United States. The national headquarters of the ACS is responsible for overall planning and coordination.

The toll-free Cancer Response System provides callers with information on cancer risks, disease sites, prevention practices, and early detection. It is a point of contact for information on ACS-sponsored programs for patients, the public, and health professionals. The ACS also sponsors a variety of support groups for cancer patients and their families (I Can Cope, International Association of Laryngectomies, Look Good . . . Feel Better, Man-to-Man, Reach to Recovery, and United Ostomy Association); information on them is included in the section of this chapter titled "Major Nationwide Direct-Help Services and Organizations." For local units of the ACS, consult the white pages of your local telephone directory under "American Cancer Society."

Cancer Information Service
National Cancer Institute
Office of Cancer Communications
Bethesda, MD 20892
(800) 4-CANCER
TTY: (800) 332-8615
http://rex.nci.nih.gov and http://cancernet.nci.nih.gov

The Cancer Information Service (CIS), a national information and education network, is the voice of the National Cancer Institute (NCI), the nation's primary agency for cancer research. Established in 1975, the CIS is the source for the latest, most accurate cancer information for patients, their families, the public and health professionals. The CIS operates based on a model for health communications that utilizes two main, complementary channels to provide vital information on cancer prevention, detection, treatment, and supportive care: a toll-free telephone service and an outreach program that focuses specifically on reaching minority and underserved audiences.

The telephone service has professional information specialists who provide individualized, confidential information about cancer to callers through 19 regional offices. By calling (800) 4-CANCER, the caller is automatically connected to the regional CIS office serving his or her area. Information specialists use PDQ, the NCI computer data base that provides the latest information on state-of-the-art treatment for each type and state of cancer, along with more than 1,000 active treatment studies under way in the country. CIS also gives information on cancer sites, cancer risks, prevention practices, and early detection. Spanish-speaking staff members are available.

The NCI is part of the Department of Health and Human Services, National Institutes of Health, and is responsible for federally funded cancer research and control programs. Within the NCI, the Office of Cancer Communications is responsible for providing the public, cancer patients, and the news media with accurate, up-to-date information about cancer. The Office of Cancer Communications also develops and distributes special informational and educational programs about cancer to health professionals, cancer patients, and the public.

Governmental Computer Resources for Cancer

CancerNet
National Cancer Institute
http://cancernet.nci.nih.gov/

CancerNet provides links to cancer information for the public, health professionals, and basic researchers. CancerNet contains portions of the PDQ database including information about ongoing clinical trials. In addition, NCI fact sheets and publications, CancerNet news and CANCERLIT (a database with more than 1 million citations on all aspects of cancer from books, government reports, presentations, theses, and scientific journals), abstracts, and citations are provided online. An index of CancerNet statements also is available through e-mail via CancerMail. Send a message to cancernet@icicc.nci.nih.gov with the word "help" in the body of the message. CancerMail will send back a contents list with instructions for ordering the documents through e-mail.

National Library of Medicine
8600 Rockville Pike
Bethesda, MD 20894
(301) 594-5983
(888) FIND-NLM
http:///www.nlm.nih.gov/

The National Library of Medicine (NLM) is the world's largest scientific research library. The NLM is open to the public, and its databases can be used to search for journal articles and abstracts. The NLM also provides access to its databases through its online network of more than 140,000 institutions and individuals in the United States. MEDLARS is composed of several NLM databases—MEDLINE (abstracts to medical journals), PDQ (advances in cancer and clinical trials), CANCERLIT (citations from books, reports, presentations, theses, scientific journals on cancer), TOXLINE and TOXLIT (pharmacological, biochemical, physiological and toxicological effects of drugs and other chemicals), RTECS (toxic effect of chemical substances), and HeathSTAR (health care delivery information). MEDLARS is available through many university and medical libraries and some public libraries. It is also available for home computers, through Grateful Med, a fee service (http://igm.nlm.nih.gov), or through PubMed (http://www.ncbi.nlm.nih.gov/PubMed/), an information retrieval service that provides free access to MEDLINE).

Healthfinder
U.S. Department of Health and Human Services
http://www.healthfinder.gov/

Healthfinder provides users with information on selected online publications, clearinghouses, databases, Web sites and support and self-help groups. The Web site also provides links to government agencies and non-profit organizations that provide reliable information for the public.

Combined Health Information Database
U.S. Public Health Service
Available through Ovid Technologies
(800) 289-4277
http://www.ovid.com

The Combined Health Information Database (CHID) is a computerized bibliographic database developed and managed by agencies of the U.S. Public Health Service. It is composed of 25 subfiles that contain references to health information and health education resources. Cancer-related subfiles include cancer patient education and cancer prevention and control and are intended to serve health professionals, health educators, patients, and the general public. The CHID provides citation to and abstracts of journal articles, books, reports, pamphlets, audio- and videotapes, product descriptions, and low-literacy and non–English-speaking resources. It also has hard-to-find information sources, such as health promotion and education programs in state and local health departments and other locations. It is available through Ovid Technologies, a commercial database vendor, which charges a user fee per hour. CHID is also available in many medical, university, and public libraries.

Major Nationwide Direct-Help Services and Organizations

American Brain Tumor Association
2720 River Road, Suite 146
Des Plaines, IL 60018
(847) 827-9910
(800) 866-ABTA
info@abta.org
http://www.abta.org

The American Brain Tumor Association supports research, offers printed materials about research and treatment of brain tumors and provides resource listings of physicians, treatment facilities, and support groups throughout the country.

Cancer Care, Inc.
1180 Avenue of the Americas, 2nd Floor
New York, NY 10036
(212) 302-2400

(800) 813-HOPE
cancercare@aol.com
http://www.cancercareinc.org

Cancer Care offers counseling, support groups, and financial assistance for nonmedical expenses, home visits by trained volunteers, and referrals to services such as housekeeping, nursing care and health aides.

Candlelighters Childhood Cancer Foundation
7910 Woodmont Avenue, Suite 460
Bethesda, MD 20814
(301) 657-8401
(800) 366-2223
info@candlelighters.org
http://www.candlelighters.org

The Candlelighters Foundation is an international organization whose goal is to help families of pediatric and adolescent cancer patients cope with the emotional stresses of their experiences. A survivors' network and an ombudsman program are also available. Candlelighters now includes 400 groups throughout the world.

Children's Hospice International
2202 Mount Vernon Avenue, Suite 3C
Alexandria, VA 22301
(703) 684-0330
(800) 242-4453
chiorg@aol.com
http://www.chinline.org

Children's Hospice International provides a network of support for dying children and their families. It serves as a clearinghouse on research programs, support groups, and education and training programs for the care of terminally ill children. It also offers publications on topics such as home care for seriously ill children and pain management.

EncorePlus
YWCA of the USA
Office of Women's Health Initiative
624 Ninth Street NW
Washington, DC 20001
(202) 628-3636
(800) 95E-PLUS
HN2205@handsnet.org
http://www.ywca.org

EncorePlus, a national program offered by the YWCA and sponsored by local YWCAs, targets medically underserved women in need of early detection education, breast and cervical cancer screening, and support services. The YWCA program also offers discussion and exercise programs for women presently under treatment for breast cancer, designed to help restore physical strength and emotional well-being. Phone the local YWCA branch for additional information.

Help for Incontinent People
P.O. Box 8310
Spartanburg, SC 29305
(800) BLADDER

This organization gives information on the benefits and drawbacks of various treatments for incontinence. It maintains a referral service of physicians and therapists to treat incontinence.

I Can Cope
1599 Clifton Road
Atlanta, GA 30329-4251
(404) 320-3333
Cancer Response System: (800) ACS-2345
http://www.cancer.org

I Can Cope is a course designed to address the educational and psychological needs of people with cancer. It is run locally, usually by nurses and social workers. Information about local courses is available through the American Cancer Society.

International Association of Laryngectomies
c/o American Cancer Society
1599 Clifton Road
Atlanta, GA 30329-4251
(404) 320-3333
Cancer Response System: (800) ACS-2345
http://www.cancer.org

The International Association of Laryngectomies, sponsored in cooperation with the American Cancer Society (ACS), assists people who have lost their voices as a result of cancer. It provides information on the skills needed by laryngectomies and works toward total rehabilitation of patients. A local chapter might be listed in the telephone directory, also contact the local ACS.

Hospice Link
Hospice Education Institute
190 Westbrook Road, Suite 3-B
Essex, CT 06426-1510
(860) 767-1620
(800) 331-1620

Hospice Link offers information about hospice care and can refer cancer patients and their families to local hospice programs.

Leukemia Society of America
600 Third Avenue, Fourth Floor
New York, New York 10016
(212) 573-8484
(800) 955-4LSA (publications only)
http://www.leukemia.org

This national voluntary health agency provides supplementary financial assistance to patients with leukemia, the lymphomas, and Hodgkin's disease, as well as referrals to other sources of help in the community. The program is administered through society chapters located in most of the United States. Further information is available by calling a local chapter listed in the white pages of the telephone directory.

Look Good, Feel Better
American Cancer Society
1599 Clifton Road
Atlanta, GA 30329-4251
(404) 320-3333
(800) 395-LOOK
http://www.cancer.org

This program was developed by the Cosmetic, Toiletry, and Fragrance Association Foundation in cooperation with the American Cancer Society (ACS) and the National Cosmetology Association. It focuses on techniques that can help people undergoing cancer treatment improve their appearance. Local ACS units can provide more information about this program.

Man to Man
American Cancer Society
1599 Clifton Road
Atlanta, GA 30329-4251
(404) 320-3333
Cancer Response System: (800) ACS-2345
http://www.cancer.org

For men with prostate cancer and their families, the Man to Man program provides education and support. The group component offers an opportunity for men and their families to talk with each other and with health professionals about their disease and related concerns. Some groups might offer "side by side" sessions for women partners with the men meeting separately.

National Alliance of Breast Cancer Organizations (NABCO)
9 East 37th Street, 10th Floor
New York, NY 10016
(212) 719-0154
(800) 719-9154
nabcoinfo@aol.com
http://www.nabco.org

NABCO is a nonprofit organization that provides information about breast cancer and acts as an advocate for the legislative concerns of breast cancer patients and survivors. It provides phone numbers for approximately 350 cancer support groups nationwide. Information on support groups by state can be accessed through http://www.nabco.org/index.html.

National Brain Tumor Foundation
785 Market Street, Suite 1600
San Francisco, CA 94103
(415) 284-2080
(800) 934-CURE
nbtf@braintumor.org
http://www.braintumor.org

The National Brain Tumor Foundation provides patients and families with information to cope with their brain tumors. This organization conducts national and regional conferences, publishes printed materials for patients and family members, provides access to a national network of patient support groups, and assists in answering patient inquiries. It also awards grants to fund research.

National Coalition for Cancer Survivorship
1010 Wayne Avenue, Fifth Floor
Silver Spring, MD 20910
(301) 650-8868
(888) 650-9127

The National Coalition for Cancer Survivorship is a network of groups and individuals that offers support to cancer survivors and their loved ones. It provides information and resources on support and life after a diagnosis of cancer.

National Hospice Organization
1901 North Moore Street, Suite 901
Arlington, VA 22209
(703) 243-5900
(800) 658-8898 (for hospice referral)
drsnho@cais.com
http://www.nho.org

The National Hospice Organization is an association of groups that provide hospice care. It was established to promote and maintain hospice care and to encourage support for patients and family members.

National Kidney Cancer Association
1234 Sherman Avenue
Evanston, IL 60202
(847) 332-1051
(800) 850-9132
office@nkc.com
http://www.nkca.com

The National Kidney Cancer Association supports research, offers printed materials about the diagnosis and treatment of kidney cancer, sponsors support groups, and provides physician referral information.

National Lymphedema Network
2211 Post Street, Suite 404
San Francisco, CA 94115-3427
(425) 921-1306
(800) 541-3259
lmphnct@hooked.net
http://www.hooked.net/~lymphnet

The National Lymphedema Network is a nonprofit resource center established in 1988. It disseminates information and guidance about lymphedema to patients and health professionals.

National Marrow Donor Program
3433 Broadway Street, NE, Suite 500
Minneapolis, MN 55413
(612) 627-5800
(800) MAR-ROW2
http://www.marrow.org

The National Marrow Donor Program, which is funded by the federal government, was created to improve the effectiveness of the search for bone marrow donors so that a greater number of bone marrow transplants can be carried out. It keeps a registry of potential bone marrow donors and provides a free packet of information on bone marrow transplants.

Skin Cancer Foundation
245 Fifth Avenue, Suite 1403
New York, NY 10016
(212) 725-5176
(800) SKIN-490
info@skincancer.org

The Skin Cancer Foundation conducts public and medical education programs to help reduce skin cancer. Major goals are to increase public awareness of the importance of taking protective measures against the damaging rays of the sun and to teach people how to recognize the early signs of skin cancer.

Reach to Recovery
1599 Clifton Road
Atlanta, GA 30329-4251
(404) 320-3333
Cancer Response System: (800) ACS-2345
http://www.cancer.org

The American Cancer Society's Reach to Recovery program offers assistance to breast cancer patients. Trained volunteers who have had breast cancer lend emotional support and furnish information to women before and after breast surgery. Additional information can be obtained from a local unit of the American Cancer Society listed in the telephone directory.

United Ostomy Association
36 Executive Park, Suite 120
Irvine, CA 92714-6744
(714) 660-8624
(800) 826-0826
uoa@deltanet.com
http://www.uoa.org

The United Ostomy Association (UOA) works in cooperation with the American Cancer Society. It is organized and administered by people with ostomies and provides mutual aid and emotional support. The UOA, which has local chapters across the country, provides information to patients and the public. In addition, the UOA sends volunteer ostomates to visit with new ostomy patients.

US TOO, International, Inc.
930 North York Road, Suite 50
Hinsdale, IL 60521
(630) 323-1002
(800) 82-USTOO
ustoo@ustoo.com
http://www.ustoo.com

US TOO is a prostate support group organization. It has chapters across the country to increase awareness of prostate cancer in the community, educate men newly diagnosed with prostate cancer, offer support groups, and provide the latest information about treatment for this disease.

Cancer Centers

There are 26 comprehensive cancer centers designated by the NCI. These medical research centers meet rigorous criteria in order to achieve their NCI designation. The Comprehensive Cancer Centers investigate new methods of diagnosis and treatment of cancer patients and provide new scientific knowledge to physicians who are treating cancer patients. Call (800) 4-CANCER (the Cancer Information Service) for the names and locations of these centers.

There also are clinical and laboratory cancer centers and medical centers that meet the requirements for support from the NCI for clinical programs to investigate promising new methods of cancer treatment or for laboratory research programs. For information about these centers call the Cancer Information Service.

The NCI conducts research programs to which patients are admitted at the Warren Grant Magnuson Clinical Center, the National Institutes of Health's research hospital in Bethesda, Maryland. To learn whether a cancer patient is eligible to participate in a research study at the Clinical Center, the patient's doctor can send a complete medical report to the Clinical Director, National Cancer Institute, Bldg. 10, Room 12N216, Bethesda, MD 20892. Additional information about the center and the investigational protocols being conducted there can be obtained by calling the Cancer Information Service.

More than 16,000 cancer research physicians at 2,200 institutions in the United States and abroad are members of the Clinical Trials Cooperative Group Program, supported in part by the NCI. Each cooperative program studies one or more kinds of cancer and assists the NCI in the clinical evaluation of new anticancer drugs and other investigational approaches to treatment. Patients admitted to these studies receive expert medical care from specially trained teams of physicians. Information about clinical cooperative groups and protocols being investigated by them is available through PDQ or the Cancer Information Service.

The Community Clinical Oncology Program (CCOP) provides an opportunity for community physicians to participate in cancer treatment research by means of clinical trials. Sponsored by the NCI, the CCOP encourages community physicians to work with scientists conducting NCI-supported clinical trials. For names of local participants and the protocols they are involved in, call the Cancer Information Service.

7

Coping with Cancer over the Course of Illness

Laurel L. Northouse
Suzanne Mellon

FRAMEWORK

Stress is an integral part of life. How individuals cope with stress depends on the meaning they give to a particular stressor. Because a diagnosis of cancer is a source of stress to both the client and family, a framework for stress and coping can help the nurse to understand, assess, and more effectively manage the care these clients require (see Figure 7–1).

Stress

Stress has been defined as a force, strain, or pressure that causes tension on an object or person. Although stimulus-response definitions of stress were once popular, they have proven to be inadequate. According to Lazarus and Folkman (1984), stress is defined more accurately in terms of the transactions that occur between individuals and their environments rather than just in terms of one or the other.

A stressor is a tension-producing stimulus that has the potential to disrupt an individual's equilibrium. Neuman (1995), a nurse theorist, contends that stressors can be viewed as intrapersonal, interpersonal, and/or extrapersonal in nature.

Intrapersonal stressors are those that occur within a person, such as a genetic factor or factors that predispose a person to cancer. These stressors are generally not under an individual's control.

Interpersonal stressors are forces in the client's external environment that involve more than one other person. Examples include breakdowns in communication patterns and/or changes in role expectations among patients and their families that occur as a result of a cancer diagnosis. As a result of hospitalization, cancer patients might be unable to assume their usual social, work, and/or family roles, and the roles of their family members could change as well.

Extrapersonal stressors are external environmental forces over which

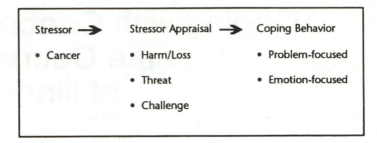

Figure 7-1. Framework for stress and coping.

the individual can usually exert some control. For clients and families living with a cancer diagnosis, one common example is the added financial strain related to loss of employment, expensive treatments, medications, and therapies.

Appraisal of Stressors

Neuman maintains that a stressor itself is a neutral entity. Whether the stressor is noxious or beneficial depends on how the client perceives it. Stressor appraisal is an evaluative cognitive process that occurs when an individual is confronted with a stressor that gives a situation meaning.

Lazarus and Folkman define three broad categories of stressor appraisals: harm or loss; threat; and challenge. *Harm or loss* appraisals are to be expected among clients living with cancer who know that the situation (cancer) they are dealing with has already caused them harm.

Threat appraisals involve seeing *potential* harm or loss in a situation. For example, the daughter of a breast cancer patient might perceive her own risk of developing breast cancer as a threat to her current health. A threat appraisal tends to be characterized by negative emotions such as anxiety, anger, worry, and fear.

Challenge appraisals focus on the potential for gain or growth from a situation. Because mastery or gain is perceived as a possible result, these situations tend to be characterized by positive emotions such as excitement, eagerness, and hopefulness. Thus, if a woman with a family history of breast cancer perceives this as a situation over which she has some control and could thus master, the stressor could result in prevention of future illness (gain).

Coping

After the appraisal of a stressor has been made, the individual must determine what can be done to manage and cope with the situation. According to Folkman and Lazarus, coping has been referred to as the ongoing cognitive and behavioral efforts that are used to manage specific external and/or internal demands that are appraised as taxing or exceeding a person's resources. Of the two major types of coping efforts that follow stressor appraisal, one is problem-focused and attempts to alter the stressful relationship between person and environment; the other, emotion-focused, tries to regulate the emotional reaction to that relationship.

Although it is not unusual for people to use both problem- and emotion-focused modes of coping, problem-focused behaviors tend to predominate in situations that the person believes are amenable to change. Some examples of problem-focused coping are obtaining additional information about a cancer diagnosis, obtaining a yearly breast or testicular exam from a health care provider, decreasing the amount of fat in the diet, and avoiding excessive exposure to the sun.

People tend to use more emotion-focused behaviors to cope with stressful situations that they believe must be accepted. Praying for a cure, displaying emotions such as anger or crying, and denying that one has been diagnosed with cancer are some emotion-focused coping behaviors that cancer patients and families could exhibit. This type of coping regulates emotions by making a person feel better about the situation. Unlike the problem-focused approach, it causes no actual change in the situation itself.

This theoretical framework for coping with stressors is drawn from the work of Neuman and Lazarus. It differs from more mechanistic views of stress and coping by emphasizing the client's perception of the stressor and the role that appraisal plays in the selection of effective coping responses.

COPING OVER THE COURSE OF ILLNESS

Coping and living with cancer is a process that extends over the course of illness. With improved health care through early detection and successful cancer treatments, cancer survivorship rates continue to increase. Surviving and coping with a cancer illness can take on many different forms, from living cancer-free after initial treatment, to living with recurrent and intermittent periods of disease, to living with continuous disease with the threat of impending death. As patients move from one phase of illness to another, they frequently confront new issues and concerns that might be unique to that phase. The following section is divided into four major phases of illness—initial, adaptation, recurrent, and terminal—and discusses the concerns that patients and their family members experience in each phase (see Table 7–1).

The Initial Phase

The initial phase of illness encompasses the period of diagnosis and early treatment of the disease. This phase is considered one of the most

Table 7-1
Issues Confronting Cancer Patients over the Course of Illness

Phase	Issue
Initial	Managing emotional upheaval Obtaining information
Adaptation	Adjusting to role changes Balancing family members' needs
Recurrent	Maintaining hope Establishing supportive relationships
Terminal	Providing care and support Dealing with loss and separation

stressful because of the high anxiety and apprehension that patients and family members experience as they wait for important diagnostic information and undergo various treatments for the cancer. Given the emotional turmoil that typically characterizes this period of time, perhaps it is not surprising that women awaiting a breast biopsy report nearly three times more anxiety and two times more depression than has been reported for the normal population (Northouse et al. 1995).

During the initial phase of illness, patients confront the emotional upheaval brought on by the uncertainty surrounding the diagnosis. In a study of newly diagnosed mastectomy patients, Northouse (1989) asked which period was most stressful: the time prior to surgery, just after surgery, or when they first returned home. The majority of the women (85 percent) reported that the time just before surgery was most stressful. They said that they experienced a tremendous amount of emotional turmoil and uncertainty as they waited for the results of mammograms, ultrasounds, and breast biopsies. Many women said that *not knowing* whether they had cancer was worse than knowing that they had it. These women found themselves in a state of limbo and uncertain about how to appraise their situation.

Typically, patients and family members move through the diagnostic phase with little help from professionals. Because most of the diagnostic workups are conducted on an outpatient basis, patients are not connected to a team of health care professionals who can offer consistent support; therefore, patients rely a great deal on family and friends during this time. Many patients have reported, however, that a supportive link with a health professional would be helpful during the diagnostic period.

After the diagnostic workups are completed, patients are often hospitalized for surgical treatment of the cancer, aggressive therapies, or further staging procedures to determine the extent of the disease. New stressors emerge when patients are hospitalized. Reports indicate that the period of hospitalization can be especially difficult for family members, who often experience stress and exhaustion as they try to juggle jobs with added home responsibilities while spending time at the hospital supporting the patient. Even though hospital stays are becoming shorter (in some cases less than 24 hours for a mastectomy), family members are still expected to take on many complex caregiving responsibilities as soon as the patient returns home. It is not uncommon for family members to report physiological manifestations of tension such as insomnia or loss of appetite during this time. Family members, like patients, need support. It is helpful when professionals take a few minutes to ask family members how they are coping and to provide them with assistance as needed.

A second major issue that confronts patients and family members is obtaining information. Both patients and family members eagerly await information that will reduce their uncertainty and give them some sense of what lies ahead. In a classic study of how much information cancer patients want, Cassileth and her associates (1980) found that most patients want as much information as possible. The investigators also found that the patients who wanted the most detailed information tended to be younger, more educated, and more recently diagnosed with cancer. Investigators who have compared the coping strategies used by early-stage and late-stage cancer patients report that seeking information is a more common coping strategy for patients in the initial phase of illness (see Chapter 6A).

Although information is important to patients, it is not always available. Time spent waiting for the results of bone scans or pathology reports can seem endless. Breast cancer patients in one study talked about the difficulty they had while waiting for the results of pathology reports on their axillary nodes, which typically took three days. Women described the experience as "being on needles and pins" or "waiting for the death knell" because the report would tell them about the extent of their cancer and their odds of surviving the disease. Given the importance of information, patients and family members should be given the results of diagnostic tests and other laboratory reports as soon as they are available, and they should also be told when to expect the information.

What helps patients and family members to cope with the emotional turmoil during the initial phase of illness? When mastectomy patients in one study were asked this question, the majority reported that emotional support, information, and religious beliefs were the most important factors. Although husbands and close family members were their major sources of support, some women identified nurses and physicians as important sources of support while they were hospitalized. Information was also helpful in getting their questions answered, understanding procedures, and knowing what to expect in the hospital. Religious beliefs, especially faith, were important because they provided the patients with another source of strength and helped them to find purpose and meaning in the illness.

Adaptation Phase

The adaptation phase of illness occurs as patients and families shift their focus from getting a diagnosis to adjusting to the illness. The specific issues faced during this period can vary a great deal from one patient to another. Some patients will be recuperating from surgery and trying to accept body image changes brought on by a mastectomy or colostomy. Other patients will be undergoing months of chemotherapy to help arrest the disease. In spite of the different challenges, both patients and family members in this phase attempt to restore some normalcy in their lives.

During the adaptation phase family members confront and learn to adjust to changes in roles and lifestyles. Recuperation from surgery and ongoing treatments can limit the extent to which patients can resume previous roles, and their responsibilities must often be reallocated in order to maintain family stability. Stetz, Lewis, and Primomo (1986) examined the coping strategies that family members used to deal with day-to-day problems following the diagnosis of cancer and other chronic diseases in the mother. They found that the three most commonly used management strategies were problem-focused: making alterations in household management, seeking assistance or information from outside sources, and mobilizing family members to take action. Coping strategies used less frequently by family members were passive acceptance, taking no action, and withdrawing from the situation.

Although reallocating roles among family members is often useful, it is not always easy. In some families "who does what" is firmly established, and there is little shifting of roles among members. It might be difficult for patients to recover in families where they experience many stereotypic role demands at the same time that they are grappling with the physical and emotional demands of the illness.

Another task that confronts patients and family members during the adaptation phase of illness is learning to balance the needs of the ill member with the needs of the well members. Early in the patient's convalescence, the family is often preoccupied with the patient's illness and might direct all of its energy toward the patient's recovery. As the illness continues, however, other family members can become resentful as their own needs go unmet. They could send subtle messages to the patient that the allotted time for recovery is up and that it is time to return to life as usual. Balancing the personal needs of well family members with the ongoing needs of the ill member is a challenge, especially if the recovery takes longer than anticipated.

Concerns about the meaning of the cancer illness and existential/spiritual needs often surface during this time. In a study of men and women receiving active treatment for their cancer illness, Post-White and colleagues (1996) examined patients' meaning of hope while facing cancer and how it was related to their spirituality and quality of life. Finding meaning in their illness through spirituality and faith was an important part in sustaining a sense of hope. In addition, focusing on day-to-day living; relying on personal inner resources; valuing relationships with family members, friends and health care providers; and looking toward surviving cancer also contributed to patients' sense of hope.

Recurrent Phase

The recurrent phase of illness refers to a period of time when the cancer returns. Until recently there was little discussion of this phase, because the return of the cancer was synonymous with death and the terminal phase of illness. However, with recent advances in the treatment of cancer, new protocols are now available to treat the recurrent cancer aggressively and cause a remission of the disease. It is not uncommon for patients to experience of series of recurrences and remissions over an extended number of years.

The recurrent phase of illness is often a disappointing time for patients and family members. The return of the cancer shatters hopes that the initial cancer was cured and raises the fear that this time the cancer will be fatal. In a study by Mahon, Cella, and Donovan (1990), the majority of patients (78 percent) reported that the recurrence was more upsetting than the initial diagnosis. These patients said that at the time of recurrence the threat of death was more real, the decisions regarding treatment more difficult, and the side effects of treatment more severe. This is also a difficult period of time for family members, who report feelings of anger and injustice at the disease's repeated assault.

Maintaining hope is one challenge that patients and family members face during a recurrence. When the cancer returns, hope fades as patients and family members realize that the potential for cure is gone. Patients in the Mahon, Cella, and Donovan study said that they were much less hopeful about their chances of recovering at the time of recurrence compared with the time of initial diagnosis. Some of the patients questioned why the cancer returned and reported feeling guilty that they may have made the wrong choice of treatment. Other patients thought the recurrence was some form of punishment. According to some researchers, patients who feel hopeless or sense hopelessness in their health care providers are more likely to turn to unconventional forms of treatment. Health professionals need to help patients maintain positive expectations in the face of highly uncertain circumstances.

Establishing supportive relationships with others is another issue that patients confront during the recurrent phase of illness. Although patients and family members need support, they report strained or ineffective relationships with health professionals during this phase. Patients in one study reported that health professionals seldom asked them how they were coping and seemed to assume that patients were coping better than they actually were. In other studies, patients have reported communication problems with professionals that leave them feeling isolated and alone as they attempt to cope with the ramifications of the recurrence. Although no definitive information is available on why patient–professional relationships are less effective during this period, the research indicates that health professionals need to devote more energy to assessing the emotional concerns of patients and family members and to communicating empathy and understanding during the recurrent phase.

In addition to supportive relationships with professionals, patients need to maintain supportive communication with family and friends. There are mixed reports on how supportive family members are during this time. In one study, more than half of the patients reported that family relationships became less supportive at the time of the recurrence because family members were more fearful and had greater difficulty providing support. Other investigators have reported no change in the nature of family relationships, suggesting that by the time the recurrence occurs, the supportive relationships have already been developed. Given these inconsistencies in the literature, it is important to assess the nature of the patient's relationship with family and professionals during this phase of illness.

Thus, it appears that coping with a recurrence can be more difficult for some patients than others. In one study, patients who had the most difficulty adjusting to the recurrence had more symptom distress (due to treatments or progressive disease), less optimism, more uncertainty, and less support from others (Northouse, Dorris, and Charron-Moore 1995). The research suggests that how patients and their family members appraise the recurrence, as well as the resources that they use to cope with it, are important factors that affect their adjustment.

Terminal Phase

The terminal phase of illness occurs as the patient's condition worsens and death appears inevitable. For many years, research on coping with cancer focused primarily on this phase of illness because cancer was so often equated with death. In recent years with increasing cancer survivorship rates, this phase has been considered one of many in the course of the illness.

During this time, families face the need to provide care and support to the dying family member. Family members, either by default or by choice, often assume the primary caregiving role. In doing this, family members often experience considerable strain trying to provide care to the dying family member while also meeting household, child care, and/or work responsibilities. The strain on family members intensifies when the dying family member's condition worsens and he or she needs assistance with daily activities such as eating or bathing.

Not all families feel that they have the emotional stamina or knowledge to assist the dying family member. Family members in one study said that they needed more information about how to provide care in areas such as controlling pain and coping with the emotional demands of the illness. Visiting nurses or members of a hospice team are important sources of information and emotional support to dying patients and their family members.

During the terminal phase, patients and family members must deal with feelings of separation and loss. A sense of powerlessness can pervade the family, due in part to the helplessness experienced by the dying family member and also to the helplessness felt by the family caregivers who are unable to ease the dying family member's helplessness or alter the course of illness. Although some family members might postpone their own grief while they assist the dying family member, others commonly have feelings of abandonment, loss, and confusion during this time. Surviving spouses often need to help children or aging parents cope with impending loss at the same time that they are trying to cope with the situation.

Several investigators have studied the communication patterns between dying cancer patients and their family members, and they found that very little discussion of death takes place. Although it is a commonly held belief that open communication during terminal illness is essential, it does not always happen. For example, in a study by Krant and Johnson (1978), 78 percent of the family members reported that they had not discussed death with the dying family member. For some families the conscious or unconscious decision to avoid discussing death is an important coping mechanism and the continuation of a long-standing pattern not to discuss emotionally charged issues in the family. As health professionals try to help families through the terminal phase of illness, the families who might be most in need of assistance are not those with comfortable, agreed-upon patterns of communication (either to discuss or not discuss). Rather, they are those that are uncertain about how to communicate about death or those in which the communication preferences of one or more members are not compatible with the preferences of other members.

An important challenge facing health care professionals during this terminal phase is assessing and intervening in such quality-of-life concerns. In a study by Greisinger and colleagues (1997), patients reported that while they received good physical care, the spiritual, existential, emotional, or family relationship issues that most concerned them were rarely addressed. Having the opportunity to discuss or work toward resolution of spiritual and psychosocial concerns was a critical issue brought out by this group of terminally ill patients.

NURSING CARE MANAGEMENT OF PATIENTS AND FAMILIES

Assessment

Assessment of the cancer patient's coping abilities needs to be family focused and ongoing. Though playing an integral role in helping patients cope with illness, families, like patients, also experience the accompanying stress. Table 7–2 provides a series of assessment questions that could be asked during each phase of illness. Obviously, neither time nor circumstances permits using all of the questions.

During the initial phase of illness, it is important to determine what information patients and family members have about the illness and also what information they want but have not received. Preferences for information can vary considerably from one patient to another, so it is often helpful to ask them about their particular desires. For example, a nurse might say to a patient, "Some people want a lot of information about their illness and various procedures while others want just the minimum. I would like to know what your preferences are, so I can keep them in mind as I plan your care." Assessment questions such as these not only provide valuable information but also convey to the patient the nurse's desire to tailor nursing care to meet the patient's needs.

Table 7–2
Assessment Questions for Cancer Patients and Family Members

Initial Phase

What information do you have about the diagnosis?
What kind of information would be helpful to you at this time?
Do you understand the procedures or tests?
How are you feeling about the diagnosis?
What particular aspect of the illness is most distressing?
What is helping you to cope right now?
Do you have any spiritual concerns?

Adaptation Phase

How much energy or fatigue are you experiencing?
To what extent are you able to carry out your previous roles?
What kind of help are you receiving from family and friends?
To what extent has life returned to normal for you?
What is the meaning of the cancer illness to you?

Recurrent Phase

How are you feeling about the recurrence?
How surprised were you by the recurrence?
Have you been able to maintain a hopeful attitude?
Are you getting the information that you need?
Are you getting the support that you need?

Terminal Phase

How are you feeling physically and emotionally?
How much stress are you experiencing in your caregiving role?
What resources are available to you?
Are you satisfied with how family members are relating?
What is most important for your quality of life now?
Do you need a referral to a social worker, chaplain, or someone else?

It is also important to assess how patients and family members are coping with the new diagnosis and stressful ramifications of the illness. For example, a nurse might say to the husband of a cancer patient, "Hospitalizations are stressful for husbands as well as wives. How are you managing your work, with the added time that you are spending at the hospital? Are you getting enough rest?" These assessment questions not only elicit important information but also convey empathy to family members, who often feel like outsiders when the patient is hospitalized.

During the adaptation phase, it is important to assess patients' energy levels and the extent to which they have resumed their normal roles and lifestyles. Patients who report more fatigue than anticipated or continuing disability should be asked about the kind of help that they might or might not be receiving from other family members. Finally, it might be helpful to determine the extent to which life has returned to normal for the patient and for the rest of the family.

In the recurrent phase of illness, nurses and other health professionals need to elicit the feelings of patients and family members about the recurrence. By asking whether they were surprised by the recurrence, the nurse can determine the extent to which they considered the possibility of the cancer recurring. Because maintaining hope is such an important factor during this phase, patients' levels of hope must be assessed. Questions such as "Have you been able to maintain a hopeful outlook since the recurrence?" or "How hopeful are you feeling about your situation?" can offer patients an opportunity to discuss their feelings.

Finally, given the reports that patients' relationships with health professionals are strained during this time, it is essential to ask patients and family members about these relationships and the extent to which they are getting the support and information they need.

During the terminal phase, health care professionals need to assess the emotional well-being and physical health of both patients and family members. Because the demands on family caregivers are high during this time, it is important to assess their stress and the resources that they have to cope with it. The effectiveness of family relationships, especially communication among family members, also needs to be determined. Throughout all phases of the illness, it is important to elicit any spiritual concerns that patients might have. Questions addressing patients' spirituality go beyond religious preferences to existential concerns regarding the purpose and meaning in life elicited by confronting a cancer illness. Openly raising these questions can assist patients and families to maintain hope and create potential new ways to cope with the illness.

Management

On the basis of the data obtained during the assessment, nurses can formulate individualized plans of care. Table 7–3 lists nursing diagnoses

Table 7-3
Nursing Diagnoses and Interventions during Various Phases of Illness

Nursing Diagnoses	Interventions
Initial Phase	
A. Fear related to potential diagnosis of cancer and its treatment.	Assist patient and family to list specific questions that they would like answered about cancer and its treatment. Provide information about diagnostic procedures and when results of procedures can be expected. Maintain consistent, supportive contact with patient and family while awaiting test results. Be optimistic when discussing possible outcomes with patient and family but support a realistic assessment of the situation.
B. Ineffective patient and/or family coping related to hospitalization secondary to cancer diagnosis.*	Determine the effectiveness of current coping strategies and suggest alternatives, if necessary. Determine the amount and type of information that would be helpful to patient/family. Teach patients and families about the disease process, medications, and pre- and postoperative routines.
Adaptation Phase	
A. Disturbance in body image/self-concept related to loss of a body part or function.	Assist patient and family to identify concerns regarding perceived body image changes. Encourage family to provide positive feedback regarding changes to patient. Emphasize patient's remaining strengths and abilities. Arrange a role model from ACS to visit with patient when appropriate.
B. Alteration in patient/family roles/lifestyle patterns secondary to cancer diagnosis.	Encourage patient and family to verbalize their feelings regarding perceived changes in roles. Assist family members to alter current household responsibilities as necessary. Provide family members with a safe outlet for expression of anger and guilt regarding role changes that may otherwise be directed at patient. Consult other departments/support personnel as needed.
Recurrent Phase	
A. Ineffective communication patterns between patient and family and/or health care providers.	Encourage patient and family to express their fears or concerns about the recurrence. Use facilitative communication techniques—e.g., open-ended questions, reflective statements, rephrasing of patient's and family's statements— that promote expression of feelings. Consult with social service, psychiatric clinical nurse specialist (CNS), or clergy, as needed.

Table 7-3 *(Continued)*
Nursing Diagnoses and Interventions during Various Phases of Illness

Nursing Diagnoses	Interventions
Recurrent Phase	
B. Spiritual Distress**	Encourage patient to discuss spiritual and religious concerns and support activities that meet these needs. Assist patient/family in exploring purpose and meaning in the cancer illness. Foster a sense of hope during current phase of illness. Respect patient's right to follow own spiritual beliefs and/or religious practices. Facilitate patient and family in expression of feelings and resolution of family concerns. Include referrals to others as needed (clergy, social workers, psychiatric CNS).
Terminal Phase	
A. Powerlessness related to loss of control over situation.	Give patient and family as much control over the environment as possible. • Allow patient to make decisions re: a.m. care, walks, naps, turning, and so on. • Encourage family not to unnecessarily restrict patient's activities. • Support and encourage family members to participate in patient's care. • Provide patient and family with pertinent information regarding basic care needs, e.g., pain management techniques. • Allow patient and family to talk about their feelings about lack of control over the situations. • Assist patient and family to identify their own strengths and provide positive reinforcement to enhance self-esteem. • If appropriate, refer to hospice setting to allow family and patient increased control over environmental factors.

* A diagnosis of ineffective coping is common to all phases of illness; the etiology could change as patient and family move through the stages of illness.

** A diagnosis of spiritual distress can occur during all phases of illness.

and interventions for each phase of illness. Generally, the focus of care centers around the following broad areas:

1. **Providing support:** Many research studies have documented that support from others is one of the most important factors that helps patients and family members cope with cancer. As patients receive support, they realize that they are not alone but that there is a network of people who are ready and willing to help them. Support from oth-

ers bolsters the courage of cancer patients and gives them a sense that they will be able to cope with the ramifications of the illness.

Support can come in various forms. Tangible support provides patients with assistance such as preparing meals, providing transportation, or caring for children. Emotional support allows patients to vent feelings, receive encouragement, and feel understood. Whether patients and family members will need tangible support, emotional support, or both depends on the nature of the illness and the demands it places on them.

One of the most important ways that nurses can provide support is by listening to the concerns of patients and family members and by showing empathic understanding. It is helpful when nurses take a few minutes out of their busy schedules to "be with" patients and to try to understand their feelings. Empathic communication helps patients verbalize their concerns to nurses and helps nurses show their support to patients.

2. **Providing information:** Information is a powerful factor that reduces patients' feelings of uncertainty and enables them to cope with illness. Nurses can play an important role in educating patients about cancer, the side effects of treatments, and ways to manage the disease. It is helpful to teach patients not only about the physical aspects of the disease but also about its emotional aspects. Family members need to be included in teaching sessions so that they can learn more about the disease and ways to help the patient. Rather than assume that patients and family members have the information that they need, nurses need to ask what they have been told and what additional information would be helpful (see Chapter 6A).

3. **Finding meaning:** Finding meaning in illness is an important dimension in living with illness or in providing care that crosses psychosocial and spiritual dimensions. A cancer diagnosis raises questions about the meaning and purpose of life, creates uncertainty regarding the future, and highlights the importance of maintaining hope. Establishing a trusting relationship, being responsive to each individual's cues, supporting individual religious beliefs, and assisting in relationships with family members and others can be critical interventions. To promote spiritual and emotional health, nurses need to explore with patients their existential concerns about the meaning and purpose of their life and foster a sense of hope.

4. **Mobilizing resources:** At times patients and family members will need additional resources to facilitate their adjustment to illness. Fortunately, there are many resources available such as I Can Cope patient education groups, hospital-based support groups, Meals on Wheels, Reach to Recovery volunteers, and so on (see Chapter 6B). Although there are many resources, patients might be

unaware of or hesitant to use them. Nurses are in a key position to inform patients and their families about what resources are available and which might be most helpful.

In summary, this chapter provides information on coping with cancer and specifically on how patients and family members cope over the course of illness. Nurses can play a major role in helping patients and family members cope by assessing their needs during each phase of illness and by providing them with support, information, meaning, and resources.

BIBLIOGRAPHY

1. Cassileth, B. R., R. Y. Zupkis, K. Sutton-Smith, and Y. March. Information and participation preferences among cancer patients. *Ann Intern Med* 92: 832–836. 1980.

   Investigators studied the amount of information preferred by cancer patients and found that the majority of patients wanted the maximum amount of information. Younger, newly diagnosed patients wanted the most information.

2. Greisinger, A. J., R. J. Lorimor, L. A. Aday, R. J. Winn, and W. F. Baile. Terminally ill cancer patients: Their most important concerns. *Cancer Practice* 5: 147–154. 1997.

   This article describes interviews with terminally ill patients and the critical issues affecting their quality of life. Open discussion and assessment of spiritual, existential, family relationship issues, and emotional aspects of their cancer illness are cited as priority concerns.

3. Johnston Taylor, E., M. Highfield, and M. Amenta. Attitudes and beliefs regarding spiritual care: A survey of cancer nurses. *Cancer Nurs* 17: 479–487. 1994.

   This article reports on a survey of oncology nurses' definitions, attitudes, and beliefs about spiritual care. Major themes included respecting and supporting patients' spiritual beliefs and supporting relationships with others.

4. Krant, M. J., and L. Johnson. Family members' perceptions of communication in late stages of cancer. *International Journal of Psychiatry in Medicine* 8: 203–216. 1978.

   Investigators studied the communication between dying patients and family members and found that little discussion of death took place. Not only was family communication guarded, but family members often felt uncomfortable visiting their dying family member.

5. Lazarus, R. S., and S. Folkman. *Stress, Appraisal, and Coping.* Springer Publishing Company, New York. 1984.

   This text explores a research-based theory of stress and coping that focuses on the importance of cognitive appraisal.

6. Mahon, S. M., D. F. Cella, and M. I. Donovan. Psychosocial adjustment to recurrent cancer. *Oncol Nurs Forum Supplement* 17(3): 47–52. 1990.

   This article describes the psychosocial adjustment of patients to various types of recurrent cancer. Subjects reported that the recurrence was more stressful than the initial diagnosis of cancer.

7. Neuman, B. *The Neuman Systems Model, 3d Ed.* Appleton & Lange, Norwalk, CT. 1995.

   This nursing theory text presents an overview of the Neuman systems model and describes its application to educational and practice settings. The major concepts included in the stress and coping model are stressor (inter-, intra-, and extrapersonal), stressor appraisal, levels of intervention (primary, secondary, tertiary), reconstitution, lines of defense, and lines of resistance.

8. Northouse, L. L. The impact of breast cancer on patients and husbands. *Cancer Nurs* 12(5): 276–284. 1989.

   This article describes the emotional reactions of patients and their husbands at two different times after a mastectomy. Both immediately after surgery and one month later, survival was the most prominent concern of patients and husbands.

9. Northouse, L. L., M. Jeffs, A. Cracchiolo-Caraway, L. Lampman, and G. Dorris. Emotional distress reported by women and husbands prior to a breast biopsy. *Nursing Research* 44: 196–201. 1995.

   This article describes a research study conducted with 300 women and a majority of their husbands prior to a breast biopsy. Women reported high emotional distress prior to biopsy; their husbands reported mild distress.

10. Northouse, L. L., G. Dorris, and C. Charron-Moore. Factors affecting couples' adjustment to recurrent breast cancer. *Social Science and Medicine* 41: 69–76. 1995.

    This study explored factors that affected women's and husbands' adjustment to the first recurrence of breast cancer. Symptom distress and hopelessness accounted for the most variance in women's and husbands' adjustment scores.

11. Post-White, J., C. Ceronsky, M. J. Kreitzer, K. Nickelson, D. Drew, K. Watrud Mackey, L. Koopmeiners, and S. Gutknecht. Hope, spirituality, sense of coherence, and quality of life in patients with cancer. *Oncol Nurs Forum* 23: 1571–1579. 1996.

    Investigators explored the meaning of hope and its relationship to spiritual beliefs, sense of coherence and quality of life of cancer patients and found that spiritual/religious beliefs helped them sustain hope and find meaning in their illness. Reliance on relationships with family members and significant others and personal inner resources were also important in maintaining hope.

12. Stetz, K. M., F. M. Lewis, and J. Primomo. Family coping strategies and chronic illness in the mother. *Family Relations* 35: 515–522. 1986.

    This article describes the coping strategies that families used to manage the day-to-day problems when a mother was diagnosed with cancer or another chronic disease. The investigators found that families used a variety of internal strategies and external resources.

Comfort

A. Pain

Patricia Manda Collins

INTRODUCTION

In 1965, Ronald Melzack and Patrick Wall published an article in the journal *Science* titled "Pain Mechanisms: A New Theory," which revolutionized the field of pain research. Prior to this, experts accounted for the mechanisms of pain according to one of two diametrically opposed theories: the specificity theory and the pattern theory. Melzack and Wall's Gate Control Theory partially explains why the ultimate response and perception of pain can be modulated in the periphery, spinal cord, and brain. This new understanding of the pain mechanism is based, in part, on their research on the interaction between large- and small-diameter afferent nerves, which transmit impulses from the peripheral toward the central nervous system. This mechanism provides the rationale for increasing large fiber activity via counterirritants such as transcutaneous nerve stimulation, massage, and cold applications, which can modify an individual's perception of pain. The Gate Control Theory includes the concept of descending control, providing support for behavioral medicine's role in pain assessment and management.

Despite the intricacies of how human beings perceive pain and the differing opinions about basic pain science, most experts agree that pain is a biopsychosocial experience. Not only do neuroanatomy, neurophysiology, and neurochemistry influence the pain response, but a complex interplay of physical, psychosocial, and environmental factors can increase or decrease pain perception. These factors include genetics, conditioning responses, emotional responses, prior learning history, environment, religion, ethnicity, race, age, and sex. Individual differences not only affect how a person perceives and processes sensory information, but ultimately, how he or she will respond to treatment. It is precisely for these reasons that our approach to managing pain demands that we carefully assess pain and employ a variety of treatment strategies, focusing on each patient as a unique individual.

DEFINITION OF PAIN

The complexity of the pain experience makes it difficult to present a good working definition. The International Association for the Study of

Pain defines pain as "an unpleasant sensory and emotional experience associated with actual or potential tissue damage or described in terms of such damage." In contrast, pain expert Margo McCaffery emphasizes the subjective nature of pain: "Pain is whatever the experiencing person says it is, existing whenever (and wherever) the experiencing person says it does." This view of pain removes the nurse from a judgmental position and assumes the credibility of the patient. The focus of care then becomes eliminating the cause of pain and/or treating the symptoms.

PAIN IN THE PERSON WITH CANCER

A person with cancer often experiences pain or discomfort for numerous reasons, some of which might not be directly related to the tumor (see Table 8A–1). Most patients will feel pain of varying duration and degree at some point in their cancer experience, during diagnosis, treatment, remission, cure, or at end of life. The pain could be acute, chronic, or both (see Table 8A–2) and have somatic, visceral and/or neuropathic components (see Table 8A–3). Furthermore, patients often have more than one pain at a time. In addition, numerous physical, psychosocial, and environmental factors can negatively influence the pain experience (see Table 8A–4).

Tumors cause pain by invading, destroying, or compressing the affected area. The most common cause of cancer-related pain is bone metastases from cancers of the breast, lung, or prostate. Other pain syndromes seen in persons with cancer include postherpetic neuralgia, incidental pain, post-surgical or -procedural pain, headache, and brachial plexopathy and lumbosacral plexopathy, which might be due to radiation therapy. Certain chemotherapeutic agents such as cisplatin, paclitaxel, and the vinca alkaloids can cause painful peripheral neuropathies. Pre-existing, nonmalignant conditions such as arthritis or migraines can be present concomitantly.

Determining the type of pain is essential when considering treatment. *Nociceptive pain* results when nociceptors (A delta and C fibers) are activated by noxious chemical, mechanical, or thermal stimulation. Nociceptive pain is either somatic or visceral and continues as long as the noxious stimulus persists or until healing occurs. For example, touching a hot stove or cutting oneself results in somatic pain. The pain is typically localized and initially is sharp but then becomes dull and aching. Visceral pain is usually poorly localized and is perceived as a deep, crampy, squeezing pain. The patient could have referred pain and autonomic symptoms such as diaphoresis, nausea, and vomiting. Patients with intestinal obstruction have visceral pain due to distention of the intestines. *Neuropathic pain* continues after the noxious stimulus is thought to have dissipated. There might be a dysfunction in the peripheral or central nervous system that leads to persistent activation of peripheral nerves. The

Table 8A-1
Causes of Pain in Cancer Patients

Source	Cause of Pain
Tumor	Release of pain-causing substances produced by the tumor or by the immune system in response to the presence of tumor. Invasion of tumor into bone, nerves, pleura/peritoneum, viscera, blood vessels, mucous membranes, soft tissue.
Treatments	Surgery: Acute postoperative pain, chronic pain syndromes (e.g., post-thoracotomy, post-mastectomy, post-surgical neuromas, post-surgical adhesions/scarring, phantom limb). Chemotherapy: extravasation, phlebitis, mucositis, neuropathy, diarrhea, constipation, aseptic bone necrosis, sepsis. Radiation therapy: skin desquamation, mucositis, diarrhea, implants, gastric ulcer, fat necrosis, fibrosis, myelopathy, nerve plexopathies, scarring, osteo-radionecrosis. Biotherapy: myalgia/arthralgia, neuropathy. Miscellaneous: insertion of central lines.
Diagnostic Tests	Bone marrow aspiration. Biopsy. Invasive radiologic procedure. Venipuncture. Lumbar puncture. Positioning on hard table.
Nursing Procedures	Injection. Venipuncture. Dressing change. Movement of painful body parts.
Co-morbid Conditions	Diabetic neuropathy. Low back pain. Headache. Arthritis. Pressure ulcer. Muscle spasms/cramps. Peripheral vascular disease. Postherpetic neuralgia. Prolonged immobility.

pain is perceived as burning, numbing, stabbing, shooting, or electric-like. Normally innocuous stimuli such as light touch can produce pain (allodynia). There might be color or temperature changes at the site. Patients often use colorful analogies to describe this type of pain. For example, a woman with postmastectomy syndrome said that it felt like a four-inch

Table 8A-2
Characteristics of Acute and Chronic Pain

Type	Description	Management
Acute	Recent onset.	Management directed to underlying cause.
	Results from noxious stimuli: recent surgery infection fracture	Usually involves standard doses of analgesics administered parenterally or orally on a PRN basis.
	Visible expression of pain common (e.g., grimace).	
	Physiologic changes often present: tachycardia diaphoresis hypertension pallor mydriasis	
Chronic	Duration >6 months.	Management directed toward symptom control.
	Pathology persists or is difficult to identify.	Analgesics are usually administered orally around the clock in doses titrated for the individual.
	Absence of physiologic signs due to adaptation.	Adjuvant drugs and nonpharmacological therapies might be indicated.
	Visible expression of pain might be absent.	
	Depression and fatigue is likely.	

copper wire was imbedded in her chest. She could even imagine the diameter of the wire. Another patient likened his pain to being stabbed by a branding iron. This type of pain can be very distressing to patients not only because of its seemingly never-ending, sickening quality, but because managing this type of pain is difficult and frustrating.

Breakthrough pain is a transitory increase in pain over usually well-controlled baseline or persistent pain. The pain intensity is usually moderate or severe and occurs either suddenly or progressively over time. Its origin could be nociceptive, neuropathic, or both and is related to the disease, treatment, or some unknown cause. Breakthrough pain can occur sponta-

Table 8A–3
Types of Pain

Nociceptive

Somatic
  Injury to cutaneous or deep tissue (e.g., bone metastasis)
  Well-localized
  Acute or chronic
  Aching or throbbing

Visceral
  Stretching or distension of thoracic or abdominal viscera (e.g., bowel obstruction)
  Poorly localized
  Acute or chronic
  Crampy, pressure, deep aching, squeezing

Neuropathic

  Injury to nerves and nerve structures (e.g., post-thoracotomy, post-mastectomy, post-herpetic neuralgia)
  Acute or chronic
  Sharp, cutting, burning, aching, shooting, electric shock-like, numbness, tingling, prickling

neously or be precipitated by activity. Typically, the person experiences several episodes a day, each lasting about 30 minutes. The ideal treatment for breakthrough pain would have a quick onset and short duration of effect. It is important to distinguish breakthrough pain from that pain caused by inadequate dosing of the around the clock (ATC) medication for baseline or persistent pain.

Treating persons with cancer- or treatment-related pain often requires an intense effort and frequently involves help from a variety of experts. While there have been tremendous advancements in treating cancer, many patients continue to suffer from unrelieved pain. Some of the reasons for this situation and the possible solutions are discussed throughout this chapter.

PAIN ASSESSMENT

Ideally, the purpose of pain assessment is to learn as much as possible about the pain so that one can identify and subsequently eliminate its cause and, in the process, provide measures to relieve the discomfort. In reality, however, it is not always easy to identify clear-cut reasons for pain, so the suffering patient then tries to "prove" that he or she indeed has pain. Reassuring patients that we believe their report of pain is an essential part of pain assessment.

Table 8A–4
Factors Which Negatively Influence the Pain Experience

Physical	Psychosocial	Environmental
Anorexia	Age (young/elderly)	Noise
Taste changes	Culture (taboos, pain	Light (too bright or dark)
Mucositis	behavior, communication	Temperature (too hot or
Dry mouth	difficulties)	cold)
Dehydration	Sex (pain behavior,	Sensory stimulation
Dysphagia	expectations of care,	—overload
Nausea and	attitudes of caregiver)	—deprivation
vomiting	Religion (meaning of pain	Poor architectural design
Abdominal	and suffering)	Restraints
bloating	Past negative pain	Dislike of facility
Constipation	experience	(hospital, nursing home)
Diarrhea	Poor economic status	Caregivers (attitude,
Incontinence	Unwanted role changes	attention, knowledge)
Urinary retention	Poor self-concept	Lack of privacy
Wounds	—body image	Presence of unpleasant
Pruritis	—self-esteem	tubes, equipment
Lymphedema	Social isolation	Important items out of
Cough	Poor coping ability	reach
Shortness of	Affective state	
breath	—anxiety	
Hiccups	—anger	
Muscle	—depression	
spasms/cramps	—fear	
Immobility	—negativism	
Insomnia	—hopelessness	
Fatigue	—loss of control	
Confusion	Poor social support	
Perspiration	Lack of knowledge about	
Indigestion	disease/treatment	
Thirst	Restricted access to	
Presence of co-	family/friends	
morbid conditions	Poor cognitive functions	
	Lack of access to care	

One of the first stages of a pain assessment is listening to the patient's pain story. Attention to this part of the assessment will provide valuable clues for the remainder of the evaluation. Additional components of the assessment include obtaining a medical history, performing a physical examination, and reviewing diagnostic studies. Many people with cancer pain have several pains, and each pain can have its own etiology. Questions about each pain should focus on location, onset, frequency, radiation, pattern, severity, and exacerbating/relieving factors, as well as analgesic uses, effectiveness, and side effects and the patient's choices regarding pain management methods. Because pain is more than a biochemical event, its evaluation must include not only the sensory aspect of the experience but the psychosocial aspects as well.

Although the patient is the best source of information, family members and caregivers can also provide information helpful in the assessment process.

Some barriers to adequate assessment are language differences, cultural issues, economic disadvantages, and limitations due to age. The health care provider can become a barrier as well when personal beliefs, attitudes and values conflict with those of the patient. Many institutions, physician offices, and clinics have instituted use of pain assessment tools. Some of these tools are cumbersome and too repetitive for frequent assessments. Nurses report being too busy to complete long assessment tools; thus, compliance is often poor. All disciplines should use consistent pain severity scales. If nurses use a 0 to 5 pain scale and physicians use a 0 to 10 scale when asking patients to rate their pain severity, this lack of consistency will create confusion for both staff and patients. Health care teams can choose among several excellent assessment tools or create their own (see Bibliography).

The initial, comprehensive pain assessment should be performed by an interdisciplinary team. If the setting does not provide for the team approach, nurses or doctors trained in pain assessment should be considered. After an initial pain evaluation is completed, briefer, follow-up assessments can be carried out effectively (Table 8A–5). The nurse should obtain, at the very least, information about the location and severity of the pain. The patient should be asked to point to where the pain is and to rank the pain on a scale of 0 to 10. Ascertaining location is important because, despite the presence of an obvious source of pain (e.g., abdominal surgery), the patient could be experiencing other incidental or concomitant pains (e.g., headache). The 0 to 10 scale gives the nurse a framework

Table 8A–5
Quick Pain Assessment*

Subjective Assessment
Ask the patient the following questions:
Location: "Show me where it hurts."
Frequency: "When does it hurt?" "Is it constant or intermittent?" "When did it start?"
Description: "What does the pain feel like?" "Does it radiate or move?"
Severity: "On a scale of 0 to 10, with 0 being no pain and 10 being the worst possible pain, what number would you give your pain now?"
Aggravating factors: "What makes your pain worse?"
Relieving factors: "What makes your pain better?"
Etiologic factors: What do you think is causing the pain?"

Objective Assessment
Always examine the painful area.
Check recent x-ray and laboratory reports for clues about the etiology of the pain.

* This quick assessment is not a substitute for a complete pain assessment.

to understand the patient's perception of pain intensity and assists in assessing the efficacy of interventions. The 0 to 10 scale is easy to remember and does not require that nurses carry a device in their pockets. Zero to 10 is also more practical than other numerical scales, including 0 to 5 and 0 to 100. The former has too few numbers to choose from and the latter has too many. Other pain severity scales such as the Wong-Baker Faces Scale and the terms *mild, moderate,* and *severe* might be helpful for patients who cannot use the 0 to 10 scale. When the location and the severity of the pain have been determined, the nurse must examine the site of pain. For example, the nurse might discover the beginnings of a shingles outbreak in a patient with flank pain, signs of intestinal perforation in a patient with abdominal pain, or ischemia in a diabetic patient with a sore toe.

Assessment must be an ongoing process because of the changing nature of pain, disease, and patient response. A sudden change in pain intensity or location could indicate a worsening of disease or development of a new problem such as spinal cord compression, an oncologic emergency. A new onset of pain could indicate tumor recurrence.

THE NURSE'S ROLE IN CANCER PAIN MANAGEMENT

Achieving pain control is a team effort. As part of this team, nurses have the following responsibilities: identifying the causes of many types of pain by skilled assessment; decreasing or eliminating nursing care-related pain; treating physical symptoms; recognizing psychosocial factors and intervening where appropriate; modifying environmental conditions that contribute to discomfort; recommending specific analgesics, routes, and dosing frequencies based on observations of pain and patient's response to treatment; preventing and/or managing the side effects of analgesics; suggesting the use of adjuvant drugs and nonpharmacological interventions as indicated; and educating colleagues and the public about pain and pain management.

Nursing actions can be the source of discomfort or comfort to patients in pain. Those that cause discomfort include using restraints; putting important items outside the patient's reach; isolating the patient from other people; and being careless, rude, or inattentive. Nursing actions that promote comfort include explaining ways to reduce pain; sitting with the patient; repositioning as needed; providing for hygiene; giving massages and warm or cool soaks; attending to environmental needs, such as lighting, noise, and temperature regulation; and facilitating visits from loved ones. Evaluation of care to identify sources of discomfort and comfort can be utilized to improve care in institutions or at home.

PHARMACOLOGICAL TREATMENT OF CANCER PAIN

Analgesics are useful in all phases of cancer care, from reducing the discomfort of a diagnostic procedure to providing comfort for the dying patient. The ideal analgesic is effective, easily administered, inexpensive, and well tolerated. Unfortunately, such a drug does not exist for every type of pain; the pharmacological treatment of cancer pain is not only a science but an art. Choosing the right drug, dose, and route for each patient requires careful assessment, competent management, and continuing evaluation. There are three main categories of analgesics: nonopioids, opioids, and adjuvant medications.

Nonopioid Analgesics

Nonopioid analgesics act primarily in the peripheral nervous system to block the transmission of chemicals that sensitize nerve endings; however a central mechanism is thought to exist as well. These analgesics include aspirin, acetaminophen, and nonsteroidal anti-inflammatory drugs (NSAIDs). Indomethacin (Indocin®) suppositories and ketorolac (Toradol®) are reported to relieve immediate postoperative pain as effectively as opioids. NSAIDs are also indicated for patients with tumor-related bone pain. However, aspirin and NSAIDs have potential side effects, such as gastric irritation, platelet effects, and hepatic and renal consequences, making their use restricted in some patients. Ketorolac carries a high risk for bleeding. For this reason ketorolac should not be administered for more than three days. Choline magnesium trisalicylate (Trilisate®) and nabumetone (Relafen®) reportedly affect platelet aggregation less than any other drug in this class. Some clinicians prescribe misoprostol (Cytotec®) to help prevent NSAID-induced gastritis. Because of the potential for hepatotoxicity, the maximum daily dose of acetaminophen should not exceed 4 grams (4,000 milligrams).

Opioid Analgesics

Opioid analgesics alter the perception of pain by binding to specialized receptor sites and preventing release of neurotransmitters. Several types of receptors have been identified—mu, kappa, and delta, as well as several subtypes. These receptors are located in the central nervous system, smooth muscle, and other sites. The endogenous opioid peptides—enkephalins, endorphins, and dynorphins—also bind to these receptors. Morphine-like drugs are called agonists and primarily bind to mu receptors to cause analgesia. These receptors, especially mu, are also partly responsible for some of the side effects of opioids such as respiratory depression and sedation. Pentazocine, nalbuphine, and butorphanol are agonists-antagonists. They attach to kappa but block mu; therefore, these drugs should not be administered to an opioid-dependent person as this could precipitate a withdrawal crisis. These drugs are rarely prescribed for oncology patients. Naloxone (Narcan®) is an antagonist with a great affinity for mu and will therefore displace the morphine-like drugs at this receptor. This property makes it a good drug for treating opioid overdoses.

Morphine

This drug is very effective when taken in appropriate doses and is available in many forms: liquid, long-acting tablet, suppository, and parenteral. Although morphine is considered inexpensive, the actual formulation used, dosage requirements, and the patient's financial situation might reduce the cost-effectiveness of this drug. A major advantage of morphine is the availability of long-acting, oral preparations (MS Contin®, Oramorph SR™), which can be taken every 8 to 12 hours, allowing uninterrupted sleep. Patients should be instructed not to break, crush, or chew time-released medication, because doing so makes the entire dose of the drug available immediately, which could be a potentially toxic dose.

In conjunction with long-acting morphine preparations, patients often rely on "rescue" doses of short-acting drug, such as morphine or another opioid, to alleviate breakthrough pain, which is defined as a brief increase in pain over baseline. It is important to distinguish breakthrough pain from uncontrolled baseline pain. If a patient requires frequent PRN doses of the breakthrough medication, the dose of the time-released morphine preparation should be increased or a nonopioid or adjuvant medication added.

Codeine, Hydrocodone, or Oxycodone with Acetaminophen or Aspirin (e.g., Percodan®, Percocet®, Tylox®, Tylenol #3®, Vicodin®)

Because they are formulated with aspirin or acetaminophen to enhance analgesia, these combination drugs are subject to dose limitations, making them suitable only for moderate pain. Patients who are using combination analgesics such as Percocet®, Tylenol #3®, Vicodin®, or Tylox® should be instructed to limit the number of tablets taken per day. Note that Tylox® and Vicodin® contain more acetaminophen than does Percocet® (see Table 8A–6). Codeine doses above 65 mg are not recommended because higher doses do not bring significantly greater relief and side effects might be increased. Oxycodone is approximately 10 times more potent than codeine. Oxycodone without the added acetaminophen or aspirin is now available in both immediate and extended-release preparation; when used to treat more severe pain, higher doses can be used.

Oxycodone (Roxicodone®, Oxy IR®, OxyContin®)

Long-acting oxycodone (OxyContin®) is rapidly replacing long-acting morphine as the preferred long-acting opioid in many oncology practices. Its advantages include a more rapid onset of action and less stigmatization than morphine. Earlier equianalgesic tables listed oxycodone as

Table 8A–6
Ingredients Contained in Selected Analgesics

Advil® = 200 mg ibuprofen	Nuprin® = 200 mg ibuprofen
Darvon® = 65 mg propoxyphene	OxyContin® = controlled-release oxycodone (12 hr) (Available in 10, 20, 40, 80 mg tablets)
Darvon® Compound-65 = 65 mg propoxyphene, 389 mg aspirin, & 32.4 mg caffeine	Percocet® = 5 mg oxycodone & 325 mg acetaminophen
Darvon®-N = 100 mg propoxyphene napsylate	Percodan® = 5 mg oxycodone & 325 mg aspirin
Darvocet-N® 50 = 50 mg propoxyphene napsylate & 325 mg acetaminophen	Roxicet® = liquid Percocet 5cc = 1 Percocet
Darvocet-N® 100 = 100 mg propoxyphene napsylate & 650 mg acetaminophen	Roxicodone® & OXY IR = immediate release oxycodone
Duragesic® = fentanyl (Available in 25, 50, 75, 100 & 200 mcg topical patches which last for 2–3 d)	Tylenol®-1 tab = 325 mg acetaminophen
	Tylenol ES®-1 tab = 500 mg acetaminophen
Ecotrin® = 325 mg enteric coated aspirin	Tylenol #2® = 15 mg codeine & 300 mg acetaminophen
Excedrin® = 250 mg acetaminophen, 250 mg aspirin, & 65 mg caffeine	Tylenol #3® = 30 mg codeine & 300 mg acetaminophen
Fioricet® = 50 mg butalbital, 325 mg acetaminophen, & 40 mg caffeine	Tylenol #4® = 60 mg codeine & 300 mg acetaminophen
Fiorinal® = 50 mg butalbital, 325 mg aspirin, & 40 mg caffeine	Tylenol PM® = 500 mg acetaminophen & 25 mg diphenhydramine
Kadian® = sustained-release (24 hr) morphine	Tylox® = 5 mg oxycodone & 500 mg acetaminophen
Lortab® = contains hydrocodone and acetaminophen. Available in the following strengths: 2.5/500, 5/500, 7.5/500, 10/500 (Hydrocodone dose is the first number and acetaminophen dose is the second number)	Vicodin® = 5 mg hydrocodone & 500 mg acetaminophen
	Vicodin® ES = 7.5 mg hydrocodone & 750 mg acetaminophen
Lorcet® 10/650 = 10 mg hydrocodone & 650 mg acetaminophen	Vicodin® HP = 10 mg hydrocodone & 660 mg acetaminophen
MS Contin® & Oramorph SR® = controlled-release (12 hr) morphine (Available in 15, 30, 60, 100, 200 mg tablets)	Zydone® = 5 mg hydrocodone & 500 mg acetaminophen

Note: Total daily dose of acetaminophen should not exceed 4 grams (4,000 mg)

being equal to morphine, milligram for milligram (e.g., 30 mg of morphine equals 30 mg of oxycodone). However, with more experience prescribing oxycodone, experts suggest that oxycodone might be slightly stronger; for instance, 15–20 mg of oxycodone is now thought to equal 30 mg of morphine.

Hydromorphone (Dilaudid®)

Hydromorphone has a short half-life and therefore might cause less confusion than other opioids in the elderly. Often, hydromorphone is prescribed for patients who are allergic to morphine.

Transdermal Fentanyl

Many characteristics of transdermal fentanyl (Duragesic®) make it ideal for chronic pain in cancer patients. One major advantage is its simple method of administration: a patch is applied to the skin every 72 hours. Fentanyl is an effective analgesic, provided that the pain maintains the same intensity from one hour to the next and that the dose is appropriate for the patient. In the treatment of breakthrough pain, the same principles that apply to long-acting morphine and oxycodone pertain. The transdermal delivery system requires subcutaneous fat, so absorption might be decreased in cachectic patients.

Methadone

This drug is used less frequently than other opioids because its prolonged plasma half-life can lead to drug accumulation, with resulting sedation and possible respiratory depression. Despite its potential problems, methadone can be very effective when the patient is closely monitored.

Meperidine (Demerol®)

This drug is frequently prescribed for patients with severe, acute pain. Meperidine is not recommended for relief of chronic pain primarily because the body accumulates normeperidine, a toxic metabolite, which can cause seizures, anxiety, and tremors. Seizures have been reported after the administration of just a few doses of the drug. Other problems include painful tissue irritation from intramuscular injections and a short duration of action (as short as 1½ hours).

Meperidine can be poorly absorbed when administered orally. Oral (PO) meperidine 50 mg is equivalent in potency to 1 Darvon® 65 or 2 acetaminophen tablets; therefore, its use is restricted to instances of mild pain. The equianalgesic dose of 300 mg PO to 75 mg intramuscular (IM) is not recommended. Because of the drug's limitations, some hospitals have removed the oral preparation from their formularies. Despite its problems, meperidine continues to be the most frequently prescribed analgesic for severe, acute pain in the United States.

Dose, Route, and Scheduling of Opioids

The dose, route, and scheduling of analgesics depend on individual patient characteristics. Assuming that the drug chosen is an effective analgesic for that patient, the right dose is that which provides analgesia without causing unacceptable side effects. It is important that a drug be given enough time to take effect before its performance is evaluated.

It is helpful to consult equianalgesic tables (see Table 8A–7) when switching drugs or routes; however, these charts have limitations. The conversions are intramuscular to oral, and in most clinical settings the IM route is not appropriate for chronic pain management. (Note: Because there is delayed absorption following intramuscular injections, studies show that the onset of analgesia after the administration of an equianalgesic (bioequivalent) oral dose of morphine is comparable to morphine administered IM.) When consulting equianalgesic charts, experts recommend using one-half the IM dose for the intravenous route. Also, a patient might not necessarily tolerate an equivalent dose of a substitute opioid; therefore, when switching opioids, a lower-than-equianalgesic dose could be effective. Finally, there is variability from drug to drug. Equianalgesic tables should be used as rough measures

Table 8A-7
Equianalgesic Chart—Adults

Drug	Equianalgesic Dose	Duration (Hours) (Median)	Comments
Morphine			
Oral	30 mg	2–4	Available in many forms. Controlled-release (8–12 hr) and sustained-released (24 hr) formulations. Not for acute pain.
IM/SQ	10 mg	4	
IV	10 mg	2–4	
Fentanyl (Duragesic®) Transdermal Patch	—	72	Not for acute pain. Patches available in the following strengths: 25, 50, 75, 100, or 200 mcg/hr. Steady-state concentration is not reached until at least 12–18 hr after initial application.
Hydromorphone (Dilaudid®)			
Oral	7.5 mg	3–4	Drug has a faster onset but shorter duration than morphine.
Parenteral	1.5 mg	2–3	
Meperidine (Demerol®)			
Oral	300 mg	3–4	This dose is not recommended. PO meperidine is poorly metabolized. Not to be used for moderate or severe pain. Meperidine 50 mg PO is equal in strength to Darvon® 65 or acetaminophen 650 mg.
IV/IM	75 mg	2–3	Repeated administration can lead to CNS toxicity (e.g., tremors, seizures).
Levorphanol (Levo-Dromoran®)			
Oral	4 mg	4–6	Drug has long plasma half-life (12–16 hr), and its metabolites accumulate, potentially causing increased incidence of side effects.
IM/SQ	2 mg	4–5	
IV	1 mg	3–4	
Oxycodone			
Oral	15–20 mg	3–4	Percocet® contains 5 mg of oxycodone with 325 mg acetaminophen.
Hydrocodone			
Oral	30 mg	3–4	
Codeine			
Oral	200 mg	3–4	Codeine doses >65 mg cause increased side effects. Tylenol #3® contains only 30 mg codeine with 300 mg acetaminophen.

Cautions When Using Equianalgesic Tables: Doses reflect averages only. There is great variability from person to person in opiate efficacy and occurrence of side effects. There could also be incomplete cross tolerance meaning a lower dose of a new drug might be just as effective. Use caution and follow patients closely when switching to another drug or route. Drug selection and doses must be carefully considered in patients with bronchial asthma, increased intracranial pressure, and renal or hepatic insufficiency.

when converting drugs. Patients must always be carefully monitored for drug effects.

The correct route or method of drug administration varies from person to person, and each regimen has advantages and disadvantages (see Table 8A–8). The administration of an intravenous analgesic will break the cycle of sudden, severe pain; oral medication can then be used. Generally, the oral route is preferred for most persons experiencing chronic cancer pain. If the oral dose is not effective, the following procedures should be used before resorting to a more complex mode of administration: increase the dose or decrease the interval between doses; switch to another drug; add an adjuvant drug; and/or use nonpharmacological interventions. Because breakthrough pain can occur suddenly and unexpectedly, the intravenous route will give the fastest relief. However, this route might be inconvenient and costly. Oral analgesics usually take at least 20 minutes to induce analgesia. Oral transmucosal fentanyl citrate is noninvasive and convenient, and has an analgesic onset within 5–10 minutes that equals intravenous morphine. Though liquid morphine is commonly administered via the sublingual route, data show that morphine is poorly absorbed in this manner and that any drug effect occurs because it is swallowed and eventually metabolized through the gastrointestinal system.

Analgesics are scheduled ATC in order to keep pain at a low level and prevent the peak-and-trough effect seen with as needed (PRN) administration. However, PRN scheduling is appropriate in the following situations: in the initial dosing of an opioid-naive patient; when the pain fluctuates in intensity; and when the pain is intermittent. Ongoing assessment is important, whether the patient is on an ATC or PRN schedule.

Analgesic Ladder

The analgesic ladder approach to pain management was developed by a panel of experts for the World Health Organization and is often described in the pain literature. In many countries, opioids are not readily available and/or prescribed for severe pain. The originators of the analgesic ladder hoped to advance pain management practice by asserting that severe pain requires strong medicine, such as morphine. The ladder outlines analgesics based on severity of pain. The steps of the ladder are:

Mild Pain	Use nonopioids with or without adjuvants
Moderate pain	Use opioids with or without adjuvants With or without nonopioids
Severe pain	Use opioids with or without adjuvants With or without nonopioids

Table 8A–8
Advantages and Disadvantages of Routes of Opioid Administration for Patients with Cancer Pain

Route	Advantages	Disadvantages
Oral	Convenient.	Slow onset if used PRN.
	Can be self-administered.	Cannot use if patient GI obstructed, vomiting or cannot take oral medications.
	Requires no special device or equipment.	If drug prescribed is an opioid, patients may have difficulty obtaining the drug from a pharmacy due to regulatory and safety concerns. Stigma may be associated with use.
	Generally less expensive than administration by invasive routes.	
	Long-acting forms available.	
	Painless administration.	
Intramuscular or subcutaneous injections	Requires no venous access.	Unpredictable absorption.
		Trauma to tissues. Painful.
	Can provide more rapid pain relief than oral administration.	Risk for abscess formation.
		Increased risk of bleeding and infection.
		Lack of suitable injection sites in some patients.
		Peak and trough effect.
		Dependent on someone else to administer.
Intravenous bolus	Rapid onset.	Requires nursing and pharmacy support.
	If used in PCA mode, allows for dose titration and patient control.	Requires venous access which can be painful.
		Potential for nausea and vomiting in opioid-naive patients.
		Potential for infection, sepsis.
		Shorter duration than other routes.
		Peak and trough effect.
		More expensive than some other routes.

Continued

Table 8A–8 *(Continued)*

Advantages and Disadvantages of Routes of Opioid Administration for Patients with Cancer Pain

Route	Advantages	Disadvantages
Continuous intravenous infusions	Provides steady blood level of medication. Not limited by infusate volumes.	Requires nursing and pharmacy support. Requires maintenance of IV line. Potential for infiltration, infection, sepsis. Requires special infusion pump. Need for greater patient monitoring. Increased cost. Cumbersome.
Continuous subcutaneous infusions	Provides steady blood level of drug. Less potential for complications than continuous intravenous route. Venous access not required. Avoids need for repeated injections.	Requires nursing and pharmacy support. Potential for infection, induration and irritation at site. Requires special infusion pump. Need for greater patient monitoring. Increased cost. Cumbersome. Only a limited volume of infusate can be administered.
Intrathecal/ epidural administration	Lower doses of drug required. Longer duration of analgesia. Selective analgesia with intrathecal route. Fewer side effects than with systemic opioids. Research shows improved recovery from surgery when used for acute postoperative pain management.	Rostal redistribution of drug limits selective analgesia. Possible presence of cross tolerance; patients tolerant to systemic opioids may not benefit. Invasive procedure; requires special expertise. Requires special subcutaneous implantable reservoir or rebolus device for chronic administration. More expensive than other routes when used for chronic pain. Tolerance can occur sooner than with oral administration. Pruritus and urinary retention are more common than with oral or parenteral administration.

Table 8A-8 *(Continued)*

Advantages and Disadvantages of Routes of Opioid Administration for Patients with Cancer Pain

Route	Advantages	Disadvantages
Rectal	Convenient alternative when no other route available. Less expensive than invasive routes. Requires no special expertise, devices, or equipment.	Cannot be used if diarrhea, fecal impaction, or thrombocytopenia present. Slow onset if used PRN. Unpredictable absorption. Route disliked by some patients/caregivers.
Transdermal (e.g., fentanyl patch)	Convenient, easier for caregivers than other routes. 72 hr duration. Can be self-administered. Less constipation with this route than with oral. Indicated for constant level of pain. Requires no special devices or equipment.	Requires 12–18 hrs to establish blood level; therefore not suitable for rapid dose titration. Not for acute pain. Drug continues to be released 17 hrs or more after patch removed. Breakthrough medication required if level of pain changes. More difficulty in managing overdoses. Drug absorption increased when fever or heat sources present. Drug absorption decreased when edema, ascites, or cachexia present. One may forget patch is present and neglect to inform new health care providers.
Oral transmucosal (e.g., oral transmucosal fentanyl citrate)	Provides rapid onset of analgesia. Short-acting. Convenient. Noninvasive. No special equipment required.	The product must be administered correctly to be absorbed (e.g., the hard matrix on a handle must be rubbed against the buccal mucosa until it is thoroughly dissolved in order for the fentanyl to pass through the mucosa into blood stream).

For example, morphine should not be prescribed for a person who has a superficial laceration. Many people with cancer pain begin with a drug from the mild to moderate pain step; then, as the cancer worsens, progress to the second, moderate pain step and eventually to the third or severe pain step. The ladder assumes that the patient progresses in a stepwise fashion from mild to moderate to severe pain; however, the ladder approach is not applicable to every situation. For example, a patient's first cancer-related pain experience could be so severe that an opioid should be prescribed immediately, as in the case of a bone fracture or spinal cord compression. The patient undergoing induction chemotherapy for leukemia might require continuous intravenous opioids to relieve severe pain from mucositis.

The drugs on the second rung of the ladder are called "weak" opioids, since there was a ceiling on the dose because they contain acetaminophen. Without acetaminophen, oxycodone is dosed as needed for severe pain, and it is useful for treating pain from the moderate through the severe level. As a result, the terms "weak" opioids and "strong" opioids are no longer useful. Furthermore, the second rung of the ladder might be obsolete now that single-drug oxycodone is available.

Side Effects of Opioids

The most common side effects of opioids are sedation, constipation, nausea, and vomiting. Other adverse effects include delayed gastric emptying, urinary retention, pruritus, dysphoria, depressed cough reflex, hypotension, dry mouth, and allergic reactions.

Sedation

Management of sedation caused by opioids requires careful assessment of the patient. The nurse must determine if sedation is, in fact, a problem. Sedation might be desired if the patient is in his or her last hours of life or if he or she needs rest. The sedating effects of opioids usually decrease in several days. It is important to rule out other possible causes of sedation such as metabolic problems or central nervous system (CNS) disease. If sedation creates problems for the patient, the dosage might be decreased, the time between doses lengthened, or another analgesic prescribed. Stimulating activities, such as exercise and playing board games, and the use of stimulants, such as coffee, tea, colas, caffeine tablets, or amphetamines, can also reduce sedation.

Nausea and Vomiting

These distressing side effects might disappear after the first few days of taking opioids, but this fact is of little comfort to the person experiencing them. Antiemetics help but will increase the sedating effects of the opioid. Changing to another opioid or to a nonopioid could eliminate nausea and vomiting. Other causes of nausea and vomiting related to disease or treatment must be ruled out, such as hypercalcemia, bowel obstruction, or CNS disease.

Patients taking morphine who have continued nausea and vomiting could be experiencing an accumulation of 6-glucuronide, a metabolite of morphine. Patients with impaired renal function are especially at risk for this problem, which can also cause prolonged respiratory depression.

Information about the nursing management of nausea and vomiting is found in Chapter 9. Commonly used antiemetics are prochlorperazine (Compazine®), thiethylperazine (Torecan®, Norzine®), haloperidol (Haldol®), metoclopramide (Reglan®), granisetron (Kytril®), and ondansetron (Zofran®). Scopolamine and dimenhydrinate (Dramamine®) are not commonly prescribed for this patient population, but they have been effective when other agents have failed, especially if nausea and vomiting is related to activity.

Constipation

Sedation, nausea, and vomiting usually disappear after a few days, but constipation increases with time. All patients taking opioids should be on a bowel program to prevent constipation (see Chapter 12B). The most conservative approach is to increase fluid and fiber intake. However, most patients require daily stool softeners and laxatives such as Senokot® or lactulose.

Respiratory Depression

Although the rate of normal respirations varies from person to person, a rate of 16 to 20 breaths per minute is considered normal in the alert person at rest. When a person is asleep or in a relaxed state, respirations usually drop to 8 to 12 per minute.

Respiratory depression can occur in the following situations:

- When opioids are prescribed for a patient who has not recently received an opioid, surprisingly low doses can cause respiratory depression.
- When the cause of the pain is no longer present, yet the patient continues to receive the same amount of medication taken for severe pain. Severe pain is an antagonist to respiratory depression.
- When the pain, especially acute pain, is under control or when the cause for pain is gone.
- When the dose of the opioid is significantly escalated within a short time in a patient who reports no increase in the severity of pain.

Fear of respiratory depression is not a justifiable reason for allowing patients to remain in pain or to inadequately treat pain. Respiratory depression can be rapidly reversed with naloxone (Narcan®), as described in Table 8A–9.

Table 8A–9
Guidelines For Administering Naloxone (Narcan®)

Purpose: To reverse opioid-related respiratory depression

Procedure: Assess patient's respiratory rate. Normal respirations vary from person to person, but generally a rate of 16–20 breaths per minute is considered normal in the alert individual at rest. When a person is asleep or in a relaxed state, respirations usually drop to 8–12 per minute. If the patient's respirations are less than 8–10 per minute, instruct the patient to breathe deeply and frequently. Often, this might be all the patient requires. Assess oxygen saturation with a pulse oximeter. If reading is less than 94, administer 3 liters O_2 via nasal cannula. If the patient is not responsive or cannot be coached to breathe regularly, naloxone should be administered. Notify patient's physician immediately.

Procedure	Rationale
Dilute 1 ampule of naloxone 0.4 mg (1 cc) with preservative-free normal saline solution in a 10 cc syringe. Gently rotate syringe to mix drug with saline.	This permits a more controlled administration of the drug because abrupt reversal of respiratory depression can result in nausea, vomiting, sweating, increased oral secretions, increased blood pressure, tachycardia, tremulousness, seizures and cardiac arrest. In postoperative patients, a larger than necessary dosage of naloxone can result in significant reversal of analgesia, and in excitement. Hypotention, hypertension, ventricular tachycardia and fibrillation and pulmonary edema have been associated with the use of naloxone.
For the initial reversal of respiratory depression, naloxone should be injected IV in 1–3 cc increments at two- to three-minute intervals to the desired degree of reversal (i.e., adequate ventilation and alertness without significant pain or discomfort).	
Repeat doses of naloxone could be required within one- to two-hour intervals depending upon the amount, type (i.e., long-acting opioids) and time interval since the last administration of opioid. IM doses of naloxone produce a longer lasting effect and may be indicated after the initial IV dose.	Long-acting opioids (MS Contin®, OxyContin®, Duragesic®, methadone and Levorphanol) usually cannot be reversed with one dose of naloxone. For this reason, these drugs are not recommended for patients with acute pain or for opioid-naive patients.

Notes:
1. Naloxone will not reverse sedation caused by benzodiazepines such as lorazepam and diazepam. Flumazenil (Mazicon®) should be given.
2. Naloxone should not be given to patients who experience seizures related to meperidine toxicity as it will aggravate the neuroexcitability problem. Lorazepam or diazepam is recommended.

References:
Acute Pain Management Guideline Panel. *Acute pain management: Operative or medical procedures and trauma.* Clinical practice guideline. AHCPR Pub. No. 92-0032. Agency for Health Care Policy and Research, Public Health Service, U.S. Department of Health and Human Services, Rockville, MD. 1992.
American Pain Society. *Principles of Analgesic Use in the Treatment of Acute Pain and Cancer Pain.* American Pain Society, Skokie, IL. 1993.
Salerno and Willens. *Pain Management Handbook.* Mosby Co., St. Louis. 1996.
Du Pont Pharmaceuticals, Medical Division.

Tolerance, Dependence, Pseudoaddiction, and Addiction

The popular association of opioids with drug abuse continues to be a factor in inadequate pain management. The "Say No to Drugs" campaign has sensitized the public, with the result that patients and families fear addiction to opioids. Education is required to explain situations in which it is appropriate to "Say Yes to Drugs." Understanding tolerance, physical dependence, and addiction (psychological dependence) is essential in helping both health care professionals and patients manage pain.

Tolerance is an involuntary decrease in response to a drug, which necessitates more frequent or larger doses to maintain the drug's original pain-relieving effects. When a dose of an opioid that previously provided pain relief for three hours now does so for only two, tolerance might have developed. For patients with chronic cancer pain, either tolerance or the progression of the disease can cause the patient to require more medication. Because neither situation qualifies as addiction, increasing the dose is appropriate. Tolerance can occur faster with epidural and bolus intravenous administration of drugs than with other methods. Central nervous system side effects do not usually result from increasing dosages in the tolerant patient. Tolerance for respiratory and CNS effects develops at essentially the same rate as tolerance for analgesic effects.

Physical dependence is a physiological response that occurs when a person has been on an opioid for a period of time. If administration of the drug stops suddenly, withdrawal can occur. Withdrawal symptoms consist of cramps, diarrhea, agitation, goose flesh, lacrimation, perspiration, yawning, coryza, nausea, and vomiting. These physiological responses can also occur if a person has been taking an agonist opioid such as morphine and then takes pentazocine (Talwin®) or another agonist-antagonist drug. Giving naloxone to reverse narcotic-induced respiratory depression can also cause withdrawal symptoms. When a patient has been taking an opioid for a period of time and then no longer requires it, the drug should be tapered off rather than abruptly terminated.

Pseudoaddiction denotes a pattern of drug-seeking behaviors to achieve pain control in a person who is not addicted. The person is experiencing unrelieved pain and is desperate for relief. For example, patients who have had a mastectomy or a thoracotomy might experience severe pain longer than expected after surgery due to intraoperative nerve injury. Such pain syndromes could go unrecognized. If patients fail to receive relief, they might resort to pseudoaddictive behaviors, such as taking more of their oral analgesic than prescribed, or "doctor shopping." Their efforts to obtain relief might be misinterpreted, and they risk being inappropriately identified as addicts. Other causes of pseudoaddiction are drug doses that are too low, and intervals between drug doses that are too long. For example, the effect of mepiridine lasts an average of two to three hours, and it is typically prescribed every four to six hours. Medication should be prescribed in accordance with its action and based on each patient's response to and experience of pain.

In contrast, *addiction* (psychological dependence) is a compulsive need to use drugs for their mood-altering effects rather than for pain. Addicts use drugs despite risk of serious harm. Addiction is a biopsychosocial disorder caused by a biological predisposition combined with certain environmental factors. According to research, people who are not at risk for addiction will not become addicted when they take opioids for relief of pain. Requiring opioids to relieve physical pain is no different from needing antibiotics to treat an infection or insulin to treat diabetes.

In the rare situation when drug abuse is a problem, help can be obtained from an addiction specialist. Persons with a past history of drug abuse will require higher-than-average doses of opioids in order to control pain. It is important to remember that all people deserve relief from pain. The potential to cause addiction is not a reason to deny people drugs that can relieve their suffering. Studies of patients using opioids in hospital settings have shown that addiction occurs in less than 1 percent of persons with no history of drug or alcohol abuse. A far greater problem than possible addiction is the unrelieved suffering that continues, despite the knowledge and resources available to manage pain.

Adjuvant Medications

Adjuvant medications include a variety of drugs, some of which were originally intended for uses other than analgesia. There are some pains, such as neuropathy, muscle cramps, several types of headaches, and bone pain, for which adjuvants are recommended (see Table 8A–10).

Amitriptyline (Elavil®), a tricyclic antidepressant, is a proven analgesic for neuropathic pain; however, this drug is associated with more anticholinergic effects and sedation than are other tricyclics such as doxepin, desipramine, and nortriptyline (Pamelor®). The anticonvulsants carbamazepine (Tegretol®), valproate (Depakene®), gabapentin (Neurontin®), and clonazepam (Klonopin®) are helpful for lancinating (shooting) neuropathic pain. Baclofen might be helpful for tic-like pain and muscle spasms. Corticosteroids, especially dexamethasone, are helpful when treating spinal cord compression and other pains caused by nerve compression. Osteoclast inhibitors such as calcitonin and bisphosphonates have been shown to reduce the pain from bone metastases due to breast and prostate cancers. Strontium 89 and samarium 153 are radiopharmaceuticals indicated for treating bone pain in selected patients. Two chemotherapeutic agents are specifically indicated for cancer-related pain: gemcitabine for

Table 8A–10
Types of Cancer-Related Pain and Interventions

Problem	Intervention
Neuropathic pain Burning, aching, dysesthetic type	Antidepressants (amitriptyline, desipramine, nortriptyline) Oral local anesthetics (e.g., mexiletine) Corticosteroids (e.g., desamethasone, prednisolone) N-Methyl-D-Aspartate blockers (e.g., ketamine, dextromethorphan) Alpha-2 adrenergic agonists (e.g., clonidine) Calcitonin (phantom limb pain) Topical agents (e.g., capsaicin) TENS Physical therapy
Neuropathic pain Shooting, stabbing, electric shock-like	Anticonvulsants (carbamazepine, clonazepam, valproate) GABAergic drugs (e.g., gabapentin, baclofen especially for trigeminal neuralgia) TENS Physical therapy
Postherpetic neuralgia	Tricyclic antidepressants Anticonvulsants TENS Topical agents (e.g., capsaicin)
Nerve compression	Corticosteroids Radiation therapy
Muscle/cramps	Muscle relaxants Moist heat Massage Correction of electrolyte disturbances
Smooth muscle spasms (tenesmus)	B&O suppository Anticholinergics (e.g., atropine, scopolamine)
Bone pain	Mechanical stabilization NSAIDs Corticosteroids Radiation Radioisotopes (strontium 89, samarium 153) Calcitonin Bisphosphonates (e.g., pamidronate)
Bowel obstruction pain	Anticholinergics (e.g., atropine, scopolamine) Corticosteroids Octreotide
Activity- or procedure-related pain	Nitrous oxide Intravenous opioids and/or benzodiazepines

NSAIDs—non-steroidal anti-inflammatory drugs; TENS—transcutaneous electrical nerve stimulation

pancreatic cancer and mitoxantrone for prostate cancer. Antitussives are indicated for pain precipitated by coughing.

NONPHARMACOLOGICAL TREATMENT OF CANCER PAIN

Nurses play a tremendous role in using nonpharmacological measures to reduce pain perception. The pain-relieving power of a back rub should not be underestimated, because this or any form of massage can be as effective as an opioid, is easily administered, inexpensive, and well tolerated by most patients. Distraction techniques, such as instructing the patient to take a breath or to count to ten during an injection, are effective pain-reducing strategies, as is holding a patient's hand during a painful procedure. Proper positioning of patients is one of the most important pain-relieving measures a nurse can employ. These methods are often used to reduce pain but are poorly documented in the patient record, so they are not recognized by other health care providers as effective interventions.

Some oncology units offer patients videotape players with humorous and motivational videotapes; portable tape players with relaxation and motivational audiotapes; games and puzzles; books and magazines; meditation classes; and support groups to use for pain or other symptom relief. Table 8A–11 lists the many nonpharmacological methods that can help with pain management. McCaffery and Beebe's book *Pain: Clinical Manual for Nursing Practice* (1989) gives detailed information about many of these techniques.

Table 8A–11
Nonpharmacological Methods for Pain Control

Heat
Cold
Recreation therapy
Massage
Distraction
Acupressure
Positioning
Acupuncture
Transcutaneous electrical nerve stimulation
Exercises
Cognitive/behavioral therapy
Biofeedback
Imagery
Hypnosis
Meditation
Prayer
Laughter

ANESTHETIC AND NEUROSURGICAL INTERVENTIONS

The goal of an anesthetic procedure is to interrupt the pain pathway either temporarily or permanently. Temporary interruption of the pain pathway during painful procedures or surgeries is commonly achieved with local anesthetics. Permanent nerve blocks are achieved by destroying nerves with agents such as phenol or alcohol. In the case of nerve blocks, "permanent" means anything that lasts from weeks to months. One indication for nerve blocks is pain due to cancer. Celiac plexus blocks for pancreatic cancer and superior hypogastric plexus blocks for pelvic malignancies can be very effective in reducing pain.

The most common invasive procedure performed for cancer pain is the placement of intraspinal catheters for the administration of opioids. These drugs are administered by either bolus or continuous infusion using an external or internal pump.

Common neurosurgical procedures include rhizotomy and cordotomy. The former destroys spinal nerve roots; the latter interrupts pain transmission in the lateral spinothalamic tract. On occasion, severe, intractable pain is relieved with cordotomy. Procedures such as neurectomy, hypophysectomy, tractotomy, and spinal cord and deep brain stimulation have been employed with varying degrees of success and require further study.

In most cases, attempts should be made to control pain with systemic analgesics before resorting to invasive procedures. The ultimate goal is maximum pain control with a minimum of side effects and complications.

NEUROSTIMULATORY INTERVENTIONS

Acupuncture, transcutaneous electrical nerve stimulation (TENS), peripheral nerve stimulation, dorsal column stimulation, and deep brain stimulation are some of the techniques used for specific situations. Some of these neurostimulatory techniques reduce pain perception by activating endorphins and/or modulating inhibition systems.

PHYSIATRIC INTERVENTIONS

Physical and occupational therapy play important roles in pain management, either by preventing problems that can lead to pain or by treating existing pain. Possible therapies include exercises, orthotic devices to support painful body parts, applications of heat or cold, massage, biofeedback, TENS, and electrical stimulation.

Some patients with chronic, stable pain related to complications from cancer therapies benefit from enrollment in a pain clinic where physiatric interventions are a major part of the treatment.

PSYCHOLOGICAL INTERVENTIONS

Studies have shown that affective symptoms such as depression, anxiety, and feelings of powerlessness can make pain worse. These feelings intensify as the patient becomes more disabled from the pain. Patients might be reluctant to report these feelings; the nurse must include questions about mood in his or her assessment. Interventions include antidepressant medications and supportive and cognitive-behavioral therapies such as hypnosis and relaxation techniques, which can help control pain and lessen feelings of helplessness. Research supports the use of music, imagery, and laughter to reduce pain and to improve the patient's sense of well-being.

MANAGING PAIN AT THE END OF LIFE

When cure is out of reach and death is imminent, the nursing focus changes. Rather than performing extensive diagnostic tests and aggressive interventions, the goal of nursing is to promote comfort and reduce suffering. This shift is sometimes difficult for nurses who work in acute care settings, where the primary focus of care is curing or controlling the cancer. It can be difficult for a nurse to provide optimal end-of-life care if hospital policies and procedures do not address the needs of dying patients. Fortunately, a growing number of hospitals are correcting this situation as a result of the involvement of hospital ethics committees, hospices and other interested groups (see Table 8A–12).

One of the most difficult aspects of pain management at end of life is the confusion surrounding the use of pain medication. Nurses have expressed concern that administering pain medication to a dying patient could hasten death. If there are no safer treatment options and the patient and family agree, it is acceptable to administer drugs such as morphine at doses titrated to the patient's comfort, even if in so doing, death is hastened. This action is supported by the American Nurses' Association's Position Statement on Promotion of Comfort and Relief of Pain in Dying Patients:

> Nurses should not hesitate to use full and effective doses of pain medication for the proper management of pain in the dying patient. The increasing titration of medication to achieve adequate symptom control, even at the expense of life, thus hastening death secondarily, is ethically justified.

Table 8A-12
Guidelines for End of Life Care

Factor	Intervention
Code status	Ascertain patient/family's understanding regarding what will happen when the patient stops breathing. Does the patient have a living will? Cardiopulmonary resuscitation (CPR) inappropriate for the majority of patients dying as a result of advanced, untreatable disease. These patients should have a "NO CPR" order. Respirations will naturally decrease over time and should not be of concern when death is imminent.
Spiritual, social, emotional, and cultural needs	Respond sensitively and respectfully while facilitating patient/family/loved ones expression of these needs. Notify Pastoral Care and Social Work Services. Involve the patient and, where appropriate, the family/loved ones in every aspect of care.
Family visits	Inquire whether family members are on their way to see the patient. Ascertain whether the patient/family wish that sedation, if prescribed and needed, be withheld until other family members arrive.
Unfinished business	Facilitate patient completing unfinished business if appropriate.
Comfort measures	Perform only those care procedures that promote comfort. If death is imminent (hrs) and turning the patient every two hrs causes pain, then do not turn the patient. If death is imminent and the patient is fighting the O_2 mask prescribed yet would tolerate a nasal cannula, get the orders changed.
Pain medication	Manage pain aggressively and effectively. Titrate analgesics to the point of comfort, using appropriate parameters prescribed by the physician. If the patient is suffering pain and the appropriate drug/dose is not prescribed, seek the advice of an experienced nurse, supervisor, the Ethics Committee, Medical Director.
Air hunger	Morphine via inhalation or intravenously should be administered for severe dyspnea.
Audible respiratory congestion	Suction PRN if appropriate. Robinul® or Levsin® may be helpful. Overhydration (IV fluids, PN and tube feedings) may contribute to pulmonary congestion and other problems such as vomiting, edema, and urinary urgency. There are benefits to dehydration when death is imminent.
Restlessness/agitation	Massage, music, meditation, or anxiolytics may be helpful.
Myoclonus (tremors, jerking of extremities)	May indicate accumulation of analgesic metabolites. Administer lorazapam, decrease analgesic if pain can still be controlled and/or change to another analgesic.
Tests/procedures	Assure that no unnecessary tests or procedures are ordered.

Pain medication should be titrated to achieve comfort. Giving an abnormally large dose of morphine to a patient who reports little or no pain should raise concern, but giving boluses of morphine to a patient experiencing sudden, severe pain is appropriate. When the patient achieves some relief, the dose can be titrated incrementally. The optimal approach is to adequately assess the patient and to treat on the basis of the patient's analgesic requirements (see Table 8A–13). The patient's disease or condition will ultimately cause death. The patient and family should be informed that

Table 8A–13
Guidelines for the Management of Continuous Intravenous Infusion of Opioid Drugs in the Patient at End of Life

Suggested drugs: morphine, hydromorphone (Dilaudid®)

- All infusions must be administered via an infusion pump.
- If the drug to be used for the infusion is the same one the patient is currently receiving parenterally (IV or IM), and has been effective, divide by 24 the total amount the patient has received in the past 24 hrs. This amount will be the hourly rate.
- If the drug to be used for the infusion is different than the one patient is presently receiving, use an equianalgesic chart to calibrate the conversion dose.
- The opioid must be prescribed using specific dose parameters (e.g., "morphine via continuous infusion 1–10mg/hr, titrate to patient's comfort"). If, after titration, the current dose becomes ineffective, the drug should be increased (e.g., "morphine via continous infusion 10–20mg/hr").
- If the patient is in severe pain or dyspnea, bolus doses of the opioid drug will be required initially in order to break the cycle of pain or dyspnea. Bolus doses of the drug may also be required on occasion due to a sudden increase in severe pain. Use 25%–50% of the hourly dose. If frequent bolus doses are needed, the hourly rate should be increased.
- Patients may develop myoclonus when receiving high doses of opioids. This symptom is due to CNS hyperactivity and may lead to seizures. Decrease the analgesic dose, change to another drug or administer lorazapam 1–2 mg IV q 2–4 hr PRN to alleviate this distressing symptom.
- It is easier to titrate analgesics if only one opioid is prescribed. Rarely is there anything to be gained by using a transdermal fentanyl patch plus IV morphine or hydromorphone.
- If the patient has an excess of respiratory secretions, Robinul® or Levsin® and suctioning might help.

General Principles:

- Opioid tolerant patients require higher than average doses of an analgesic to achieve effect. It would be difficult to standardize analgesic doses and routes because of the extreme variability of patient conditions. The optimal approach is to adequately assess the patient and treat based on the individual's analgesic requirements.
- The first application of a transdermal fentanyl patch requires at least 8 hrs for it to begin its analgesic effect; therefore if this mode is going to be used, the patient will require another drug given orally, rectally or parenterally until the fentanyl begins to take effect.
- Titrate an analgesic to a level of comfort. It is safer to administer morphine via continuous infusion and increase in increments rather than as a huge bolus dose. If the patient is in extreme pain, a bolus to start is appropriate, then titrate the infusion. IV or rectal administration is indicated when the patient cannot take analgesics PO. The most important principle is to get the patient's pain under control quickly.
- Meperidine IM or IV carries an increased risk for seizures, especially if high doses are administered. Meperidine PO should never be prescribed for moderate/severe pain as its potency is equivalent to two aspirin or acetaminophen.
- Patients who are elderly and/or who have renal disease might experience less toxicity with hydromorphone than with morphine due to the shorter half-life of hydromorphone.
- Patient/family/loved ones should be involved in discussions about end of life issues so that they have a clear understanding of the situation and can participate in planning care.
- Comfort is the primary goal when death is imminent and there is no hope of recovery.

the goal is comfort and the patient is dying from disease and not from pain medication. Hospice and pain management specialists recount anecdotal reports of patients who, when pain, agitation, or dyspnea are relieved, are able to complete important tasks at the end of life. Barbiturates should never be the only drug used when a person is experiencing severe pain. If administered, the patient will still feel the pain but will be too sedated to report it.

USE OF PLACEBOS IN PAIN MANAGEMENT

The use of placebos in pain management is inappropriate, unethical, and possibly illegal, except in clinical trials for which patients have given informed consent. This position is supported by the American Pain Society, the Oncology Nursing Society, and the American Hospital Association. Typically, placebos have been used in an attempt to prove that patients are fabricating their pain. Testing a patient's report of pain by administering a placebo and getting a positive response only shows that placebos have profound physiological and psychological effects. This mechanism is poorly understood. Policies and procedures in patient care settings should reflect this standard.

HIGH-TECH PAIN MANAGEMENT

Eighty to 90 percent of cancer-related pain can be managed with proper administration of oral analgesics that are safe, convenient, non-invasive, and inexpensive. Financial and ethical problems arise when analgesics are administered by unnecessary high-tech methods when a simpler approach would be just as effective. Examples are epidural catheters/pumps, intravenous catheters/ports, and internal or external pumps. These devices are expensive, invasive, and burdensome, and carry a risk of complications.

The following factors can contribute to the inappropriate prescription of high-tech pain control:

- Inadequate pain assessment;
- Inadequate trial of oral analgesics in the right dose and frequency;
- Lack of knowledge about pain management;
- High-powered sales pitches by company representatives;
- Pressure to use hospital- or physician-owned equipment;
- Reimbursement issues (some insurance carriers will only pay for parenteral administration of analgesic drugs);
- Pressure from the patient and/or family.

There are instances when parenteral pain management is indicated for chronic pain: When the oral/rectal/transdermal routes cannot be used; when unacceptable side effects occur using these routes; and when administration of analgesics via these routes is ineffective, despite dose escalations and use of adjuvant drugs.

ACCOUNTABILITY

Caring for patients who are experiencing pain is an exceedingly important responsibility. This task is often a difficult one due to the complexity of the pain mechanisms, lack of knowledge among professionals about pain management, regulatory concerns, and numerous other reasons (see Table 8A–14).

Table 8A–14
Pain Management Barriers and Improvement Strategies

Barriers to Adequate Pain Management	Suggestions to Improve Pain Management
Health care professionals: Inadequate knowledge	Teach pain management in nursing, medical, and pharmacy schools.
Poor assessment of pain	Distribute the AHCPR guidelines to staff.
Lack of interdisciplinary focus	Provide educational conferences, videos, computer programs.
Concerns about regulatory issues	Organize an interdisciplinary pain team or task force.
Concerns about reimbursement for services	Offer a variety of pain reduction methods.
Low priority given to pain management	Create a video- and audio-tape collection. Form classes on meditation and relaxation.
	Provide pain management guidelines (e.g., end-of-life care, opioid infusion protocols, equianalgesic charts).
	Join professional pain associations and state cancer pain initiatives.
	Make pain management a priority. Form a continuous quality improvement team. Conduct patient satisfaction surveys.
Patient/Family/Community: Inadequate knowledge about analgesics (e.g., indications, administration, side-effect management, addiction issues)	Participate in community education programs about pain management.
	Display patient education materials. Ensure that educational materials are appropriate for the age, education, and culture of the patient.
Communication problems with health care professionals	Specifically ask about pain. Perform a comprehensive assessment. Listen to patient/family concerns and respond appropriately.
Unable to locate pharmacy that carries prescribed analgesic	Direct patient to pharmacy, if appropriate. (Be aware that pharmacies are concerned about being scrutinized by regulatory agencies and burglarized by drug seekers).
Unable to obtain optimal care because of inadequate funds or reimbursement problems	Provide information on financial assistance.

AHCPR—Agency for Health Care Policy and Research

Persons with pain have a right to pain relief, yet many continue to suffer. Lack of education is a major cause of poor pain management. The World Heath Organization is addressing this problem by publishing educational materials and working to make appropriate analgesics available. A panel of experts has written standards for pain management that are available from the Agency for Health Care Policy and Research (see Bibliography), and most states have established cancer pain initiatives. Table 8A–14 also lists some ways to make pain management more visible in hospitals, clinics, hospices, and home nursing agencies. These steps are help-ing to bridge the gap between practice and the latest advances in pain management.

While nurses receive very little formal education about pain manage-ment, they are increasingly being held more accountable for pain control. Joining state initiatives and pain associations, attending seminars on pain, reading books and journals, and learning from colleagues, patients, and fam-ilies will assist the nurse in maintaining competence in pain management.

BIBLIOGRAPHY

1. American Nurses Association Board of Directors. *Position Statement on Pro-motion of Comfort and Relief of Pain in Dying Patients.* Washington, DC. 1991.

   This document supports the role of nursing in maximizing comfort through ad-equate management of pain in dying patients.

2. American Pain Society. *Principles of Analgesic Use in the Treatment of Acute Pain and Chronic Cancer Pain.* American Pain Society, Glenview, IL. 1989.

   This is a concise guide to analgesic agents.

3. Cushing, M. Pain management on trial. *AJN* (February): 21–22. 1991.

   This article reviews a case in which a dying patient received inadequate pain relief.

4. Jacox, A., D. B. Carr, R. Payne, et al. Management of Cancer Pain. *Clinical Practice Guideline No. 9. AHCPR Pub # 94-0592.* Agency for Health Care Policy and Research, Rockville, MD. March 1994.

   This guideline was developed by an interdisciplinary panel of clinicians, pa-tients, researchers, and experts in health policy. The guideline provides a syn-thesis of scientific research and expert judgment to make recommendations on pain assessment and management.

5. McCaffery, M., and A. Beebe. *Pain: Clinical Manual for Nursing Practice.* Mosby Co., St. Louis. 1989.

   This must-have comprehensive manual, designed to be used in the clinical set-ting, includes very helpful patient/family teaching points and assessment tools that the authors have generously approved for duplication.

6. Melzack, R. The tragedy of needless pain. *Scientific American* (February): 27–33. 1990.

   This is a treatise on the subject.

7. Melzack, R., and P. D. Wall. Pain mechanisms: A new theory. *Science* 150: 971. 1965.

   This is the article that revolutionized the field of pain pathophysiology.

8. Portenoy, R., Guest Editor. Cancer pain management: Update on breakthrough pain. *Seminars in Oncology* 24: 5, Suppl 16. 1997.

   This is a collection of six articles on the subject written by cancer pain experts.

9. Portenoy, R. *Management of Cancer Pain: Opioid and Adjuvant Pharma-cotherapy.* American Pain Society monograph, Glenview, IL. 1997.

   This is an excellent overview by an expert.

10. Portenoy, R. Neuropathic pain. In *Pain Management Secrets.* R. Kanner, ed. 122–144. Hanley & Belfus, Philadelphia. 1997.

    Clinicians and scientists from a number of disciplines contributed to this concise text written in question and answer format.

11. Porter, J., and H. Jick. Addiction rare in patients treated with narcotics. *N Engl J Med* 302: 123. 1980.

    This study discusses the infrequent development of addiction in patients treated with narcotics.

12. Salerno, E., and J. Willens. *Pain Management Handbook: An Interdisciplinary Approach.* Mosby Co., St. Louis. 1996.

    This is a succinct yet comprehensive handbook on pain.

B. Sleep

Paula Anderson
Marcia Grant

On the list of American's most frequent health complaints, difficulty sleeping is second only to the common cold (Lamberg 1994). It is estimated that there are 60 million people in the United States who perceive themselves as having trouble sleeping. In a study by Vitiello in 1996, it was found that as many as 50 percent of older adults complain about their sleep, and one-third of all elderly report having chronic problems with sleep. One-half of community-dwelling older people use either over-the-counter or prescription sleeping medications. Sleeping difficulties are known to increase as people grow older, affecting 90 percent of those over the age of 60 years.

A simple behavioral definition of sleep, used by Carskadon and Dement in 1994, is a reversible behavioral state of perceptual disengagement from and unresponsiveness to the environment. Sleep has also been described as a state of reduced responsiveness to external stimuli, an altered state of consciousness from which a person can be aroused if the stimulus is of sufficient magnitude.

Insomnia is defined as difficulty in initiating or maintaining sleep, or unrestorative sleep. The definition includes the perception or complaint of inadequate or poor quality sleep because of one or more of the following:

This project was supported by an Oncology Nursing Foundation Grant titled "Quality of Life and Fatigue: A Multicultural Approach."

- Difficulty falling asleep or sleep latency;
- Waking up frequently during the night with difficulty returning to sleep;
- Early morning awakening;
- Unrestorative sleep.

Three types of insomnia are known to occur. *Initial insomnia,* also know as sleep latency, is difficulty in falling asleep and is a frequent sleep disorder reported by adults. *Intermittent insomnia* is the inability to stay asleep, with frequent or prolonged premature awakenings during the night. *Terminal insomnia* occurs after being in bed most of the night with disruption by early morning awakenings, daytime napping, and early retiring.

Insomnia can be transient in nature, lasting from a few days to three weeks. Situational stressors such as major life changes (e.g., new job, upcoming tests, medical illnesses, changes in medications, jet lag) fall into this category. Sleep medications are effective in producing desired sleep when the insomnia is of short duration. Chronic insomnia lasts longer than three weeks and requires detailed evaluation. Assessment of chronic insomnia should include predisposing factors (personality type), precipitating factors (new job), and perpetuating factors (alcohol, sleeping pills). Chronic insomnia sets the stage for the occurrence of major depression, requiring treatment for both the sleep disorder and the depression.

Mild insomnia can consist of an almost nightly complaint of insufficient sleep or not feeling rested after sleeping. There is little or no evidence of impairment of social or occupational functioning. Mild insomnia often is associated with feelings of restlessness, mild anxiety, and daytime fatigue. *Moderate* insomnia is associated with a nightly complaint of sleep disturbance, mild impairment of social or occupational functioning, and feelings of restlessness and anxiety. *Severe* insomnia occurs when there is a nightly complaint with a severe disruption of functioning and is always associated with feelings of restlessness and anxiety.

PHYSIOLOGY

Sleep is an extremely complex combination of both physiological and behavioral processes. Within the process of sleep, two states exist that have distinct manifestations: nonrapid eye movement (NREM) and rapid eye movement or REM sleep.

Within NREM sleep, four progressively deepening stages exist and can be measured using an electroencephalogram (EEG) and other instruments such as the electro-oculogram (EOG) and electromyogram (EMG). When using the EEG, the four NREM stages are shown to have distinct characteristics and are described as being synchronous, having sleep spindles, K complexes, and high voltage slow waves (Figure 8B–1). As the NREM stages of sleep progress from Stage 1 through Stage 4, increasing

8B

Figure 8B-1. The stages of NREM sleep. The four electroencephalographic (EEG) tracings depicted here are from a 19-year-old female volunteer. Each tracing was recorded from a referential lead (C3/A2) recorded on a Grass Instruments Co. Model 7D polygraph with a paper speed of 10 mm/sec, time constant of 0.3 sec, and 1/2 amplitude high-frequency setting of 30 Hz. On the second tracing, the arrow indicates a K complex, and the underlining shows two sleep spindles.

Reprinted with permission from Carscadon, M. A., and W. C. Dement. Normal human sleep: An overview. In Principles and Practice of Sleep Medicine. *2nd edition. (M. H. Kryger, T. Roth & W. C. Dement, eds.). WB Saunders Co., Philadelphia. p. 16. 1994.*

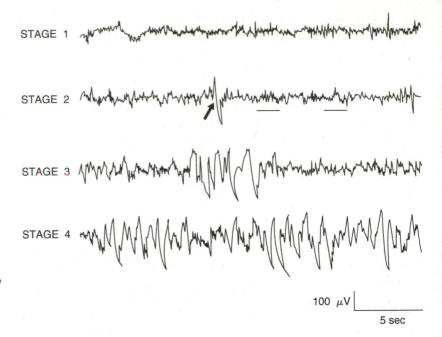

depth of sleep occurs. The arousal response of the sleeper decreases as the stage of sleep increases. Arousal is easiest in Stage 1 and most difficult in Stage 4. In NREM sleep, less mental activity is evident on the EEG, yet the brain continues its regulatory functions in a *movable* body. NREM regulatory functions include decreased blood pressure, decreased heart rate, and decreased respiratory rate.

REM sleep, in contrast, is characterized by marked activation on the EEG, muscle flaccidity (atonia), and episodes of rapid eye movements. While in REM sleep, dreaming occurs. Eighty percent of sleepers awakened during REM sleep will remember their dreams. One short definition of REM sleep is a highly activated brain in a paralyzed body. REM sleep regulatory behaviors include increased blood pressure, increased heart rate, increased respiratory rate, and increased gastric secretions. It is during REM sleep that the cardiovascular demands of the body increase suddenly. In a normal person, this occurrence results in no untoward effects. As noted by Roberts in 1986, in a patient with any compromise in the cardiovascular system, the sudden jump in sympathetic stimulation during REM sleep can result in a cardiac incident. The physiologic differences between NREM sleep and REM sleep are identified in Table 8B–1. The physiologic changes experienced by the body during sleep categorized by system are listed in Table 8B–2.

Stages of sleep can be differentiated on the EEG. The normal adult enters sleep through NREM sleep and progressively descends from Stage 1 to Stage 4 sleep. The sleeper then ascends quickly back up through Stage

Table 8B–1
Descriptions of Physiologic Systems During Sleep

Cardiovascular Physiology

- Blood pressure decreases during sleep.
- Heart rate slows during sleep.
- Cardiac output decreases and peripheral conductance increases during sleep.
- Vasoconstrictions might occur in association with phasic REM events.
- Sinoaortic reflexes prevent severe vasodilation during REM sleep.
- Baroreflexes might be diminished during REM sleep.

Cerebral Blood Flow, Intracranial Pressure, and Cerebral Metabolism

- Cerebral blood flow increases during REM sleep.
- Phasic increases in cerebral blood flow are superimposed on tonically increased cerebral blood flow in REM sleep.
- The mechanisms for the changes in cerebral blood flow in sleep are unknown.
- Some evidence indicates that there is a neurogenic cerebral vasodilation.
- Intracranial pressure increases in REM sleep.
- Brain temperature increases in REM sleep.
- Total body oxygen consumption is greater in REM sleep than in NREM sleep, but lower in REM sleep than in wakefulness.

Temperature Regulation

- Body temperature falls throughout the night.
- Increases in body temperature that coincide with REM sleep periods are superimposed on this decline.
- Thermoregulatory sweating is suspended during REM sleep.
- Temperature regulation is absent in REM sleep.

Respiration

- Respiration rate and minute ventilation decrease during NREM sleep.
- Respiration is rapid and irregular in REM sleep.
- The ventilatory response to carbon dioxide decreases in slope and shifts to higher CO_2 pressures during NREM sleep.
- Some upper airway dilating muscles are hypotonic during sleep.
- Snoring is more frequent in males than in females and the incidence of snoring increases with age.
- Lung secretions are retained during sleep.
- Airway reflexes are altered in sleep.
- Airway smooth-muscle tone changes during sleep.
- Pulmonary stretch receptor reflexes are intact in NREM sleep, but they are altered in REM sleep.
- The arousal response to airway occlusion, hypoxia, hypercapnia, laryngeal stimulation, and airway and intrapulmonary irritation is delayed in REM sleep.

Endocrine Functions

- Growth hormone is secreted during NREM sleep early in the night.
- Prolactin secretion peaks during late sleep.
- Secretion of thyroid-stimulating hormone peaks in the evening and is inhibited in sleep.
- Gonadotropin secretion occurs during sleep in puberty.
- Sleep inhibits the ACTH-cortisol circadian rhythm.

Continued

Table 8B-1 *(Continued)*
Descriptions of Physiologic Systems During Sleep

Renal Function

- Urine volume and the excretion of sodium, potassium, chloride, and calcium decrease during sleep.
- Variations in the level of antidiuretic hormone do not account for the sleep-related changes in renal function.
- Plasma aldosterone levels increase during sleep and may account for the reduced urine sodium excretion.
- The sleep-related increase in plasma prolactin concentration may potentiate the actions of aldosterone.
- Increases in parathyroid hormone might be a factor in the reduced calcium excretion during sleep.
- Variations in autonomic activity might account for REM-related decreases in urine volume and increases in urine osmolality.

Alimentary Function

- Gastric acid secretion might increase during sleep in patients with duodenal ulcer disease.
- Esophagitis is associated with reflux during sleep.
- Swallowing frequency and esophageal motility decrease during sleep.
- Studies of intestinal motility during sleep show conflicting results.

Penile Tumescence

- Penile tumescence occurs during sleep.
- Tumescence during sleep varies with age.

Reprinted with permission from Orem J., Barnes, C. D. *Physiology in Sleep.* Academic Press, Orlando. 1980.

3, Stage 2, and sometimes Stage 1. REM sleep then occurs and is followed by descent to Stage 4, and the cycle is repeated. REM sleep does not occur until 80 minutes or longer after NREM sleep begins. NREM and REM sleep alternate cyclically through the night about every 90 minutes. As sleep continues throughout the night, the NREM Stages 3 and 4 decrease in length, and the REM Stage becomes progressively longer. One sleep cycle consists of both NREM and REM sleep (see Table 8B–3):

- Stage 1: This stage has a role in the wake-to-sleep transition. Sleep is easily discontinued during this stage by softly calling the person's name, touching him or her lightly, or quietly closing a door. Stage 1 is associated with a low arousal threshold and lasts 1–7 minutes.
- Stage 2: NREM sleep is signaled by sleep spindles or K complexes on the EEG. It follows Stage 1 and continues for 10–25 minutes. A more intense stimulus is required to produce arousal.

Table 8B-2
Physiological Characteristics of NREM and REM Sleep

NREM	Baseline REM	During Phasic REM Activity
Hypotension	Hypotension	Increased blood pressure
Bradycardia	Bradycardia	Tachycardia
Decreased cardiac output	Decreased cardiac output	Decreased cardiac output
Vasodilation	General vasodilation Vasoconstriction of red muscle	Vasoconstriction
Intact baroreflexes	Intact baroreflexes (human); impaired baroreflexes (cat)	Intact baroreflexes (human)
Cerebral blood flow changes, heterogeneously	Cerebral blood flow increases Increased intracranial pressure	Further increases in cerebral blood flow
Brain temperature decreases	Brain temperature increases	
Total body O_2 consumption decreases	Total body O_2 consumption increases	Total body O_2 consumption increases
Thermoregulatory mechanisms are functional: sweating, shivering, tachypnea, and thermoregulatory vasomotion occur when needed	Thermoregulation is impaired: sweating, shivering, tachypnea, and thermoregulatory vasomotion do not occur	Thermoregulation is impaired: sweating, shivering, tachypnea, and thermoregulatory vasomotion do not occur
Respiratory rate decreases	Respiratory rate increases	Further increases in respiratory rate
Minute ventilation decreases	Minute ventilation is variously reported to increase or decrease	Minute ventilation is variously reported to increase or decrease
Respiratory muscles maintain their tone or show a small decrease in tone	Diaphragmatic activity persists; intercostals are atonic; genioglossus and other upper airway muscles are atonic or hypotonic	Transient inhibition of diaphragmatic activity; other respiratory muscles show twitches
Ventilatory responses to hypoxia intact; slope of the response to CO_2 levels	Ventilatory responses to hypercapnia and hypoxia are intact	Ventilatory responses to hypercapnia and hypoxia are impaired
Mucocilliary clearance is reduced; coughing does not occur; laryngeal stimulation produces apnea	Mucocilliary clearance is reduced; coughing does not occur; laryngeal stimulation produces apnea	Mucocilliary clearance is reduced; coughing does not occur; laryngeal stimulation produces apnea
Airway smooth-muscle tone decreases	Airway smooth-muscle tone generally decreases	Airway smooth-muscle tone increases

Continued

Table 8B–2 *(Continued)*
Physiological Characteristics of NREM and REM Sleep

NREM	Baseline REM	During Phasic REM Activity
Pulmonary stretch receptor reflexes are intact	Pulmonary stretch receptor reflexes are intact	Pulmonary stretch receptor reflexes are absent
Arousal response to airway occlusion hypoxia, hypercapnia, laryngeal stimulation, and airway and intrapulmonary irritation occurs with a shorter latency than during REM sleep	Arousal response to airway occlusion hypoxia, hypercapnia, laryngeal stimulation, and airway and intrapulmonary irritation has a longer latency than during NREM sleep	Arousal response to airway occlusion hypoxia, hypercapnia, laryngeal stimulation, and airway and intrapulmonary irritation has a longer latency than during NREM sleep
Growth hormone is secreted in the early part of the night		
Prolactin secretion peaks in the early morning hours; circadian episodes of thyrotropin secretion are inhibited by sleep; gonadotropin secretion occurs during sleep in puberty; sleep inhibits the ACTH-cortisol circadian rhythm; plasma aldosterone levels increase		
Parathyroid hormone concentration increases. Gastric acid secretion, water secretion, and fractional rate of emptying decrease; swallowing and esophageal motility decrease		
Penile tumescence occurs infrequently	Penile tumescence; clitoral tumescence	Penile tumescence; clitoral tumescence
Glomerular filtration rate, renal plasma flow filtration, fraction, and excretion of Na^+, Cl^-, K^+, and Ca^{2+} decrease	Excretion of smaller amounts of more concentrated urine	Excretion of smaller amounts of more concentrated urine

Reprinted with permission from Orem, J., and C. D. Barnes. *Physiology in Sleep.* pp. 330–334. Academic Press, Orlando. 1980.
ACTH—adrenal corticotropic hormone; Ca^{2+}—calcium; Cl^-—chloride; K^+—potassium; Na^+—sodium

- Stage 3: Stage 3 is entered as high-voltage slow waves gradually appear on the EEG. This stage lasts only a few minutes and transitions to Stage 4 as high-voltage slow wave activity increases.
- Stage 4: This stage generally lasts for about 20–40 minutes in the first cycle, with decreasing amounts of time in subse-

Table 8B-3
Typical Night's Sleep

Time	Process
	Fatigue sets in.
Midnight	Typical 20–40 year old drifts to sleep in about 7 minutes. During sleep onset thoughts wander, bizarre hallucinations may occur or one may have the sensation of falling or floating. Occasionally some muscles relax sooner than others, and this may trigger a sudden jerk of the arm or leg.
12:07–12:30	NREM Episode 1. The pattern of brain waves resembles small closely spaced peaks and valleys and most people, if awakened, will insist they were "just thinking".
12:30–1:00	Brain waves became farther apart, larger and more regular with bursts of high voltage brain activity (sleep spindles) that last 1–2 seconds. This marks entry into Stage 2. With deepening sleep, heart rate and breathing slow; there is a decrease in both body temperature and blood pressure.
1:00–1:45	NREM progresses to Stage 3–4. If roused abruptly while in Stage 3–4 an individual may be disoriented or confused, may not have his/her usual coordination or judgment. Normal sleepers almost never awaken spontaneously during Stage 3–4 sleep.
1:45–1:55	REM Episode 1 occurs about 90 minutes after the beginning of sleep. Adults will rise from Stage 3–4 NREM into the light sleep of Stage 2, then enter their first REM episode. Here, they experience their first of 4 or 5 nightly dreams. In REM sleep the brain waves are fast, irregular and simulate the brain at wakefulness. Heart rate slows and blood pressure shows great variability. The person is virtually paralyzed in REM sleep. People may awaken at the end of a REM episode, but have no memory of it.
1:55–3:30	NREM Episode 2. REM episodes grow longer over the night. The sleeper travels through Stage 2, returns to Stage 3–4, and the cycle repeats.
3:30–3:45	REM Episode 2. REM episodes grow longer over the night.
3:45–5:00	NREM Episode 3. This will contain more Stage 2 and Stage 1 sleep and less Stage 3–4 than the earliest NREM episodes.
4:00	People who are awakened experience the highest degree of sleepiness and thus the poorest performances. Body temperature is at its lowest point. It is also a time when one is most sensitive to the effects of bright light. If an insomniac turns on a light to read, they may train their body to wake up consistently at that time.
5:00–5:30	REM Episode 3.
5:30–6:30	NREM Episode 4—increasingly lighter sleep.
6:30–7:15	REM Episode 4.

Reprinted with permission from Lamberg, L. *Bodyrhythms Chronobiology and Peak Performance*. William Morrow and Co., New York. 1994.

quent sleep cycles. An incrementally bigger stimulus is required to produce arousal from Stage 3 or 4. Stage 3 and 4 are often referred to as "slow wave" sleep, delta sleep, or deep sleep.

Body movement usually signals an ascent to the lighter NREM sleep stages and then into REM sleep. REM sleep in the first cycle of the night is usually short (1–5 minutes), lengthening throughout the night.

Sleep Problems in Oncology Patients

Nurses and physicians working with oncology patients report that insomnia is a common clinical problem for patients with cancer. However, few research studies focus on the prevalence and nature of sleep disturbance in cancer patients. A 1983 study by Kaye and colleagues found that 45 percent of the cancer patients studied reported difficulty staying asleep, as compared with 14 percent of the controls. In another study done by Beszterezey and Lipowski in 1977, questionnaires were administered to 47 cancer patients. Findings revealed that patients had significant difficulties both falling asleep and staying asleep. In addition, the degree of insomnia was not associated with unrelieved pain but rather with symptoms of anxiety and depression. In the 1977 Holland and Plumb study of 97 patients with advanced cancer, the degree of insomnia was noted to be as high as is found in patients who are suicidally depressed, although symptoms of depression in the cancer population were no more than that which was found in the control group. A survey of 1,600 cancer patients by Derogatis and colleagues revealed that 44 percent had received a prescription for sleeping medication. In most instances, the prescription was written for a hypnotic. When Silverfarb, Hauri, and Oxman (1993) studied sleep architecture and psychologic state in breast and lung cancer patients, findings indicated that lung cancer patients slept as poorly as did insomniacs but under-reported their sleep difficulties. The breast cancer patients in this group slept similarly to normal-sleeping volunteers but reported having a slight sleep disturbance in some measures (sleep efficiency, sleep latency, and awake after first sleep epoch).

When Monro and Potter (1996) quantified distress from more than 400 assessments of breast, lung, and head and neck cancer patients, those with breast cancer reported difficulty concentrating, pain, and sleep disturbances as significantly troublesome problems.

These research findings give support to the clinical observation that sleep difficulties occur with frequency in the cancer population and warrant keen assessment as well as precise intervention. The extent of sleep problems span a wide range of cancer diagnoses and include difficulty falling asleep, difficulty staying asleep, and awakening too early. Sleep difficulties occur in approximately 45 percent of the patients studied across a wide number of cancer diagnoses. The causes of the sleep disruption in this population are likely multifactorial.

Sleep Disturbances Related to Sleep Cycles

When a person is deprived of REM or NREM sleep either by being awakened or by chronic use of sleeping medications, a disruption in the normal sleep pattern occurs. When natural sleep resumes, a preferential rebound to the last stage of sleep will occur. For example, chronic restriction of sleep, an irregular sleep schedule, or frequent disturbance of sleep—as would occur for the hospitalized cancer patient—can result in premature REM sleep. These sleep onset REM episodes do not allow the normal cyclic NREM/REM pattern, setting the framework for significant sleep disruption or sleep deprivation.

Circadian rhythm is the internal clock that controls sleep. The circadian phase at which sleep occurs affects the distribution of sleep stages. REM sleep, in particular, occurs with a circadian distribution that peaks in the early morning hours (4 a.m.) when the body temperature is at its lowest. Studies of adults sleeping in laboratories free of all environmental cues have shown that the timing of sleep onset and length of sleep occurs as a function of circadian phase. Therefore, if sleep onset is delayed until early morning (when REM is peaking), REM sleep will tend to dominate and can occur at the onset of sleep. This gives rise to nonrestorative sleep and progresses to sleep deprivation. Consideration should be given as to whether the patient's 24-hour internal clock has been affected in some way by surgery, hospital schedules, or the treatment itself.

The exact function of sleep is not precisely known, although some theories promote sleep as having restorative functions both physically and mentally. Negative effects of sleep deprivation may include enhanced nocturnal plasma interleukin 1- and 2-like activities, delay in lymphocyte response to stimulation, and prolonged decline in natural killer cell activity. The greatest amount of growth hormone is released during sleep; therefore, disrupting, delaying, or prohibiting sleep reduces circulating levels of this hormone. The disruption of sleep also impairs physical and mental performance in both the healthy and ill, will lower the pain threshold, and will heighten emotional reactivity.

Sleep deprivation is a common occurrence in both the hospitalized and nonhospitalized patients. The environment of the clinical unit, absence of cues for sleeping (e.g., dim light, silence, normal sleep routine, evening shower, brushing teeth, personal sleep clothes), medications, age, psychological stress, and individual response to surgery and treatments all contribute to sleep disruption and deprivation. Deprivation of total sleep needs or of different sleep stages produces observable signs. For the person with initial sleep deprivation, signs and symptoms include a feeling of fatigue, headache, nausea, anxiety, depression, burning eyes, and signs of somno-lence: irritability, restlessness, apathy, lassitude, periods of inattention, puffy eyelids, reddened conjunctiva, and dark areas around the eyes.

As total sleep deprivation continues, more pronounced signs and symptoms include difficulty concentrating, decreased attention span, mis-perceptions, auditory or visual hallucinations, and muscle weakness. Ob-jective signs of prolonged total sleep deprivation include muscle tremors, decreased coordination and reaction time, disorientation, slurred speech, and behavior changes such as aggression or withdrawal. Recovery from sleep deprivation of this type requires more hours of sleep than were previ-ously lost, in terms of both total sleep time and individual sleep stages. Physiologically, sleep loss affects the body's ability to regulate tempera-ture and hormone production, cardiac and respiratory function, brain activ-ity as measured by EEG, and control of eye musculature.

It is possible for a person to be deprived of a particular sleep stage without total sleep deprivation. Deprivation of REM sleep poses a par-ticular problem to hospitalized patients. Symptoms of REM deprivation include irritability, anxiety, difficulty concentrating, hyperactivity, in-creased appetite, and difficulty coping with stress. Several factors inher-ent in the hospitalization experience can contribute to this kind of sleep deprivation. Hospitalized patients can develop day/night sleep reversal or not get enough total sleep (e.g., 3–4 hours of sleep in a 24-hour pe-riod). Such patients frequently sleep for only short periods (up to one hour) at a time, totally eliminating periods of REM, which occurs at the end of a normal 90-minute sleep cycle. At a time when the patient is most in need of rallying all defenses to combat the effects of cancer treatment, sleep deprivation works to deny the patient the restorative benefits of sleep.

Sleep over the Life Span

The strongest factor affecting the pattern of sleep stages across the night is age. As growth occurs, sleep characteristics change significantly (see Figure 8B–2).

In infancy, the cyclic alteration of NREM and REM sleep is present; however, instead of 90-minute cycles, the infant moves through the stages of sleep in 50- to 60-minute cycles. In childhood, slow-wave (deep or delta) sleep is at its highest level. Slow-wave sleep in young children is both quantitatively and qualitatively different from adults. Children have been found to be much more difficult to awaken with noise than adults. Measurements in young adults show that slow-wave sleep quantitatively decreases by 40 percent sometime during the second decade, even when length of nocturnal sleep remains constant. In general, no consistent male/female distinctions have been found when measuring sleep in normal young adults.

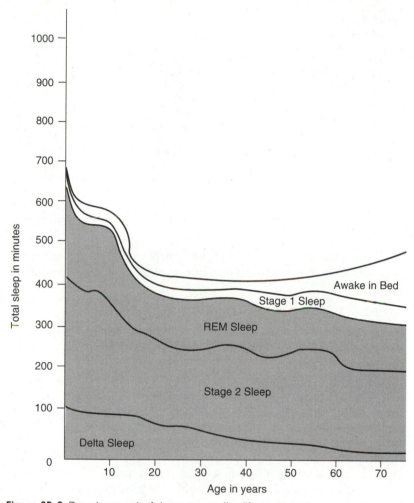

Figure 8B-2. Development of sleep across the life span.
From Hauri, P. The Sleep Disorders. Current Concepts, p. 14. Upjohn, Kalamazoo, MI. 1982.

REM sleep as a percentage of total sleep is maintained well into old age. Women appear to maintain slow-wave sleep later into life than do men. Both extended awakenings and brief unremembered arousals during sleep increase with age.

ASSESSMENT

When a complaint of sleep disruption is reported by the patient or family member, a brief initial assessment can help determine whether the problem is chronic or transient in nature. The use of several initial questions (Table 8B–4) will give the patient an opportunity to discuss the prob-

Table 8B–4
Initial Sleep Questions

1. Are you satisfied with your sleep?
2. Does sleep or fatigue intrude in your daytime activities?
3. Does your bed partner or others complain of unusual behavior while you sleep (such as snoring, interrupted breathing or leg movements)?
4. Do you have an irregular schedule of sleep?
5. Do you find yourself lying in bed and ruminating about stressful events prior to sleep?
6. Do you spend excessive amounts of time in bed?
7. Do you have any habits (such as smoking, caffeine intake, lack of exercise, dark rooms, alcohol, self-medication, late evening meals) that could adversely affect your sleep?
8. Do you worry excessively about not sleeping?

lem. Patients with severe sleep difficulties may require comprehensive assessment and a more extensive plan of care with physician referral (Table 8B–5).

Educational and Behavioral Interventions

Sleep is an active process, is fragile, and changes over the life span. Nurses can teach patients about areas of their lifestyle that are affecting good sleep. These can include dealing with stress, and physical factors such as pain, frequent urination during night, hormonal shifts, and medications that might interfere with sleep. Patients will benefit from understanding that any change in sleep habits requires patience and that chronic sleep problems require a longer time to resolve. A basic teaching guide using the rules of sleep hygiene (Table 8B–6) will help patients make sound decisions when dealing with insomnia.

PHARMACOLOGIC TREATMENT

The ideal medication for insomnia should have a rapid onset, be effective with continued use, not interfere with daytime activities, produce no hangover effects, produce no insomnia when stopped, not alter sleep stages, and have a limited potential for abuse. No medication currently available meets these recommendations. Medications currently used to promote sleep have side effects related to one or more of these characteristics, diminishing their value as a sedative/hypnotic. Therefore, pharmacologic management of insomnia should only be used when behavioral and cognitive approaches have been exhausted. Medication use should be im-

Table 8B–5
Factors that Influence Sleep and Assessment of Sleep Disturbance in Cancer Patients

Factor	Assessment	Intervention
General (age and developmental level)	What are the patient's age and developmental level (infant, school age, adolescent, young adult, middle age, elderly)? How has the patient been sleeping (describe sleep habits, usual amount of sleep)?	Observe the patient's own sleep routines as much as possible. Discuss changes and plan alternatives with the patient. Remind the patient that total sleep time decreases with advanced age.
Time to bed	What time does the patient usually go to bed?	Have the patient retire only if sleepy, not just when the time seems appropriate.
Patterns of insomnia Initial	How long does it take the patient to fall asleep? Does the patient fall asleep right away? How does the patient feel before falling asleep? How often does the patient have trouble falling asleep?	Help the patient establish a relaxing, quiet period before sleep. Prevent excitement in the evening before bedtime.
Intermittent	Does the patient wake up during the night? What causes awakening? How often does the patient awaken during the night? What helps the patient get back to sleep?	If unable to sleep, have the patient get up and pursue some relaxing activity to produce drowsiness.
Terminal	What time does the patient wake up? What wakes the patient up early? How often do early awakenings occur? Is the patient depressed? What does the patient do upon awakening early?	With early awakening, have the patient get up and accomplish some useful activity (e.g., morning hygiene).
Patient's response to quality of sleep	Does the patient feel rested after a night's sleep? How does the patient feel after getting up? Does the patient appear to be well rested? Validate patient versus nurse perceptions.	Encourage discussion of the patient's subjective experience of sleep.
Naps	Does the patient nap during the day? How long? Does the patient have day/night reversal (sleeps more during the day than at night)? Does the patient have excess daytime sleepiness (e.g., due to brain tumor)?	Establish regular times to go to sleep and wake up. Increase stimulation and provide activities (e.g., after meals).
Recreation/exercise	Does the patient exercise? What sort of activity is involved? When does the patient have exercise in relation to bedtime?	Help the patient exercise during the day. Promote self-care and provide group participation as appropriate. Have the patient exercise for a brief period at least two hours before retiring to promote Stage 4 sleep.
Emotional factors Anxiety	Is the patient worried about the outcome of the illness? Is there an inability to manage normal responsibilities?	Explore potential causes of anxiety (e.g., financial problems, family situation, fear of death).

Continued

Table 8B–5 *(Continued)*
Factors that Influence Sleep and Assessment of Sleep Disturbance in Cancer Patients

Factor	Assessment	Intervention
Emotional factors		
Depression	What is the patient's mood (cheerful, depressed)?	Offer presence, and counsel if appropriate.
Stress	Has the patient received a recent diagnosis of cancer or recurrence? Are there any other obvious sources of stress in the patient's life (e.g., a new course of treatment)?	Promote receptive atmosphere for expression of fears and questions. Provide adequate answers. Allow for more sleep time. Provide massage, back rub, and relaxation techniques if desired. Discourage focusing on sleep problems, because it will aggravate them.
Sleep environment	What is the patient's usual sleep environment? What have been the previous experiences when sleeping in an unfamiliar place?	Obtain a baseline on the patient's usual sleep environment, and then adapt it to the patient's needs if possible.
Lighting	Does having a light on at night disturb the patient?	Dim lighting.
Ventilation	Does the patient like to sleep with a door or window open?	Adjust ventilation. Leave door open or closed.
Bedding	How many and what type of pillows does the patient use? Is any special bedding used (blankets, mattress, or pads)?	Ensure clean linens. Smooth any wrinkles in bedding. Provide adequate covering.
Temperature	Does the patient need the room warm or cool to sleep well?	Adjust thermostat. Provide extra blankets for the elderly.
Noise	Do noises wake the patient or keep the patient awake? Does the patient need quiet to sleep?	Restrict noise from staff, roommates, phones, radio, television, intercom, and visitors. Direct equipment noise (e.g., infusion pumps) away from patient.
Positioning	What is the patient's usual sleep position? Does the patient need to be turned every two hours?	Assist the patient to a preferred position if possible. Determine which movements or positions are not tolerated.
Social factors	Does the patient usually sleep alone, share a room, or share the bed? Does the patient have increased social stimulation before bedtime?	Provide a compatible roommate if the room is shared. Provide a safe environment (side rails up, call bell in reach). Monitor the effect of visitors in relation to bedtime.
Presleep routine	What does the patient do immediately before going to bed?	Learn about the patient's normal routine. Assist and adapt as needed.

Table 8B–5 *(Continued)*
Factors that Influence Sleep and Assessment of Sleep Disturbance in Cancer Patients

Factor	Assessment	Intervention
Beverages	Does the patient like a beverage before going to bed?	Avoid caffeinic beverages late in the day. Withhold fluids in the evening if nocturia is a problem. (See Table 8B-7.)
Hygiene	Does bathing at bedtime help the patient sleep?	Offer a bath and oral care.
Food	Does the patient like to eat something at bedtime?	Avoid large meals in the evening. Offer a high-protein snack at bedtime. (Most protein foods contain L-tryptophan, an amino acid precursor of serotonin).
Medication	What medications is the patient receiving? Is the patient on steroids (which can produce chronic insomnia)? Does the patient take any medications (including alcohol) to produce sleep?	Use nondrug measures to promote sleep as much as possible. Use sleep medications on a short-term or intermittent basis, and use agents that do not alter REM sleep (or withdraw REM-suppressant drugs gradually). Observe the sleep effects of a new or current medication routine.
Personal beliefs about sleep	How much sleep does the patient think is necessary? What does the patient feel are the consequences of insufficient sleep?	Explore concerns about sleep, and correct misconceptions.
Disease/treatment factors	What is the patient's diagnosis, disease status, and course of treatment?	Be familiar with medications, other treatments, and expected side effects.
Pain/discomfort	What is the source of any pain (e.g., recent surgery, mucositis)? Is the pain control adequate? Is the patient febrile? Is pain preventing sleep or causing awakening?	Reposition the patient for comfort. Medicate for pain (give before sleep medication). Provide soothing irrigations, heat, cold, and mental diversion.
Fatigue	Does the patient have a balance of activity and rest during the day? Has the patient undergone a late evening test or treatment?	Prevent late evening overstimulation. Gradually increase exercise tolerance to overcome fatigue.
Impaired nutritional status	Is the patient NPO? Is there nausea or vomiting?	Provide oral hygiene and/or antiemetics if nausea/vomiting occurs.
Dyspnea/cough	Does the patient need oxygen or suctioning? Is coughing disrupting sleep?	Provide extra pillows and elevate the head of the bed; offer respiratory treatment and medications as needed.
Urinary frequency/ incontinence	Is the patient receiving IV therapy or diuretics? Is the patient aware of the urge to void? If present, is the bladder catheter patent?	Have the patient void at bedtime. Limit fluid in the evening unless a high urine flow is necessary.

Continued

Table 8B-5 *(Continued)*
Factors that Influence Sleep and Assessment of Sleep Disturbance in Cancer Patients

Factor	Assessment	Intervention
Disease/treatment factors		
Diarrhea	What are the frequency and consistency of stools?	Medicate to slow peristalsis and eliminate odors.
Nighttime confusion	Does the patient's mental status undergo changes from day to night? Does the patient have an electrolyte imbalance?	To prevent nighttime confusion, reorient the patient frequently. Keep the patient's environment and the staff as consistent as possible.
Altered skin integrity	Are there pressure ulcers? Are there draining wounds or lesions that require frequent dressing changes?	Perform wound care and dressing changes before bedtime. Eliminate odors and provide clean linens.
Disruptive caregiver routines (tests, treatments, routine care, health team rounds)	What procedures are absolutely necessary (e.g., antibiotic administration), and which can be eliminated or postponed until the patient is awake (e.g., every-two-hour mouth care)?	Observe the sleeping patient's condition in a nondisturbing way (minimal physical contact, no overhead light). Use any spontaneous awakening by patient to complete tasks and make assessments when possible. Awaken the patient only when necessary, and, if possible, observe for REM sleep and awaken after the sleep cycle is completed. Organize nursing activities so they can be completed during one awakening (e.g., midnight vital signs, patient voiding, pain medication, antibiotic). Discuss with the physician the possibility of changing times of medication, treatments, etc., to allow for sleep. Plan with the patient procedures that will necessitate awakening.

Reprinted with permission from Kaempfer S. H. and B. L. Johnson. Sleep. In Gross, J. and B. L. Johnson, eds. *Handbook of Oncology Nursing,* 2nd Ed. 314–316, 323–325. Jones & Bartlett, Sudbury, MA.

plemented with caution. In 1997, Kupfer and Reynolds identified these principles of use for medications:

- Control symptoms that could be causing insomnia, such as pain, nausea, and/or diarrhea.
- Use the lowest dose possible to prevent drug intoxication.
- Use intermittent doses (e.g., two to three times per week) to minimize tolerance and prevent accumulation of toxic metabolites.
- Use for short periods of time only (e.g., three to four weeks).
- Discontinue gradually to prevent insomnia from rapidly returning.

Table 8B-6
Rules for Sleep Hygiene

Rule	Rationale
Sleep just long enough.	Each patient should sleep as much as needed to feel refreshed during the following day. Some people just seem to need more sleep than others. But sleep no longer than is necessary. Limiting time in bed seems to solidify sleep; excessively long times in bed seem to be related to fragmented and shallow sleep.
Wake up and go to bed at the same time every day.	Regulating the sleep schedule seems to strengthen circadian cycles and will help lead to regular sleep onset. Weekends should not be an exception to the schedule (Riedel 1995).
Create a routine for going to bed; use bed only for sleep and sex (avoid other activities such as eating).	Comfortable bed clothes; light snack, bath, same routine each night will facilitate sleep response. A light snack and something warm to drink helps many people sleep. Resolve personal disputes before sleeping.
Exercise regularly.	A consistent amount of daily exercise helps to deepen sleep over time, but occasional sporadic exercise may not. Do not exercise right before retiring as this will interfere with sleep onset (Browman 1976).
Get light exposure every day (open shades, walk, work outdoors).	This sets the circadian clock.
Eliminate noise (no TV in bedroom; use white noise). The use of ear plugs may be helpful.	Occasional loud noises (e.g., aircraft flyovers, sirens, others up and moving about, dogs barking) disturb sleep even when people do not awaken because of them and do not remember them in the morning.
Regulate room temperature.	Excessive cold or heat disturb sleep. Regulate the temperature for comfort.
Know the effect that daytime napping has on you.	Some people sleep better at night and others have sleep disruption following daytime napping. The time used to take a nap should be limited to 30 minutes in the early afternoon (Hu 1991).
Avoid stimulants; chronic use of tobacco can be disruptive to sleep.	Many poor sleepers are sensitive to stimulants. Caffeine takes at least 8 hours to metabolize. No stimulant drinks should be taken after lunchtime. (See Table 8B-7.) Nicotine acts as a stimulant.
Limit alcohol consumption.	Alcohol initially helps stressed people to fall asleep, but the sleep is fragmented and not restful or restorative.
Do not try too hard; if unable to fall asleep after 15–20 minutes, get out of bed and go into another room.	Relaxation techniques include: visualization; cognitive strategies such as writing mental letters; multiply by 7's; recall pleasant memories. Read with a dim light and avoid watching TV (light exposure). Return to bed only when sleepy.

Adapted from Hu, D. and P. M. Silverfarb. Management and sleep problems in cancer patients. *Oncology* 5:23–28. 1991.

Table 8B–7
Caffeine Content

Brewed coffee	135 mg
Instant coffee	90 mg
Decaffeinated coffee	3–5 mg
Black tea	50 mg
Cola	45 mg
Orange soda	40 mg
Mountain Dew®	50 mg
Dark chocolate	31 mg
Milk chocolate	9 mg

The decision to use a medication for insomnia involves careful consideration. Selection criteria include the history of the sleeping disorder, length of time the disorder has been present, patient age, co-morbid conditions, and history of medication use, focusing especially on those that are associated with insomnia. For cancer patients receiving chemotherapy, insomnia could be associated with use of pentostatin, daunorubicin, interferon, cortisone, and progesterone. Long-term sleep disorders lead to sleep deprivation and can lower a person's tolerance for sedatives. Therefore, a smaller dose might be effective in producing the desired effect.

Most sedatives/hypnotics cause disturbances in the sleep stages, especially Stage 4 and REM. When deprived of REM sleep, persons can become chronically fatigued and lose their ability to concentrate. When sedative/hypnotics are discontinued, REM rebound can continue for several weeks. REM rebound occurs when a patient is finally able to have uninterrupted sleep and spends a greater proportion of sleep time in REM. This can be problematic for patients with coronary problems, because of the increased physiological demands during REM sleep. Pain, arrhythmias, and heart failure can occur. Gradual discontinuation of sedatives/hypnotics is essential in this setting.

Classes of medications recommended for use as sedatives/hypnotics for insomnia are listed in Table 8B–8. Generic and trade names are followed by the usual dose, the onset of action, half life, and the effect on the sleep cycle. A section on comments is used to identify precautions and complications. A medication with a short half life is recommended in order to avoid daytime drowsiness.

The benzodiazepines constitute one category of currently used sedatives/hypnotics. Table 8B–8 includes some of the most common medications in this category. These medications should be prescribed in small amounts (only enough for three to four weeks at a time). Refills should be avoided, as the effects of long-term use have not been studied. Patients must be cautioned about daytime sleepiness; thus, driving and operating heavy equipment should not be permitted. Although they are safe in lower doses, use of the benzodiazepines can lead to impaired judgment and aggressive behavior. When mixed with alcohol, fatal overdoses can occur. Onset of action differs among the medications in this category, ranging from 20–30 minutes for flurazepam to one hour for clorazepate. All of the benzodiazepines interfere with the sleep cycle, most commonly causing suppression of Stage 4.

Chloral hydrate, a chloral derivative, is a popular, relatively inexpensive, and effective medication for sleep for short-term use. Physical and psychological dependence is common with prolonged use. It does not cause confusion and has little effect on the sleep cycle. Chloral hydrate does cause gastrointestinal irritation and is toxic when combined with alcohol.

Zolpidem (imidazopyridine) acts similarly to the benzodiazepines but does not suppress Stage 4 or REM sleep. It is a newer hypnotic in the United States and is the most expensive of all the sedatives/hypnotics.

Antidepressants represent another category of medications used to treat insomnia. Because of both a concern for dependence and the side effects of benzodiazepines and the need for triplicate prescriptions for benzodiazepines, the use of antidepressants has increased dramatically. Few clinical trials of antidepressants as treatment for insomnia have been conducted, and the dose and efficacy of these agents for insomnia has not been tested. In addition, this group of medications produces side effects such as orthostasis and cardiac arrhythmias. Both overdose with alcohol and dependency can occur with the antidepressants. The most appropriate use for this group of medications is probably insomnia associated with depression.

Additional medications that have traditionally been used for insomnia, but are no longer recommended, include alcohol, the barbiturates, and antihistamines. Alcohol works quickly to induce sleep but then causes fragmentation of the sleep cycle. It can also affect performance the next day, and it potentiates other sedative hypnotics, a combination that can be lethal.

At one time barbiturates were the most common group of medications used to induce sleep; however, insomnia is common when discontinuing barbiturates, and this resulting insomnia is accompanied by dreaming and nightmares. In addition, physical and psychological dependence are common. These problems are accentuated in the elderly.

The most common group of medications available over the counter to enhance drowsiness are the antihistamines. This group includes diphenhydramine (Benadryl®), hydroxine (Vistaril®, Atarax®), and promethazine (Phenergan®). However, persistent drowsiness and feelings of hangover are common with these medications. There is no evidence that they are as safe or effective as other sleep medications. Because they are not specifically formulated as medications for insomnia, antihistamines are considered an alternative therapy and should not supplant more specific sedatives/hypnotics.

Table 8B–8
Medications Used to Promote Sleep

Drug Category	Medication	Dose (Route)	Onset (Duration of Action)	Effect on Sleep Cycle	Half Life (Hours)	Comments
Benzodiazepines*	Chlordiazepoxide (Librium®)	50–100 mg (capsule, tablet)	30–60 min (6–8 hr)	Suppression of Stage 4.	5–30	
	Clorazepate (Tranxene®)	15 mg (capsule, tablet)	1 hr (24 hr)	Suppression of Stage 4.	18–50	
	Diazepam (Valium®)	5–10 mg (tablet)	30–60 min (3 hr)	Shortening of Stage 4.	20–70	
	Flurazepam (Dalmane®)	15–30 mg (capsule)	20–30 min (7–8 hr)	Marked Stage 4 reduction. Little or no suppression of REM.	50–240	Elderly more prone to residual effects.
	Lorazepam (Ativan®)	2–4 mg (tablet)	Highly individual	Highly individual.	10–24	
	Oxazepam (Serax®)	10–30 mg (capsule, tablet)	Shorter than diazepam	Fewer effects on sleep stages than chlordiazepoxide.	5–15	
	Temazepam (Restoril®)	15–30 mg (capsule)	30 min (6–8 hr)	Marked Stage 4 reduction. Little or no suppression of REM.	10–24	
	Triazolam (Halcion®)	0.25–0.5 mg (tablet)	15–30 min (6–8 hr)	Decreased sleep latency. Increased duration of sleep.	1.6–5.4	
	Estazolam (ProSom™)	1–2 mg	60–120 minutes (10–15 hr)		10–24	Moderate half life so fewer daytime sedation effects.

Class	Drug	Dose	Onset (duration)	Effect on sleep stages	Half-life (hr)	Comments
	Quazepam (Doral®)	7.5–15 mg	30 minutes (10–30 hr)		25–75	Rapidly metabolized but accumulates with chronic use.
Chloral derivative	Chloral hydrate (Noctec®)	0.5–1.0 g (capsule, syrup, suppository)	30–60 min (4–8 hr)	Suppression of Stage 4 in high doses.	8–10	Short term—7–10 d. Tolerance occurs.
Imidazopyridine	Zolpidem (Ambien®)	10 mg	30 min (2–4 hr)	No suppression of Stage 4 or REM.	1.4–4.5	Short half life so fewer daytime sedation effects.
Tricyclic antidepressants	Amitriptyline (Elavil®)	75–200 mg (tablet)	Highly variable	Suppression of REM.	10–50	Dependence common.
	Nortriptyline (Pamelor®)	75–100 mg (tablet)	Highly variable	Suppression of REM.	18–28	Elderly susceptible to adverse effects.
	Doxepin (Sinequan®)	75–150 mg (capsule, syrup)	Highly variable	Suppression of REM.	8–25	Dependence common.
	Imipramine (Tofranil®)	100–200 mg (capsule)	Highly variable (10–25 hr half-life)	Suppression of REM. Decrease in number of awakenings from sleep.	8–16	Overdose toxicity with alcohol. Dependence common.
Serotonin antagonists	Trazodone (Desyrel®)	150 mg (tablet)	Variable	Suppression of REM.	5–9	Preferably for sleep disturbances associated with depression.

*General comments: Recommended use for 1 month only. Caution with liver metastases because of decreased ability to metabolize drug. Dependence can occur. Insomnia might recur quickly when stopped. Mixing with alcohol can be lethal.

NURSING ASSESSMENT AND INTERVENTION

The responsibility of the nurse includes careful assessment of the sleeping disorder, implementation of cognitive and behavioral interventions first (Tables 8B–5 and 8B–6), followed by cautious use of prescribed medications. The dose should be selected carefully and based on the patient's age, body mass, other medications, and probable cause of insomnia. For cancer patients at home, careful teaching about principles of use and side effects to monitor is required. Written instructions and regular monitoring by professional staff are essential components of the nursing care plan for patients using medications to induce sleep. When discontinuing these medications, the dose should be tapered gradually to avoid recurrent insomnia. Medications should be used for the shortest period of time necessary.

BIBLIOGRAPHY

1. Beszterczey, A., and Z. J. Lipowski. Insomnia in cancer patients. *Canadian Medical Association Journal* 116: 355. 1977.

   A study of 47 cancer patients whose questionnaires revealed difficulty with both falling asleep and staying asleep is presented.

2. Carskadon, M. A., and W. C. Dement. Normal human sleep: An overview. In Kryger, M. H., T. Roth, and W. C. Dement, eds. *Principles and Practice of Sleep Medicine*, 2d Ed. 16–25. WB Saunders, Philadelphia. 1994.

   This is a thorough discussion of normal human sleep with emphasis on the physiology of sleep. This chapter is one of many "must-reads" for those interested in the complexities of sleep mechanisms. The entire book can be used as a sleep bible.

3. Derogatis, L. R., M. Feldstein, G. Morrow, et al. A survey of psychotropic drug prescriptions in an oncology population. *Cancer* 44: 1919–1929. 1979.

   This is a retrospective study of 1,600 cancer patients in five major cancer centers that examines the use of psychotrophic drug prescriptions over a six-month period.

4. Farney, R. J., and J. M. Walker. Office management of common sleep-wake disorders. *Medical Clinics of North America.* 79(2): 391–402. 1995.

   A comprehensive review of the range of common sleep-wake conditions encountered by primary care practitioners is presented in a framework of sleep physiology and current diagnostic technology.

5. Holland, J., and M. Plumb. A comparative study of depressive symptoms in patients with advanced cancer. *Proceedings of the American Association Cancer Research* 18: 201. 1977.

   This is a classic research study that set early ground with patients with advanced cancer, depression, and insomnia.

6. Hu, D., and P. M. Silverfarb. Management and sleep problems in cancer patients. *Oncology* 5: 23–28. 1991.

The article clearly outlines sleep hygiene recommendations for the oncology patient.

7. Kaye, J., K. Kaye, and L. Meadow. Sleep patterns in patients with cancer and patients with cardiac disease. *Journal of Psychology* 114: 107–113. 1983.

This study compares sleep problems in cancer patients with a control group of patients with cardiac problems.

8. Kupfer, D. J., and C. F. Reynolds. Management of insomnia. *New England Journal of Medicine* 336(5): 341–346. 1997.

The review article thoroughly documents the medical evaluation of insomnia and places emphasis on the pharmacotherapeutic management.

9. Lamberg, L. *Body Rhythms Chronobiology and Peak Performance*, 1st Ed. William Morrow and Company, New York. 1994.

This textbook-style overview of circadian rhythm theory presents the effects of sleep deprivation on performance, and steps to be taken to obtain better sleep. Format flows well with excellent documentation.

10. Munro, A. J., and S. Potter. A qualitative approach to the distress caused by symptoms in patients treated with radical radiotherapy. *British Journal of Cancer* 74: 640–647. 1996.

A study of 110 breast, head and neck, and lung cancer patients with 400 assessment points reveals sleep disturbances as a significant problem.

11. Naitoh, P., T. Kelly, and C. Englund. Health effects of sleep deprivation. *Occupational Medicine* 5: 209–236. 1990.

This research study discusses the impact that sleep disruptions have on the amount of growth hormone released during sleep.

12. Roberts, S. Sleep deprivation. In Roberts, S., ed. *Behavioral Concepts and the Critically Ill Patient*. 63–94. Appleton-Century-Crofts, Norwalk, CT. 1986.

This well-referenced chapter on sleep deprivations focuses on the effects in the critically ill patient.

13. Robinson, C. R. Impaired sleep. In Carrieri-Kohlman, V., A. Lindsey, and C. M. West, eds. *Pathophysiological Phenomena in Nursing*. 490–528. WB Saunders, Philadelphia. 1993.

This comprehensive chapter contained in a physiology-guided textbook thoroughly addresses all aspects of impaired sleep.

14. Silverfarb, P. M., P. J. Hauri, and T. Oxman. Assessment of sleep in patients with lung cancer and breast cancer. *Journal of Clinical Oncology* 11: 997–1004. 1993.

Sleep architecture and psychologic state of 32 patients with lung or breast cancer compared with 32 age- and sex-matched normal sleeping volunteers and 32 otherwise healthy insomniacs is presented. Findings indicate that lung patients sleep as poorly as insomniacs but under-report sleep difficulties.

15. Vitiello, M. V. Sleep disorders and aging. *Current Opinion in Psychiatry* 9: 284–289. 1996.

This is classic with a focus on the elderly, this article discusses sleep disorders and various solutions to sleep disturbances.

16. Zarcone, V. P. Sleep hygiene. In Kryger, M. H., T. Roth, and W. C. Dement, eds. *Principles and Practice of Sleep Medicine*, 2d Ed. 542–546. W.B. Saunders, Philadelphia. 1994.

This is a very informative chapter on not only the fundamentals of sleep hygiene, but the effects of caffeine, ethanol, and nicotine on sleep.

C. Fatigue

Grace E. Dean
Betty R. Ferrell

INTRODUCTION

Fatigue, a symptom of acute and chronic illnesses, has been identified as the seventh most common reason for seeing a primary care physician and estimated as the cause of more than 7 million office visits per year (Epstein 1995). Fatigue is also reported to be a widely prevalent and significantly distressing symptom of cancer; however, its treatment has been largely ignored because it is usually self-limiting and not life threatening. Fatigue can be a symptom of the cancer itself and precede diagnosis, or result from surgery, radiation therapy, chemotherapy, or biotherapy. In advanced cancer, fatigue is rated as moderate to severe in 60 percent to 80 percent of cases.

Few studies (Dean et al. 1995; Rhodes et al. 1988; Camarillo 1991) have been conducted that describe patients' experiences with fatigue and its impact on quality of life (QOL). These studies focus on the lack of knowledge about fatigue and its relationship to other symptoms, energy levels, livelihood, relationships, roles, and leisure activities. This lack of knowledge stems from the complex nature of fatigue and its occurrence in both healthy and ill populations. There is no agreement in the literature on the definition of fatigue, its causes, indicators, effects, or remedies. To date, a precise definition and means of valid and reliable measurement are lacking.

Although studies demonstrate that fatigue is a significant problem in and of itself, other aspects of the patient's life, such as sleep, pain, and the ability to socialize and carry on daily activities, are affected (Grond et al. 1994; Donnelly and Walsh 1995; Ferrell et al. 1996). In addition, the multidimensional nature of fatigue adds complexity to clinical assessment.

This project was supported by an Oncology Nursing Foundation Grant titled "Quality of Life and Fatigue: A Multicultural Approach."

Disease-related factors such as stage, co-morbid conditions, symptoms, anemia or infection, overall physical condition, age, and gender can also influence the fatigue experience.

Grant and colleagues (1998) have proposed a definition of cancer-related fatigue as:

> A subjective perception and/or experience related to disease or treatment [which] . . . is multidimensional, is not easily relieved by rest, and has a profound impact on the dimensions of QOL including physical, psychological, social, and spiritual well-being. This fatigue is influenced by the cultural context of the individual and is associated with a reduced capacity to carry out expected or required daily activities.

PATHOPHYSIOLOGY

Physiologists view fatigue as a safety mechanism to prevent changes in metabolism that could result in irreversible damage to muscles and even to other organs such as the brain. However, just as with other safety mechanisms, if there is a malfunction, normal processes can become pathological.

Examples of models to explain the cause of fatigue have been developed predominantly by muscle physiologists (Table 8C–1). The *central-peripheral model* suggests an integration between central and peripheral mechanisms that lead to fatigue (Gandevia et al. 1995). At the peripheral nervous system (PNS) level, a decline in intracellular calcium in peripheral nerves, for example, leads to the failure to maintain required or expected muscle force leading to reduced performance. The chemoreceptors in fatigued muscles send sensory impulses back to the reticular formation in the central nervous system (CNS). These impulses can inhibit motor pathways anywhere from the voluntary centers in the brain to the spinal motor neurons.

Another model designed to explain the pathophysiology of fatigue is the *accumulation-depletion model* (Aisters 1987). The accumulation mechanism involves a buildup of waste products (e.g., undue accumulation of lactate or by-products of cell death) that interfere with normal cellular functioning. Anemia, a deficiency of red blood cells or lack of hemoglobin that leads to a reduction in the oxygen carrying capacity of the blood, is an illustration of the depletion mechanism.

The *cellular nutrition model* suggests that there are at least five metabolic causes of fatigue (Newsholme et al. 1992). One in particular, proton accumulation, could be an important factor in patients who are physically inactive for prolonged periods. In these patients, the aerobic capacity markedly decreases so that ATP must be synthesized by the much less efficient anaerobic system.

8c

Table 8C–1
Pathophysiology of Fatigue

I. Central-Peripheral Model

A. Impairment at the brain/psyche level
  1. Lack of motivation
  2. Impaired recruitment of motor neurons
  3. Inhibition of voluntary effort
  4. Malfunction of nerve cells
  5. Increase in branched chain amino acids ratio resulting in increased synthesis of 5-HT, a central neurotransmitter
  6. Increased levels of brain ammonia (NH_3) that can occur during skeletal muscle exercise
B. Impairment at the neuromuscular junction
  1. Impaired peripheral nerve function
  2. Impaired neuromuscular junction transmission
  3. Impaired fiber activation

II. Accumulation or Depletion Model

A. Accumulation of certain metabolites (lactic acid, pyruvic acid) that results in acidosis which causes fatigue by reducing enzyme activity
B. Depletion of energy substrates (i.e., nutrition/oxygen)

III. Cellular Nutrition Model

A. Depletion of the phosphocreatine concentration in muscle
B. Accumulation of protons in muscle
C. Depletion of glucogen in muscle
D. Decrease in the blood glucose concentration
E. Increase in plasma concentration ratio of free tryptophan to branched-chain amino acids

---

Whether fatigue is the result of a central neuroendocrine mechanism or caused by the interaction of several factors is not clear. What is clear is that fatigue is not simply a physical symptom or physiological event, but rather a multicausal, multidimensional phenomenon that demands further study.

A useful way to examine fatigue is to evaluate its impact on QOL. The following discussion summarizes the impact of fatigue using a model that identifies four domains of well being that comprise QOL, proposed by Ferrell (1996) (Table 8C–2).

Physical Well-Being

Physical well-being is defined as the control or relief of symptoms and the maintenance of function and independence. Decline in physical function or ability to engage in a variety of day-to-day activities are common indicators of fatigue. Decreased functional status has been identified as a predictor of diminished QOL (Buccheri et al. 1995; Bergman et al.

Table 8C-2
The Impact of Fatigue on Quality of Life

I. Physical Well-Being

A. Decreased level of energy
B. Inability to perform usual/previous activities
C. Inability to be useful/active
D. Inability to exercise
E. Negative impact on work/employment
F. Negative impact on leisure
G. Interference with ordinary tasks/household tasks
H. Impaired mobility
I. Life focused on decreased function
J. Increased demands for sleep
K. Interaction of fatigue with other symptoms such as pain

II. Psychological Well-Being

A. Negative impact on happiness
B. Insufficient energy for a balanced life
C. Interruption in life satisfaction
D. Interaction of the physical and psychological effects of fatigue
E. Indication of time limitations
F. Lack of appreciation by others of impact on well-being
G. Feelings of uselessness
H. Difficulty coping
I. Depression
J. Anxiety/frustration
K. All consuming nature of fatigue

III. Social Well-Being

A. Limitation in social activities
B. Interruption in family roles
C. Impact on sexuality
D. Demanding effect on spouse/marriage
E. Decreased participation in activities which define "being alive"
F. Increased dependence
G. Difficulty maintaining a sense of normalcy

IV. Spiritual Well-Being

A. Change in spirituality/priorities
B. Limitation in meaningful activity
C. Creation of hopelessness
D. Increased meaning/appreciation for life
E. Impact on all domains of QOL

1994; Hollen et al. 1994). Functional limitations have been linked with increased psychological distress for patients and their caregivers (Given et al. 1994). Many of the limitations in day-to-day activities could be due to decreased energy from disease and the side effects of treatment. Fatigue, and therefore continued limitations in function, can continue even after disease is in remission and treatment has ended.

Changes in activity level can include (1) limitations in day-to-day activities, (2) difficulties in accomplishing normal activities, and (3) decreased satisfaction with the ability to participate in the activity and the quality of that participation. Patient perceptions can be influenced by concomitant symptoms such as pain, dyspnea, nausea, and insomnia. Change in function can vary widely, depending on the baseline activity level of the person as well as upon environmental, social, and gender related demands. For example, limitations in household chores was identified as one of the most prevalent disruptions of fatigue in a study of women with lung cancer (Sarna et al. 1993).

Psychological Well-Being

Psychological well-being is determined by a sense of control in a life-threatening illness characterized by emotional distress, altered life priorities, and fears of the unknown as well as positive changes in life.

Fatigue affects mental, emotional, and physical activity and influences psychological well-being. The inability to focus attention or to meet activity expectations causes stress that adversely affects psychological well-being. Prolonged physical and mental stress is a principal cause of fatigue, which in turn influences perceived psychological well-being.

Studies link attributes of psychological well-being such as anxiety, depression, and attention to fatigue (Christensen et al. 1992; Pickard-Holley 1991; Oberst and James 1985). Irvine and colleagues report that mood and perceived symptom distress are strongly associated with fatigue. A study by da Silva (1993) provides evidence of a strong relationship between fatigue and psychological well-being as measured by feelings of tension, irritability, worry, and depression in men with prostate cancer.

Social Well-Being

Social well-being is defined as a way to view not only the cancer or its symptoms, but also the person surrounding the tumor; it is the means by which we recognize persons with cancer, their roles, and relationships. Studies reveal the strong impact of fatigue on roles and relationships and on the family caregivers (Irving et al. 1994). In a study of family caregivers of cancer patients, Jensen and Given (1993) document a positive relationship between the hours of daily care provided by the caregiver and severity of fatigue experienced by the patient. In addition, 53 percent of caregivers in this study report their own fatigue as being moderate or severe.

Studies have examined demographic characteristics of the patient or the family caregiver in relation to fatigue. Similar to other symptoms in cancer, age is generally negatively associated with fatigue, indicating that older patients could experience or report less severe fatigue (Pickard-Holley 1991; Bloom et al. 1990). The association of age and fatigue might be due in part to fewer daily activity demands, expectations of aging, and social beliefs about reporting symptoms.

Camarillo (1991) uses case studies to describe perceptual meanings of fatigue experienced during chemotherapy. Fatigue is viewed as a negative experience that influences normal physical and social activities. Camarillo concludes that fatigue often disrupts the patient's ability and desire to accomplish desired role functioning, ultimately diminishing QOL.

In a study conducted on the experience of fatigue during treatment with alpha interferon, Dean (1995) asked patients about their perceptions of the causes, descriptions, and remedies for fatigue. Results support the belief that fatigue interferes with the ability to work or engage in enjoyable activities. Fatigue also interferes with sexual activity and intimacy. Cancer patients have reported that fatigue experienced during cancer treatment intensifies the stress on the marital relationship and greatly diminishes sexual activities.

Many patients describe having to reprioritize activities as a result of diminished energy to save energy for only the most essential. For example, family members and relationships become the focus of their limited time and energy.

Spiritual Well-Being

Spiritual well-being is defined as the ability to maintain hope and derive meaning from the cancer experience characterized by uncertainty. Spiritual well-being involves issues of transcendence and is enhanced by one's religion and other sources of spiritual support. Spiritual well-being has been described as including aspects of hope, transcendence beyond life, and meaning derived from illness experiences (Ferrell and Dean 1995). In the study of cancer survivors described previously, subjects were able to describe the existential impact of fatigue in terms such as how this symptom made them feel "mortal." Some reported feeling abandoned by their bodies because of overwhelming fatigue. Others were able to report positive coping by seeking meaning through the contemplation and quiet time imposed by the fatigue. Fatigue also heightened feelings of uncertainty or hopelessness. A powerful emotion expressed was that fatigue wastes time, and time is precious.

The area of spirituality in oncology has received greater attention in recent years. This field of inquiry has extended beyond aspects of religiosity to include aspects such as deriving meaning from the illness and the existential aspect of cancer survivorship. Studies have explored fatigue as a symptom that embodies significant meaning to patients, depending on its cause, timing, and severity. Fatigue can also be seen as a sign of worsening illness, and thus may be a reminder of death (Glaus 1996).

Table 8C–2 summarizes the impact of fatigue on all domains of QOL. In physical well-being, fatigue has a significant effect on function, work at home, and the employment setting. The areas of psychological well-being influenced by fatigue include happiness, coping, life satisfaction, and symptoms such as anxiety or depression. Patients describe the frustration of wanting to do more when confronted with life-threatening illness yet being able to do much less. The areas of social well-being cited by patients include aspects of family life, dependence, and sexuality.

Research provides insightful descriptions of the influence of fatigue on aspects of spiritual well-being such as hopelessness, altered priorities, and a change in appreciation for life. Patients describe feeling that fatigue wastes precious time, and that having cancer is a time "when life is in high speed, but you are in slow motion."

CLINICAL ASSESSMENT OF FATIGUE

Conceptual models developed by Piper and Winningham are commonly used to guide fatigue research and are valuable for use in the clinical assessment of fatigue. Assessment of fatigue requires collection of subjective information to evaluate the impact of this symptom on the person's QOL. The Piper Fatigue Scale (PFS) measures fatigue in four dimensions: cognitive/mood, behavioral/severity, affective meaning, and sensory. Within these dimensions, the PFS measures perception, performance, motivation, and change in mental and physical activities. The PFS is limited

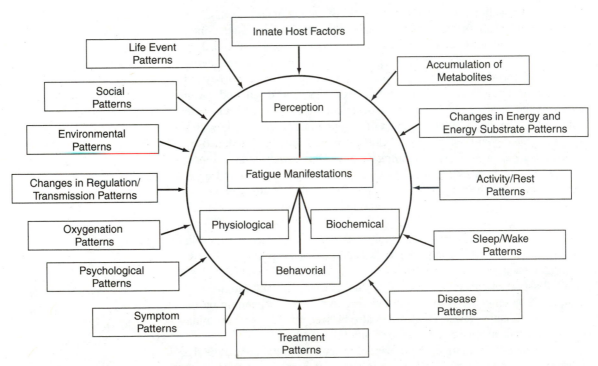

Figure 8C-1. Piper's Integrated Fatigue Model

Reprinted with permission from Piper, Lindsey, and Dodd. Fatigue Mechanisms in Cancer Patients: Developing Nursing Theory. Oncology Nursing Forum 14(6): 17–22. 1987.

to subjective data; thus, alteration in neuromuscular/metabolic processes is not measured.

Piper's Integrated Fatigue Model (Figure 8C–1) is used to define fatigue, its etiologic factors (causes or correlates), its manifestations or indicators, and its effects. Winningham's Psychobiologic Entropy Model (Figure 8C–2) provides the basis for exploring the potential interaction between fatigue and its etiologic factors and whether this interaction exacerbates each, leading to a spiraling increase in fatigue. Symptoms such as pain and depression lead to fatigue, which in turn causes further pain and depression, which then further exacerbates fatigue.

Table 8C–3 includes a summary of the synonyms used for fatigue by patients derived from several studies (Ferrell 1996). Table 8C–4 provides a

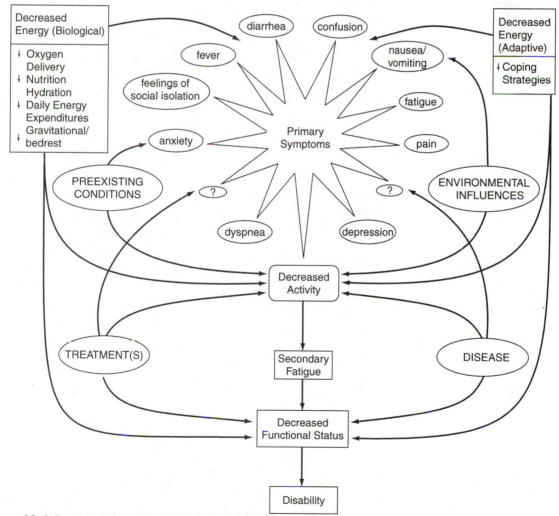

Figure 8C–2. The Winningham Psychobiologic-Entropy Model
Reprinted with permission. © 1998 by Maryl L. Winningham.

Table 8C–3
Patient Terms Related to Fatigue

Ability to function well	No ambition
Annoyed	No enthusiasm
At the end of my rope	Not able to do what I used to
Bone tired	Out of energy
Burnout	Physical strength
Can't keep up	Priorities changed
Collapsed	Rubber knees
Consumes all trains of thought	Run down
Disoriented	Saddened me
Drugged	Sense of urgency
Exhaustion	Sleepy
Extreme stress	Slowed me down
Fatigue wave	Three and a half cylinders instead of four
Feel vulnerable/mortal	Tire(d)
Grumpy	Wastes time
Hit the wall	Weak
I was a lump	Weary
Irritable	Wet cement
Lack of stamina	Wiped me out
Laziness	Wreck, apathetic
Less mobile	

Table 8C–4
Adjectives Related to Fatigue

Angry	Grateful
Anxious	Guilty
Cautious	Healing
Chronic	Humbling
Debilitating	Isolating
Dependency	Mortal
Depression	Nervous
Devastating	Overwhelming
Difficult	Painful
Difficult to accept	Restrictive
Difficulty concentrating	Sadly tolerated
Distressing	Selfish
Dysfunctional	Severe
Egocentric	Stressful
Exhausting	Stupid
Extreme	Transient
Feel terrible	Uncomfortable
Feel bad	Unproductive
Feel less adequate	Useless
Forgetful	Time-wasting
Frightened	Weakest
Frustrating	Worrisome

list of adjectives these patients used to describe their fatigue. These words provide insight to the meaning of fatigue and to the impact of fatigue on QOL.

While the patient's perception of fatigue is central to assessment, there are many physiologic components of fatigue. Objective biochemical or instrumental (e.g., muscle strength, activity monitor) indicators of cancer-related fatigue need to be identified. To date, no biological fatigue markers have been identified, although physiological parameters such as hemoglobin and hematocrit levels are thought to be important indicators.

MEDICAL MANAGEMENT

Medical management of fatigue involves a history, complete physical examination, and psychological assessment. When an etiology is determined, such as anemia, infection, or depression, treatment of the underlying condition is indicated (see also Chapters 7 and 10A). Treatment can include red blood cell transfusions, use of the growth factor erythropoietin, systemic antibiotics, or an antidepressant. When the source of fatigue cannot be determined, there is often a belief that nothing can be done, and the common treatment approach is to advise rest and wait for improvement.

Health care providers view fatigue as a common symptom of cancer and as a common side effect of treatment. Evaluation of the symptom is often conducted only when patients volunteer complaints of fatigue. Patients who are persistent with their complaints might persuade their health care provider to conduct laboratory evaluations of their nutritional status, electrolytes, and oxygenation status. If an abnormality is detected, intervention to correct any imbalance or deficiency is recommended. More often, there is no obvious or treatable cause for cancer-related fatigue. Many patients will experience fatigue as a chronic problem, and care is directed toward supportive measures that ameliorate the impact of fatigue on QOL.

NURSING MANAGEMENT

To date, several nursing interventions have been tested in cancer populations. Johnson and colleagues (1988) evaluated the effect of providing objective descriptions of common patient experiences during radiation therapy to new patients in an effort to reduce reported fatigue. The intervention group reported significantly less disruption in usual activities during and after radiation therapy compared to a control group. By simply informing patients what to expect during radiation therapy, these researchers were able to reduce the amount of fatigue their patients experienced (see also Chapter 6A).

Cimprich (1992) examined mental fatigue (inability to direct attention) in postoperative patients with breast cancer. Patients were instructed to se-

Table 8C–5
Nursing Management of Cancer-Related Fatigue

Problem	Intervention	Rationale

Lack of information: Fatigue (Chapter 6A)	Explain complex nature of fatigue and importance of communication with health care professionals
	Explain causes of treatment-related fatigue
	  Fatigue can increase during treatment
	  Cancer cells can compete with body for essential nutrients
	  Treatments, infection, fever increase body's need for energy
	  Worry or anxiety can cause fatigue as well as depression, sadness, or tension
	  Changes in daily schedules, new routines, or interrupted sleep schedules contribute to the development of fatigue
	Prepare patients for diagnostic and treatment-related procedures
		Preparatory sensory information reduces anxiety and fatigue

Disrupted rest/sleep patterns (Chapter 8B)	Establish or continue regular bedtime and awakening Obtain sufficient, not excessive, amount of sleep Brief rest periods or naps during the day, if needed; do not interfere with nighttime sleep	Curtailing time in bed helps patient feel refreshed and avoids fragmented sleep; strengthens circadian rhythms
Deficient nutritional status (Chapter 9)	Monitor weight to avoid significant weight loss Recommend nutritious, high protein meals Suggest more small, frequent meals Use protein supplements to augment diet Encourage adequate intake of fluids Recommend 8–10 glasses of water/day unless medically contraindicated	Food will help energy levels; less energy is needed for digestion with small frequent meals

Symptom management (Chapters 9, 12)	Control other symptoms (nausea, vomiting, pain, diarrhea, constipation)	Managing other symptoms requires energy; other symptoms might interfere with restful sleep
Distraction/ restoration	Encourage activities to restore energy: Spending time in the natural environment Gardening Listening to music Meditating, praying Engaging in hobbies Spending time with family and friends	Pleasant activities might reduce/ relieve mental (attentional) fatigue
Decreased energy	Plan activities: Utilize optimal times of the day Save energy for most important events Delegate responsibilities for household chores and child care as needed Learn to listen to the body; if fatigued, rest	Energy conservation helps to reduce burden and efficiently use energy available
Physical limitations	Engage in an individually tailored exercise program approved by the health care team Enjoy leisure activities (e.g., walking, golf, bicycling, swimming)	Exercise reduces the deleterious effects of immobility and deconditioning

lect activities that restore directed attention for 20 minutes at least three times per week. These activities involved sitting in a park or tending to flowers or plants (primarily spending time in the natural environment). Patients randomized to the treatment group had increased attentional capacity and function compared with the randomized control group. Activities that involved creative aspects of life tended to restore energy in this study.

Winningham (1992) demonstrated an increase in functional capacity and reduction in fatigue through the use of aerobic training in a select group of patients receiving chemotherapy for breast cancer compared to nonexercising control patients. Similarly, Mock and colleagues (1997) recently reported the results of a walking exercise program conducted with women receiving radiation therapy for breast cancer. The exercise group scored significantly higher than the control group on physical functioning and reported less fatigue, anxiety, and difficulty sleeping.

Patients have learned to accept fatigue as a companion of illness, and are reluctant to mention it unless they are asked. When patients do voluntarily complain of fatigue, it is either very prominent or interfering with an important aspect of their lives. The health care team needs to provide patients with cancer-related fatigue an environment that is receptive to their symptomatic complaints. Patients also need to be assured that their symptoms are taken seriously and that interventions to help relieve their fatigue will be offered.

Currently, interventions that are the mainstay of nursing management for cancer-related fatigue are based on individual nursing preference. Table 8C–5 incorporates research-based interventions with those commonly used to help patients prevent, alleviate, or combat fatigue.

Identifying barriers to effective assessment of fatigue is of paramount importance. Because fatigue is not perceived as life threatening, patients as well as clinicians often believe that little can be done to resolve it, and proper assessment and possible treatment is ignored. Research and clinical experience demonstrates that patients need to express and define the impact of symptoms on their overall QOL, by talking about their experiences. Documenting fatigue and its presence, intensity, and impact will enable clinicians to validate patients' concerns and bring fatigue to the attention of the entire health care team.

BIBLIOGRAPHY

1. Aisters, J. Fatigue in the cancer patient: A conceptual approach to a clinical problem. *Oncology Nursing Forum* 14(6): 25–30. 1997.

   An overview of fatigue in the cancer patient is presented, including discussions on definition, mechanism, assessment, intervention, and implications for future research.

2. Bergman, B., N. K. Aaronson, S. Ahmedzai, S. Kaasa, and M. Sullivan for the EORTC Study Group on Quality of Life. The EORTC QLQ-LC12: a modular

supplement to the EORTC core quality of life questionnaire (ALA-C#) for use in lung cancer clinical trials. *European Journal of Cancer* 30A: 635–642. 1994.

This is a report on the evaluation of the EORTC Quality of Life Questionnaire, covering general aspects of health-related QOL and additional disease- or treatment-specific questionnaire modules in 883 patients before and during treatment.

3. Bloom, J. R., R. D. Gorsky, P. Fobair, R. Hoppe, R. S. Cox, A. Varghese, and D. Spiegel. Physical performance at work and at leisure; validation of a measure of biological energy in survivors of Hodgkin's disease. *Journal of Psychosocial Oncology.* 1: 49–63. 1990.

This article examines the concurrent validity of a measure of use of biological energy. The measure consists of the individual activity patterns at work and at leisure and is weighted by a factor associated with the expenditure of biological energy.

4. Buccheri, G. F., D. Ferrigno, M. Tamburini, and C. Brunelli. The patient's perception of his own quality of life might have an adjunctive prognostic significance in lung cancer. *Lung Cancer* 12: 45–58. 1995.

This study analyzes 11 items of the Therapy Impact Questionnaire, assessing both disease and therapy impact on physical condition, functional status, concomitant emotional and cognitive factors and social interactions and how they are associated with prognosis.

5. Camarillo, M. A. The oncology patient's experience of fatigue. In M. Whedon, ed., *Quality of Life A Nursing Challenge.* 39–44. Meniscus Ltd., Philadelphia 1991.

Case studies on cancer patients undergoing chemotherapy provide the patient's perspective on the experience of fatigue.

6. Christensen, T., N. Hjorts, E. Mortensen, M. Riis-Hansen, and H. Kehlet. Fatigue and anxiety in surgical patients. *British Journal of Surgery* 72: 63–65. 1992.

This article presents a prospective study measuring fatigue and anxiety in non-cancer patients undergoing abdominal surgery.

7. Cimprich, B. Attentional fatigue following breast cancer surgery. *Research in Nursing & Health* 15: 199–207. 1992.

This study evaluates the effect of exposure to a natural environment on attentional fatigue resulting from surgery for breast cancer.

8. Da Silva, F. C. Quality of life in prostatic cancer patients. *Cancer* 72(12 Suppl.): 3803–3806. 1993.

This study describes a first effort to introduce a quality of life assessment in prostate cancer clinical trials.

9. Dean, G. E., L. Spears, B. R. Ferrell, W. Q Y. Quan Jr, S. Groshen, and M. S. Mitchell. Fatigue in patients with cancer receiving interferon alpha. *Cancer Practice* 3(3): 164–172. 1995.

This article describes the experience of fatigue over time in patients with malignant melanoma receiving treatment with interferon alpha.

10. Donnelly, S., and D. Walsh. The symptoms of advanced cancer. *Seminars in Oncology* 22(2 Suppl. 3): 67–72. 1995.

The authors describe a prospective study of symptom prevalence and severity in 1,000 patients with advanced cancer.

11. Epstein, K. R. The chronically fatigued patient. *Medical Clinics of North America* 79(2): 315–327. 1995.

    An overview of the diagnosis and management of the patient presenting with chronic fatigue is provided.

12. Ferrell, B. R. The quality of lives: 1,525 voices of cancer. *Oncology Nursing Forum* 23(6): 907–916. 1996.

    The author presents a review and synthesis of 25 studies involved in quality of life research in different cancer diagnoses that include: pain, bone marrow transplantation, cancer survivors, breast, thyroid and ovarian.

13. Ferrell, B. R., and G. Dean. The meaning of cancer pain. *Seminars in Oncology Nursing* 11(1): 17–21. 1995.

    This article presents a review of the literature on the meaning of pain and provides case examples and analysis of the search for meaning in cancer pain.

14. Ferrell, B., M. Grant, G. E. Dean, B. Funk, and J. Ly. "Bone tired": The experience of fatigue and impact on quality of life. *Oncology Nursing Forum* 23(10): 1539–1547. 1996.

    This article describes the impact of fatigue on the quality of life of cancer survivors, and patients under treatment for breast, ovarian, and thyroid cancer.

15. Gandevia, S. C., G. M. Allen, and D. K. McKenzie. Central fatigue: Critical issues, quantification and practical implications. In *Fatigue*. S.C. Gandevia, ed. 281–294. Plenum Press, New York. 1995.

    This chapter describes proposed physiological mechanisms that contribute to the development of central fatigue.

16. Given, C. W., B. A. Given, and Stommel. The impact of age, treatment, and symptoms on the physical and mental health of cancer patients. *Cancer* 74, 2128–2138. 1994.

    To describe continuing care and rehabilitation needs of cancer patients, a longitudinal design was performed among patients 50 years of age and older with solid tumors.

17. Glaus, A., R. Crow, and S. Hammond. A qualitative study to explore the concept of fatigue in cancer patients and in healthy individuals. *Support Care Cancer* 4: 82–96. 1996.

    The authors present a qualitative study that explores fatigue in cancer patients inductively and compares experiences of fatigue and tiredness with those of healthy individuals to identify cancer-specific fatigue and related concepts.

18. Grant, M., P. Anderson, M. Ashley, G. Dean, B. Ferrell, M. Kagawa-Singer, G. Padilla, M. Bradshaw-Robinson, and L. Sarna. Fatigue and quality of life: A multicultural approach. *Oncology Nursing Forum*. 1998.

    This paper describes the process of developing a multi-institutional, multicultural team of investigators with the common goal of studying fatigue and quality of life.

19. Grond, S., D. Zech, C. Diefenbach, and A. Bischoff. Prevalence and pattern of symptoms in patients with cancer: A prospective evaluation of 1635 cancer patients referred to a pain clinic. *Journal of Pain and Symptom Management* 9(6): 372–382. 1994.

This study examines the prevalence of 15 physical symptoms and symptom groups in 1,635 patients with cancer referred to a pain clinic.

20. Hollen, P.J., R. J. Gralla, M. G. Kris, and C. Cox. Quality of life during clinical trials: Conceptual model of the Lung Cancer Symptom Scale (LCSS). *Supportive Care in Cancer* 2: 213–222. 1994.

This is a presentation of a conceptual model of the Lung Cancer Symptom Scale following the evaluation of the tool in several studies.

21. Irvine, D. M., L. Vincent, J. E. Graydon, N. Bubela, and L. Thompson. The prevalence and correlates of fatigue in patients receiving treatment with chemotherapy and radiotherapy. *Cancer Nursing* 17(5): 367–378. 1994.

This study investigates the prevalence of fatigue among patients receiving treatment with radiation therapy and chemotherapy over two measurement points and compares them with a healthy control group.

22. Johnson, J. E., L. M. Nail, D. Lauver, K. D. King, and H. Keys. Reducing the negative impact of radiation therapy on functional status. *Cancer* 61: 46–51. 1988.

This study evaluates a cognitive intervention of preparing patients with prostate cancer for the experience of radiation therapy to improve functional status.

23. Mock, V., K. Hassey Dow, C. J. Meares, P. M. Grimm, J. A. Dienemann, M. E. Haisfeld-Wolfe, W. Quitasol, S. Mitchell, A. Chakravarthy, and I. Gage. Effects of exercise on fatigue, physical functioning, and emotional distress during radiation therapy for breast cancer. *Oncology Nursing Forum* 24(6): 991–1000. 1997.

This study tests the hypothesis that women participating in a walking exercise program during radiation treatment for breast cancer would demonstrate increased levels of physical functioning and decreased levels of symptom intensity than women who did not participate in the exercise program.

24. Newsholme, E. A., E. Blomstrand, and B. Ekblom. Physical and mental fatigue: Metabolic mechanisms and importance of plasma amino acids. *British Medical Bulletin* 48(3): 477–495. 1992.

This article describes the five metabolic causes of fatigue: a decrease in phosphocreatine, proton accumulation in muscle, depletion of glycogen stores in muscle, hypoglycemia, and an increase in plasma concentration of free tryptophan.

25. Oberst, M., and R. James. Going home: Patient and spouse adjustment following cancer surgery. *Topics in Clinical Nursing* 7(1): 46–56. 1985.

This exploratory study describes the psychological adjustments patients with urogenital cancers and their spouses make after discharge from the hospital.

26. Pickard-Holley, S. Fatigue in cancer patients: A descriptive study. *Cancer Nursing* 14(1): 13–19. 1991.

This study examines the relationships between fatigue and various physical and psychological factors in women undergoing chemotherapy for ovarian cancer.

27. Piper, B. F., S. L. Dibble, and M. J. Dodd. The revised Piper Fatigue Scale: Confirmation of its multidimensionality and reduction in number of items in women with breast cancer. *Oncology Nursing Forum* 23(2): 352. 1996.

This is an abstract that describes the psychometric evaluation of the revised 22-item Piper Fatigue Scale in women with breast cancer.

28. Rhodes, V. A., P. M. Watson, and B. M. Hanson. Patients' descriptions of the influence of tiredness and weakness on self-care abilities. *Cancer Nursing* 11(3): 186–194. 1988.

This study examines the relationship between self-reported symptoms and self-care ability perceived by patients undergoing chemotherapy.

29. Sarna, L., A. M. Lindsey, H. Dean, M. L. Brecht, and R. McCorkle. Weight change and lung cancer: Relationships with symptom distress, functional status, and smoking. *Research in Nursing & Health* 17: 371–379. 1993.

An evaluation of the influence of several factors (symptoms, smoking and functional status) on the disease prognosis and weight loss in patients with lung cancer is presented.

30. Winningham, M. L. How exercise mitigates fatigue: Implications for people receiving cancer therapy. In *The Biotherapy of Cancer*. R. M. Johnson, ed. 16–21. Oncology Nursing Press, Pittsburgh. 1992.

This chapter describes the concept of energetics (Psychobiologic-Entropy Hypothesis=PEH) and how it relates to patients with cancer. The PEH theory defines fatigue as energy deficit.

Nutrition

Mary E. Ropka

INTRODUCTION

Diet, nutrition, and cancer are related in at least three ways. Nutrition, specifically the diet we consume, is being investigated as a factor in causing some cancers. In addition, cancer and its treatment affects the nutritional status of the patient. Evidence suggests that nutritional status is related to morbidity, mortality, and response to treatment, thus influencing both the quality and quantity of life. Finally, nutrition is used as an adjunct modality during cancer treatment, especially in the perioperative period.

This chapter reviews the framework of normal physiology related to nutrition; the pathophysiology of nutritional deficiencies and the consequences of cancer, both disease-related and treatment-related; nutritional assessment; and nursing management of nutritional problems occurring in cancer patients.

PHYSIOLOGY

The ultimate goal of the nutritional processes is to supply the body with fluids, electrolytes, and nutrients in quantities sufficient to meet individual requirements. Various parts of the gastrointestinal (GI) tract (Figure 9–1) are structured and adapted for specific functions, including (1) intake and transportation of food between areas; (2) storage of food in different stages of digestion; (3) digestion of food, including the secretion of digestive juices; and (4) absorption of fluids and nutrients during the various stages of the digestive process. The GI system (stomach and intestines, especially the small intestine) breaks down complex carbohydrates, protein, and fats into materials that are absorbable. Minerals, fluids, vitamins, and nonessential nutrients are also digested. Following digestion, absorption occurs mainly in the small intestine. The absorbed nutrients then enter the circulation in a variety of ways. Fat-soluble nutrients enter the lacteal or lymphatic system and empty into the systemic blood circulation at the thoracic duct. Other nutrients enter the hepatic portal vein, pass through the liver, and eventually enter the blood stream.

9

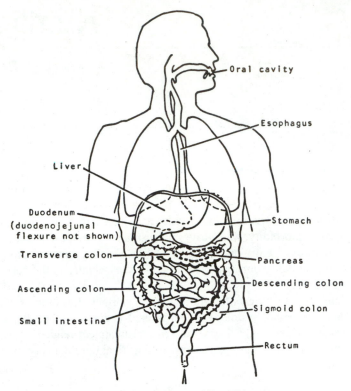

Figure 9-1. Anatomy of the GI tract.

Ingestion

Ingestion of food and fluids involves appetite, hunger, mastication, and deglutition (or swallowing). Intake of food is regulated by the body's stores of nutrients, as well as by the effects of eating on the digestive tract. Ingestion is a complicated process with many interrelated psychological and physiological factors.

The desire for specific types of food, rather than food in general (hunger), is determined by appetite. Although appetite is controlled in cortical areas of the brain higher than the hypothalamus, it is still closely connected to hypothalamic functioning. Food intake should ideally match caloric expenditure and nutrient needs.

Defined as the intrinsic desire for food resulting from the basic need for energy, hunger is the primary mechanism for control of food intake. It is currently believed that the lateral nuclei of the hypothalamus contain *the feeding center*, whose stimulation is related to nutritional status and is involved in the awareness of hunger and desire for food. The *satiety center*, thought to be located in the ventromedial nucleus of the hypothalamus, inhibits the feeding center, which is continually activated, resulting in a decreased desire for food. The brainstem controls the actual mechanism of eating, such as chewing and swallowing. The cortical regions of the limbic system are also involved in feeding and preference for food.

Chewing breaks large food particles into smaller particles so that they can pass through the entire GI tract without damaging it, particularly the mucosa. Food is mixed with oral secretions, which provide limited initial digestive activities and moisten the food particles for easier movement. Chewing is especially important for most fruits and raw vegetables because it increases the total surface area of the food exposed to digestive intestinal secretions.

Swallowing is a complex act that involves three stages: oral, pharyngeal, and esophageal. During the oral stage of swallowing, which is the only stage under voluntary control, the contents of the mouth are moved to the back of the pharynx, where the swallowing reflex is initiated. The pharyngeal stage, which is involuntary, involves moving food from the pharynx to the upper esophagus. The glottis closes during this time and respirations are inhibited through the medulla in order to prevent aspiration. During the esophageal phase (also involuntary), food travels through the esophagus to the stomach by primary and secondary peristalsis. Relaxation of the lower esophageal sphincter allows food to pass into the stomach and prevents reflux of gastric contents into the esophagus.

Digestion and Absorption

Digestion involves mechanical and chemical processes in the GI tract that break food down into particles of a size and chemical composition that the body can absorb. Secretions from specialized cells and the motility of the GI tract are involved in the process of digestion. Absorption by special cells transfers the digested nutrients into the body fluids. The nutrients are then transported to tissues for storage, further processing, or utilization. Most absorption occurs in the small intestine. Nutrients are stored, further metabolized for energy or excretion (catabolism), or synthesized to form new materials for cellular growth, maintenance, or repair (anabolism), when they are within the body's cells. Each nutrient, including the three major nutrients—protein, fat, and carbohydrates—requires different metabolic processes.

Food is chewed and prepared for swallowing in the mouth, assisted by the saliva, which is secreted in amounts of 1,000–1,500 ml daily. Saliva contains ptyalin, an enzyme that aids in starch digestion; mucin, which lubricates; and large amounts of water and small amounts of sodium, chloride, and bicarbonate (HCO_3^-). Excessive loss of saliva (xerostomia) can result in dental caries and mouth sores or make it difficult to swallow or chew because saliva provides moisture and lubrication.

Food moves through the esophagus from the oropharynx to the stomach by primary and secondary peristalsis. Primary peristalsis originates from the pharynx and moves toward the stomach during the pharyngeal stage of swallowing. If food remains in the esophagus, secondary peristalsis arises from the esophagus itself under vagal control. Mucus is secreted by glands along the length of the esophagus to provide lubrication for swallowing.

The stomach consists of four anatomic parts: the cardia, the fundus, the body, and the antrum. The fundus is functionally part of the body of the stomach. In the stomach, food is chopped and mixed into chyme by constrictor waves, or weak peristaltic waves, which move the chyme distally from the antrum toward the pylorus. This partially digested food is stored in the stomach until it moves along into the duodenum. Stronger peristaltic waves move the chyme into the duodenum when the pyloric valve relaxes.

Nervous control of the stomach occurs through the autonomic and intrinsic nervous systems. Gastric secretion mechanisms are stimulated by the vagus nerve and by food in the stomach. They are inhibited by the enterogastric reflex, which is initiated in the duodenum by the presence of food in the small intestine, and by hormones released by the small intestine—especially cholecystokinin and secretin.

Four major types of secretory cells, found in the mucosa of the fundus and greater curvature of the stomach, provide secretions that compose the 1,000–3,000 ml of gastric juice produced daily: (1) chief cells that secrete pepsinogen; (2) parietal cells that secrete hydrochloric acid and intrinsic factor; (3) mucus-producing cells; and (4) gastrin-producing G cells. Electrolytes—including sodium, potassium, magnesium, chloride, and bicarbonate—are produced. Gastric juice also contains small quantities of enzymes, including gastric lipase, gastric urea, lysozyme, carbonic anhydrase, gelatinase, and gastric amylase. Little absorption occurs in the stomach (only lipid-soluble substances) because of the absence of an absorptive membrane.

Motility of the three segments of the small intestine—the duodenum, jejunum, and ileum—consists of mixing contractions and propulsive contractions. Mixing contractions, or segmentation, are local contractions of small segments of the wall of the gut that chop chyme and help move food forward slightly. Propulsive contractions, or peristalsis, move chyme toward the ileocecal valve and spread chyme along the intestinal mucosa. Distension is the usual stimulus for this contractile ring of peristalsis to arise. Effective peristalsis requires a functional myenteric nerve plexus to operate, and its intensity and velocity are altered by parasympathetic stimulation. Villi, which are finger-like folds of the mucosa that greatly increase the absorptive surface of the small intestine, contract to increase absorption further. The ileocecal valve, located between the small intestine and proximal large intestine, prevents the reflux of fecal contents of the colon and controls emptying of the small intestine.

In addition to its absorptive functions, the small intestine secretes about 2,000 ml per day of almost pure extracellular fluid from the crypts of

Lieberkuhn, which are located in the grooves between the villi on the entire surface of the small intestine, except where Brunner's glands are located. Mucus is secreted from Brunner's glands and goblet cells on the surface of the intestinal mucosa and from the crypts of Lieberkuhn. Enzymes, secreted from the brush border of the epithelium to aid breakdown of nutrients, include sucrase, maltase, isomaltase, and lactase. In addition, cholecystokinin (CCK) is secreted and absorbed into the bloodstream, where it stimulates the gall bladder and pancreas.

The specialized anatomy of the small intestine permits most GI absorption to occur here, with absorptive capacity to spare. Absorptive mechanisms include pinocytosis, diffusion, and active transport.

The large intestine, which includes the ascending, transverse, descending, and sigmoid areas of the colon, absorbs water and sodium; stores fecal material; forms vitamins K, B_{12}, thiamine, and riboflavin; and carries out some secretion. Digestive enzymes are not secreted by the large intestine. Water and electrolytes are secreted when the large intestine is irritated, such as by infection or laxatives. Large numbers of goblet cells secrete mucus to protect the mucosa from trauma, cause the feces to be self-adherent, and protect the bowel from bacteria.

Motility of the large intestine consists of mixing movements (haustrations) and propulsive movements (mass movements). Haustrations are a result of large circular constrictions and contraction of the tinea coli so that greater exposure of the mucosa for absorption and mixing occurs.

The large intestine absorbs large quantities of water and electrolytes, especially the ascending and transverse colons. All ions are absorbed. Sodium (Na^+) moves by active transport, taking chloride (Cl^-) along with it. Water is absorbed passively as a consequence of the osmotic gradient from absorption of the Na^+ and Cl^-.

Feces consist of inorganic material, undigested plant fiber, fat, bacteria, water, and protein. Its brown color is from stercobilin and urobilin (bilirubin) and can vary with the food eaten and bacterial flora of the colon.

The pancreas contains exocrine acinar cells that secrete digestive juices and endocrine cells of the islets of Langerhans that secrete hormones essential for glucose metabolism. When acid chyme from the stomach enters the duodenum, secretin is released along with CCK. Secretin stimulates the pancreas to release water and HCO_3^- from the ductal epithelium, while CCK causes the release of pancreatic enzymes from the acini. These include the proteolytic endopeptidases, trypsin and chymotrypsin; the proteolytic exopeptidases, carboxypolypeptidase and aminopeptidase; the ribonucleases, deoxyribonuclease and ribonuclease; amylase; and the lipolytic enzymes, lipase and cholesterol esterase. Bicarbonate, released to neutralize the acid chyme from the stomach when it is in the duodenum, protects the mucosa of the duodenum from damage and provides an appropriate pH for pancreatic enzyme function. Pancreatic enzymes include (1) amylase, to hydrolyze carbohydrate to disaccharide; (2) preproteolytic enzymes, primarily trypsinogen and chymotrypsinogen, to hydrolyze protein to amino acids; and (3) pancreatic lipase, which hydrolyzes fats to glycerol and fatty acids. Pancreatic polypeptide, an endocrine pancreas GI hormone, is involved in postprandial exocrine secretion regulation, gallbladder emptying, and gut contraction.

The liver carries out many functions, including bile production, carbohydrate storage, control of carbohydrate metabolism, reduction and conjugation of adrenal and gonadal steroid hormones, drug and toxin detoxification, plasma protein manufacture, formulation of urea and ketones, and fat metabolism. Bile is secreted by the liver cells into the intrahepatic bile caniculi. Bile is then carried from the liver through the common bile duct, which drains into the duodenum at a site close to or the same as the pancreatic duct. Discharge of bile from the common bile duct into the duodenum is controlled by the Sphincter of Oddi. Between meals this path is closed, and bile is stored in the gallbladder. When food is eaten, the Sphincter of Oddi relaxes, and when gastric contents enter the duodenum, the hormone CCK causes the gallbladder to contract and empty concentrated bile into the duodenum.

Bile, made by the hepatocytes, contains bilirubin, bile salts, bile pigments, cholesterol, fatty acids, plasma electrolytes, and water. Bilirubin and biliverdin are bile pigments that are formed from hemoglobin and give bile its characteristic golden color. Bile acids are formed in the liver from cholesterol. Some bile acids are converted by bacterial action in the intestine to secondary bile acids. Some bile acids are conjugated in the liver and are then known as bile salts. Bile salts perform several functions: (1) emulsifying fat-globules to aid digestion; (2) joining with lipids to form micelles for transport to the intestinal villi for absorption by the lymphatics; (3) activating lipases in the intestine; and (4) stimulating re-esterification of fatty acids and glycerol synthesis from glucose. Bile salts are required for absorption of fat-soluble vitamins A, D, E, and K. Most of the bile acids are absorbed in the terminal ileum, transported back to the liver in the portal vein, and re-excreted in the bile (the enterohepatic circulation).

Excretion

Excretion of contents of the colon occurs as a result of the complex act of defecation. Defecation involves reflexes that are cord mediated and those that are intrinsic through the myenteric plexus of the sigmoid colon. The long rectal muscles contract and shorten the rectum in concert with relaxation of the anal sphincter. Involuntary mass movement of the colon moves the feces into the rectum, producing the desire to defecate. Under voluntary control, the external anal sphincter relaxes when intra-abdominal and intrathoracic pressures increase, allowing expulsion of stool (see Chapter 12B).

CHANGES IN NUTRITIONAL STATUS

Protein-Calorie Malnutrition

Three major types of protein-calorie malnutrition (PCM) that are often discussed are (1) marasmus, or cachexia; (2) kwashiorkor, or acute visceral attrition; and (3) mixed, a combination of both. Marasmus results from chronic depletion of muscle or fat that occurs over a prolonged period of inadequate intake. The protein-calorie ratio in the intake might be acceptable, but the total dietary intake is inadequate. Fat and muscle stores are used as energy reserves. Marasmus can occur in the person with anorexia, partial intestinal obstruction, chronic illness, or old age. Usually the person will look wasted, but marasmus can be covered up in muscular or heavy-set persons.

The second type of PCM is kwashiorkor, when the person's intake of protein is insufficient, although carbohydrate intake might be adequate. Kwashiorkor can occur from fad diets, from overall decreased intake, or when patients are maintained for prolonged periods on dextrose and water infusions without protein supplements. Kwashiorkor is easily overlooked in the obese person or the person who appears well nourished, or when laboratory data are not evaluated carefully.

The third type of PCM, a combination of the two previously described, occurs most commonly in hospitalized patients or those with a prolonged illness, such as cancer or AIDS.

To assist with nutritional assessment, the body can be thought of as having two major components: fat and fat-free mass. Fat-free mass is composed of skeletal muscle, nonskeletal muscle and soft lean tissues, and the skeleton. Body muscle, largely composed of protein, is a major component of fat-free mass and provides an indication of protein reserves of the body. These can become depleted during prolonged undernutrition and result in muscle wasting. Fat or adipose tissue is a rich source of energy as an alternative to carbohydrates. In contrast, skeletal mass is inert and does not produce energy.

NUTRITIONAL CONSEQUENCES OF CANCER

Weight loss and other nutritional problems are a frequent, but not inevitable, consequence of cancer. The incidence of malnutrition varies widely in persons with tumors depending on site, extent of disease, and treatment approaches. When it does occur, malnutrition indicates a poor prognosis for both children and adults and can predict increased likelihood of complications such as delayed wound healing and infection. Malnutrition can become the most disabling aspect of the disease, resulting in decreased quality of life as well as increased morbidity and mortality. Cancer cachexia, a syndrome that occurs as a late effect in one-half to one-third of all cancer patients, is manifested by anorexia, malaise, weight loss, and wasting. Development of malnutrition from cancer involves many factors, both physiological and psychological.

For ease of understanding, the major nutritional consequences of cancer are divided into three main areas: inadequate ingestion, impaired digestion and absorption, and systemic metabolic alterations.

Inadequate Ingestion

Inadequate ingestion can result from the inability to eat, as well as from changes in the body's ability to use nutrients when ingested. Many physiologic or psychosocial factors can affect ability to eat, including fatigue, nausea and vomiting, depression, pain, or poverty, as well as such problems as (1) anatomical and mechanical alterations, (2) anorexia, and (3) altered taste perception.

Anatomical and mechanical barriers to eating can result from anatomical and physiological changes. Patients with cancer of the head and neck are most likely to experience such problems; patients with brain tumors are likely candidates also. Tumors involving the oral cavity and supporting structures can cause difficulties in chewing and swallowing. Painful lesions of the gastrointestinal mucosa can impair ingestion and swallowing. Facial or jaw pain also interferes with eating. Brain tumors, depending on the location, can affect chewing ability. Esophageal tumors can cause alterations in motility that manifest as odynophagia (painful swallowing). Obstruction of the esophagus can prevent passage of food or liquids. Some gastric tumors cause pain and gastric distension, resulting in feelings of early satiety (feeling full after eating small amounts) that can decrease a person's intake of nutrients. When the type or quality of foods and liquids consumed changes, malnutrition can develop, as can fluid and electrolyte disturbances.

Anorexia, or decreased appetite, results from a complicated process involving numerous physiologic and psychologic factors. Anorexia is frequently one of the earliest manifestations of cancer. The degree of anorexia is not necessarily related to size or type of tumor, although it generally increases in frequency and severity in the more advanced stages of disease. It has been shown to decrease with successful anticancer treatment, which supports the idea that it is a paraneoplastic process. Possible psychological components include the distress of being diagnosed with cancer, discouragement or depression, anxiety, interruption of normal lifestyle patterns, or isolation from support people and family. Taste changes, fatigue, and respiratory problems and other disease complications also contribute to anorexia.

The specific physiologic mechanisms that cause anorexia in cancer patients are not known, although many suggestions have been made regarding mechanisms of appetite control. Most of the theories about anorexia involve decreased hunger or increased satiety, which are regulated primarily by the hypothalamus. Delayed digestion and prolonged stimulation of the volume receptors of the GI tract can decrease feelings of hunger or cause prolonged stimulation of the satiety center. Another theory suggests that anorexigenic metabolites from the tumor (peptides and oligonucleotides) are released into the bloodstream, altering metabolic patterns or feeding by their effects on the peripheral receptors and brain centers. Malignant processes might cause abnormal neuronal or hormonal signals from the gastrointestinal tract that directly influence the hypothalamic appetite centers.

Altered taste perception can profoundly affect the patient's appetite. Taste is a complex sensation that is also highly dependent on smell. Normally the four primary taste sensation receptors, located on four different areas of the tongue, combine to give hundreds of taste sensations. Sweet receptors are located on the anterior surface and tip of the tongue. Salty and sour receptors are located on the lateral sides of the tongue. Bitter receptors are located posteriorly on the circumvallate palate.

In general, changes in taste have been found to be associated with the extent but not the type of tumor. Decreased taste acuity is called hypogeusia, and dysgeusia means a perverted sense of taste. For instance, a lowered urea recognition threshold is thought to result from an increased response of the taste buds to amino acid, which is manifested as an aversion to meat. A decreased response of the taste buds to sweets is believed to result in an elevated sucrose recognition threshold. In other words, food and drink must be sweeter to taste sweet to the consumer. Taste changes are thought to result from a chemical, rather than physiologic, alteration because taste sensations frequently return to normal as the tumor responds to treatment.

In addition, treatments themselves can cause permanent or temporary taste alterations. Surgery of the oral cavity, tongue, nasal area, or olfactory nerve can alter the perception of taste. Radiation therapy of more than 1,000 cGy can destroy taste buds or cause xerostomia. Changes in taste that are frequently reported following chemotherapy administration include a metallic taste in the mouth, a bitter taste, an increased threshold for sweet, or an aversion to sweet foods.

Impaired Digestion and Absorption

Obstruction of the lower GI tract, diarrhea, and external nutrient losses are three major nutritional problems that impair digestion and absorption in patients with cancer.

Intestinal obstruction of the lower GI tract occurs when, as a result of mechanical or neuromuscular alterations, its contents fail to progress. Obstruction can result from intrinsic involvement by tumor, extrinsic compression by metastatic cancer, or obstruction from benign lesions accompanying a metastatic process. Obstruction of the distal GI tract can occur from lymphomatous invasion of the small bowel, primary tumor of the colon or rectum, or diffuse carcinomatosis secondary to ovarian, colonic, pancreatic, or breast tumors. Peritoneal carcinomatosis is the most frequent cause of obstruction from metastatic disease.

When obstruction of the distal GI tract occurs, the symptoms and sequelae vary with the location of the blockage and can result in severe metabolic difficulties. If the obstruction is high, such as in the pylorus, metabolic alkalosis can result from losing gastric hydrochloric acid from vomiting or nasogastric intubation. When obstruction is high in the small bowel, dehydration is rapid. Dehydration is less likely in obstruction of the distal large bowel because most of the fluids will have already been absorbed. Neuromuscular obstructions, or adynamic ileus, occur after general anesthesia, abdominal surgery or trauma, electrolyte imbalance (particularly hypokalemia), certain chemotherapy agents, metabolic imbalances, peritoneal irritation, or severe pain. When mechanical obstruction occurs, replacement of fluids and electrolytes is essential and surgical correction is frequently required (see Chapter 15E).

Diarrhea implies a change in bowel habits. There is tremendous variation among individual persons in normal bowel function. Diarrhea can be defined as "too much of a too liquid stool." It involves increased frequency, volume, or fluidity, or abnormal constituents (blood, pus, or mucus) in the stools. Clinically, major changes in fluidity, frequency, or constituents are the usual hallmarks of diarrhea, but stool weight greater than 250 grams per day is the definitive criterion.

Diarrhea is a result of cancer in the following instances: (1) in association with hormone-secreting tumors (carcinoid syndrome, villous adenoma of the colon); (2) in deficiency of pancreatic enzymes or bile salts; (3) with infiltration of the small bowel by lymphomas or carcinomas; (4) due to blind loop from a partial upper bowel obstruction; and (5) in malnutrition.

Diarrhea involves different physiologic mechanisms in these circumstances. An understanding of the physiologic mechanism causing the diarrhea helps in its identification and management. Three major physiologic mechanisms have been identified: (1) excess fluid in the stools as a result of decreased net absorption in the intestines, causing an osmotic diarrhea; (2) increased net secretion by the intestines, resulting in a secretory diarrhea; and (3) these two mechanisms in combination, as in hypermotility states. Table 9–1 contains a summary of the differences in these three pathophysiologic processes. Fluid status, electrolytes, acid-base balance, and the availability of nutrients for energy and nutritional needs are all at risk for disturbance when diarrhea occurs.

Hormone-secreting tumors are usually associated with a secretory diarrhea. Pancreatic enzyme deficiencies and bile salt deficiency or excess result primarily in impaired digestion of fats and some decrease in protein digestion, ultimately causing an osmotic diarrhea. Abnormalities of the wall of the intestine from the infiltration of the tumors, such as lymphomas, involve atrophy or destruction of the microvilli, thus decreasing absorptive surfaces. In addition, protein-losing enteropathies result from loss of protein-rich substances when lymph channels are obstructed and when lym-

Table 9-1
Pathophysiology of Diarrhea

Type of Diarrhea	Mechanism	Characteristics of Diarrhea and Composition of Diarrheal Fluid	Examples
Osmotic	Unabsorbable (e.g., oligosaccharide) or poorly absorbable (e.g., Mg^{2+}, SO_4^{2-}) solute in the alimentary tract	24-hr stool volume usually <1 L. Stool volume decreases with fasting. Stool pH decreased <7	Lactose intolerance; cathartic abuse; excessive antacid use; postgastrectomy or partial gastrectomy
Secretory	Increased secretory activity of the alimentary tract, with or without inhibition of absorption of intestinal contents: may also result from inhibition of electrolyte and water absorption	24-hr stool volume usually >1 L. Stool volume does not decrease with fasting. Stool pH ~7	Non beta islet cell tumors of the pancreas; Zollinger-Ellison syndrome; villous adenoma; medullary carcinoma of the thyroid
Mixed	Increased rate of transit as in hypermotility states; osmotic effect of ingested solute may result from rapid intestinal transit and decreased net absorption	Variable	Carcinoid syndrome; cholinergic drugs

Adapted by permission of Mosby-Year Book, Inc. from Greenberger, N.J. *Gastrointestinal disorders: A pathophysiologic approach*, 4th ed. Year Book Medical Publishers, Inc., 1989.

phatics within the intestinal villi are dilated. Even with the extra-alimentary tract malignancies, the PCM that ultimately occurs is associated with histologic abnormalities of the mucosa, epithelial cell loss, and decreased lactose utilization. Thus, the ability of the intestine to digest or absorb is decreased. Bacterial overgrowth occurring in the upper small bowel when it is partially obstructed can cause steatorrhea and vitamin B_{12} deficiency.

External nutrient losses occur primarily through repeated vomiting or diarrhea. Nausea is the subjective feeling of the imminent need to vomit. It is the conscious psychic recognition of subconscious physiologic excitation in an area of the medulla closely associated with or a part of the true vomiting center (TVC). Nausea is frequently a precursor to vomiting, or emesis, the forceful expulsion of gastric contents. A complex act physiologically, vomiting is controlled by the lower brain stem, which is closely associated with respiration, to preserve safe respiration while preventing aspiration. The three elements of the act of vomiting—nausea, retching, and expulsion—can occur separately or in combination. Anticipatory nausea and vomiting result from psychogenic or cerebral and limbic mechanisms. They can occur as a conditioned response to tactile, olfactory, or other stimuli associated with illness or treatment.

The physiologic mechanisms by which nausea and vomiting occur are coordinated by the emetic center, which lies in the lateral reticular formation of the medulla oblongata near the vagus. It is composed of the TVC and the chemoreceptor trigger zone (CTZ). The TVC is located in the lateral region of the reticular formation of the medulla. All neurologic input for vomiting occurs here, making it the final common pathway mediating all vomiting. Both peripheral and central nervous system pathways are involved. The TVC efferent pathways involved with the act of vomiting include the phrenic nerve to the diaphragm, the spinal nerves to the abdominal muscles, and the visceral nerves to the stomach and esophagus. The afferent pathways leading to the TVC include the CTZ through vagal and other spinal sympathetic nerves from the viscera, midbrain receptors for elevated intracranial pressure, the labyrinth apparatus in the middle ear, and the cerebral cortex and higher central nervous system (CNS) structures.

The CTZ is believed to be in the area postrema, a medullary center located in the floor of the fourth ventricle. It is responsive to chemical stimulation and is connected to the emetic center through the faciculus solitarius. Toxic substances, including some drugs and possibly radiation therapy, stimulate the CTZ, which in turn stimulates the TVC. Irritation of the CTZ is thought to be the mechanism by which chemotherapy-induced nausea and vomiting occurs. The CTZ appears to be accessible by blood and cerebral spinal fluid. It works with the TVC, probably mediated by several neurotransmitters. Consideration of the types of neurotransmitter receptors present in the CTZ, the TVC, or the GI tract is important in developing and selecting effective antiemetic treatment.

GI tract fistulas result in the loss of gastric and small bowel fluids. External losses of protein can also occur as a result of repeated taps for the relief of malignant effusions or from dilution of albumin in abnormally large extracellular fluid compartments of malignant and ascitic effusions.

Systemic Metabolic Alterations of Cancer

Systemic metabolic alterations of cancer are believed to include at least three aspects: (1) alterations in the metabolism of carbohydrates, proteins, and fats, which can also contribute to increased energy expenditure; (2) competition for nutrients between tumor and host; and (3) ectopic hormone secretion. Knowledge in this area is based on preliminary evidence that is at times conflicting. In addition, cancer comprises a multitude of diseases. The many different types of cancer depend pathologically on the tissue of origin and the specialized cells within that tissue. Varying degrees of malignancy also exist.

Altered carbohydrate metabolism is a major systemic consequence of cancer. Tumors are believed to rely heavily on carbohydrates for energy, but the metabolic processes used are inefficient. Cancer cells are thought to have an imbalance in carbohydrate metabolism, using anaerobic glycolysis more than respiration. Anaerobic glycolysis is a biochemical process (the Embden-Meyerhof pathway) that converts sugars, primarily glucose, to pyruvic and lactic acids in order to obtain energy. Glycolysis yields four molecules of adenosine 5-triphosphate (ATP) from every one molecule of glucose after lactic and pyruvic acids enter the systemic circulation. Respiration is an aerobic biochemical process to metabolize carbohydrates. Glucose molecules are oxidized to create acetic acid, which is activated by an enzyme and further metabolized into carbon dioxide (CO_2) and hydrogen (H^+). The hydrogen is then oxidized in order to release energy. In contrast to glycolysis, this efficient process produces 34 molecules of ATP from one molecule of glucose.

The person with cancer responds to this increased demand for glucose with a high rate of gluconeogenesis. This is the synthesis of glucose by the liver and renal cortex from noncarbohydrate sources such as lactate, glycerol, and amino acids. Increased Cori Cycle activity, in which muscle glycogen is converted to lactic acid and then glucose, drains normal tissue for energy and stimulates significant gluconeogenesis. When protein in the form of lean body mass is broken down to provide amino acids for this process, the muscle wasting of PCM is thought to result.

The usual control or feedback mechanisms that function in the non-cancer patient during periods of starvation do not seem to work in cancer patients. Normally, during starvation, the body increases the mobilization of fatty acids from adipose tissue, decreases gluconeogenesis from amino acids, lowers oxygen consumption, and reduces energy requirements for ATP. Thus, total body protein and lean tissue mass are conserved during starvation. One possible explanation is that malignant cells grow continuously rather than follow the usual diurnal pattern of metabolic activity found in normal cells. Cancer patients seem less able to utilize tissue-conserving mechanisms and decreased gluconeogenesis from protein stores. Instead, they are thought to have inappropriately elevated energy expenditure, increased basal energy consumption, increased CO_2 production, and accelerated gluconeogenesis.

Another abnormality that has been postulated about carbohydrate metabolism is an abnormal glucose tolerance curve in patients with malignant tumors. Cancer patients who are losing weight have been shown to be glucose-intolerant, which can result from decreased sensitivity to insulin and/or a decreased insulin response. These patients are unable to utilize available glucose for energy.

Table 9–2
Endocrine Paraneoplastic Syndromes

Syndrome (Hormone)	Tumor	Clinical Manifestations with Nutritional Consequences
Ectopic adrenocorticotrophic hormone syndrome [Ectopic ACTH] (ACTH)	Small cell lung Carcinoid Pancreas	Hypokalemia, hyperglycemia, muscle weakness and atrophy, hypertension, and metabolic alkalosis
Diarrhea (catecholamine)	Neuroblastoma Pheochromocytoma	Secretory diarrhea
Nonmetastatic hypercalcemia (PTH)	Lung cancer—all types Other tumors	Fatigue, weakness, lethargy, renal insufficiency, anorexia, nausea, vomiting, constipation, abdominal pain
Diarrhea (Gastrin, VIP)	Zollinger-Ellison syndrome Pancreas, villous adenoma	Secretory diarrhea
Syndrome of inappropriate antidiuretic hormone [SIADH] (AVP)	Lung—small and non-small cell Head & neck cancer	Hyponatremia, serum hypo-osmolarity, inappropriate urine hyperosmolarity; and urinary concentration of sodium, euvolemia
Calcitonin	Medullary carcinoma of thyroid Breast cancer Small cell lung Carcinoid	Elevated serum calcitonin levels

ACTH—adrenocortical hormone; AVP—arginine vasopressin; PTH—parathormone; VIP—vasoactive intestinal peptide.

Adapted with permission from DeVita, V. T., S. Hellman, and S. Rosenberg. *Cancer: Principles and practice of oncology.* 5th ed. J. B. Lippincott, Philadelphia. 1997.

Protein metabolism is thought to be altered, so that muscle tissue is used to obtain protein to meet energy needs rather than the usual mechanisms in which protein is spared and carbohydrates are utilized as an energy source. Progressive muscle wasting, one of the hallmarks of cancer cachexia, is the result. In the tumor, protein synthesis continues at the expense of the host's nitrogen balance. The tumor becomes a "nitrogen trap," holding nitrogen and using it to produce protein that would ordinarily be used to produce protein for normal body growth and maintenance. Furthermore, the cancer patient can have decreased albumin and protein synthesis as well as an altered insulin regulatory mechanism. An altered insulin regulatory mechanism affects the metabolism of protein as well as carbohydrates. Elevated corticosteroids and catecholamine production from fever, infection, surgery, or other physiologic stress also contribute to increased protein catabolism.

Fat metabolism is altered in cancer patients, although the exact mechanisms are not known. Fatty acids (stored fat) are believed to be mobilized from adipose cells and released into the bloodstream for use as fuel for energy production because tumor tissue produces lipolytic substances that increase mobilization of fat. This process is controlled by the inhibitory effects of insulin, which are compromised in cancer patients. Body stores of fat are depleted as the disease progresses.

It has been suggested that tumor cells might use glucose preferentially so that normal cells must use other mechanisms to obtain nutrients. Reports conflict as to whether increased basal metabolic rate (BMR) is present in patients with cancer, with some found to be hypermetabolic, some normal, and some hypometabolic regardless of location or extent of tumor. It is believed that although the tumor competes effectively for nutrients when they are limited in availability, it is not capable of inhibiting normal body growth. It is emphasized, however, that feeding must occur simultaneously with effective tumor treatment.

Some tumors abnormally synthesize biochemical substances that have undesired systemic effects. The substances produced are hormones or hormone-like, can be metabolically active, and are often produced normally in other body organs. Such "paraneoplastic syndromes" can cause severe metabolic imbalances when physiologic feedback systems are not operating. Table 9–2 lists some paraneoplastic syndromes that have nutritional consequences, including information about the hormone secreted and the tumor.

NUTRITIONAL CONSEQUENCES OF CANCER TREATMENT

The primary modalities for treating cancer are surgery, radiation therapy, and chemotherapy. These approaches are used alone or in simultaneous or sequential combination depending on the location, type, and extent of the disease. When used in combinations, the effects can be synergistic. Many of the effects of cancer treatment that affect nutrition are similar to those of the disease itself. Frequently, the nutritional status of patients is already compromised by the disease at the time they are diagnosed, thus complicating the effects of treatment. Effects of each of the three treatment modes are described in the following sections.

Surgery

Surgery can be used as a curative treatment, totally removing tumor from the body, or as a palliative treatment, decreasing the bulk of the tumor or relieving obstruction or pressure. In any patient, surgery has immediate general metabolic systemic effects, including increased energy expenditure after surgery, utilization of visceral protein stores, and elevated catecholamines from the physiologic trauma of surgery.

Specific surgical procedures can have chronic effects on nutrition that are related to the organs resected and the degree of resection. Table 9–3 provides detailed information about the nutritional sequelae of surgical oncology procedures.

Radiation Therapy

Radiation therapy (RT) has a direct cytotoxic effect on tumor cells, as well as undesired effects on normal cells. Like chemotherapy, RT does not work selectively on cancer cells but affects all cells located within the treatment field. The patient's nutritional status when RT is begun will be a factor in the patient's tolerance of subsequent cancer treatment. Nutritional status will in turn be affected by RT. Patients most likely to develop nutritional problems from RT are those being radiated in the oral cavity, larynx, pharynx, and abdomen. Development of nutritional problems depends on numerous factors: the part of the body involved in the field, intensity of radiation, the period over which RT is administered, the volume of tissue radiated, the nutritional status of the patient at initiation of treatment, the sensitivity of the tissue to radiation, and the person's general physical and psychological status.

Fatigue and anorexia are two common side effects experienced by people receiving radiation therapy. Immediate and long-term consequences of RT that influence nutritional status are outlined in Table 9–4. Immediate consequences usually begin two to four weeks after the RT begins and resolve within six weeks of the end of RT. Late damage can be extensive and irreversible, occurring several months to years after RT is administered (see Chapter 2B).

Chemotherapy

Antitumor chemotherapy can cause impaired nutritional status as a result of decreased intake of nutrients, GI toxicity from systemic effects of the chemotherapy, and dysfunction of specific major organ sys-

Table 9-3
Nutritional Consequences of Cancer Surgery

Surgery	Consequences with Nutritional Implications
Radical resection of oropharynx	Difficulty chewing or swallowing Dependence on tube feedings when unable to eat Inadequate intake to support healing and health Altered taste perception
Esophagectomy, esophagogastrectomy, esophageal reconstruction	Gastric stasis and achlorhydria from vagotomy Diarrhea Steatorrhea Fistula or stenosis
Gastrectomy (partial or complete)	Dumping syndrome (cramps, diarrhea, fullness) Achlorhydria and megaloblastic anemia secondary to absence of intrinsic factor and vitamin B_{12} Malabsorption of fats, iron, vitamin B_{12}, calcium Delayed gastric emptying (with vagotomy) Early satiety secondary to decreased size of reservoir Post-gastrectomy syndrome (anemia, malnutrition, steatorrhea)
Intestinal resection Duodenum	Malabsorption of fat Low iron
Jejunum	Vitamin B_{12} deficiency, hyperoxaluria, bile salt losses
Ileostomy and colostomy	Fluid and electrolyte disturbance
Massive bowel resection	Malabsorption Metabolic acidosis Malnutrition
Blind loop syndrome	Diarrhea Steatorrhea Weight loss and malnutrition Anemia Multiple vitamin deficiencies
Pancreatectomy	Exocrine insufficiency leading to malabsorption Endocrine insufficiency leading to diabetes mellitus

tems (Table 9–5). When the functioning of major organ systems is disturbed by chemotherapy, further nutritional deterioration can occur. Systemic effects of chemotherapy that can have nutritional consequences include fever and chills, electrolyte imbalance, and weight loss.

Table 9–4
Nutritional Consequences of Radiation Therapy

Site	Consequences	
of RT	Immediate	Late
Head and neck	Dry mouth (xerostomia) Taste change or loss (hypogeusia) Difficulty swallowing (dysphagia) or painful swallowing (odynophagia) Loss of appetite (anorexia) Sore mouth or throat (mucositis) Fatigue	Taste change (dysgeusia) Osteoradionecrosis Xerostomia Dental caries Trismus
Esophagus	Dysphagia Sore throat Fistulas Obstruction Esophagitis Indigestion Nausea	Esophageal fibrosis Esophageal stenosis
Lung	Anorexia Shortness of breath Sore throat Nausea	
Upper abdomen	Nausea/vomiting Weight loss	
Whole abdomen	Nausea/vomiting Cramping and gas Diarrhea	Chronic enteritis Obstruction Fistula Stricture
Pelvis	Diarrhea	Ulcer perforation Malabsorption
GI tract	Diarrhea Nausea/vomiting Anorexia	

NUTRITIONAL ASSESSMENT OF THE ADULT WITH CANCER

Nutritional status is determined by the degree to which a person's need for nutrients is met by his or her intake. Good nutritional status of the cancer patient has been correlated with decreased morbidity and mortality, as well as with improved response to treatment.

Nutritional assessment can be performed for different purposes, including (1) to screen for potential problems and provide a complete base-

Table 9-5

Nutritional Consequences of Chemotherapy Resulting in Decreased PO Intake and GI Toxicity

Problem	Comments
Anorexia and taste changes	Complex physical and psychological causes. Most likely with methotrexate, cyclophosphamide, fluorouracil, mechlorethamine, and dactinomycin. Results in decreased intake and food aversions.
Nausea and vomiting	Intensity, duration, onset vary with drugs and doses (cisplatin, cyclophosphamide, dacarbazine, dactinomycin, methotrexate, mitomycin, mechlorethamine, nitrosoureas have severe emetic action). Results in decreased intake, fluid and electrolyte imbalances, general weakness, and weight loss. Thought to be caused by stimulation of the true vomiting center, the chemoreceptor trigger zone.
Stomatitis and esophagitis	Very common; alimentary tract is one of the most vulnerable targets of chemotherapy because of rapid cell proliferation. Results in inflammation and ulceration of the oropharynx and esophagus, cheilosis, glossitis (7–14 d after administration). Common with antibiotics, fluorouracil, vinca alkaloids, methotrexate.
Diarrhea	Similar causes as for stomatitis and esophagitis. Occurs most frequently with fluorouracil, methotrexate, hydroxyurea, nitrosoureas. If severe, proctitis, muscosal ulceration, bleeding, and perforation can occur. If prolonged and uncontrolled, can result in dehydration, electrolyte imbalance, inanition.
Constipation and adynamic ileus	Major toxicity of vincristine. Result of autonomic neuropathy. Occurs with vinblastine, hydroxyurea.

line data base for people at high risk; (2) to identify, work up, and plan interventions for existing problems; and (3) to determine response to and efficacy of interventions. Examples of factors that can be used to identify those at risk for PCM are as follows:

1. Inadequate oral intake for greater than 7 days;
2. Weight loss of 1 percent to 2 percent in one week, 5 percent in one month, and more than 10 percent in six months;
3. Recent major surgery, trauma, or infection;
4. Radiation therapy within the past six months;
5. Persistent symptoms, such as nausea, vomiting, diarrhea, dysphagia, odynophagia, mucositis, depression, anorexia, or fatigue, persisting for longer than two weeks or that recurs;

6. Inability to chew or swallow;
7. Diminished self-care ability in a person with inadequate home care support;
8. Recent medications, including catabolic steroids, immunosuppressants, antitumor agents, antibiotics, antacids, and opioids;
9. Illness lasting more than three weeks during the past six months;
10. Dementia;
11. Poverty.

Although PCM is frequently experienced by cancer patients, it is also important to consider vitamin, mineral, and fat intake and electrolyte imbalance. The current use of megavitamin therapy and other nontraditional cancer treatment approaches, in addition to the popularity of fad diets, makes it necessary to consider excesses of nutrients as well as deficits.

Unfortunately, malnutrition is not an uncommon problem in hospitalized patients in general and patients with cancer in particular. A surprisingly large proportion of hospitalized patients have been found to be malnourished. As an initial step in providing for patient's nutritional and metabolic needs, assessment of nutritional status must include psychosocial as well as physiologic parameters. Family members and friends can be additional sources of information.

Assessment Methods

Nutritional assessment can include clinical observation, anthropometric techniques, biochemical analysis, and dietary evaluation. The specific methods used in assessing the nutritional status of patients with cancer will vary according to the assessment goals, patient setting and population, and other concurrent diseases or health conditions. A combination of measurements might be necessary to provide a complete survey of the various body components.

This includes consideration of the physical condition of the patient, psychological factors, socioeconomic status, medication, and other health problems. A complete physical examination will reveal a person's overall nutritional status. Careful attention to skin, hair, mouth, teeth, and general muscle tone can provide early clues to nutritional deficiencies. Psychological factors that must be considered include the existence of depression, anxiety, or isolation. Ability to purchase and prepare foods should be appraised. Evaluation of the potential impact of current medications should include information about vitamins, prescriptions, over-the-counter medications, and recreational drugs. Additional health problems that can affect nutrition—such as diabetes, renal disease, thyroid disorders, or malabsorption syndromes—should be identified. Much of this information is contained in any thorough nursing history.

Among the measurements that can be obtained are mid-arm muscle circumference (MAMC), triceps skin-fold thickness (TSF), subscapular skin-fold thickness (SST), and weight for height. The purpose and process for these and other measurements are shown in Table 9–6. When measurements are obtained, they should be compared with age- and sex-specific reference values or standards. When tables of standards are applied in order to make clinical judgments about patients, it is important that they not be interpreted too rigidly, thus losing sight of the wide range of normal variation that occurs among people.

Serum albumin and transferrin indicate visceral protein levels, but have varying half-lives; total lymphocyte count is an indicator of immune function and also reflects visceral protein stores; creatinine height index reflects skeletal or lean body mass (somatic protein); recall skin testing shows cell-mediated immunity; and urinary urea nitrogen or total nitrogen indicates degree of protein catabolism.

Dietary history and intake can be evaluated by using various approaches alone or in combination, including (1) 24-hour recall, (2) food frequency questionnaire, (3) complete dietary history, (4) food diary or record, (5) direct observation, and (6) evaluation of nutrient intake according to standard nutritional criteria, such as the Basic Four Food Groups or Recommended Dietary Allowances. Assessment of the person's knowledge about nutrition can be an alternative or a complement to other methods. This approach, however, assumes that a direct relationship exists between what people know about nutrition and what they eat.

In the 24-hour recall approach, the person completes a questionnaire or is interviewed to determine what he or she recalls eating in the past 24 hours or on the previous day. Food frequency questionnaires collect information on the number of times per day, week, or month particular foods are eaten. Content of the 24-hour recall can be specific or general. The method provides additional information that can be used to validate the accuracy of what is gathered from other sources. The dietary history, collected by the nurse or nutritionist, provides the most complete account of nutritional intake; it can utilize 24-hour recall and the food frequency questionnaire as part of data-gathering procedures. The history includes information about activity, economics, home life (or hospital life), eating patterns, ethnic background, health history, medication, and appetite. If the person is keeping a food record or diary, he or she is asked to record all intake of food or fluids for a given period. The period covered depends on the regularity of the person's food patterns. Accuracy is increased if the person records the intake immediately after eating. Observation of food intake is the most precise assessment method, but it is also the most demanding in time and energy; the hospitalized patient is more easily observed than the person at home.

These methods are discussed in detail in many nutrition textbooks. Potential problems in evaluating dietary intake include the following: (1) recording influences intake; (2) the patient might be unable to remember types and amounts; (3) nutrient composition of food varies with prepara-

Table 9-6
Anthropometric Measurements for Nutritional Assessment

Measurement	Purpose	Process	Advantages	Limitations
MAC	Reflects muscle and fat	Measure circumference of arm at midpoint from between acromial process of scapula and olecranon process of ulna using metal tape measure	Simple Easily accessible	No limits for overnutrition
MAMC	Reflects skeletal muscle protein mass	Indirectly from mid-arm circumference (MAC)—(0.314 × TSF mm); interpret in light of usual weight percentiles	Simple Easily accessible Not affected by edema	No standards for elderly
TSF	Estimates subcutaneous fat stores and energy reserves (not degree of malnutrition)	Caliper measurement of nondominant arm at midpoint; measure and sum with subscapular skin-fold thickness; interpret in light of usual weight percentiles	Easily accessible Not usually affected by edema Variability of caliper brands	Changes occur slowly Requires expensive calipers Requires tables of normal values for sex, age, and site Tables of norms not fully developed IV fluid administration affects pliability of skin Reliability varies with examiner and technique
SST	Estimates subcutaneous fat	Caliper measurement 1 cm below tip of right scapula		Does not reflect acute changes

Parameter	Significance	Formula/Method	Advantages	Limitations
Weight	Represents total of all body constituents; indicates changing nutritional reserves; basis for other anthropometric measures	Same scale, clothing, time of day; Measure, don't accept report; Interpret using percentiles	Inexpensive; Easily obtained; Noninvasive nature; Quick	Proper scales required; Trained personnel needed; Influence of third-spacing; Underestimated loss of body mass secondary to increased ECF with starvation; Normal daily variation for individuals of up to 1 kg
% IBW	Compares real weight to suggested norms	$\%IBW = Wt/IBW \times 100$		IBW standards for Metropolitan Life; Insurance of questionable validity
% UBW	Reflects weight change	$\%UBW = Current\ wt/Usual\ wt \times 100$	Avoids need for table norms	Assumes usual weight is his or her "ideal" weight
Weight change	Identifies risk factor	$Usual\ wt - Actual\ wt/Usual\ wt \times 100$		

ECF—extracellular fluid; IBW—ideal body weight; IV—intravenous; MAC—mid-arm circumference; MAMC—mid-arm muscle circumference; SST—subscapular skin-fold thickness; TSF—triceps skin-fold thickness; UBW—usual body weight; Wt—weight.

Patient-Generated Subjective Global Assessment (PG-SGA) of Nutritional Status

(To the patient: please check the box or fill in the space as indicated in the next four sections)

A. History

1. Weight change

   Summary of my current and recent weight:

   I currently weigh about _____ pounds
   I am about _____ feet _____ inches tall
   A year ago I weighed about _____ pounds
   Six months ago I weighed about _____ pounds
   During the past 2 weeks, my weight has
   ❑ decreased　❑ not changed　❑ increased

2. Food intake:

   As compared to normal, I would rate my food intake during the past month as either:

   ❑ unchanged
   ❑ changed:　❑ more than usual
   　　　　　　❑ less than usual

   I am now taking:

   ❑ little solid food　　❑ only nutritional supplement
   ❑ only liquids　　　　❑ very little, if anything

3. Symptoms: During the past 2 weeks, I have had the following problems that kept me from eating enough (check all that apply):

   ❑ no problems eating
   ❑ no appetite, just did not feel like eating
   ❑ nausea　　　　　　❑ vomiting
   ❑ constipation　　　　❑ diarrhea
   ❑ mouth sores　　　　❑ dry mouth
   ❑ pain (where?) _____
   ❑ things taste funny or have no taste
   ❑ smells bother me
   ❑ other _____

4. Functional capacity:
   Over the past month, I would rate my activity as generally:

   ❑ normal, with no limitations
   ❑ not my normal self, but able to be up and about with fairly normal activities
   ❑ not feeling up to most things, but in bed less than half the day
   ❑ able to do little activity and spend most of the day in bed or chair
   ❑ pretty much bedridden, rarely out of bed

(The remainder of this form will be completed by your doctor, nurse or therapist. Thank you.)

5. **A. History** (continued)
   Disease and its relationship to nutritional requirements
   Primary diagnosis (specify) _____
   (Stage, if known) _____
   Metabolic demand (stress)　❑ no stress　　❑ low stress　　❑ moderate stress　　❑ high stress

   B. Physical (for each trait specify: 0 = normal, 1 = mild, 2 = moderate, or 3 = severe)
   _____ loss of subcutaneous fat (triceps, chest) _____ muscle wasting (quadriceps, deltoids)
   _____ ankle edema _____ sacral edema _____ ascites

   C. SGA rating (select one)
   ❑ A: well nourished
   ❑ B: moderately (or suspected) malnourished
   ❑ C: severely malnourished

Figure 9–2. Patient-Generated Subjective Global Assessment (PG-SGA) of Nutritional Status.

Reprinted with permission from Ottery, F. D. Nutritional Oncology: A proactive, integrated approach to the cancer patient. In Shikora and Blackburn, eds. Nutrition Support. Chapman & Hall, New York. 1997.

Table 9–7

Guidelines for Subjective Global Assessment Categories

Stage A— Well Nourished	Stage B— Moderately Malnourished	Stage C— Severely Malnourished
Well-nourished or Recent nonfluid weight gain and/or Improvement in components of history, e.g., improved symptoms, intake	> 5% weight loss within a few weeks No weight stabilization or weight gain Definite decrease in intake Mild subcutaneous tissue loss	Obvious signs of malnutrition (e.g., severe loss of subcutaneous tissue, possible edema) Clear and convincing evidence of weight loss

Reprinted with permission from Ottery, F. D. Nutritional Oncology: A proactive, integrated approach to the cancer patient. In Shikora and Blackburn, eds. *Nutrition Support*. Chapman & Hall, New York. 1997.

tion; (4) accuracy varies with interviewing skills; (5) cooperation and honesty is necessary; and (6) the recorded intake might be atypical.

One approach to evaluation of nutritional status that has received more attention recently is the Subjective Global Assessment (SGA) which was originally developed in 1987 by Jeejeebhoy and colleagues. It was modified for use in oncology patients by Ottery in 1993. A later modification, the Patient-Generated Subjective Global Assessment (PG-SGA), is displayed in Figure 9–2. The PG-SGA, which is filled out by the patient, is useful for any clinican in inpatient or outpatient settings. The clinician finishes it by adding brief information from the physical exam. Finally, the patient is categorized as Stage A—well nourished; Stage B—moderate or suspected malnutrition; Stage C—severely malnourished. Table 9–7 gives the guidelines for each category. This category is used to place the patient at a specific point in the algorithm displayed in Figure 9–3. This algorithm guides interventions for cancer patients who are at risk for nutritional complications.

MANAGEMENT OF PROBLEMS RELATED TO NUTRITION

Diarrhea

Knowledge about the mechanisms and etiology of the diarrhea helps provide a basis for rational therapy. For the patient with cancer, diarrhea has numerous potential causes. The tumor itself can cause diarrhea, as can malabsorption, fistulas, or pancreatic insufficiency. More commonly,

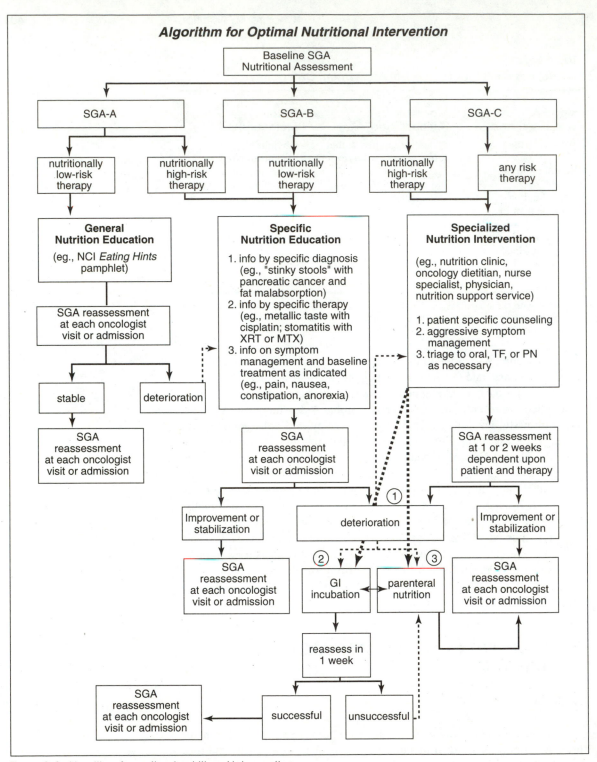

Figure 9–3. Algorithm for optimal nutritional intervention.

diarrhea results from surgical or medical interventions. Surgery, such as pyloroplasty, gastrectomy, and intestinal resections, can cause dumping syndromes or malabsorption. Radiation therapy to the abdomen or pelvis can damage the intestinal cells located in those fields. Cells of the intestinal epithelium are inherently sensitive to the toxic effects of radiation therapy and chemotherapy because of their rapid cell turnover. Such medications as antitumor chemotherapeutic agents, antibiotics, laxatives, and antacids also cause diarrhea in cancer patients. Other potential etiologies for diarrhea in this group of patients are bowel infections, fecal impaction, tube feedings, and anxiety and stress.

The medications available for treating diarrhea include bulk-forming agents, adsorbents, opioids, antidiarrheals, and antacids. Adsorbents such as kaolin powder and pectin are not very effective except when diarrhea is caused by an excess of bile salts. Bulk-forming agents such as methylcellulose and psyllium (Metamucil®) are helpful, especially with RT patients. Various agents are available: opium derivatives (codeine, paregoric, tincture of opium, and belladonna); diphenoxylate (Lomotil®); and loperamide (Imodium®). Most antacids contain magnesium and act as osmotic agents to stimulate elimination. Those that contain aluminum instead of magnesium, such as Basogel® and Amphogel®, can be used to alleviate loose stools in those patients who require frequent antacids.

When diarrhea is severe, the person might need to rest the bowel by restricting all oral intake except fluids containing electrolytes and sugars that will facilitate absorption of water as well as simply provide fluid replacement. Dietary intake is gradually increased, avoiding high fiber and other stimulants of the bowel. Further suggestions for the care of the cancer patient with diarrhea are found in Table 9–8.

Nausea and Vomiting

Control of nausea and vomiting is necessary to enhance the physical and psychologic comfort of the patient; to prevent pronounced physical debilitation from malnutrition, impaired mobility, and fatigue; and to allow anticancer therapy to continue. Other reasons that nausea and vomiting should be minimized are to avoid dehydration; metabolic alkalosis from loss of potassium, chloride, and hydrogen ions; straining of abdominal muscles; and danger of aspiration.

Nausea and vomiting in cancer patients can result from the presence of the tumor itself, but more frequently they occur following chemotherapy or RT. Patterns of nausea and vomiting include anticipatory nausea or vomiting, acute post-therapy nausea or vomiting, and delayed nausea or vomiting. Among the factors that must be considered in antiemetic therapy are (1) patient characteristics, including emesis control during prior chemotherapy, history of alcohol use, and age; (2) the cancer treatment, including emetic potential, dosage, schedule, and route of administration of

Table 9–8
Nursing Considerations for the Management of Diarrhea

Factor	Nursing Intervention
Health perception, health management	Explore the implications of having diarrhea for each patient. Determine usual practices to maintain health and cooperation with health promotion plans and care. Assess response to current treatment measures and adjust as needed. Evaluate knowledge about diarrhea and its treatment.
Nutritional, metabolic status	Assess nutritional status, paying particular attention to hydration and electrolytes. Determine nutritional needs. Weigh daily. Evaluate dietary intake, including intake and output of fluids. Encourage avoidance of food and medication that aggravates the bowel. Appraise tube feedings as cause of diarrhea. Try frequent low-residue feedings if able to tolerate (bananas, applesauce, rice) and high carbohydrate and high protein intake. If hypokalemia is evident, include foods high in potassium (baked potatoes, bananas, halibut). Supplementation or IV repletion might be necessary if prolonged. Drink 2–3 quarts of fluids daily. Koolaid®, Jell-O®, apple juice, bouillon, Gatorade®, and weak tea are good sources when served at room temperature. Carbonated beverages should be allowed to flatten before drinking. Avoid foods that are too hot or cold. Extreme temperatures may stimulate gastrointestinal activity. Avoid milk and milk products to prevent lactose intolerance symptoms. Lactose-free products may be substituted such as Dairy Rich®, and non-dairy creamer. Lact-aid® can be used to break down the lactose in milk. Administer antidiarrheal medications about $\frac{1}{2}$ hr before meals to minimize diarrhea.
Activity, exercise	Assess a person's ability to care for him/herself, including obtaining and preparing food. Determine energy levels and tolerance of activity and exercise.
Sleep, rest	Evaluate usual and current sleep/rest patterns. Encourage resting and naps to conserve energy. Plan medication administration and treatments to avoid interrupting sleep.
Comfort	Evaluate discomfort caused by diarrhea (abdominal cramping, soreness around anus). Apply heat to abdomen for comfort.
Elimination	Assess usual patterns of elimination for each individual. Evaluate for fecal impaction. Record frequency, amount, and appearance of stool. Evaluate bowel sounds. Clean rectal/anal area after each bowel movement and dry carefully. Apply substances for protection of skin and mucous membranes and to promote healing such as A & D® Ointment, Desitin®, Nupercainal®. Apply a local anesthetic (ointment or spray) such as Tucks®. Use sitz baths. Avoid anal/rectal stimulation.
Coping, stress	Assess family and support systems. Identify sources of stress and anxiety (finances, family, illness, fears). Encourage measures to decrease or cope with stress and anxiety (medication, counseling, relaxation training, biofeedback).
Role relationship	Assess ability to carry on usual role relationships. Assess patient's and family's perceptions of impact of diarrhea on work and social relationships.

the chemotherapy agent(s), or the radiation dose and field; (3) the antiemetic itself, including dosage and schedule, route of administration, and the use of antiemetic agents in combination.

The cancer chemotherapeutic agents that have the highest emetogenic potential are cisplatin, dacarbazine, dactinomycin, mechlorethamine, streptozotocin, and cyclophosphamide. It is believed that different classes of chemotherapeutic agents initiate vomiting by directly or indirectly stimulating different sites—either the TVC or CTZ. The occurrence of nausea and vomiting is also influenced by psychological factors such as anxiety and fear, expectations based on the patient's past experience or that of others, the environment's sights and smells, and conditioned responses. Other less common emetic stimuli include fluid and electrolyte abnormalities, bowel obstruction or peritonitis, CNS metastases, hepatic metastases, uremia, local infections and septicemia, and opioids. Careful determination of the etiology of the symptoms by history and physical examination is essential in order to plan appropriate interventions. Two major approaches to relieve nausea and vomiting involve pharmacologic measures and the use of behavioral approaches.

Pharmacologic Therapy

Metoclopramide (Reglan®) is a procainamide derivative with peripheral and central antiemetic action. It increases GI motility and gastric emptying. Metoclopramide appears to have two sites of action, including dopamine antagonist activity in the CNS, and in the GI tract, where it promotes gastric emptying. When administered orally after chemotherapy, it is ineffective. To avoid the risk of mucosal tears in the GI tract, its use is contraindicated following resection or anastomoses. Side effects include extrapyramidal symptoms, fatigue, insomnia, anxiety or agitation, which can be alleviated by concurrently administering diphenhydramine (Benadryl®).

Cannabinoids are the active ingredients of marijuana that have proven to have antiemetic properties. Delta-9-tetrahydrocannabinol, or dronabinol (Marinol®), has been effective for both chemotherapy- and RT-induced nausea and vomiting. Cannabinoids are not without significant toxicities, including sedation, severe dysphoria, hallucinations, and orthostatic hypotension. Their use should be avoided with the naive user and the elderly.

Glucocorticoids have been suggested for use as antiemetics following anticancer therapy. Dexamethasone, available in oral and parenteral forms, and methylprednisolone are used. It is postulated that they work by blocking the synthesis or release of prostaglandins.

The more traditionally used antiemetic medications include the phenothiazines, butyrophenes, and antihistamines. Phenothiazines are potent dopamine agonists (blockers) that are believed to act on the CTZ. Phenothiazines are of limited use as single agents with strongly emetic agents. Phenothiazine tranquilizers are classified on the basis of their chemistry and pharmacology into three groups: the aliphatic class, the piperazine class, and the piperidine class. Chlorpromazine (Thorazine®), an aliphatic compound, has limited antiemetic action during chemotherapy. Phenothiazines such as prochlorperazine (Compazine®), a piperazine compound, have a pronounced antiemetic effect, including use for delayed nausea and vomiting. Potential side effects include sedation, orthostatic hypotension, extrapyramidal symptoms, and elevated prolactin levels.

The butyrophenes, including haloperidol (Haldol®) and droperidol, are among the most potent inhibitors of the CTZ through dopamine antagonism. Because hypotension or other cardiorespiratory effects are not likely, these drugs are useful for patients who are elderly or debilitated.

Antihistamines, such as dimenhydrinate (Dramamine®) and diphenhydramine (Benadryl®), are helpful in increasing effectiveness and decreasing toxicity when given with other antiemetics. The primary site of these histamine (H_1) blockers is the CTZ. The antihistamine, diphenhydramine, is used to minimize extrapyramidal symptoms.

A new class of antiemetic, the serotonin antagonists has become the standard of care in managing nausea and vomiting associated with moderate to severe emetogenic cancer treatments. Chemotherapy induces the release of serotonin from the enterochromaffin cells of the intestine, evidenced by an increase in one of its metabolites, 5-hydroxyindoleacetic acid ($5\text{-}HT_3$), in the urine; elevated levels of this metabolite correspond to the onset of postchemotherapy nausea and vomiting. Ondansetron (Zofran®) and granisetron (Kytril®), $5\text{-}HT_3$ antagonists, have demonstrated significant antiemetic activity, particularly against the nausea and vomiting caused by cisplatin. Because ondansetron is metabolized in the liver, caution must be taken for use in patients with liver dysfunction.

The recommended intravenous dose of ondansetron is .15 mg/kg, given 30 minutes before and four and eight hours after chemotherapy, or as a single 32 mg infusion 30 minutes before chemotherapy. Ondansetron is available in oral form as 4 or 8 mg tablets. The recommended adult dose is one 8 mg tablet given twice per day, beginning 30 minutes before chemotherapy with the next dose 8 hours later. Patients can continue to take ondansetron two times per day for one to two days following chemotherapy. The most common side effects are dizziness, diarrhea, headache, and constipation. These effects respond well to symptomatic treatment. Granisetron is given as a single oral dose of 2 mg within one hour before chemotherapy or 10 mcg/kg intravenously given 30 minutes before chemotherapy. No subsequent doses are recommended. Side effects are similar to those experienced with ondansetron. As for other antiemetics, ondansetron and granisetron can be combined with other effective agents to further reduce the nausea and vomiting caused by chemotherapy.

Behavioral Approaches

Many nonpharmacologic behavioral approaches have been suggested for the alleviation of post-treatment nausea and vomiting. These include hypnosis, behavior modification, deconditioning or desensitization, guided

Table 9-9
Nursing Management of Nausea and Vomiting

Factor	Nursing Intervention
Activity intolerance	Assess the effects of movement and activity on symptoms of N/V. Encourage activity to the extent it does not aggravate N/V and provides diversion and exercise. Avoid sudden rapid movements.
Anxiety	Assess nature and extent of anxiety as a contributing cause of N/V. Administer antianxiety medications, if indicated. Inquire about past experiences of patient and others to determine if they contribute to increased anxiety. Instruct patient about various relaxation techniques if interested and appropriate.
Breathing (aspiration)	Assess risk of aspiration. Position and monitor patient to prevent aspiration during vomiting. Remove dentures or partial plates.
Comfort	Assess sources of discomfort or pain. Promote comfort measures, using an individualized approach based on patient needs. Control the environment to remove unpleasant sounds, sights, and smells and reduce stimulation of the vomiting center. Administer antiemetic at appropriate dosages and intervals. Prevent N/V from occurring initially, especially related to chemotherapy. Provide mouth care after vomiting and as needed to freshen mouth.

Fluid volume
  Deficit from
  active loss or
  decreased
  intake
	Assess fluid and electrolyte status by history, physical examination, and review of laboratory work.
	Observe and record intake and output of fluids, including the amount and character of emesis.
	Monitor weights, blood pressure, skin turgor, urine concentration.
	Administer antiemetic medications as prescribed, paying particular attention to patterns of N/V and dosage and administration schedule of drugs.
	Provide fluids that reduce nausea and do not induce vomiting.

Sleep/rest	Determine present and usual sleep patterns. Medicate with antiemetics and provide uninterrupted rest. Sedatives may be used if desired by patient to induce sleep during periods of N/V.
Inadequate nutrition	Assess nutritional status by dietary evaluation, physical examination, history, and laboratory tests. Evaluate food preferences and tolerance. Determine past measures that have been effective. Record the pattern of N/V and the amount and appearance of emesis. Evaluate ability to obtain and prepare food. Encourage small, frequent feedings of food that is tolerated well and of high nutritional value. Avoid intake of "empty calories" or food with low nutritional value. Use foods that have been tolerated well in the past to provide positive reinforcement. Medicate prior to meals so that antiemetic effect is active during and immediately after meals. Avoid fat, spicy, or highly salted foods or foods with a strong odor. Remove food covers outside of the room where food will be eaten. Minimize stimuli that aggravate nausea (sights, smells, overstimulation). Provide distraction and relaxation opportunities.

Continued

Table 9-9 *(Continued)*
Nursing Management of Nausea and Vomiting

Factor	Nursing Intervention
Injury/safety	Evaluate the potential for injury as a result of weakness or changes in mental status. Guard against aspiration. Arrange for necessary assistance to maintain safe and healthful environment in home or hospital.
Knowledge deficit	Assess knowledge about the causes of N/V and measures recommended to treat them. Review signs and symptoms to report to the health care provider.
Immobility	Assess ability to tolerate activity, strength, and endurance. Provide assistance if needed to get about safely.

N/V—nausea and vomiting

mental imagery, biofeedback, relaxation techniques, diversion, and meditation. Suggested advantages of nonpharmacologic approaches are numerous. They can (1) potentiate the placebo effect of medications; (2) improve patient/provider relationships; (3) transform passive patients into active patients; (4) improve patient compliance; and (5) promote an increased sense of well-being. For the most part, they are without side effects and are inexpensive and portable. Among the most significant potential problems with these nonpharmacologic approaches are difficulties providing a conducive environment in institutional settings, time needed to practice and perform these measures, and the requisite patient motivation to carry them out. Decisions regarding which approach to implement for any individual require trial and error.

Table 9–9 contains further considerations for the care of the cancer patient experiencing nausea and vomiting.

Increasing Oral Intake

Oral intake by patients with cancer can be decreased as a result of numerous symptoms, side effects, and conditions associated with cancer or its treatment. Anorexia, fatigue (Chapter 8C), pain (Chapter 8A), nausea or vomiting, stomatitis (Chapter 10B), anxiety, depression (Chapter 7), and changes in environment or lifestyle can result in decreased intake of food and nutrients. Table 9–10 incorporates several approaches to encourage increased oral intake.

Enteral nutrition (tube feeding) is used for cancer patients who have functioning GI tracts but for whom oral feeding methods are either contraindicated, inadequate to meet needs, or not tolerated. This situation can occur when the patient is unable to take adequate amounts (less than

Table 9-10
Nursing Protocol to Increase Oral Intake

Factor	Nursing Intervention
Activity	Encourage activity appropriate to abilities and energies of individual in order to increase appetite and utilization of nutrients.
Fatigue	Assess ability to obtain and prepare food. Arrange for necessary assistance. Teach to expend minimal energies on food preparation. Encourage frequent rest periods, particularly before meals. (See Chapter 8C.)
Bowel elimination Constipation Diarrhea	Evaluate alterations such as constipation or diarrhea. Relieve constipation by appropriate diet and medication (see Chapter 12B). See Table 9–7 for interventions for diarrhea.
Pain/comfort	Evaluate nature and extent of discomfort or pain. Encourage wearing apparel that is loose and comfortable. Provide pain relief measures prior to meal times (see Chapter 8A). Plan care so that unpleasant or painful procedures do not take place before meals.
Knowledge/information	Assess knowledge about appropriate nutritional intake and measures to encourage it. Provide verbal and written information for patient and family regarding nutrition.
Anorexia	Evaluate circumstances of anorexia. Encourage eating foods that are appealing at times when appetite is best. Instruct about nutritional supplements, methods for adding protein and calories to diet. Assist to obtain. Serve foods attractively and in a pleasant environment. Provide companionship while eating. Remove all unpleasant stimuli from eating environment. Encourage "freshening up" before meals by washing hands and face and mouth care. Eat frequent small meals rather than three large meals. If not contraindicated, try a glass of wine or sherry prior to meals. When hospitalized, have friends and family bring in favorite foods. Keep nutritious snacks handy for nibbling. Avoid eating or drinking foods low in calories or other nutrients. Limit the amount of liquids consumed with meals. Serve foods at appropriate temperatures.
Nausea and vomiting	Assess patterns of N/V. Plan feedings around predictable times. Medicate prior to eating. Avoid lying down flat for at least two hours after eating.
Oral mucositis	Evaluate condition of oral cavity. Provide measures to relieve oral discomfort prior to eating (see Chapter 10B). Maintain good oral hygiene.
Powerlessness	Allow the opportunity to choose meal times and food.
Sensory-perceptual alteration	Provide assistance with eating required as a result of weakness, paralysis, visual disturbances. Assess taste changes and alter available foods to accommodate.
Social isolation	Provide companionship and a pleasant environment for eating.

N/V—nausea and vomiting.

50 percent of required amounts) of food and fluids by mouth (anorexia, oral or esophageal abnormalities) or when the GI tract is not functioning normally (malabsorption, short bowel syndrome, fistulas). Hypermetabolic states, such as postsurgery, or sepsis might also require that tube feedings be initiated in order to meet the increased demands for nutrients. Enteral feeding is also used in the transition between parenteral nutrition and oral feeding.

Tube feedings can be administered through various routes—orogastric, nasogastric, nasoduodenal, nasojejunal, esophagostomy, gastrostomy, or jejunostomy. The appropriate route, formula, and delivery method are selected based on the patient's nutritional requirements and medical condition. To avoid the development of sores or fistulae, any of the routes that utilize a tube passing through the nose are limited to a maximum of three weeks. Gastrostomy tubes can be temporary or permanent. New techniques have been developed to decrease the demands of their insertion.

Enteral nutrition through a tube is a relatively safe and simple procedure that can be carried out at home. If the patient has a working gut, it should be used in preference to parenteral (intravenous) routes. The mechanical, gastrointestinal, or metabolic complications that can occur with tube feedings include fluid and electrolyte disturbances, such as dehydration and tube feeding syndrome (dehydration, hypernatremia, hyperchloremia, azotemia); aspiration; gastric or abdominal distension; constipation; and, most commonly, diarrhea. Feedings can be administered continuously, intermittently, or by bolus, except into the small bowel, where bolus methods of administration are not appropriate. Whenever bolus feedings are tolerated poorly, continuous feedings will need to be considered. The key to patient tolerance of tube feedings is the rate of administration, usually over 20 to 30 minutes. Advantages of intermittent or bolus feedings are increased mobility and freedom, independence, ease of maintenance, and its similarity to the physiologic aspects of normal food consumption. For optimal safety and accuracy, continuous infusions require a pump. Alternatively, a gravity system including an in-line solution administration set can be used. The maximum flow rate should be around 125 cc/hour. The rate of administration and concentration of the solution should be increased gradually to decrease side effects. The rate is usually increased before the concentration.

Various types of formulas are available for tube feedings. Decisions about which to use will depend on the patient's nutritional needs. Formulas vary in digestibility; osmolality; viscosity; content of fat, carbohydrate, protein, lactose, vitamins, and minerals; and expense. Blenderized and milk-based feedings are relatively inexpensive and easy to use. Because they contain intact protein and lactose, they can only be used with a normally functioning GI tract. Their osmolality is relatively high (500–800 mOsm/kg). Lactose-free formulas are available with standard calorie content (1 kcal per cc) or as high-density formulas (1.5–2 kcal per cc). Osmolality of these formulas is low (300–400 mOsm/kg). Chemically defined or elemental formulas contain nutrients in partially digested forms so that they can be used for patients with impaired GI function, such as malabsorption or short bowel syndrome, or with metabolic disorders. Modular formulas designed specifically to supplement carbohydrate, fat, or protein are also available. Nursing concerns for administering tube feedings are outlined in Table 9–11.

Parenteral nutrition is a process by which carbohydrate, fat, and protein, along with trace elements, vitamins, and electrolytes, are infused into the venous system to correct nitrogen balance, allow weight gain, and help tissue repair. Parenteral nutrition can be accomplished through a large peripheral vein (peripheral parenteral nutrition, PPN) or through central venous access (central parenteral nutrition, CPN) using veins such as the cephalic, subclavian, or jugular. It is indicated when the patient (1) has a dysfunctional gastrointestinal tract; (2) needs bowel rest; (3) is severely malnourished or hypermetabolic and unable to meet energy and/or protein needs via the enteral route; or (4) requires an alternative to enteral feeding in critical situations to avoid uncertainties of nutrient uptake or utilization.

Peripheral parenteral nutrition is used on a short-term (five to ten days) basis to supplement oral intake when requirements are higher than normal or when the risk of using central approaches is too great. Peripheral routes are useful only for short-term repletion of mild to moderate malnutrition and when anabolic requirements are greater than normal but not excessive. Peripheral parenteral nutrition can be used as a boost in conjunction with oral feedings or when central line insertion is contraindicated. It requires a high percentage of calories from fat (30 percent to 60 percent) and a high fluid volume (3 liters) to reach the upper calorie limit (2,000 kcal/day).

Central parenteral nutrition should be considered for long-term support (longer than seven to ten days). Indications for CPN include the following: (1) oral intake or enteral intake is impossible, potentially hazardous, or insufficient; (2) the patient has short gut or short bowel syndrome, resulting in decreased absorption in the small intestine; (3) the patient has hypermetabolic states (sepsis); (4) the patient is unable to eat as a result of severe nausea, vomiting, anorexia, or obstruction; (5) a suitable peripheral vein is unavailable; and (6) long-term parenteral repletion is required.

Composition of the solutions administered by a central route are different from those administered peripherally. More hypertonic solutions can be administered centrally; thus solutions given peripherally are 5 percent to 10 percent dextrose and those given centrally are 20 percent to 35 percent dextrose. When very hypertonic solutions (20 percent to 35 percent dextrose) are administered, they must be given centrally through a large

Table 9-11
Nursing Protocol for Enteral Nutrition (Tube Feeding)

Factor	Nursing Intervention
Sleep/rest	Provide opportunity for sleep free of interruptions by procedures or equipment changes.
Skin integrity	Assess condition of skin around esophagostomy, gastrostomy, or jejunostomy. Change dressing at least daily and clean around tube with half-strength H_2O_2. Do not use alcohol.
	Evaluate for signs of essential fatty acid deficiency (dry scaling over distal lower extremities).
	Encourage activity and changing positions to avoid skin breakdown.
	Check nose for irritation, erosion, or necrosis if nasal tube is in place. Reposition tube.
Diarrhea	Evaluate frequency, consistency, and volume of stools.
	Adjust formula type and rate of administration to avoid diarrhea.
	Administer formula at room temperature (not cold).
	Change administration set and tubing q 24 hrs.
	Discard intermittent feeding syringes after each feeding.
	Rinse with hot water when refilling set.
	Hang supply for 4 hrs only.
Comfort/pain	Regulate the rate and select formula to prevent abdominal cramping, distension, vomiting, or diarrhea.
	Position patient comfortably during administration.
	Check for gastric residual every 4–8 hrs. If >125 cc over 4 hrs temporarily discontinue.
Family coping	Provide an opportunity for the patient and family to discuss the impact of enteral hyperalimentation feeding techniques.
Fear	Provide opportunity to discuss fears regarding tube feeding and nutrition.
	Give information to help alleviate fears and provide support and practice opportunities.
Fluid volume	Evaluate for dehydration or fluid overload.
	Maintain accurate records of intake and output, including fluid used to flush.
Body image	Determine the patient's usual and current body image.
	Provide opportunity to talk about body image and self-concept.
Oral hygiene	Encourage or provide mouth care at least every 3–4 hrs when awake.
Aspiration	Check placement of the tube in the stomach before initiating any feeding and at least every 8 hrs during continuous feeding.
	Elevate head of bed at least 30° during feeding and for 1 hr after completed unless the tube is in the jejunum, to prevent reflux or aspiration.
Nutrition	Assess nutritional status.
	Irrigate the tube with 20–30 cc of water prior to and following administration of feeding or medications, and every 3–4 hrs.
	Select feeding type and amount based on individual needs and condition.
	Regulate rate and volume based on individual needs and condition.
	Check serum or urine q 6–8 hrs for sugar for the first 3 days.
	Watch for Tube Feeding Syndrome.
	Evaluate electrolyte and serum chemistry status.
	Check residuals 1 hr before tube feedings through NG tubes, gastrostomy, and PEG tubes.
Knowledge	Evaluate knowledge level and learning abilities and preferences.
	Provide information as patient demonstrates readiness.
Mobility	Encourage activity and independence.

H_2O_2—hydrogen peroxide; NG—naso-gastric; PEG—percutaneous endoscopic gastrostomy.

vein such as the subclavian in order to provide rapid dilution and to prevent irritation and thrombophlebitis. Usually 2,000–3,500 ml of fluid are required daily.

Calories are usually provided by a carbohydrate source, such as dextrose. Adequate calories are required so that the amino acids infused for synthesis of protein into muscle mass can be utilized (usually 150–280 calories per gram of nitrogen). Some calories can be provided from fat sources. The Harris Benedict equation can be used to estimate basal energy expenditure (BEE) or energy needs for men, BEE (kcal) = 66.5 + (13.7 × Weight in kg) + (5 × Height in cm) − (6.8 × Age in years); and for women, BEE (kcal) = 65.5 + (9.6 × Weight in kg) = (1.7 × Height in cm) − (4.7 × Age in years). Final estimation of caloric requirements of individual persons involves multiplication by an activity or injury factor.

Protein needs are supplied by amino acid compounds. Free crystalline amino acids are frequently used. The normal adult requires about 0.8–2.0 grams protein / kg daily. These basic requirements might be exceeded during the physiologic stress of illness or surgery. The balance between nitrogen from protein that is consumed and that which is required is evaluated by nitrogen balance studies.

Fat is provided by infusion of commercial fat emulsions (10 percent or 20 percent). Administration of fats is useful as an additional concentrated calorie source to provide for increased calorie needs. It is also necessary to avoid essential fatty acid deficiencies in patients receiving CPN for prolonged periods (more than two weeks).

Minerals, trace elements, multivitamins, and electrolytes are added to individualized parenteral nutrition solutions at the time of preparation by the pharmacy. The electrolytes sodium, potassium, chloride, calcium, magnesium, and phosphorus are added because they are important in maintaining osmotic pressure in body fluids. Endogenous insulin supplies might be inadequate when hypertonic glucose solutions are administered. Insulin supplies are best augmented by administering insulin in the parental nutrition solutions, rather than administering subcutaneously on a sliding scale basis. Salt-poor albumin might be needed to restore visceral protein levels.

Complications occurring from parenteral nutrition can be categorized as technical, metabolic, and septic. Potential technical complications are related to the method of venous access (see Chapter 3B). Metabolic complications that can occur are hyperglycemia, hypoglycemia, hyperglycemic hyperosmolar nonketotic dehydration and coma, hypophosphatemia, essential fatty acid disturbances, hypomagnesemia, or electrolyte and fluid imbalance. Septic complications are serious potential dangers when parenteral nutrition is administered, especially through central access in immunocompromised cancer patients.

Major considerations for nurses administering central parenteral nutrition (CPN) are outlined in Table 9–12. Additional detailed instructions should be sought in institutional procedure manuals and nursing or nutrition textbooks.

Table 9–12
Nursing Protocol for Parenteral Nutrition Administration

Factor	Nursing Intervention
Infection	Check the in-line fittings frequently. Refrigerate solutions until one-half hour prior to use. Additions to solutions should be done in pharmacy under laminar flow hood. Check clarity and expiration date on bottles before hanging. Notify physician of signs of inflammation, purulence, thrombosis, or extravasation at insertion site. Use final micropore .22 micron filter. Change IV tubing (except high-pressure tubing) daily using aseptic technique. Use sterile technique in handling catheter site. Change dressing at catheter insertion every other day, using aseptic technique (see Chapter 3B). Apply an occlusive dressing, looping the tubing to prevent dislodgement.
Fluid balance	Initiate and discontinue gradually. Infusion rate should never exceed prescribed rate by 10%. Infuse with a volumetric pump. Check rate at least hourly. Record intake and output, weight. Warm solution to room temperature prior to administering to increase viscosity, allowing correct calculation of flow rate. Evaluate fluid balance of patient (including vital signs) every four hours.
Nutrition	Test urine glucose every six hours. Report 3+ or 4+ readings. Use appropriate urine testing products (i.e., Clinitest® tablets vs Clinistix® strips) to avoid inaccurate results from other medications. Evaluate serum electrolytes, glucose, intake and output, weight. Allow opportunity to talk about changes in eating activities.
Oral hygiene	Examine the oral areas for dryness, mucositis, or infection. Evaluate condition of the teeth. Provide mouth care on a regular basis every four hours while awake. Obtain artificial saliva if needed.
Information	Instruct patient and family about purpose and procedure of PN. Ensure that patient and family have knowledge and experience to care for PN if going home.
Anxiety	Evaluate feelings about PN. Provide information and support during PN. Instruct regarding relaxation and diversion measures.
Activity	Develop exercise program to improve utilization of nutrients and improve/maintain strength. Offer diversional activities.
Body image	Provide opportunity for discussion of feelings about appearance.
Role change	Assess the impact on usual responsibilities and role activities.

PN—parenteral nutrition.

BIBLIOGRAPHY

1. Bergerson, S. L. Nutritional support in bone marrow transplant recipients. In R. K. Burt, H. J. Deeg, S. T. Lothian, & G. W. Santos, eds. *On Call In . . . Bone Marrow Transplantation.* 343–356. R. G. Landes Company, 1996.

   This chapter is an excellent overview of aspects of nutritional support in bone marrow transplant (BMT) recipients including nutritional requirements, modified bacteria diet for BMT patients, parenteral and enteral nutrition in BMT, nutritional assessment, eating problems with suggested interventions, and posttransplant complications affecting nutritional status.

2. *Eating Hints: Recipes and Tips for Better Nutrition During Cancer Treatment.* NIH Publication No. 81-2079. U. S. Department of Health and Human Services, National Cancer Institute, Bethesda, MD. 1981.

   This book provides an excellent resource for practical approaches to common nutrition problems experienced by cancer patients and has many recipes contributed by cancer patients and their families.

3. Grant, M. M., and L. M. Rivera. Anorexia, cachexia, and dysphagia: The symptom experience. *Seminars in Oncology Nursing* 11(4): 266–271. 1995.

   Alterations in nutrition can lead to nutritional compromise from symptoms such as anorexia, cachexia, and dysphagia. Nutritional assessment, pharmacological and nonpharmacological interventions, and patient and family teaching are included in the management of these nutrition-related problems.

4. Herrington, A. M., J. D. Herrington, and C. A. Church. Invited review: Pharmacologic options for the treatment of cachexia. *Nutrition in Clinical Practice* 12: 101–113. 1997.

   This article provides a review of cancer cachexia etiology, clinical trials in cancer cachexia, appetite stimulants, metabolic inhibitors and anticytokine therapy, and anabolic agents, and recommendations for the treatment of cancer and AIDS-related cachexia and anorexia.

5. Kalman, D., and L. Villani. Nutritional aspects of cancer-related fatigue. *Journal of the American Dietetic Association* 97: 650–654. 1997.

   This article reviews fatigue models useful in understanding fatigue associated with cancer and its treatment, physiologic concerns, and the links between cancer therapy and fatigue. The authors suggest nutrition intervention to improve fatigue experienced by cancer patients.

6. Klein, S., J. Kinney, K. Jeejebhoy, D. Alpers, M. Hellerstein, M. Murray, P. Twomey, et al. Nutrition support in clinical practice: Review of published data and recommendations for future research directions. *Journal of Parenteral and Enteral Nutrition* 21(3): 133–156. 1997.

   This article reports the work of an advisory committee that performed a critical review of the current medical literature evaluating the clinical use of nutrition support. The following areas were evaluated: nutritional assessment, nutrition support in patients with gastrointestinal diseases, nutrition support in wasting diseases, nutrition support in critically ill patients, and perioperative nutritional support.

7. Smith, S. A. N. Theories and intervention of nutritional deficits in neoplastic disease. *Oncol Nurs Forum* 9(2): 43–46. 1982.

This article provides a classic review of cachexia from neoplastic diseases in terms of deficit factors, assessment parameters, and the interventions of psychosocial modification, dietary modification, nutritional supplements, tube feeding, and parenteral nutrition.

8. Sokal, J. E. Measurement of delayed skin test responses. *N Engl J Med* 293(10): 501–502. 1975.

Issues and procedures for performing and evaluating delayed skin tests as a clinical tool are presented, including practical suggestions.

Protective Mechanisms

A. Bone Marrow

Patricia Jassak
Douglas Haeuber

INTRODUCTION

Hematopoiesis is the process by which the components of the blood are formed and made available in the circulation. This process has three primary components: proliferation, differentiation, and maturation. Circulating blood cells are terminally differentiated with life spans ranging from several hours to many years.

Blood cell formation consists of the production of white blood cells or leukocytes (granulocytes, also called neutrophils, monocytes/macrophages, eosinophils, basophils), and lymphocytes, erythrocytes, and platelets. In humans, the process of hematopoiesis is initiated in the bone marrow and provides for the important functions of immunity, hemostasis, oxygen transport, and protection from infection.

For a variety of reasons that will be discussed, the person with cancer is at risk for disruption of hematopoiesis due to bone marrow depression (BMD), leading to granulocytopenia (also called neutropenia), lymphocytopenia, thrombocytopenia, and anemia. At the least, BMD can severely affect the quality of life of the person with cancer and at worst can place him or her in a life-threatening situation. The nurse caring for the patient experiencing BMD must have a clear understanding of the pathophysiology underlying BMD and appropriate assessment skills, medical management, and supportive care to address the threats posed by BMD.

10A

ANATOMY AND PHYSIOLOGY

The formation of blood cells is a highly structured, complex process. Hematopoiesis involves the production of blood cells whose levels and functions are regulated through an elaborate system of molecular signals. The structural architecture of the bone marrow, known as the hematopoietic inductive microenvironment (HIM), provides a setting conducive to hematopoiesis in which the early, most primitive cells in the hematopoietic hierarchy are either exposed to or protected from influences leading to pro-

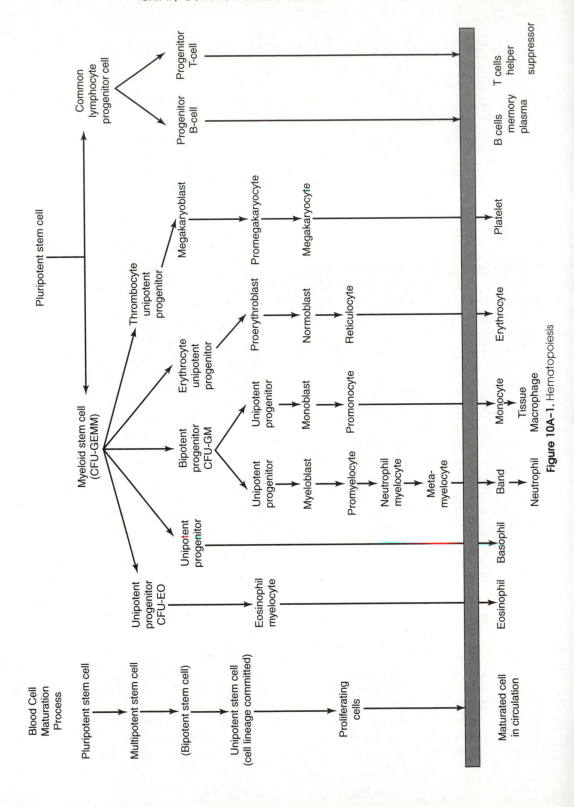

Figure 10A–1. Hematopoiesis

liferation and differentiation. It is clear that the structural (stromal) elements of the marrow—including fibroblasts, endothelial cells, and fat cells, along with so-called accessory cells (macrophages and lymphocytes) present in the marrow—can have either a direct effect on early marrow cells through contact adherence or an indirect effect through the release of substances known as hematopoietic growth factors (HGF). These HGFs form complex signaling networks and function as positive or negative regulators of blood cell proliferation and differentiation.

Figure 10A–1 provides a schematic diagram of the hematopoietic hierarchy, demonstrating the various levels of cells involved in the process of blood formation. The cells at the top of the figure are the most primitive of the blood cells, and those at the bottom are the most mature functional cells found in the peripheral blood circulation. All blood cells have their origin in a common source, the pluripotent stem cell. The pluripotent stem cell possesses three vital characteristics: a high self-renewal capacity; a capacity to give rise to all blood cell lineages; and a low degree of mitotic activity. The pluripotent stem cell has the unique ability to divide asymmetrically, yielding either two identical progeny or one stem cell and a committed multipotential cell. The pluripotent stem cell will return to the resting state (G_o) while the multipotential cell is subject to the influences in the HIM that will cause it to begin the process of differentiation. These abilities to self-replicate and return to a G_o phase are fundamentally intriguing features. Resting cells are less vulnerable to genetic damage; hence, this return to a resting phase accounts for the characterization of the pluripotent stem cell as "immortal" and forms the foundation for hematopoiesis throughout life.

The immediate progeny of the pluripotent stem cell have a more limited ability to self-replicate yet retain the capability of differentiating into one of two developmental pathways, the myeloid or lymphoid cell line. One example of this multipotential stem cell is the colony forming unit–granulocyte erythrocyte monocyte megakaryocyte (CFU-GEMM), which has lost the ability to differentiate into the lymphoid cell line but retains the ability, depending on the stimuli to which it is subject, to differentiate into any of the myeloid cell lines. With subsequent divisions, increasing differentiation occurs, and the cells undergo an irreversible commitment to a specific cell line.

BLOOD CELL LINEAGES

Granulocytes/Monocytes

The committed stem cell for both the granulocyte and monocyte/macrophage lines is the colony forming unit–granulocyte macrophage (CFU-GM), which possesses the ability to differentiate into either type of cell. Specific hematopoietic growth factors regulate differentiation into a particular cell line. The HGFs will be discussed separately, but those that influence granulopoiesis and monocytopoiesis are interleukin 3 (IL-3), granulocyte macrophage–colony stimulating factor (GM-CSF), granulocyte–colony stimulating factor (G-CSF), and monocyte–colony stimulating factor (M-CSF). The release of HGFs regulating leukocyte formation can occur as a consequence of infection and inflammation in the body, the circulation of bacterial endotoxin, exercise, stress, and the presence of glucocorticoids. When these conditions are present, accessory cells such as tissue macrophages and T-lymphocytes release HGFs that increase the presence of mature granulocytes and monocytes in two ways: (1) by stimulating proliferation and maturation of these leukocytes; and (2) through *demargination*, which is the release into circulation of a preexisting pool of granulocytes fixed to endothelial cells, such as those lining blood vessels.

The functions of granulocytes and monocytes are listed in Table 10A–1. The primary function of granulocytes is to act as the body's first defense against microorganisms on the skin, gastrointestinal mucosa, and

Table 10A–1
Functions of Leukocytes

Leukocytes	Function
Granulocytes Neutrophil (segs and bands)	Chemotaxis, moves to locus of inflammation, produces lysosomes, pus formation. Phagocytosis of bacteria (first line of defense).
Basophil	Release of histamine, heparin, and enzymes in acute inflammation; can prevent clot formation and growth.
Eosinophil	Phagocytosis and release of enzymes in allergic reactions; contribute to fibrin clot digestion.

Monocytes
  Blood monocyte
  Tissue monocyte (histocyte or tissue macrophage)
	Phagocytosis of cellular debris, fungi, tumors.
	Phagocytosis, filtration of particles (tumor, cellular and noncellular debris).

Lymphocytes
  B cell (humoral immunity)
  Plasma cell
  T cell (cellular immunity)
    Helper cell
    Suppressor cell
 	
  Cytotoxic or "killer" cell
	Role in lymphocyte antibody activity.
	Antibody production; complement fixative.
	Regulate function of other lymphocytes.
	Mediate antibody production.
	Diminish B cell and T cell activity; mediate cellular-humoral immunity.
	Specific effector function (e.g., delayed hypersensitivity reaction, graft-vs.-host disease, tumor cell kill).

lung tissue. Granulocytes have the ability to phagocytize and destroy bacteria, forming pus in the process. Monocytes and macrophages also possess bacteriocidal and phagocytic abilities, in addition to the role they perform in presenting antigens to lymphocytes to initiate the immune response. They function as mechanical barriers and can play a feedback role in increasing neutrophil proliferation in the presence of infection. The life span of circulating granulocytes is quite brief, about 12 hours; monocytes live substantially longer while circulating and can survive for several months if they become fixed-tissue macrophages. The normal laboratory values for all blood cells are provided in Table 10A–2.

Lymphocytes are a product of the same pluripotent stem cell that gives rise to all of the myeloid cell lines (erythrocytes, granulocytes, platelets, and so on). Under the influence of specific growth factors, the precursors of mature lymphocytes migrate from the bone marrow to specialized sites where proliferation and maturation occur. In the case of T-lymphocytes, this site is the thymic endothelium; for B-lymphocytes, the development of precursor cells seems to occur in lymphoid tissue. Lymphocytes are long-lived (measured in years) and recirculate throughout the

Lymphocytes

Table 10A–2
Normal Laboratory Values

Cells	Range
WBC	4,500–11,000/mm^3
Differential	
Granulocytes	
Neutrophils—segs	54%–62%
bands	3%–5%
Eosinophils	1%–3%
Basophils	0%–1%
Monocytes	3%–7%
Lymphocytes	15%–34%
Platelets	150,000–400,000/mm^3
RBC	
Female	4.20–5.40 mil/mm^3
Male	4.60–6.20 mil/mm^3
Hgb	
Female	12–16g/dl
Male	14–18g/dl
Hct	
Female	38%–47%
Male	40%–54%

Note: Values might vary slightly by laboratory.

Hct—hematocrit; Hgb—hemoglobin; mil—million; RBC—red blood cells; WBC—white blood cells

body via the blood stream, the lymphatic drainage, and the thoracic duct. They tend to concentrate in lymphoid tissues such as lymph nodes, the thymus, and the spleen, as well as in the bone marrow.

Lymphocytes are responsible for the host's ability to distinguish self from nonself (foreign antigens) and respond to the presence of foreign antigens by mounting an immune response (see Table 10A–1). Specificity refers to the ability of lymphocytes to respond to single bacterial, viral, or tumor antigen, either through surface recognition sites in the case of T-lymphocytes (cellular immunity) or immunoglobulins/antibodies produced by B-lymphocytes (humoral immunity). Memory of specific antigens is preserved by lymphocytes, allowing a more efficient response to the antigen on subsequent exposures. *Amplification* refers to the rapid expansion of lymphocytes when exposed to an immune stimulus.

Immunocompetence involves the effective defense provided by both cellular and humoral responses to foreign antigens (bacteria, viruses, and malignant cells). Host defense is a highly integrated network, involving the interaction of myeloid cells, such as granulocytes and macrophages, lymphoid cells, and the initiation of nonspecific processes such as the complement cascade.

Thrombocytes/Platelets

Like the other myeloid cell lines, platelets are ultimately derived from the pluripotent stem cell, which gives rise to a committed megakaryocytic progenitor cell (burst forming unit-megakaryocyte, BFU-Mega). As with the other cell lines, there are specific growth factors (megakaryocyte growth and development factor, MGDF; thrombopoietin, TPO; IL-11) that regulate the process of megakaryocytopoiesis and platelet production. One of these HGFs appears to act on the progenitor cell pool and the other on the cells that are recognizable as megakaryocytes. Platelets are produced when megakaryocytes, having undergone a process of internal nuclei division called *endo-reduplication*, fracture, and fragments are released into the bloodstream as platelets.

Platelets live for eight to ten days. They play a central role in hemostasis, preventing the leakage of red blood cells through capillary walls. In addition, they are involved in initiating the intrinsic clotting mechanism and in clot retraction. The liver and spleen are responsible for the removal and destruction of "old" platelets. At any one time approximately one-third of circulating platelets are sequestered in the spleen. Persons with splenomegaly might have a platelet count below normal, while a splenectomized person often has platelet counts above normal. The average platelet count in the adult is 250,000 platelets/mm^3.

Erythrocytes/Red Blood Cells

Red blood cells (RBCs) are the products of a differentiation process beginning with the multipotent stem cell, continuing through such early precursor cells as the burst forming unit–erythroid (BFU-E) and the colony forming unit–erythroid (CFU-E). The immediate precursor of the RBC, the reticulocyte, is released from the bone marrow and completes its maturation in the bloodstream. The reticulocyte count serves as a useful indicator of bone marrow function with regard to RBC production.

The primary stimulus of RBC production is tissue hypoxia, which causes certain parenchymal cells in the kidney to release a red cell growth factor known as erythropoietin (EPO). RBCs require folic acid, vitamin B_{12}, and iron to develop and function properly. Their major function is to transport hemoglobin (Hgb), which in turn carries oxygen. In addition, the RBCs transport carbon dioxide to the lungs to be expelled.

The life span of RBCs ranges from 100 to 140 days. They are removed from the blood through phagocytosis by macrophages. In the human, approximately 1 percent of RBCs turn over every day. Usually, hematocrit (Hct) and hemoglobin (Hgb) are the measures used to determine if a person is anemic. The normal range of values for RBCs, Hct, and Hgb in the adult male and female is provided in Table 10A–2.

Hematopoietic Growth Factors (HGFs)

HGFs are naturally occurring, hormone-like glycoproteins that are intrinsically involved in the regulation of every aspect of hematopoiesis. Nearly 20 HGFs have been identified, characterized, and cloned to date. There are five human myeloid HGFs and 13 cytokines that are identified as interleukins. The nomenclature of HGFs is confusing. The earliest factors derived names as colony stimulating factors (CSF) from the *in vitro* observation that progenitor cells are stimulated to form colonies of recognizable mature cells. Another group, the interleukins, derive their name from cellular sources and action on leukocytes. Recent additions are given sequential interleukin numbering.

All HGFs are defined by their ability to induce the proliferation, differentiation, maturation, and, in some cases, functional activation of the hematopoietic cells in the various lineages discussed earlier. These substances act like hormones, attaching to receptors on the target cells, setting in motion the intracellular processes involved in cell division, development, and function. Whether a specific hematopoietic cell is affected by a particular HGF is determined by the presence and number of receptors on the membrane of the target cell with affinity for that HGF.

One useful way to categorize HGFs is by their ability to affect either one or several cell lineages. Certain HGFs, such as IL-3 and GM-CSF, tend to have an impact on the earlier progenitor cells in the hematopoietic hierarchy and thus affect several cell lines. Other HGFs (G-CSF, M-CSF, EPO) might have a limited effect on more than one lineage, particularly in conjunction with other HGFs, but are primarily restricted to a single lineage.

Hematopoietic growth factors are produced by numerous cells in the body, including stromal cells in the bone marrow and accessory cells (T-lymphocytes and macrophages) in both the marrow and the circulation. In addition, certain HGFs are produced by parenchymal cells in organs such as the kidney and liver.

The identification, purification, and recombinant production of HGFs for therapeutic use has increased during the past two decades. In general, recombinant HGFs have been utilized to address many important issues related to BMD in oncology patients, such as the treatment of anemia with EPO, granulocytopenia (GCP) with G-CSF and GM-CSF, and most recently thrombocytopenia with IL-11. In addition, recombinant HGFs can be used to enhance the effectiveness of cytotoxic agents in treating cancer, such as leukemia.

PATHOPHYSIOLOGY OF BONE MARROW DEPRESSION

The factors that cause BMD are many, involving environmental and hereditary influences, disease, and treatment regimens. In patients with cancer, BMD can occur as a consequence of a single process or a combination of processes. The person with a myeloproliferative malignancy (e.g., leukemia, lymphoma) might experience BMD as an aspect of the primary disease process. Patients with solid tumors can have invasion of their bone marrow by metastatic disease (myelophthesis), causing replacement of marrow cells by cancer, with impairment of normal hematopoietic proliferation and differentiation. Solid tumors that tend to metastasize to the bone marrow include lung, breast, and prostate cancers. In these situations, the hematopoietic cells that are produced can be abnormal, immature, or less functional (e.g., less able to phagocytose foreign particles).

In addition, BMD can occur as a side effect of chemotherapy and radiation therapy, and can be acute and/or chronic. Hematopoietic cells—which, in general, are rapidly dividing cells—are quite susceptible to the effects of cytotoxic therapy. Granulocytes and platelets, both of which have relatively brief life spans, are affected most severely, although the other hematopoietic cells suffer as well.

In the myeloid cell line, chemotherapy affects cells in most stages, from myeloblast through myelocyte. Stem cells are more resistant to cell cycle-specific drugs (e.g., methotrexate) than they are to non–cycle-specific alkylators (e.g., cyclophosphamide). Cells that have matured beyond the myelocyte stage are also less susceptible to the effects of chemotherapy. Thus, granulocytic and megakaryocytic cells early in the process of differentiation are most sensitive to the effects of antineoplastic drugs.

The general pattern of chemotherapy-induced granulocytopenia (GCP) and thrombocytopenia (TCP) consists of a mild reduction in counts for a few days after treatment, a nadir (the most pronounced decrease) at 7 to 14 days post-treatment, and recovery within 14 to 18 days. This pattern is logical considering the life cycle of granulocytes and platelets. As the circulating mature granulocytes and platelets are naturally removed from the circulation through aging and death, they are not replaced because of the destructive impact of the therapy on cycling, differentiating precursor cells in the bone marrow. There is then a lag between generations of hematopoietic cells caused by the treatment, which corresponds to the period of the lowest counts. Chemotherapy can also cause lymphocytopenia, suppressing both humoral and cell-mediated immunity. This is usually a temporary effect, lasting only 2 to 3 days.

In general, BMD is affected by dose, schedule, and route of treatment; previous treatment history; concomitant therapy; and other factors such as age, nutritional status, tumor type and disease stage. Higher doses and more frequent treatments cause more severe nadirs, since hematopoietic cells have less chance to recover. (See Chapter 2C for specific drug-induced hematopoietic toxicity.)

As a systemic treatment, chemotherapy has a generalized effect on the bone marrow. Radiation therapy, on the other hand, tends to affect marrow activity only in the designated treatment field. The relative risk of bone marrow toxicity for patients undergoing radiation therapy is related to the volume of productive marrow in the treatment field. Distribution of bone marrow and percentage of bone marrow involved in common treatment fields are identified in Tables 10A–3 and 10A–4.

When radiation therapy (RT) is administered concomitantly with chemotherapy, the bone marrow toxicity is usually greater than that of either therapy alone. In addition, prior treatment with radiation therapy can increase the bone marrow toxicity of subsequent chemotherapy treatments. The reverse is also true. Therefore, in assessing a patient's risk for BMD, it is important to determine the type and extent of previous treatments. A late effect of chemotherapy and radiation therapy is atrophy and fibrosis of the bone marrow, with consequent effects on the hematopoietic inductive microenvironment and cellularity. In some cases, these therapies could also produce a second primary cancer such as leukemia. Finally, there is evidence that surgery induces a suppression of both humoral and cell-medi-

Table 10A–3

Proportion of Bone Marrow Radiated by Usual Therapeutic Fields

Radiation Field	Estimated Percentage of Bone Marrow Affected
Total body irradiation	100
Total nodal irradiation	60–70
Mantle	20–50
Para-aortic	20–25
Pelvic	15–25
Pulmonary and mediastinal	20–25
Abdominal	20–25
Cranial	25–45
Chestwall and lymphatics	15–20

Reprinted with permission from Dritschilo, A., and D. Sherman. Radiation and chemical injury in the bone marrow. *Environmental Health Perspectives* (June):62. 1981.

Table 10A–4
The Distribution of Active Bone Marrow in the Adult

Site	Percentage of Total Red Marrow
Head	13.1
Upper limb girdle	8.3
Sternum	2.3
Ribs (all)	7.9
Vertebrae	
Cervical	3.4
Thoracic	14.1
Lumbar	10.9
Sacrum	13.9
Lower limb girdle	26.1
Total	100.0%

Adapted from Ellis, R. E. The distribution of active bone marrow in the adult. *Physics in Medicine and Biology* (January):257. 1961.

ated immunity for several weeks, an important consideration for the patient receiving multimodal therapy. Figure 10A–2 depicts the major factors that affect BMD in the patient with cancer.

Complications of BMD

The most common and serious complication of BMD is infection due to GCP, a major cause of morbidity and mortality in the person with cancer. Infection in patients with GCP is difficult to evaluate. Classic signs and symptoms of redness, heat, swelling, and tenderness are absent due to decreased numbers of functional granulocytes. Fever greater than 38°C is the most reliable indicator of infection in a granulocytopenic patient.

The most common sites of infection are the gastrointestinal (GI) tract, where mucosal damage caused by antineoplastic therapy allows access by opportunistic organisms, and the skin, which can be broken by invasive procedures such as the placement and use of intravenous and central venous access devices. Other possible sites of infection in patients with cancer with BMD include the respiratory tract, genitourinary (GU) tract, central nervous system (CNS), and blood. The risk of infection can be compounded by age, drug dosage, nutritional status, ability to metabolize drug (impaired hepatic/renal function) and concomitant steroid administration. Three key factors are important in predicting the risk of infection for patients with cancer: the degree and duration of granulocytopenia, and the rate at which the absolute granulocyte count (AGC or ANC) drops. The risk of infection increases with a more rapid drop in AGC. The formula for calculating the AGC is described in Table 10A–5. The level of granulocytopenia predicts the patient's risk for infection.

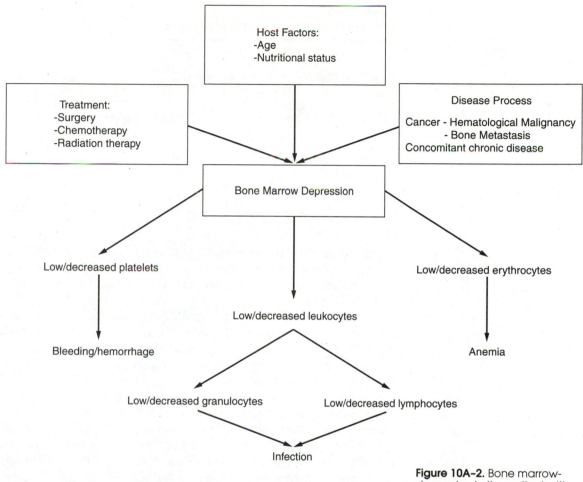

Figure 10A–2. Bone marrow-depression in the patient with cancer

A second major complication of BMD is bleeding as a result of chemotherapy- and RT-induced thrombocytopenia (TCP). TCP is often divided into three levels of suppression, which can help to predict which patients are at greatest risk for bleeding:

Mild TCP	50,000–100,000 platelets/mm^3
Moderate TCP	20,000–50,000 platelets/mm^3
Severe TCP	<20,000 platelets/mm^3

The risk for spontaneous hemorrhage especially in the GI tract and CNS increases greatly when platelets are less than 20,000/mm^3. Other factors also enter into an assessment of the potential for bleeding. These are infection, fever, tumor lysis caused by chemotherapy, splenomegaly, other

Table 10A-5
Calculation of Risk for Granulocytopenia

• Absolute Neutrophil Count (ANC)

$$\frac{\text{Total WBC Count} \times (\% \text{ Segs } + \% \text{ Bands})}{100} = \text{ANC}$$

• Level of Neutropenia	Risk of Infection
>2000 mm/$^\beta$	Not significant
1500–1900 mm/$^\beta$	Minimal
1000–1400 mm/$^\beta$	Moderate
500–900 mm/$^\beta$	Severe
<500 mm/$^\beta$	Life threatening

coagulopathies such as disseminated intravascular coagulation (DIC), and whether the platelet count is falling or rising; as the platelet count rises, the patient is likely to have younger platelets, which are known to be more effective in clotting.

Anemia, a third complication of BMD, is often discounted, because the toxic effects of chemotherapy and RT on erythropoiesis develop more slowly than GCP or TCP because of the longer life span of RBCs. Also, anemia is treated with relative ease with packed red blood cell (PRBC) transfusions and with the administration of erythropoietin. The patient with anemia is usually asymptomatic when the Hgb is above 8 g/100 ml or the Hct is greater than 25 percent; however, other factors such as underlying cardiovascular disease could affect the onset of symptoms. Severe anemia is represented as Hgb less than seven gm/dl or Hct less than 25 percent. The most common type of anemia in cancer patients is hypoproliferative normochromic, normocytic anemia, which can be due to cytotoxic treatment, myelophthesis, or the processes associated with any chronic disease. Anemia can cause or exacerbate fatigue, which has a profound impact on a person's quality of life and functional abilities (see Chapter 8C).

ASSESSMENT

Accurate assessment of patients at risk for BMD is essential to identify risk factors, to educate patient and family, and to plan and implement preventive and therapeutic nursing care. A thorough assessment can contribute to early detection of BMD before the complications related to GCP, TCP, and anemia arise.

When performing a health assessment for the person with cancer, the nurse must be alert to subtle changes that could indicate an impending complication in the bone marrow suppressed patient. For example, headache might be the first sign of an intracranial hemorrhage caused by

TCP, alerting the nurse to assess the patient for other signs of increasing intracranial pressure (see Chapter 15A). In addition, because bleeding due to TCP consists of microvascular bleeding through capillary walls, early clinical evidence can include oozing from mucous membranes or venipuncture sites, or scattered petechiae and ecchymotic areas not associated with trauma. In an elderly patient, hypotension and behavioral changes can be the initial presentation of infection and sepsis. In the absence of adequate circulating granulocytes, infected lesions might not cause pain or produce pus, and fever is an early and often the only sign of infection.

Fever in the patient with GCP is defined as a single oral temperature greater than 38.5° C, a temperature greater than 38° C over at least an hour, or three such temperatures in a 24-hour period. In the patient with an AGC of less than 500/mm^3, a fever must be considered a medical emergency, requiring prompt initiation of antibiotic therapy. It is important that the assessment include an examination of such areas as the oral cavity, pharynx, lungs, intravenous and vascular catheter sites, perineum, and skin surface. Two sets of blood cultures should be taken, including one set from a central venous catheter if present. Other cultures should include urine, sputum, and any open lesions found on physical examination. If diarrhea is present, stool should be tested for *clostridium difficile* as well as for bacterial organisms. In addition, a chest x-ray should be obtained.

After completing a health history and physical examination, the nurse should determine the relative risk for complications of BMD. This risk can be determined by preexisting factors such as a history of antineoplastic treatment, environmental exposures, or health habits; factors such as diabetes or protein-calorie malnutrition; or concurrent factors such as ongoing treatment. The latter category entails a thorough examination of serial laboratory values, including a CBC with differential, platelet count, coagulation studies, and reticulocyte count.

MEDICAL MANAGEMENT

Granulocytopenia

Several levels of protection can be implemented to prevent exposure of the granulocytopenic patient to nosocomial pathogens. Simple protective isolation involves the use of a private room, gowns, gloves, and mask. Protective precautions usually consist of a private room and strict handwashing. The most complete approach is the total protective environment (TPE) of a laminar air-flow room (LAF) with sterilization of all items brought into the room. TPE is expensive, time-consuming, and cumbersome and can be reserved for specific patients undergoing bone marrow transplantation (see Chapter 3A). The evidence is inconclusive as to which of these approaches is most effective, although the depth and expected duration of a patient's GCP could help to determine the most appropriate approach. In general, granulocytopenic patients should be cared for using the most basic precautions: a private room; the use of masks for persons entering the room who have symptoms of an upper respiratory infection, and employed for the patient when out of the room; good handwashing by patient, visitors, and staff; and the removal of all plants or cut flowers from the room. Many institutions use a low-microbial diet for patients with GCP as another method of preventing the introduction of pathogens. This diet usually allows cooked foods only, prohibiting raw fruits and vegetables in order to avoid colonization by such organisms as *E. coli* and pseudomonas, particularly in a patient receiving broad-spectrum antibiotics that can impair the normal flora of the gut. The majority of granulocytopenic infections (more than 80 percent) are attributable to the patient's own flora.

Prophylactic antibiotics (systemic and oral nonabsorbable) can be used in patients with BMD to prevent opportunistic infections such as those caused by the organisms listed in Table 10A–6. Because of the dan-

Table 10A–6
Immune Defects and Associated Infections in Bone Marrow Depression

Immune Defect	Organisms

Cellular immune deficiency	Bacteria
	    Gram-positive
	    Mycobacterium spp., Nocardia asteroides
	    Gram-negative
	    Listeria monocytogenes, Salmonella spp.
	Fungi
	    Cryptococcus neoformans, Histoplasma capsulatum
	Protozoa
	    Pneumocystis carinii, Toxoplasma gondii
	Viruses
	    Cytomegalovirus (CMV), herpes simplex, varicella zoster

Granulocytopenia	Fungi
	    Aspergillus spp., Mucor
	    Candida albicans (yeast)
	Gram-negative bacilli
	    Escherichia coli, Klebsiella pneumoniae, Pseudomonas aeruginosa
	Gram-positive cocci
	    Staphylococcus aureus, Staphylococcus epidermidis

Humoral immune dysfunction	Gram-negative bacteria
	    Hemophilus influenzae
	Gram-positive bacteria
	    Streptococcus pneumoniae

gers of superimposed infection, the emergence of resistant organisms, and the side effects of these drugs—as well as problems with efficacy, cost, and compliance—prophylactic antibiotics are used with caution. Recently, orally administered fluorinated quinolones such as ciprofloxacin, which is well absorbed by the GI tract, have been used with good effect to prevent infection in granulocytopenic patients. However, all prophylactic antibiotic regimens should be used with careful attention to risks and benefits and to nursing practices that reduce the risk of contamination and colonization of the immunocompromised host.

Evidence indicates that administering HGFs (G-CSF and GM-CSF) reduces both the depth and the duration of GCP in cancer patients undergoing antineoplastic therapy. Positive outcomes include measurable reductions in infection rates, antibiotic usage, and hospital lengths of stay. It is recommended that these agents be used prophylactically only in patients who are highly likely to experience severe BMD or with selected protocols/treatments, such as high-dose chemotherapy or bone marrow transplantation, where the BMD is likely to be severe and prolonged.

Empiric antibiotic therapy, usually based on the most likely causative agent, is initiated concurrently with assessment of fever in the granulocytopenic patient, but after cultures are obtained. The initial drug regimen will vary between institutions depending on infection control recommendations, and between patients depending upon individual circumstances (e.g., presence of a central venous catheter, severe mucositis, renal function), but consists of a broad-spectrum intravenous antibiotic regimen at therapeutic dosages. Combinations could include an aminoglycoside (gentamicin, tobramycin) with a third-generation antipseudomonal cephalosporin (ceftazidime) or a combination of these drugs with vancomycin. The latter drug is added if, for example, the patient has a central venous catheter that might be contaminated with gram-positive organisms (coagulase-negative staphylococci) or if methicillin-resistant *S. aureas* is suspected.

After the empiric antibiotic therapy is begun, the results of the various cultures at the onset of fever and the clinical condition of the patient are monitored closely. Based on culture results, antimicrobial therapy can be adjusted to include agents effective against a specific organism, although broad-spectrum therapy should be maintained. In general, it is recommended that antibiotics be continued until follow-up cultures are clear and the clinical condition of the patient indicates lack of infection for at least seven days.

If the patient's fever persists beyond three days while on broad-spectrum coverage, reassessment should occur in an attempt to determine the cause, which could be a nonbacterial organism (fungus, virus), bacterial resistance, a second bacterial infection, or such factors as inadequate serum drug level, a drug fever, or tumor fever. The antibiotic regimen might be altered as a consequence of this reevaluation, or an antifungal agent such as amphotericin B could be added, because up to a third of febrile granulocytopenic patients who do not respond to a week of antibiotics have a systemic fungal infection.

The cessation of antibiotic therapy depends on several factors. When the AGC is greater than 500/mm^3 and the patient has had at least a week of therapy and remains afebrile, antibiotics can be stopped. If the AGC remains less than 500/mm^3 but the patient is clinically well with no signs of infection, the antibiotics can be stopped after seven days and the patient closely observed. If the GCP persists (AGC less than 500/mm^3) and the patient is not clinically well, antibiotics will be continued. If amphotericin B has been initiated and no systemic fungal infection has been definitively established, it is suggested that the drug be continued for two weeks and then stopped. Some patients with persistent GCP may be on antimicrobial therapy much longer than seven to ten days. In this situation, the emergence of resistant organisms and superinfection becomes a serious concern.

Thrombocytopenia

Until recently, the treatment of choice for TCP was platelet transfusion. Three newer HGFs hold promise for treating TCP. Interleukin 11 (oprelvekin (IL 11)), thrombopoietin (TPO), and megakaryocyte growth and development factor (MGDF) have demonstrated clinical thrombopoietic activities. Oprelvekin, approved for use by the FDA in December 1997, stimulates the growth of hematopoietic stem cells in synergy with other hematopoietic growth factors, causes proliferation of megakaryocytic progenitor cells, and induces megakaryocytic maturation. Clinical experience with the use of this newest HGF will yield new approaches to the patient with TCP.

The question of when to initiate platelet transfusions remains unresolved. No definitive study indicating a specific trigger threshold for administering platelet transfusions has been undertaken. In many institutions, platelet transfusions are routinely given for a platelet count of less than 20,000/mm^3. Recently, however, it has been argued that platelet transfusions should be administered not simply on the basis of platelet counts but according to the overall clinical picture, because this therapy is not without its hazards for the patient (febrile reaction, infection, alloimmunization). Some patients might tolerate a platelet count of less than 5,000/mm^3 for prolonged periods, whereas others will experience hemorrhage with a count greater than 20,000/mm^3, particularly in the presence of infection, certain drugs, tumor lysis, and precipitously falling platelet levels.

A second area of controversy relates to the type of platelet product to be administered. In general, random multiple donor platelets (one unit of platelets from each unit of whole blood donated by individual donors) are given, because they are less expensive and readily available. Some researchers argue that alloimmunization to HLA-antigens is a dose-related phenomenon and that for specific patients (leukemia patients undergoing induction therapy, bone marrow transplantation patients) who are certain to require numerous platelet transfusions, single-donor platelets (collected from one donor through apheresis) or even HLA-matched platelets are most appropriate. Use of filters that remove up to 99 percent of leukocytes (the primary source of the antigens causing alloimmunization) have become standard practice as an effective means of forestalling alloimmunization.

The dose of platelets to be given is usually determined according to body weight (or body surface area) at about one unit of platelets per 10 kg of body mass. A normal dose for an adult would be about six units. An increment of approximately $50,000/mm^3$ ($7,000/mm^3$ for each unit) would be expected in the uncomplicated patient. Each patient should be routinely assessed following transfusion by checking the platelet count at specific intervals. A platelet count taken one hour post-transfusion is important in deciding if a patient is becoming refractory to platelets, and a 24-hour post-transfusion platelet count is useful in determining the impact of such factors as splenomegaly, fever, and infection, all of which produce increased consumption of platelets.

Other approaches to the management of TCP include avoidance of drugs that can affect coagulation, such as aspirin and nonsteroidal anti-inflammatory drugs (often found in over-the-counter pain, cold, and flu products); the diagnosis and management of other coagulopathies that could increase the risk of bleeding; the use of intravenous IgG to delay the removal of platelets by the immune system; and the use of aminocaproic acid, a drug that inhibits fibrinolysis and therefore slows thrombocytopenic bleeding.

Anemia

It is important to diagnose the cause of anemia in cancer patients to be certain that it is a treatment-related, normochromic, normocytic anemia. Other types of anemia can be treated by vitamin and mineral supplements or, in the case of anemia due to blood loss, by treating the primary cause. Commonly, the normochromic, normocytic anemia found in patients who have had chemotherapy and RT is not treated unless the patient becomes symptomatic. In the symptomatic patient, the treatment of choice has been transfusion with PRBCs, with the attendant risk of volume overload and infection.

Increasingly, however, due to the risks of multiple transfusions, the HGF erythropoietin is being utilized to prevent as well as treat anemia in patient groups where it is commonly encountered. The success of therapy with EPO depends on the level of endogenous EPO present in a patient's blood. In some cases, it appears that the endogenous EPO response in the anemia of cancer patients, for example, is inadequate to compensate for the level of anemia present. In this situation, the administration of recombinant EPO could effectively address the problem. Where appropriate EPO levels are present, however, additional EPO is usually of little value, and PRBC transfusions will be necessary.

NURSING MANAGEMENT

The nursing management of the patient with BMD is provided in Tables 10A–7 to 10A–10. For each aspect of BMD, overlapping components of nursing management exist. The nurse should take a *preventive* approach to the complications of BMD by performing a thorough initial assessment of the patient and by regular reassessments of the patient. The patient at risk for infection due to GCP should have temperature and vital signs taken on a regular basis and be assessed for other changes in clinical status including signs of local (e.g., perirectal) infection and changes in mental status that could indicate hypoxia or sepsis. The patient at risk for bleeding

Table 10A–7
Nursing Protocol for Prevention and Early Detection of Infection in Patients with Bone Marrow Depression

Problem	Intervention
General guidelines	Assess risk for infection using history and clinical examination. Monitor CBC and differential daily. Teach patient and family how to prevent and detect infection.
Need for protection from environmental risks	Private room is usually indicated. Patients with BMD should not share room with those with known infectious diseases. Restrict visitors and staff with infections. Wash hands meticulously prior to each patient contact. Teach visitors to do the same. Have patient wear mask when appropriate (e.g., when leaving room for any reason). No humidifiers. No cut or potted flowers/plants in room. Low microbial diet (e.g., no fresh fruits or vegetables). Date respiratory equipment and change per institutional policy.
Maintenance of patient's defenses	Encourage good oral hygiene. Use of soft toothbrush, low alcohol mouthwash, use of prophylactic oral antibiotics, antifungals and antivirals. Cleanse high risk sites (e.g., skin folds, perineum) on an established schedule. Lubricate dry areas (artificial tears, skin emollients). Counsel patient regarding well-balanced diet, adequate fluid intake, and importance of rest and sleep. Encourage exercise as tolerated. Turn immobilized patients q 2 hrs and encourage cough and deep breathing. Assist smokers to stop smoking. Avoid invasive procedures including rectal temps, rectal exams, enemas, suppositories, IM or SC injections, urinary catheterizations. If invasive procedures must be performed (e.g., bone marrow biopsy), inspect site periodically for signs of infection. Administer growth factors (G-CSF, GM-CSF) as ordered.
Vascular access	Use appropriate management of peripheral IV therapy (see Chapter 3B).

BMD—bone marrow depression; CBC—complete blood count; IM—intramuscular; IV—intravenous; SC—subcutaneous

Table 10A–8
Nursing Protocol for the Management of Infection in BMD Patients

Problem	Intervention
General guidelines	Implement specific isolation procedures and post on door to patient's room.
	Monitor WBC and differential daily.
	Record temperature and VS q 4 hr or more frequently; for temp >38.5 C, notify physician and implement orders for CXR and cultures. Cultures usually include blood (central and peripheral), throat, sputum, urine, open wounds.
	Observe for signs and symptoms of sepsis. See Chapter 16E.
	Administer antibiotics on time; see that peak and trough levels are drawn if ordered.
	Monitor and report side effects of antimicrobials (e.g., symptoms of nephrotoxicity with aminoglycosides).
	Observe for superinfection (e.g., candidiasis in patient receiving antimicrobials).
	Administer acetaminophen for comfort after cultures have been drawn and antimicrobial therapy initiated.
	Implement other comfort measures as indicated: cooling blanket, ice packs, tepid baths.
	In case of severe rigors, administer meperidine as ordered.
	Increase fluids if not contraindicated.
	If discharged on PO or IV antibiotics, teach patient and family importance of taking each dose, side effects, symptoms of superinfection, guidelines for correct administration (e.g., taking with or without food).
Guidelines for specific sites	
Oral	Inspect oral mucosa q shift. Encourage adherence to mouth care protocol. See Chapter 10B.
Respiratory	Monitor respiratory rate, breath sounds, skin color, presence of cough/sputum production. Assess response to oxygen therapy. See Chapter 14.
Skin	Inspect skin daily. Note and document presence, appearance, and extent of lesions. See Chapter 10C.
GI	Record quantity and quality of stool. Culture stool if GI infection is suspected. Assess bowel sounds. Note and document pain, tenderness, distention. See Chapters 9, 12B.
GU	Record I&O and evaluate fluid balance. Assess characteristics of urine (e.g., color, clarity, odor). Urinary catheter may not be appropriate in neutropenic patient. See Chapter 12C.
CNS	Monitor for changes in mental status. Record neurological vital signs q 4 hr if indicated. Assess patient for symptoms such as neck stiffness and photophobia. See Chapter 11.
Guidelines for specific medical therapies	
Antimicrobials	Note presence of allergies, sensitivities. Assess renal function. Check compatibilities of IV antimicrobials with other IV medications and fluids. Evaluate response to therapy.
Amphotericin B	Mix only in D5W. Test dose usually given. If patient reacts to amphotericin B, obtain premedication orders from physician (may include acetaminophen, diphenhydramine, and hydrocortisone). In case of rigors, meperidine may be given. Amphotericin B is usually ordered in doses that increase in increments from day to day and is administered over 4 to 6 hrs. Assess renal function and serum electrolytes.
Hematopoietic growth factors	Currently only G-CSF and GM-CSF are approved for use in granulocytopenia. May be given either SC or IV. Monitor for possible side effects: bone pain, localized erythema at injection site. Monitor WBC response to therapy.

CXR—chest xray; D5W—5% dextrose/water; I&O—intake & output; SC—subcutaneous; IV—intravenous; PO—by mouth; GI—gastrointestinal; VS—vital signs; WBC—white blood count.

Table 10A–9
Nursing Protocol for the Management of Thrombocytopenia
and Bleeding in BMD Patients

Problem	Intervention
General guidelines	Monitor platelet count daily and administer platelets if prescribed. Be aware of patient-specific requirements (e.g., reaction history, need for premedication, leukocyte filter, pooled vs. single-donor vs. HLA-matched, radiated, CMV negative platelets). Transfusion usually administered over 20–30 minutes unless contraindicated by patient's fluid status. Observe for adverse reactions: chills/rigors, fever, hives. In case of reaction, notify physician and administer diphenhydramine or meperidine as ordered. Platelet infusion is usually continued. Transfusion effectiveness may be assessed with one-hour post-transfusion platelet count if alloimmunization is suspected. Oprelvekin (Neumega® IL-11) may be prescribed for patients to prevent severe thrombocytopenia and reduce the need for platelet transfusions.
Platelets 20,000–50,000/mm^3	Avoid invasive procedures, including rectal temps, enemas, suppositories, IM injections. Post sign in room stating that patient is at risk for bleeding. If invasive procedures (such as lumbar puncture, bone marrow biopsy, arterial blood gas, or surgery) must be performed, physician may request blood bank to have platelets available. Observe site of invasive procedure frequently for signs of bleeding. Apply pressure as necessary. Test urine and stool for occult blood.
Platelets <20,000/mm^3 or >20,000/mm^3 with fever, infection, or other coagulopathy	Perform head to toe, system by system assessment daily for evidence of bleeding. Be sure that IV access is available. See site-specific interventions below.
Site specific Skin	Observe for and record presence of petechiae, bruising, and oozing from openings in the skin. Patients should be instructed to avoid trauma and use electric razor for shaving. Both patient and nurse should be prepared to inform other health care personnel (e.g., float nurses, phlebotomists) of increased risk for bleeding. For incessant oozing (e.g., at Hickman site), topical thromboplastin may be ordered.

CMV—cytomegalovirus; IM—intramuscular

Table 10A-10
Nursing Protocol for the Management of Anemia in BMD Patients

Problem	Intervention
General guidelines	Monitor Hgb and Hct daily or more frequently if active bleeding is suspected. Reticulocyte level may be obtained to assess bone marrow function.
	Assess patient for signs and symptoms of anemia: fatigue, shortness of breath, dizziness, tachycardia, and pallor of skin, mucosa, and conjunctiva.
	Evaluate effect of anemia on patient's quality of life and ability to perform ADL.
	Administer PRBCs if prescribed. RBCs are generally given if patient is symptomatic or Hct <25%. Be aware of patient-specific requirements (e.g., reaction history, need for premedication, leukocyte filter, CMV negative, washed and/or radiated cells).
	Determine patient's ability to tolerate fluid volume and possible need for diuretic before, after, or between units of RBCs.
	Observe for symptoms of transfusion reaction and stop transfusion immediately if present.
	Assist patient and family in developing strategies to cope with fatigue related to anemia (see Chapter 8C):
	• set aside adequate time for rest between activities • be realistic in expectations regarding abilities • modification of roles and responsibilities may be necessary • nutritious diet high in iron, vitamins, and minerals is indicated
	Erythropoietin may be prescribed for patients experiencing chronic anemia (e.g., cisplatin therapy, multiple myeloma, myelodysplastic syndromes).

Hgb—hemoglobin; Hct—hematocrit; ADL—activities of daily living; RBC—red blood cell; PRBCs—packed red blood cells; CMV—cytomegalovirus

due to TCP should be assessed daily (or more often) for the appearance of petechiae on the skin and/or mucosa. In addition, patients with GCP and TCP should be protected from iatrogenic hazards by such measures as infection precautions (protective environments) or prevention of unnecessary invasive procedures (rectal temperatures, intramuscular injections, excessive venipuncture).

Secondly, *prompt* and *knowledgeable* nursing management is necessary to address the complications of BMD effectively. This involves ensuring that appropriate antibiotics are delivered in therapeutic doses to an infected granulocytopenic patient with a minimum of delay, even if it requires pressing other hospital departments to make the medications available as quickly as possible. Familiarity with the platelet products to be transfused and the individual patient's transfusion history allows the nurse to predict the need for premedication to prevent febrile reactions. For the anemic client, effective nursing management could involve the careful administration of PRBCs to a patient at risk for volume overload because of a history of congestive heart failure, or the monitoring of serial reticulocyte counts and Hcts for an anemic client receiving EPO.

Education of patient and family is integrated throughout the preventive and therapeutic nursing management of the client with BMD. Educational efforts should begin prior to the administration of any antineoplastic therapy that could result in BMD. The nurse should instruct the patient at risk for BMD and family members about the signs and symptoms of the complications of BMD and the self-care measures that can be implemented to prevent and recognize these complications. When the patient is actually experiencing a complication of BMD, all therapeutic interventions should be carefully explained to the patient and family if possible before implementation in order to enhance their ability to cope with the uncertainty and threats inherent in such situations.

Summary

The effective multidisciplinary management of the patient at risk for or experiencing BMD remains the responsibility of the nurse. Knowledge of the risks for granulocytopenia, anemia, and thrombocytopenia, thorough assessment of presenting signs/symptoms, prompt therapeutic evaluation and interventions, and a consistent approach to educating patients and families about BMD will ensure appropriate care is instituted.

BIBLIOGRAPHY

1. Brandt, B. Nursing protocol for the patient with neutropenia. *Oncology Nursing Forum* 17(Suppl., January): 9–15. 1990.

   This classic article focuses specifically on the problem of granulocytopenia (neutropenia) in the cancer patient and provides an excellent protocol for nursing care of the granulocytopenic patient.

2. Dean, G., D. Haeuber, and L. Rivera. Management of major clinical nursing problems: Infection. In R. McCorkle, M. Grant, M. Frank-Stromborg and S. Baird, eds. *Cancer Nursing.* 963–978. W. B. Saunders, Philadelphia. 1996.

   This comprehensive chapter offers an overview of infection in the patient with cancer; it includes a thorough discussion of nursing management of BMD.

3. Hays, K. Physiology of normal bone marrow environment. *Seminars in Oncology Nursing* 6(1): 3–8. 1990.

   This is a review of normal bone marrow physiology and bone marrow examination.

4. Higgins, V. L. Leukocyte-reduced blood components: patient benefits and practical applications. *Oncology Nursing Forum* 23(4): 659–667. 1996.

   This review article discusses leukocyte-reduced blood components and nursing implications.

5. Kefer, C., J. Godwin, et al. Blood component therapy. In R. McCorkle, M. Grant, M. Frank-Stromborg and S. Baird, eds. *Cancer Nursing.* 485–503. W. B. Saunders, Philadelphia. 1996.

   This book chapter provides a thorough discussion of blood component therapy and nursing management.

6. Lin, E., and S. M. Beddar. Management of major clinical nursing problems: Abnormalities in hemostasis and hemorrhage. In R. McCorkle, M. Grant, M. Frank-Stromborg and S. Baird, eds. *Cancer Nursing.* 979–1008. W. B. Saunders, Philadelphia. 1996.

   This chapter provides an overview of key concepts in hemostasis and hemorrhage and implications for the patient with cancer.

7. Pavel, J. N. Red blood cell transfusions for anemia. *Seminars in Oncology Nursing* 6(2): 117–122. 1990.

   This offers a good overview of the nursing management of anemia, including a brief review of the biology of RBC compatibility, issues in RBC preparation/storage, and a useful protocol for the administration of RBCs.

8. Pizzo, P. A. Management of fever in patients with cancer and treatment-induced neutropenia. *New England Journal of Medicine* 328: 1323–1332. 1993.

   This article provides a clinical synopsis of managing fever in patients with cancer and granulocytopenia (neutropenia).

9. Rieger, P. T., et al. A new approach to managing chemotherapy-related anemia: nursing implications of Epoetin alfa. *Oncology Nursing Forum* 22(1): 71–81. 1995.

   This article reviews the clinical and scientific implications for the management of chemotherapy related anemia using erythropoietin.

10. Rostad, M. Current strategies for managing myelosuppression in patients with cancer. *Oncology Nursing Forum* 18 (Suppl., March): 7–15. 1991.

    This article provides a useful perspective on the myelosuppression of the cancer patient by categorizing GCP, TCP, and anemia according to three levels of severity, from potential to mild to severe. The author then suggests a range of nursing interventions to be employed depending on the level of BMD encountered.

B. Mucous Membranes

Reidun Juvkam Daeffler

ANATOMY AND PHYSIOLOGY

Mucous membranes line the alimentary canal from the lips to the anus, participating in digestion, absorption of food and fluids, and elimination of residue and waste products. They also serve as a protective barrier to maintain the integrity of the organs.

The mucosal lining consists of layers of epithelial cells and various structures that correlate with the function of different organs or parts of an organ. Mucus, produced by glandular epithelial cells in the mucosa, facilitates movements of the contents of the canal and protects the mucosa from abrasions. The mucosa continuously renews itself; each cell has a life span of 10 to 14 days. The mitotic index is highest in children and young individuals.

Saliva is formed by secretions of the salivary glands and the oral mucosa (Figure 10B–1). It is usually slightly acidic, with a pH of 6.0 to 7.0, and consists of water (97 to 99 percent), mucin, enzymes, and electrolytes. It also contains bacterial and fungal organisms and epithelial cells from the mucosa. Approximately 1,000 ml of saliva are secreted per day, depending on the quantity and quality of food intake and other factors. During regular conditions, about 0.5 ml of saliva is secreted each minute except during sleep, when the secretion becomes very little. Saliva production increases

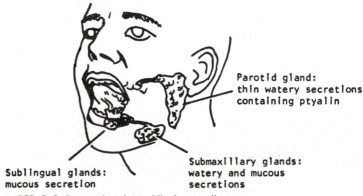

Parotid gland: thin watery secretions containing ptyalin

Sublingual glands: mucous secretion

Submaxillary glands: watery and mucous secretions

Figure 10B-1. Salivary glands and their secretions.

Reprinted with permission from Daeffler, R. Oral hygiene measures for patients with cancer. Cancer Nursing *(October 1980), p. 348.*

with the amount of food taken and with appetizing food. Factors that decrease saliva flow include general decline in health status, depression, stress such as a common cold or surgeries, diabetes, autoimmune disorders, and a variety of medications.

The functions of saliva are as follows:

1. Moistens the food and lubricates the oral cavity, pharynx, and esophagus to facilitate both swallowing and contact between dry food and the taste buds in the tongue.
2. Facilitates speech by lubricating the oral structures.
3. Reduces starches to maltose with the help of the enzyme ptyalin (an amylase).
4. Protects the structures from microbial invasion and dental caries by:
   a. Washing away pathogenic bacteria and food particles that provide their metabolic support;
   b. Destroying microbes by means of components such as thiocyanate ions, proteolytic enzymes, and lysozyme.
   c. Participating in the humoral immune response by means of protein antibodies such as secretory IgA, known to have antiviral properties.

PATHOPHYSIOLOGY

The mucosal tissues in individuals with cancer can be exposed to physical, chemical, and microbial injury. The normal local reaction of tissues to such injury is inflammation, sometimes accompanied by constitutional symptoms, such as fever. Mucosal inflammation can lead to sloughing of the cells, causing the mucosa to become thin, denuded, and ulcerated.

During inflammation, granulocytes constitute a mobile reserve for fighting infection. They destroy bacteria and liquefy cell fragments. When granulocytes are reduced in number or impaired in quality, susceptibility to infection occurs. Patients with granulocyte counts of less than 1,000 cells/mm^3 often develop opportunistic infections—bacterial, fungal, or viral (see Chapter 10A).

The factors most likely to affect mucosal integrity in the cancer patient are (1) the disease itself, (2) antitumor therapies, and (3) nutritional compromise. In the transplant patient, graft-versus-host disease (GVHD) can manifest as mucosal desquamation or oral ulcers. The complex interrelationship of factors that commonly contribute to mucosal alterations is illustrated in Figure 10B-2, which focuses on oral mucositis. The terms *stomatitis* and *oral mucositis* are used interchangeably here, although some writers distinguish between the two: *mucositis* refers to the mucosal reaction to systemic chemotherapeutic agents; *stomatitis* is sometimes referred to as an oral mucosal reaction to local factors such as trauma, while others define it simply as inflammation (mucositis) of the oral cavity.

10B

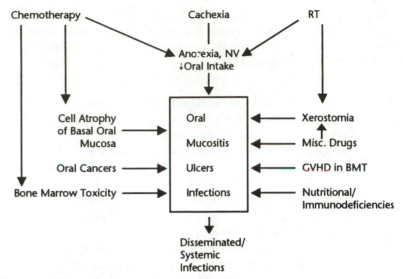

Figure 10B-2. Factors contributing to oral mucositis in cancer.

This chapter addresses oral, pharyngeal, and esophageal mucositis, as well as rectal inflammation and abscess. Oral mucositis will receive most attention, partly because the visible oral mucosa serves as a "window" to the mucous membranes of the gastrointestinal (GI) tract.

Chemotherapy

Cytotoxic drugs affect the mucosa directly through toxic effects on rapidly dividing tissues and indirectly by myelosuppression, increasing the susceptibility to infections and bleeding.

Oral mucositis is a direct consequence of damage to the dividing cells in the basal epithelial layers of the oral mucosa, which inhibits replacement of the superficial layer of cells. It occurs in about 40 percent of patients receiving chemotherapy, depending upon the type of drug administered, dosage, administration schedule, drug metabolism, rescue capability, and use of colony stimulating factors. The incidence of oral mucositis in bone marrow transplantation has been reported as high as 100% (see Chapter 3A). Cytotoxic drugs causing mucositis are listed in Table 10B–1. Mucositis can become a dose-limiting side effect; that is, the desired therapeutic dose might need to be reduced because of mucositis.

The incidence of mucositis can vary with administration schedule. It has been shown to increase with rapid infusion of high-dose fluorouracil. Doxorubicin administered over three consecutive days leads to a greater incidence and severity of mucositis.

Table 10B-1
Stomatotoxic Chemotherapeutic Agents

Classification	Drug	Comment
Antimetabolites	Cytarabine	High dose
	Fludarabine	
	Fluorouracil	Common
	Floxuridine	
	Hydroxyurea	
	Mercaptopurine	High dose
	Methotrexate	
	Thioguanine	
Plant alkaloids	Docetaxel	
	Etoposide	High dose: Severe
	Paclitaxel	
	Teniposide	
	Topotecan	Rare
	Vinblastine	
	Vincristine	
	Vinorelbine	
Alkylating agents	Busulfan	High dose
	Lomustine	
	Mechlorethamine	
	Melphalan	High dose
	Thiotepa	High dose only
Antitumor antibiotics	Bleomycin	
	Dactinomycin	Common
	Daunorubicin	
	Doxorubicin	Common. Severe with high dose
	Idarubicin	
	Mitomycin	
	Plicamycin	
Nitrosureas	Lomustine	
Miscellaneous	Mitoxantrone	
	Procarbazine	

The incidence of mucositis (and other side effects) is increased if a person cannot adequately metabolize or excrete certain chemotherapeutic agents. For example, the metabolism of doxorubicin depends on liver function. The body's ability to excrete methotrexate is decreased with renal compromise (i.e., elevated BUN and creatinine). The risk of mucositis is decreased by administering folinic acid (citrovorum factor, leucovorin) after methotrexate.

Infection is an indirect effect of chemotherapy, because cytotoxic therapy can induce granulocytopenia (see Chapter 10A). When the patient's natural barriers to infection are affected, organisms of even low virulence have a readily accessible port of entry. Preexisting periodontal and dental disease are reservoirs for hematogenous seeding of infection. The loss of an intact epithelial barrier in the mouth and in the rectum, which tend to be heavily colonized by normal flora, makes an easy entrance for systemic infection in the immunocompromised patient. Early diagnosis of oral infections is important for appropriate treatment to prevent systemic spread.

Viral mucosal infections are commonly caused by reactivation of herpes simplex virus (HSV) in the immunocompromised patient. Systemic treatment is preferable to topical application, because the virus is likely to spread locally and systemically. Effective therapy is available in acyclovir. Because viral mucositis is indistinguishable from noninfectious mucositis, these infections can go undiagnosed until secondary bacterial infections develop as a result of the mucosal breakdown. Prophylactic acyclovir can be administered to prevent HSV reactivation in immunocompromised patients. Staff or family members with active HSV infection should not have physical contact with these patients (see Chapter 10C).

Fungal invasion with candida is frequent when the mucosa is impaired in immunocompromised patients. Patients receiving long-term antimicrobial therapy against gram-negative bacilli are at increased risk for infection with candida (as well as gram-positive cocci). Candida infections can be treated locally or systemically (see Table 10B–2). Systemic fungal infections have become a leading cause of death from infection in neutropenic patients. Prevention of infection in high-risk patients can include oral ketoconazole or fluconazole. Standard treatment is fluconazole or amphotericin B (intravenous). A new liposomal amphotericin B (Abelcet®) is indicated for systemic fungal infections in patients who are refractory to or intolerant of conventional amphotericin.

Bacterial infections can be primary or superinfections originating in periodontal disease. Exacerbation of gingival infections can manifest in vague, poorly localized jaw pain, followed by bleeding and ulceration. Upon laboratory diagnosis, bacterial stomatitis can be treated successfully with antibiotics.

Thrombocytopenia occurs in association with chemotherapy-induced myelosuppression and can cause severe bleeding from mucosal surfaces. Platelet counts less than 50,000 platelets/mm^3 predispose to bleeding as a result of invasive procedures or local trauma; spontaneous oral or GI bleeding can occur when the platelet count is less than 20,000 platelets/mm^3. The risk of gingival bleeding and infection increases when meticulous hygiene is not maintained and the mucosa becomes dry and friable. Regardless of whether the patient is thrombocytopenic, gingival bleeding can indicate an underlying herpes infection.

Tables 10B–3 and 10B–4 serve as a guide in planning the care of persons at risk for mucositis after chemotherapy.

Table 10B-2
Treatment of Oral Mucositis*

Indication	Product	Administration**	Nursing Implications
Dry mouth & throat; decreased saliva	Saliva substitutes (OTC) Glandosane® MoiStir® MouthKote® OraLube® Salivart® XeroLube®	Swish 5–15 ml in a clean oral cavity; swallow or discard or apply with a swab. Administer prn.	"Synthetic saliva" consists mostly of sorbitol and carboxymethylcellulose in aqueous solution; no known side effects. Dispenser/spray bottles allow patient to squirt small amount directly into mouth. Premoistened swabs allow for easy application (e.g. MoiStir® Oral Swabsticks).
	Oralbalance Moisturizing Gel™ (OTC)	Apply $\frac{1}{2}$ inch from tube onto affected area; gently massage on gums.	Recommended by manufacturer for xerostomia, mouth breathers, ventilated patients, and denture wearers for 8 hrs of relief. Apply underneath dentures to improve retention.
	Pilocarpine tablets Solagen®	2.5–7.5 mg three times/day for prevention/ management of radiation-induced xerostomia.	Stimulates salivary glands; ineffective if salivary glands completely destroyed by RT. Therapeutic effect to be expected within 3 weeks. Sweating is the most common side effect. For contraindications, refer to drug information.
	Fluoride gel (carrier/mold/ tray/mouthguard)	Apply per dentist's directions (usually 10 minutes/day).	Effective to prevent xerostomia-associated caries in patients receiving high-dose radiation to salivary glands.
Oral Mucositis; "Sore Mouth"	Sucralfate oral suspension	Swish, swirl, and swallow/discard 15 ml every 6 hours.	Coats and protects the mucosa. Apply after other local agents to avoid blocking their effect.
	Diphen-hydramine Benadryl® elixir	Swish 5–10 ml for 2 min, gargle and discard; swallow for throat discomfort.	Used alone or in combination with local anesthetics and antimicrobials. Also used to treat motion sickness, allergic reactions, extrapyramidal reactions. May cause sedation, dizziness, or hypotension, especially in older patients.
	Kaopectate®	Mix 10 ml with pain reliever (below) to coat mucosa and keep analgesic in place.	Will decrease digoxin absorption by up to 30%; avoid within 1–2 hrs of digoxin administration.
	Mouthwash without alcohol Biotene® (OTC)	Swish oral cavity every hour prn, or swab throughout mouth.	Contains antibacterial enzymes. May dilute with water.

Continued

Table 10B–2 *(Continued)*
Treatment of Oral Mucositis*

Indication	Product	Administration**	Nursing Implications
Pain with oral mucosal lesions	Zilactin® or Zilactin®-B (Available in tubes or single packs OTC)	Apply a thin coat on dried affected mucosa; allow to dry 60 seconds.	Zilactin®-B contains 10% benzocaine. May cause a stinging sensation on first application. Forms a thin film, clear on dry skin/lips, white on moist mucosa. Claims protection 5–6 hrs, allowing food and fluid intake.
	Dyclonine 0.5%	Swish and discard 5–15 ml; may swallow for esophageal effect.	Topical anesthetic; reduces the gag reflex. Potential systemic absorption could result in CNS changes, especially in debilitated patients. Daily dose limited per MD order.
	Systemic liquid analgesics Tylenol® Lortab® elixir (acetaminophen & hydrocodone) NSAIDs	Swish and swallow for *possible* local and systemic analgesic effect.	Consider dose limitations for each drug.
	20% benzocaine topical anesthetic available in a gel and a liquid Hurricane® (OTC)	Apply to affected oral mucosa PRN.	Comes in a variety of packages, including spray, individual packages, tube, and a "dry handle applicator". Some varieties are flavored (cherry, pı̆na colada, natural). Onset 30 seconds; duration 15 minutes. Low systemic absorption.
	Oratect gel (OTC)	Use rayon swabs provided in the package to dry affected area and apply gel. Allow to dry 30–60 seconds.	Manufacturer proclaims long-lasting adhesion uncompromised by food and hot or cold beverages. Contains 15% benzocaine in hydroxypropylcellulose.
	Ulcerease® (OTC)	Swish and swallow every 2 hrs prn.	Alcohol-free buffering anesthetic.
	"Miracle Mouthwash"	Swish, gargle and swallow PRN	Nystatin,® Benadryl® Elixir, tetracycline, and hydrocortisone mixed in hospital pharmacies.
Lip lesions, cold sores, fever blisters	Zilactin®-L (OTC)	Apply a thin coat to dry affected areas of lips/skin; allow to dry 60 sec.	Non–film-forming version of Zilactin intended for extraoral use. Viricidal potential appropriate for herpes lesions. Contains 2.5% lidocaine.

Table 10B-2 (Continued)
Treatment of Oral Mucositis*

Indication	Product	Administration**	Nursing Implications
Candidiasis and other fungal infections, oral or esophageal	Fluconazole	One 100–200 mg tablet daily for 2–3 weeks	Same as ketoconazole (see following).
	Itraconazole oral solution	Vigorously swish and swallow 10–20 ml (100–200 mg) daily for a minimum of 3 weeks, or 2 weeks following resolution of symptoms.	Most effective when taken on empty stomach. Monitor liver enzymes. Refer to product insert for list of drug interactions.
	Ketoconazole	Systemic administration: 200 mg daily for 1–2 weeks.	Systemic therapy may offer improved efficacy, compliance, and better protection against systemic candidiasis, as compared to topical agents. Hepatic monitoring indicated. Effective in treating oral thrush.
	Clotrimazole or miconazole nitrate cream	Apply thin layer on oral mucosa.	This tasteless, odorless vaginal cream has been found soothing for inflamed oral tissues.
	Clotrimazole troches	Dissolve 10 mg lozenge slowly in mouth (5 troches/day for 2 weeks). May alternate with nystatin suspension every 4 hrs.	Same as for nystatin tablet following. May be ineffective in xerostomia.
	Nystatin suspension	Swish 500,000 U every 4–6 hrs; keep in mouth for 5 min, then discard/ swallow for esophageal application.	NPO for 20 min after application. Contains sucrose and may promote caries.
	Nystatin pastilles	Dissolve slowly in mouth every 6 hrs.	Use only for patients who understand instructions for administration and are able to keep troche in mouth until dissolved. Also available in tablet, cream, or ointment.
Herpes simplex viral infection	Acyclovir capsules 200/400/800 mg	Systemic administration of up to 1–2 gm daily.	Systemic therapy preferable to topical due to risk of viral spread. Also available in oral suspension 200 mg/5 ml.

BMT—bone marrow transplant; CNS—central nervous system; OTC—over-the-counter; NPO—nothing by mouth

* Prophylaxis of bacterial infections in BMT not included.

** All topical agents should be applied to clean mucosa, followed by NPO for 15–30 minutes.

Table 10B-3
Nursing Protocol for Patients at Risk for Oral Mucositis

Problem	Intervention
Potential oral mucositis related to cancer therapy	Assess oral mucosa and document baseline condition (see Figure 10B–3).
	Initiate dental referral for preexisting disease.
	Instruct patient/ significant other and evaluate outcome of instructions:
	Potential/ expected oral complications of particular treatment regimen.
	Daily oral self-exam:
	• Wash hands.
	• Use mirror and note changes from normal oral mucosa and lips.
	• Report signs and symptoms of mucositis: dryness, burning, redness, small white or yellow lesions, difficulty swallowing, swelling of gums or tongue, coating, ulcerations, blisters.
	Oral hygiene program:
	• Floss teeth daily with nontraumatic dental tape.
	• Brush teeth with soft toothbrush, using a sweeping motion from the gum toward the crown, cleaning back and front surfaces. Use horizontal motion for top surfaces of teeth.
	• Remove any prostheses during the procedure; brush, clean, and store in clean water.
	• Cleanse oral cavity after meals, at bedtime, or more frequently; vigorously rinse the mouth by swishing; use plain water, mild salt water, or a dilution of a mild mouthwash in water.
	Avoid irritating agents: commercial mouthwash containing phenol, astringents, or alcohol; harsh toothpaste; hot or spicy foods/beverages; alcohol; tobacco; poor fitting dentures; lemon-glycerin; hard candy.
Xerostomia	Oral care as above. Include oral care before meals.
	Select soft, moist foods with sauces and gravies; avoiding dry, coarse foods.
	Fluid intake as tolerated; sip frequently throughout the day.
	Apply saliva substitute prn (see Table 10B–2).
	Consider Salagen® tablet TID.
	Increase air moisture by means of humidifier or vaporizer PRN (attention to cleanliness). Consider Biotene® or other sugar-free gum.
Thick, sticky saliva	Rinse mouth with sodium bicarbonate, $\frac{1}{2}$–1 tsp. per pint of water to dissolve mucus.
	Add moisture by means of popsicles, ice chips, saliva substitutes, frequent sips of water.
Indwelling endotracheal or nasogastric tube	Apply a coating agent (Zilactin®, Oralbalance™, or sucralfate) to protect mucosa (see Table 10B–2).
	Oral hygiene TID. and at bedtime.

Table 10B-4
Timetable for Development of Chemotherapy-Induced Mucositis

Time After Treatment	Effect	Comment
5–7 days	Histologic changes: drug interference with cell division and maturation.	
7–14 days (less in children or 3–5 days prior to drop in granulocyte count	Erythema, most frequently in the soft palate, buccal mucosa, tongue, and floor of the mouth. Ulcerations most often <5 mm, multiple, and superficial. Oral ulcerations resulting from minor trauma.	Most severe mucositis prior to granulocyte nadir. Oral pain begins an average of 14 days into chemotherapy; can precede visible mucositis. Patients with ulcerations may not experience more pain than those with erythema alone.
21 days, beginning with resumption of basal cell mitotic activity and granulocyte recovery	Resolution of mucositis.	Oral ulcers lasting after granulocyte recovery could have other causes, such as GVHD in allogeneic transplants, or unusual infection with virulent microbes.

GVHD—graft versus host disease

Biologicals

Mucositis is a side-effect of some of the more commonly used biologic response modifiers (BRMs), such as interleukin 2 and interferons. It is also observed after administration of tumor necrosis factor (TNF) and lymphocyte activated killer cells (LAK). The exact pathophysiology is not known (see Chapter 2D).

Radiation Therapy

Injury to surrounding mucous membranes during radiation therapy (RT) for oral cancer can result in xerostomia, dental decay, decreased oral intake, and mucositis and predispose the person to infection and bleeding (see Chapter 2B). Xerostomia alone presents a threat to the patient's quality of life, causing difficulties in speaking, chewing, and swallowing, and diminished enjoyment of food and social functions. Osteoradionecrosis and trismus are serious late effects of RT to the head and neck.

Xerostomia (dryness of the mouth caused by decrease or loss of salivary secretions) occurs when the major salivary glands are radiated (see Figure 10B–1). It is related to dose and frequency of treatment and usually starts during the first or second week of treatment. Although radiation-induced xerostomia might be irreversible, some patients report subjective improvements in mouth dryness in the months and years after therapy.

Without the cleansing and lubricating functions of saliva, the risk for gingival bleeding and infection increases (see Table 10B–3).

Oral mucositis is seen within the first two weeks of RT to the head and neck and is related to the dose and the duration of treatment. Early signs include dryness, progressing to irritative hyperemia and edema, with the mucosa appearing red and swollen. As treatment continues, the mucosa can become denuded, ulcerated, and covered with a fibrinous exudate. This condition usually persists until two to four weeks after the last treatment, when the normal healing process begins, unless it is complicated by secondary infection.

Osteoradionecrosis can occur at the site of radiation beginning two months after therapy is completed. Necrotic ulcers develop because of fibrosis and impaired blood supply caused by the RT. These extremely painful ulcers are precipitated by trauma and are slow to heal and likely to expand.

Radiation-induced enteritis can occur any time following high-dose GI radiation. It could present as chronic diarrhea or as a bowel obstruction and result in bowel ulceration, stricture, or fistula formation. Chronic or late radiation changes include vascular thrombosis, submucosal fibrosis, necrosis, and ulceration, and obstruction or perforation can result.

Radiation recall is a reactivation of a previous epithelial radiation effect when chemotherapeutic drugs are given soon after RT. Such radiation recall can occur in the radiation field—for example skin or esophagus—upon administration of methotrexate, bleomycin, cyclophosphamide, or fluorouracil, but is most commonly caused by doxorubicin and dactinomycin.

Nutritional Status

Lack of nutrients can precipitate a nutritional-deficiency stomatitis. Nutritional deficiencies are common in cancer patients, arising from a combination of such factors as (1) anorexia caused by malignancy, RT, or chemotherapy; (2) dryness or soreness of the mouth; (3) dysphagia; (4) taste alteration/loss after chemotherapy/RT; (5) surgical procedures; (6) nausea/vomiting; (7) malabsorption; (8) GI obstruction; (9) fatigue; and (10) depression.

The condition of the mucosal membranes and nutritional status are interdependent. Malnutrition slows the growth of epithelial tissue, delays healing of local ulcerations, and increases susceptibility to infection. Figure 10B–2 illustrates some of these interrelationships. Further details are discussed in Chapter 9.

Primary Malignancies

Cancerous growths can involve the mucosa directly, causing changes in functions, inflammation, tissue sloughing, necrosis, and ulceration. Examples are (1) leukemic gingivitis and leukemic infiltrates, common in acute monocytic leukemia (leukemic infiltrates of tonsils can mimic infectious disease); (2) intestinal tumor causing partial-to-complete bowel obstruction; (3) colorectal cancer causing diarrhea and constipation; (4) leukoplakia, a painless, precancerous lesion easily confused with oral candidiasis, appearing as a grayish hyperkeratosis that can only be removed by tearing; and (5) salivary gland tumor, most commonly found in the parotid gland.

ASSESSMENT

Oral Cavity

A baseline oral assessment of all patients prior to cancer treatment should include:

1. The presenting condition of the oral cavity;
2. Identification of problems that should be dealt with prior to treatment;
3. Oral hygiene practices, personal attitudes, and knowledge of oral health and techniques;
4. Predisposing factors—denture wearers and patients with a history of oral lesions might develop mucositis sooner than average; smokers have a higher incidence of mucositis;
5. Age—reduced rate of tissue repair with increasing age;
6. Type of cancer—increased incidence of mucositis with hematologic cancers (leukemias, lymphomas) over solid tumors;
7. Treatment-related factors—chemotherapy plus radiation poses a higher risk than chemotherapy alone; total body irradiation (TBI) increases the risk of mucositis in transplant patients;
8. Drug and dose (see Table 10 B–1).

This assessment serves as a basis for an individualized teaching plan and for monitoring changes that occur over the course of treatment.

Because of the number of stressors that affect the oral mucosa, a systematic assessment should take place upon admission to a health care institution. To increase validity and reliability of documentation, a standardized assessment form should be used. Figure 10B–3 lists a selection of published assessment forms used to describe oral mucositis. Basic tools for such assessment include a tongue blade and a flashlight. Outpatients are instructed to assess themselves daily in front of a mirror with good light. They are informed that oral pain could be a late symptom of stomatitis, so visual examination is necessary for early detection.

Frequent and astute assessment facilitates early detection of infection. In the immunocompromised patient, the usual signs and symptoms

I   World Health Organization (WHO) Grading of Mucositis:
     0 = No side effects
     1 = Sore mouth; no ulcers
     2 = Sore mouth with ulcers; able to eat solids
     3 = Able to eat liquids only
     4 = Unable to eat and drink
     Several varieties of the 0–4 grading index have been published. One 0–4 grading is included in the toxicity criteria for NCI sponsored clinical trials. Some of these grading scales include more detailed descriptions of mucosal changes. The advantage of these scales is simplicity and ease of application. They are too limited to differentiate well between varieties in oral condition.

II   Oral Assessment Guide (OAG)
     • Eight categories reflecting oral health and function are given a score from 1 (normal) to 3 (2 and 3 representing problems)
     • Developed and tested at the University of Nebraska Medical Center. Interrater reliability reported as 91%.
     • Available as an attractive color chart from Halbrand's Educational Services Department, P.O. Box 272, Willoughby, OH 44094.

III Oral Cavity Assessment Form
     • Numerical ratings from 1–4 are assigned to each of five categories (lips, tongue, oral mucosa, teeth/dentures, saliva), resulting in total scores representing mild (6–10), moderate (11–15) and severe (16–20) dysfunction.
     • Available as a laminated card from Sage Products, Inc., 680 Industrial Drive, Cary, IL 60013.

IV   Visual Analogue Scale
         Directions: Make a mark on this line representing degree of oral mucositis from normal to worst possible.

     |——|

     Normal, healthy   Worst possible
     oral mucosa   oral condition

         A *numerical value* is obtained by measuring the distance from the left to right (0–10 centimeters)

         This scale can easily be modified for the patient's subjective report on oral pain, providing a subjective measure in addition to the nurses' numerical assessment.

Figure 10B–3. Oral assessment tools.

of infection might be lacking, because the inflammatory process is delayed or reduced (see Chapter 10A). Mucosal changes can occur before the patient complains of discomfort. Appearance of the mucosa could be very similar in bacterial, fungal, and viral infections, so lesions should be cultured as early as possible. Viral, fungal, aerobic, and anaerobic cultures could be necessary diagnostic tools for initiating appropriate antimicrobial treatment. However, the presence of candida in itself may not confirm candidiasis; about 50 percent of the general population show candida in oral cultures.

Esophagus

When mucositis extends from the oral mucosa to the esophagus, the patient might experience additional symptoms calling for special interventions. Early symptoms of esophagitis are difficulty in swallowing solid foods, a "lump" in the throat, and pain in swallowing. Progression can lead to severe substernal pain.

Assessment of dysphagia includes the three phases of swallowing:

1. Oral—the patient's ability to move the tongue, keep lips closed, and make a sucking movement with lips and cheek. These movements are necessary to chew and move food to the posterior tongue.
2. Pharyngeal—the patient's ability to elevate the larynx.
3. Esophageal—the patient's ability to move food into the stomach.

Rectal Area

Because the rectal area is less accessible for observation than the oral cavity, patient cooperation in assessment is especially important. The patient is taught to report signs and symptoms of infection and bleeding, including rectal and perineal pain, bleeding, itching and burning, and urinary burning and frequency.

Visual inspection of the rectal area is part of the nursing assessment in the immunocompromised patient. Perianal herpes is frequently misdiagnosed as pressure sores. Perianal abscess is suspected when the temperature is elevated more than 1 degree centigrade for more than 24 hours and when the patient experiences rectal pain. The usual signs of inflammation may be reduced or absent in the immunosuppressed patient, especially while being treated with corticosteroids and other anti-inflammatory agents.

MANAGEMENT

A healthy oral and GI mucosa is essential for emotional expression, verbal communication, comfort, nutrition, elimination, and fluid/electrolyte balance. Attention to oral health is considered a necessity in oncology, because mucositis threatens continuation of life-saving therapy, and lack of attention can allow life-threatening infections to develop.

Systematic oral hygiene protocols have been shown to reduce the incidence of oral mucositis from cancer chemotherapy. Such measures can also reduce the severity of mucositis and the incidence of life-threatening infections. Preexisting periodontal disease, as well as poor oral hygiene,

Table 10B-5
Nursing Protocol for Management of Oral Mucositis

Problem	Intervention
Impaired oral mucous membranes	Cleanse oral cavity every 4 hours, selecting a mouthwash based on specific condition: NS as a basic mouthwash; sterile if WBC less than 1,000 mm^3. Use after sodium bicarbonate or alone. Sodium bicarbonate $\frac{1}{2}$ tsp in 1 cup H$_2$O or NS to dissolve thick saliva. Avoid commercial mouthwash containing alcohol, phenol, astringents.
Inability to swish/swallow	Prevent aspiration: use side-lying or sitting position over sink or basin; use tonsil-tip suction or suction Ora-Swab® (Sage): Irrigate oral cavity using cleansing device (irrigation bag with tubing or atomizer with nozzle/tip), avoid high pressure. Remove debris using moistened foam stick (e.g., Ora-Swab® without dentifrice), soft toothbrush (e.g., Oral B® 35) or prepacked moist swabstick (e.g., MoiStir®).
Dry, cracked, or ulcerated lips	Keep lips moist with lubricating jelly or water-soluble moisturizer. Gently cleanse cracked or ulcerated lips every 2 hours with 4x4 gauze pads and NS. If lips are encrusted, may prewash with sodium bicarbonate, then NS. Pat dry and apply moisturizer.
Discomfort/pain	Select appropriate pain reliever (see Table 10B-5) in consultation with physician. For severe discomfort, use of parenteral drugs (e.g., morphine by continuous IV drip) may be necessary. Use swish and discard method if frequent local anesthetic is required. Avoid hot, acidic, coarse, spicy, and fried foods; citrus juices; and fruits. Try soft, coating foods, e.g., yogurt, sour cream, cottage cheese.
Impaired verbal communication due to increased or thickened saliva	Provide tonsil-tip suction set-up and instruct patient in suctioning technique. Rinse mouth with sodium bicarbonate solution to dissolve mucus (1 tsp in 500 ml NS or water); postrinse with NS. Respond promptly and in person to patient's call.

Potential for infection due to neutropenia

General hygiene (see Chapter 10A)	Maintain clean environment; hand-washing, care of cleaning devices, care of eating utensils. Prepare food carefully: avoid raw fruits, eggs, and vegetables; foods of questionable origin. Use sterile NS.

Table 10B–5 *(Continued)*
Nursing Protocol for Management of Oral Mucositis

Problem	Intervention
	Use individually wrapped foam sticks and discard after use. Avoid damage to mucosa: commercial mouthwashes or dentifrice, tobacco, hot food/beverages, alcohol, spicy foods, poorly fitting dentures; gently use soft toothbrush and dental tape.
Teaching of patient	Assess patient understanding of oral hygiene program and reinforce teaching as needed. Teach signs and symptoms of infection: pain, white patches, encrustation, ulcerations, coated areas, swelling.
Early detection	Assess patient's oral cavity daily using an oral assessment chart or grading (Figure 10B–3). Report signs and symptoms of infection to physician promptly. Culture oral mucosa when signs are present.
Infection of oral mucosa	Administer appropriate medication per physician order. Provide oral care prior to local administration of medication. Avoid mouthwash and oral intake for 20 min after medication to allow for effect. If patient intolerant of medication: try alternative method of administration (e.g., freeze in desired liquid and serve as popsicle); encourage patient and emphasize importance of treatment. Maintain anti-infection protocol. Measure vital signs every 2–4 hrs. Report abnormal findings promptly.
Oral bleeding	Promptly notify physician and assist: platelet infusion; topical thrombin (e.g., 5,000 units mixed in diluent, then in 50 ml NS to swab area of bleeding, repeating every 4 hrs or PRN for active bleeding).

H_2O_2—hydrogen peroxide; H_2O—water; NS—normal saline; WBC—white blood count

predisposes the patient to oral complications of cancer treatment, including gingival bleeding in those with thrombocytopenia. The purpose of oral care in cancer patients is to:

1. Prevent infections and periodontal disease;
2. Prevent gingival bleeding;
3. Improve the patient's feeling of well-being and quality of life;
4. Maintain/improve the nutritional function of the oral cavity;
5. Prevent further damage to oral structures; and
6. Reduce oral complications to allow for completion of the treatment plan.

The ideal approach to the management of oral complications of chemotherapy and RT is interdisciplinary, combining the expertise of dentists, nutritionists, oral surgeons, and infectious disease physicians with those of medical oncologists, radiation oncologists, and nurses. Management of oral infections uses this multidisciplinary approach in the high risk patient:

1. Pre-treatment dental evaluation with attention to potentially irritating teeth surfaces, underlying gingivitis, periodontal infection, and ill-fitting dentures;
2. Patient education to keep the oral cavity clean, moist, and intact and to prevent further damage to the mucosa during myelosuppressive therapy (see Table 10B–3);
3. Routine oral assessment for early diagnosis of complications;
4. Management of complications: symptomatic treatment (Tables 10B–2 and 10B–5); antimicrobial treatment (Table 10B–2).

Although there is reasonable agreement on the value of systematic oral care protocols, there is little consistency regarding agents to use. Several interventions have been tested, but no cleansing agent has been proven superior in randomized comparative studies. Granulocyte-macrophage colony stimulating factor (GM-CSF) has been shown to reduce the severity and duration of chemotherapy-induced oral mucositis. Recent evaluations

Table 10B–6
Nursing Protocol for Patients at Risk for Perirectal Infection

Problem	Intervention
Potential for rectal infection/abscess related to • neutropenia less than 1,000 mm^3 • cytotoxic chemotherapy • radiation therapy to perirectal area • steroid drugs	Assess patient's personal hygiene practices and instruct/assist as needed: • Clean perineal/perianal area after each bowel movement and PRN to a minimum of BID, using a mild soap, tepid water; rinse thoroughly and carefully; pat dry with soft cloth. • Wear clean, soft undergarments, washed with mild detergent and rinsed well. • Wash hands after procedure. Teach patient to report rectal or perineal pain, bleeding, itching, burning, urinary burning or frequency. Prevent rectal injury by avoiding enemas and suppositories, rectal thermometers, sharp fingernails. Place on prophylactic bowel regimen to avoid constipation (see Chapter 12B). Maintain integrity of perianal skin: • Avoid rubbing, scratching, or massaging area • Avoid tight clothing and medications and other chemical products • Protect irritated skin with protective barrier cream. Use sitz baths for rectal irritation after bowel movement, observing meticulous clean technique. Culture any ulcer or sign of infection.

of GM-CSF mouthwash for prevention have not demonstrated any additional benefits. Oral cryotherapy has been evaluated with inconclusive results; this treatment requires local application of ice chips to the entire oral cavity for 5 minutes prior and 30 minutes after chemotherapy; its usefulness is limited to intravenous bolus administration. Prophylaxis with local antioxidants is being studied with mixed results; topical Vitamin E has shown some promise. A pilot study showed that swish and swallow of a glutamine suspension decreased the severity of chemotherapy-induced mucositis; glutamine is an amino acid that appears to be the major energy source for intestinal epithelium. Capsaicin, the active ingredient in chili peppers, has shown promise in reducing oral mucosal pain.

Nursing protocols for the care of the patient with potential or actual alterations in mucous membranes are presented in Tables 10B–3, 10B–5, and 10B-6. Selection of tools, schedule, agents, and teaching methods should be based on the identified problem, degree of risk, and the patient's response to the interventions.

BIBLIOGRAPHY

1. Allison, R. R. et al. Symptomatic acute mucositis can be minimized or prophylaxed by the combination of sucralfate and fluconazole. *Cancer Investigation* 13: 16–22. 1995.

   The combination of sucralfate and fluconazole was prescribed to 40 patients. Half received sucralfate suspension from the first week through the completion of radiation therapy and fluconazole from the fourth week. The other half were given both drugs simultaneously after the symptoms appeared. Both cohorts experienced diminished oral pain and discomfort. Prophylactic sucralfate allowed completion of the prescribed radiation dose in all patients.

2. Blom, M. et al. Acupuncture treatment of patients with radiation-induced xerostomia. *European Journal of Cancer, Part B, Oral Oncology* 32(May): 182–190. 1996.

   In this Swedish study 20 patients with radiation-induced xerostomia received classical acupuncture twice a week for a total of 12 weeks. The patients were randomized to the experimental (acupuncture) group or a control group of 18 participants receiving "superficial acupuncture." Salivary flow was measured at intervals for one year after treatment. Salivary flow increased in both groups. Some of the patients had received radiation therapy several years earlier. The authors point out that acupuncture may give positive effects only when the function of the salivary glands has been disturbed but not completely destroyed. The report also describes factors influencing changes in salivary flow, including chemotherapy, surgery, stress, depression, the common cold, new medications, and metastases.

3. Dodd, M. J., et al. Randomized clinical trial of chlorhexidine versus placebo for prevention of oral mucositis in patients receiving chemotherapy. *Oncol Nurs Forum* 23: 921–927. 1996.

   Data from this study suggest that the use of a systematic oral hygiene program may reduce the incidence of chemotherapy-induced mucositis from an esti-

mated 44 percent to 26 percent. The program tested in this study was a nurse-initiated oral hygiene teaching program (PSMA). The researchers compared chlorhexidine mouthwash with water and concluded that water was just as effective as the more expensive chlorhexidine.

4. Ganley, B. J. Mouth care for the patient undergoing head and neck radiation therapy: A survey of radiation oncology nurses. *Oncol Nurs Forum* 23(10): 1619–1623. 1996.

   The author surveyed 192 members of the Oncology Nursing Society Radiation Special Interest Group on their practices and recommendations. The large majority of the respondents reported an ocurrance of mucositis and xerostomia in more than 80 percent of their patients.

5. Jacobs, C. D. and M. VanDerPas. A multicenter maintenance study of oral pilocarpine tablets for radiation-induced xerostomia. *Oncology* 10(3): 16–20. 1996.

   Based on an open-label study of 265 patients with head and neck cancer over 36 months, the authors conclude that oral pilocarpine effectively and safely reduces the symptoms of radiation-induced xerostomia. Pilocarpine, a parasympathomimetic agent, stimulates residual functioning tissue in damaged salivary glands. The doses averaged 5 mg TID, with adjustments from 2.5 mg to 10 mg TID or BID. The most common side effects were sweating (55 percent) and flu-like syndrome (20 percent).

6. Madeya, M. L. Oral complications from cancer therapy: Part 2—Nursing implications for assessment and treatment. *Oncol Nurs Forum* 23: 808–821. 1996.

   This article presents a good overview of oral complications and their prevention and treatment. It incorporates a review of recent studies on agents for prevention and treatment of mucositis.

7. Mueller, B. A. et al. Mucositis management practices for hospitalized patients: National survey results. *Journal of Pain and Symptom Management* 10(October): 510–518. 1995.

   The purpose of this survey was to identify the national treatment practices for oral mucositis, mucocutaneous HSV infection, and oral candidiasis, and to compare them with the NIH Guidelines of 1989. The 62 pharmacists who returned the questionnaire report a diversity of agents, including products and combinations that lack proven clinical efficacy.

8. Consensus Development Conference Statement Oral Complications of Cancer Therapies: Diagnosis, Prevention and Treatment. National Institutes of Health 7(7) (April 17–19, 1989).

   This report gives conclusions from a consensus conference that brought together biomedical investigators, dentists, oncologists, and other physicians, nurses, dietitians, and representatives of public interest groups to review scientific information on prophylactic, diagnostic, and treatment approaches to oral complications of cancer treatment.

9. Ross Laboratories. *Mouth Care Instructions for the Chemotherapy and Radiation-Therapy Patient* (patient booklet). Ross Laboratories, Columbus, Ohio.

   An 11-page pocket-sized booklet, distributed for patient education with instructions, is written in easy language and explains care of the normal as well as the sore mouth. It includes management of problems such as difficulties in eating, pain, dry mouth and lips, and bleeding.

10. Skubitz, K. M., and P. M. Anderson. Oral glutamine to prevent chemotherapy induced stomatitis: A pilot study. *Journal of Laboratory & Clinical Medicine* 127(February): 223–228. 1996.

   This article presents one of the innovative studies on prevention of mucositis. Glutamine, the most abundant amino acid in the blood, is a significant source of nitrogen and energy for the intestinal mucosa. Fourteen chemotherapy patients received a suspension of L-glutamine, 4 grams twice a day, swish and swallow. The researchers conclude that glutamine can significantly decrease the severity of chemotherapy-induced mucositis and warrants further study.

11. Toth, B. B. et al. Minimizing oral complications of cancer treatment. *Oncology* 9(September): 851–863. 1995.

   The authors describe the preventive and therapeutic oral care protocols and ongoing clinical practices at M.D. Anderson Cancer Center.

C. Skin

Ellen Sitton
Lynne Early

ANATOMY AND PHYSIOLOGY

The skin is a physical barrier that protects the body from external infectious organisms. The skin is divided into two layers: The outermost layer is the epidermis, and the inner layer is the dermis. These two layers are separated by a single layer of cells called the basement membrane. The basement membrane, at the dermal-epidermal junction, welds the epidermis and dermis layers together. Its role is the regulation of epidermal growth by diffusion of nutrients from the dermal blood vessels. It also serves as a barrier to the movement of neoplastic and inflammatory cells between layers.

10c

Epidermis

The epidermis, or the stratified (multilayered) squamous epithelium, is avascular and derived from the embryonic ectoderm. The inner layer of the epidermis, the basal layer, produces keratinocytes that are continuously undergoing cell division. As these cells mature, they are pushed to the outermost portion of the epidermis, the stratum corneum, where they are shed. This process of cell replacement occurs approximately every 15–30 days.

The basal layer contains melanocytes and Langerhans cells. Melanocytes are pigment-producing cells of the skin that synthesize melanin when activated, resulting in skin pigmentation. Langerhans cells are antigen-presenting cells.

Dermis

The dermis is the thickest skin layer located between the epidermis and subcutaneous adipose tissue. Blood vessels, nerves, skin appendages, fibers, and various cells are contained within the dermis. The dermis provides a matrix that supports the epidermis and gives the skin strength, elasticity, and softness, while protecting deeper structures from injury. Blood vessels supply oxygen and nutrients to the epidermis and regulate body temperature. The dermis consists of two protein fibers, collagen and elastin, produced by fibroblasts. Collagen provides tensile strength to the skin, and elastin gives the skin its elastic recoil property.

Skin appendages include hair and sebaceous and sweat glands. The epidermis invaginates the hair follicles and sweat ducts. Sebaceous glands empty oily secretions between the hair follicle and hair root and are found throughout the skin except on the palms of the hand and soles of the feet. Sweat glands are located throughout the body. Macrophages and mast cells are found in the dermis. These cells are a part of the skin's immunological system. The function of macrophages is to ingest and digest bacteria.

Skin Function

There are seven major functions of the skin:

1. Sensory perception of pain, touch, pressure, and temperature.
2. Body temperature regulation through vasodilation or constriction of blood flow. Sweat glands cool the body through excretion and evaporation of water, and subcutaneous adipose tissue provides insulation.
3. Fluid and electrolyte balance, providing a homeostatic environment.
4. Protection against bacteria, foreign substances such as chemicals and liquids, physical and mechanical trauma, heat, and ultraviolet (UV) rays. Hair protects the skin surface, enhances tactile senses, and provides temperature regulation by conserving body heat.
5. Vitamin D production, which participates in calcium and phosphate metabolism and is important in the mineralization of bone.

6. Immunological defense provided by dermal lymphocytes, mast cells, mononuclear phagocytes, and Langerhans cells.
7. Communication and expression of body image.

Skin changes occur as persons age; chronic exposure to the sun increases the rate of these changes. The skin becomes drier, less elastic, thinner, wrinkled, and has decreased subcutaneous fat. Changes due to aging increase the risk of injury and disease of the skin.

TISSUE INJURY AND WOUND REPAIR

Tissue injury impairs the integrity of the skin, disrupting vascular supply and perfusion of oxygen and nutrients. This leads to tissue hypoxia, delayed healing, and necrosis at the site of injury. When tissues are injured, a cascade of events for wound healing is initiated. A successfully healed wound provides approximately 80 percent of original tissue strength. The rate of healing is determined by the cause, location, and depth of the wound and the underlying condition of the patient. The process of tissue repair includes inflammation, proliferation, and maturation (see Table 10C–1). Wounds heal by primary or secondary intention. Primary intention, with simple, clean wounds, occurs when fibroblasts proliferate and migrate to the subcutaneous tissue. Epithelial cells then multiply to restore the surface area. Larger, ulcerated, or necrotic areas heal from within by secondary intention. Granulation results from fibroblast proliferation, capillary budding, and macrophage proliferation. Eventually, epithelial cells join to cover the surface defect.

Table 10C-1
Phases of Wound Healing

Phase	Completion Time	Event	Cellular Components
Inflammation	2 hours	Homeostasis	Platelets Erythrocytes Fibrin
	4 days	Phagocytosis	Leukocytes Macrophages
Proliferation	21 days	Neoangiogenesis Epithelialization Collagen synthesis Contraction	Endothelial cells Keratinocytes Fibroblasts Myofibroblasts
Maturation	21 days–2 years	Collagen synthesis and lysis (remodeling)	Fibroblasts

The *inflammatory phase* begins at the time of tissue injury and can last up to four days. During this phase, the healing cascade is initiated, bacteria is engulfed, and the immune response is triggered. The injured tissue becomes hypoxic, as bleeding occurs. The vasculature is exposed to collagen, which activates coagulation factors and causes platelet aggregation. Prothrombin coagulation factor converts prothrombin to thrombin, and thrombin converts fibrinogen to fibrin. Fibrin deposits, platelet aggregation, and red blood cell trapping mesh together to form a fibrin clot. When the fibrin clot is formed, vasodilation occurs, increasing capillary permeability. The increased fluid to the injured tissue results in edema, erythema, and pain. Leukocytes are attracted to the wound to break down the fibrin clot and phagocytize bacteria. Leukocytes are then replaced by macrophages, which debride the wound and continue phagocytosis. This mechanism of cleansing the wound attracts fibroblasts, which initiate collagen synthesis and stimulate growth factors.

The *proliferative phase* begins approximately four days after injury and continues for approximately 21 days. During this phase, neoangiogenesis extends the surface of the wound, supplying oxygen and nutrients to the migrating fibroblasts. This causes the fibroblasts to produce and secrete collagen. Collagen forms the matrix of the wound bed, also known as granulation tissue. The healthy wound bed appears red, moist, and friable. From the edge of the wound, epithelial cells migrate toward each other in order to resurface the wound. Contraction occurs by secondary intention. The myofibroblasts mobilize and pull together the tissue and skin surrounding the defect in order to reduce the size of the defect.

The final phase of wound healing is called the *maturation phase*. This phase occurs 21 days after tissue injury (or at completion of wound epithelialization) and extends up to two years. In this phase, fibroblasts continue to generate collagen and replace disorganized collagen fibers. The disorganized collagen fibers are lysed by proteolytic enzymes. The result is the reorganization of collagen fibers to increase wound strength.

PATHOPHYSIOLOGY

Many disease and treatment-related factors influence integrity of the skin in the patient with cancer. Lesions range from minor changes in skin color or texture to large, draining, malodorous ulcerations or fungating wounds. The patient could have lesions that are premalignant or malignant, as well as lesions that are characteristic of systemic cancer. Malignant lesions include primary or recurrent skin cancer or cutaneous metastases. Treatment-related skin impairment occurs with radiation therapy, chemotherapy, biotherapy, hyperthermia, and surgery (see Chapter 2). GVHD following bone marrow transplantation can also cause skin manifestations (see Chapter 3A). Debilitated patients with cancer can have additional risk factors for skin impairment related to nutrition, edema, infection, jaundice, and incontinence.

Disease-Related Causes of Skin Impairment

Actinic (solar) keratosis is a result of chronic UV radiation exposure and infrequently evolves into invasive squamous cell carcinoma (SCC) of the skin. Actinic keratosis generally occurs in sun-exposed areas of the skin in patients 40–50 years of age, and is more frequent in fair-skinned persons. Lesions are scaly and can appear unpigmented, hyperpigmented, or erythematous.

Premalignant Lesions

Bowen's disease, or SCC *in situ,* can have a prolonged course and may progress to invasive SCC. Lesions are usually found in the head and neck area but can arise in any skin region and are characterized by scaly, erythematous plaques or macules.

Dysplastic nevi (atypical moles) are larger than the usual melanocytic nevi, with variable pigmentation and irregular borders. When they are present in abnormal numbers in an individual, there is an increased risk for developing melanoma.

The most common type of skin cancer is basal cell carcinoma (BCC). The primary risk factor for BCC is chronic exposure to UV radiation from the sun. Most lesions occur in the head and neck region and in persons with fair skin. Additional risk factors include previous injury at the site (e.g., burns, trauma), exposure to arsenic, exposure to ionizing radiation, certain genetic syndromes (e.g., xeroderma pigmentosum, nevoid BCC syndrome, albinism), and immunosuppression. Lesions may appear as pearly white or erythematous macules or patches, or waxy, translucent nodules. Ulceration of nodules is frequent and is often referred to as a "rodent ulcer." Some lesions are pigmented and resemble dysplastic nevi or melanoma. BCC most often grows slowly by direct extension destroying local tissue, which can be significant. However, BCC is rarely life-threatening and metastases are rare.

Malignant Lesions
Basal Cell Carcinoma

The second most common type of skin cancer is SCC, which represents approximately 20 percent of skin cancers. SCC is more aggressive than BCC and has a faster growth rate, less well-defined margins, and greater metastatic potential. It usually arises in areas of chronic sun exposure, occurs in mid- to late-life, and is more common in fair-skinned persons. Other etiologic factors include occupational exposure to hydrocarbons, chronic arsenic exposure, and exposure to ionizing radiation. SCC can also occur in burn scars and areas of chronic inflammation. Lesions are often hyperkeratotic skin-colored papules, nodules, or plaques and could be inflamed, crusted or ulcerative. Tumor infiltration into surrounding skin

Squamous Cell
Carcinoma

causes induration around the nodule. Pain can indicate extension to nerves. Metastasis generally occurs first to regional lymph nodes. Factors that increase risk of metastasis include primary size greater than 2 centimeters, depth of invasion 4 or more millimeters, tumors with high grade histology, and underlying immunosuppression.

Treatment for nonmelanomatous skin cancer is based on tumor type, location, size, and growth pattern, and the patient's age and general health. It includes surgical excision, curettage and electrodessication, cryosurgery with liquid nitrogen, CO_2 laser ablation, radiation therapy, chemotherapy (topical, systemic), and Mohs micrographic surgery (chemosurgery: debulking + zinc chloride paste). Margins must be treated adequately to prevent recurrence.

Cutaneous Melanoma

Melanoma has a much lower incidence than nonmelanoma skin cancers but has three times the mortality rate, primarily due to its high metastatic potential. Melanoma of the skin arises in melanocytes. The incidence of melanoma in the United States has been increasing rapidly over the past 20 years. The etiology is unknown; however, known risk factors include previous melanoma, exposure to sun, family history, certain genetic influences (e.g., xeroderma pigmentosum, familial atypical multiple mole or melanoma syndrome), fair skin, nonfamilial dysplastic nevi, and immunosuppression. Blistering sunburns in children and adolescents rather than cumulative chronic sun exposure has been associated with an increased risk of melanoma in adulthood.

Melanoma can spread superficially or invade the dermis and underlying subcutaneous fat. It can appear as a new pigmented lesion or a change in an existing mole. The color can be black, pink, red, tan, or brown, and the lesion can be irregular in shape or asymmetric and have irregular borders. The irregular surface can become shiny and possibly ulcerate. Satellite metastatic lesions can appear near the primary site or near the scar from an excised melanoma.

The person's immune system can cause spontaneous regression of melanoma lesions. This might account for the inability to find a primary site in some patients with metastatic melanoma. Early recognition and treatment of melanoma is essential. Depth of invasion is the major factor in the prognosis of the person with melanoma. Tumors tend to metastasize to almost any organ, including the liver, brain, lungs, lymph nodes, other skin, and bone. Metastatic disease is rarely curable.

Melanoma Skin Cancer Treatment

Treatment of melanoma includes surgical excision and, frequently, lymph node dissection. Patients with positive lymph nodes or a thick primary lesion are at increased risk for metastatic disease and need additional therapy to prolong disease-free survival. Adjuvant programs of therapy include chemotherapy (e.g., dacarbazine, nitrosureas, cisplatin, paclitaxel), nonspecific immunotherapy (e.g., levamisole, bacillus Calmette-Guerin), interferons and interleukins, active specific immunotherapy (e.g., melanoma vaccines), chemoimmunotherapy (e.g., chemotherapy and interleukin-2), regional extremity perfusion with chemotherapy, and radiation therapy with or without hyperthermia. Recent studies have been conducted using hormonal therapy with drugs including tamoxifen, diethylstibestrol, estramustine, progesterone, and antiandrogens.

Cancers of the skin are seen in congenital immunodeficiency diseases and after organ transplantation. Nonmelanoma skin cancers are frequently diagnosed in patients who have received organ transplants. BCC and SCC in sun-exposed areas is relatively common. SCC is most common and is found much more frequently than BCC and melanoma. Melanoma is also increased in the transplant population. Skin cancers in these patients could be aggressive. Kaposi's sarcoma (KS) is not seen in patients with congenital immunodeficiency.

Immunosuppression-Related Skin Cancers: Non-HIV

Historically, Kaposi's sarcoma was a little known disease found in Africa and in immunosuppressed patients after organ transplant. Classic KS is indolent and most often found in the skin of the lower legs in elderly Mediterranean, eastern European, or Jewish men. A large increase in the incidence of KS has occurred with the AIDS epidemic. AIDS-related KS is found mostly in homosexual men, and cutaneous lesions are most often located in the oral cavity, face, trunk, penis, and lower extremities. About half of these patients develop lymph node disease. Progression of the disease often correlates with progression of AIDS. Lesions can be single or multiple and are often reddish-purple, macular or papular, or nodular. Progressive lesions can become painful, ulcerative, and infected. Lymphatic spread causes severe pain with cutaneous and subcutaneous edema, and obstructive or ulcerative lesions. Visceral spread can be fatal, possibly involving lungs, bowel, liver, spleen, and other organs. The etiology of both classic and AIDS-related KS is unknown. There is no known cure for AIDS-related KS, and therefore, treatment is palliative. Radiation therapy, systemic chemotherapy, and interferon can be used in the management of AIDS-related KS.

Immunosuppression-Related Skin Cancers: HIV

BCC is very common in patients with HIV disease, and lesions are commonly found on the trunk. SCC is also found in sun-exposed skin in these patients.

Some T-lymphocytes have antigens on the cell surface that allow them to migrate to the skin and bind to cutaneous endothelial cells. In CTCL, malignant cutaneous T-lymphocytes are found in the skin. From the skin the disease can spread to the lymph nodes, blood, and viscera. Suggested causes of CTCL include a retrovirus, and immunosuppression has been associated with the development of CTCL. Biopsies of early skin lesions might appear to be inflammatory skin disease, and definitive diagnosis can take years.

Cutaneous T cell Lymphoma (CTCL)

Mycosis fungoides (MF) is a type of CTCL in which lesions evolve from dry, scaly patches to plaques and tumors. Sezary's syndrome occurs when both skin and peripheral blood are infiltrated by malignant T cells, and causes erythroderma. This progression can take months to years. Lesions can be asymptomatic or intensely pruritic. Erythroderma usually occurs initially and is usually accompanied by intense pruritus. Factors that have a negative impact on CTCL prognosis include a large amount of skin involved, depth of invasion, loss of normal T cells, leukemia, and lymph node or visceral involvement.

Several treatments have been used for CTCL. Topical mechlorethamine or carmustine applied to the entire skin surface has been used. In photochemotherapy with ultraviolet-A light (PUVA), the patient ingests 8-methoxypsoralen and is then exposed to UV-A light. In extracorporeal photochemotherapy, the patient ingests 8-methoxypsoralen, and the blood is subsequently collected. Leukocytes are separated from red blood cells and exposed to UV-A light. Radiation therapy to specific lesions or total skin electron therapy is also used for CTCL. Electrons do not penetrate deeply and can provide relatively high doses of radiation only to the skin.

Paget's Disease

Paget's disease is a rare adenocarcinoma most often found in the epidermis. The etiology is unknown. It is most often found in the elderly. Although it is an indolent disease, it can become invasive and metastasize. The lesion is a well-circumscribed, reddish brown plaque, which can be eroded and moist. It is most often found on the nipple and the anogenital region and less often in skin of the chest, axilla, posterior knee, and ear canal. Paget's disease might occasionally be associated with an internal malignancy such as rectal, bladder, or prostate adenocarcinoma. Mammary Paget's disease is almost always associated with underlying breast cancer and appears oozing, crusted, and ulcerated.

Treatment of Paget's disease is surgical excision, with careful attention to clear margins. Moh's micrographic surgery is useful in determining the extent of the margins and can be performed with local anesthesia in an outpatient setting.

Cutaneous Metastasis

The incidence of cutaneous metastasis depends on the type and location of the primary cancer. The most common malignancies that metastasize to the skin are melanoma and breast, lung, colon, and head and neck cancers. Lesions are usually movable, firm cutaneous or subcutaneous nodules, but they can appear as plaques. Color ranges from skin colored to erythematous, violaceous, or black/brown. As they progress, they become painful and ulcerated and bleed. Metastasis from visceral cancer to the skin often indicates widespread, systemic disease and poor prognosis.

Cutaneous Paraneoplastic Syndromes

Skin lesions that are caused by tumor production of biologically active substances but are located a distance away from the tumor are considered paraneoplastic dermatoses (see Table 10C–2). When the cancer is removed, the skin lesions clear. Conversely if the cancer recurs, the skin lesions can reappear.

Table 10C-2
Paraneoplastic Syndromes

Cutaneous Manifestation	Most Common Associated Malignancies
Acanthosis nigricans. Symmetrical, gray-brown, velvety skin thickening. Increased skin fold markings. Axilla, base of neck, groin, and antecubital areas most often involved. Might have generalized skin involvement. Pruritus common.	Intra-abdominal cancers (especially gastric cancer), carcinomas of the gallbladder, liver, and lung, Hodgkin's lymphoma, cutaneous T cell lymphoma. Also seen in benign disease.
Collagen-vascular disease (dermatomyositis).	Bronchogenic cancer most common. Also breast, ovarian, cervical, and gastrointestinal cancers. Also seen in benign disease.
Erythema gyratum repens. Erythematous concentric, raised, or flat bands over body surface in "wood grain" pattern.	Breast, lung, bladder, prostate, cervix, stomach, and esophageal carcinomas and multiple myeloma.
Erythroderma. Diffuse, generalized erythema and scaling of whole skin surface.	T cell leukemia and lymphoma, lung, liver, prostate, thyroid, colon, pancreas, and stomach cancers. Most often seen in benign disease.
Flushing. Manifestation of carcinoid syndrome. Most commonly of central face and upper trunk. Numerous episodes can cause telangiectasia, chronic diffuse erythema, and cutaneous sclerosis.	Most commonly from metastatic small bowel cancer. Cancers of the bronchus, stomach, pancreas, and thyroid and teratomas.
Hypertrichosis lanuginosa acquistita. Increased growth of fine body hair.	Cancers of the colon, rectum, bladder, lung, pancreas, gallbladder, uterus, and breast and lymphoma.
Ichthyosis (acquired). Hyperkeratosis. Dryness.	Lymphoma (non-Hodgkin's, Hodgkin's, and T cell), multiple myeloma, cancers of the breast, cervix, and lung, Kaposi's sarcoma, leiomyosarcoma, and rhabdomyosarcoma.
Necrolytic migratory erythema (glucagonoma syndrome). Erythema, vesicles, pustules, bullae, and erosions generally of face and intertriginous areas.	Glucagon producing pancreatic tumor.
Paraneoplastic acrodermatosis of Bazex. Symmetrical dermatosis. Erythematous to violaceous scaling lesions. Progressive eruption. Commonly affects digits, nails, feet, ears, and nose.	Cancers of tongue, pharynx, esophagus, and lung.
Pemphigus.	Lymphoma (especially Hodgkin's disease) and Kaposi's sarcoma.
Pruritus. Skin can appear normal or dry. Usually generalized. Paroxysmal. Burning quality.	Leukemias and lymphomas most common. Also in cancers of the pancreas and stomach, and liver metastases. Can occur with benign disease.
Subcutaneous fat necrosis. Nodules or ulcers that leave scar with healing. Most common on legs, buttocks, and trunk.	Acinar cell adenocarcinoma of the pancreas.

Continued

Table 10C–2 *(Continued)*
Paraneoplastic Syndromes

Cutaneous Manifestation	Most Common Associated Malignancies
Sweet's syndrome (acute febrile neutrophilic dermatosis). Tender, red plaques with vesicles, and nodules. Most common on face and extremities.	Leukemias (especially acute myelocytic) and lymphomas. Less often with adenocarcinomas and embryonal testicular, ovarian, and gastric carcinomas.
Thrombophlebitis. Peripheral thrombophlebitis.	Gastric cancer, cancers of the pancreas, prostate, lung, liver, bowel, gallbladder, and ovary; lymphoma; and leukemia.
Xanthomas. Purpura can appear within xanthomas.	Multiple myeloma most common. Leukemias and lymphomas.

Treatment-Related Causes of Skin Impairment

Radiation Therapy

External beam radiation therapy is generally used as a localized treatment and affects tissues in the path of radiation, including the skin (see Chapter 2B). Treatment fields can be located over any part of the body. The reaction of the skin is determined by factors such as the energy and type of radiation, dose of radiation, concurrent or previous treatments, and patient characteristics (see Table 10C–3). Skin changes can occur during or for a short time after radiation therapy or months to years after treatment. Early side effects in the radiated site include alopecia, erythema, increased pigmentation, dry flaking and scaling (dry desquamation), and denuded areas with serosanguinous drainage (moist desquamation). Early reactions might be increased in skin folds such as the inframammary fold and axilla. These reactions generally heal four to six weeks after treatment. Hair loss generally begins about the fourth week of treatment and occurs locally within the treatment field. With the exception of very high doses of radiation, hair loss is usually temporary. Regrowth of hair occurs after two to three months. New hair might have a different texture and slightly different color. Late effects include telangiectasia, or dilated small blood vessels seen at the skin surface, occurring one to two years after radiation. The epidermis in the treated area often becomes atrophied and thin with pigmentation changes. Fibrosis in the radiated field might also be observed, especially following high doses of radiation therapy.

When chemotherapy is combined with radiation therapy in the treatment of cancer, an additive effect can occur, which can decrease the skin tolerance to a given dose of radiation or chemotherapy. Radiation recall is an inflammatory reaction in previously radiated sites upon administration of certain chemotherapy drugs (e.g., doxorubicin, dactinomycin).

Table 10C–3
Possible Factors in Radiation-Induced Skin Reactions

Factors	Effect
Radiation factors: Electron beam, tissue equivalent (bolus) material placed on skin surface during treatment, large doses of radiation, and large treatment fields.	Increased skin reactions
Radiation factors: High energy x-rays, small doses, flat field surface, and small treatment fields.	Decreased skin reactions
Patient-related factors: skin folds in treated area, sloping skin surface, poor nutritional status, use of skin irritants, and concurrent disease that increases radiosensitivity (e.g., ataxia-telangiectasia).	Increased skin reactions
Patient-related factors: minimizing all types of skin irritants (e.g., sun exposure, chemical irritants, mechanical irritants, thermal irritants).	Decreased skin reactions
Combination therapy with certain chemotherapy agents or hyperthermia.	Increased skin reactions • Radiation recall • Enhancement of reactions

Chemotherapy

Chemotherapy affects rapidly proliferating cells such as those in the skin, causing alopecia, erythema, rash, pruritus, pigmentation changes, and nail changes (see Table 10C–4). Chemotherapeutic agents affect the skin in different ways. Several drugs (e.g., fluorouracil with leucovorin, paclitaxel, plicamycin) cause temporary facial flushing. Painful or tender erythema of the palms and soles is known as acral erythema. Dry desquamation of these areas can follow erythema. Drugs associated with acral erythema include fluorouracil, doxorubicin, high-dose cytarabine, and floxuridine. Other agents can cause alterations in sense of touch. Chemotherapy also inhibits wound healing. Extravasation of agents that are vesicants causes severe skin and tissue damage (see Chapters 2C and 3B).

Some chemotherapy, especially alkylating agents and antitumor antibiotics, induce skin hyperpigmentation. Increased pigmentation might be focal or generalized and can affect skin, nails, hair, and/or mucosa. Skin color changes can be temporary or permanent.

Photosensitivity is a skin reaction caused by UV radiation exposure. It can also be caused by agents including fluorouracil, dacarbazine, vinblastine, and high-dose methotrexate.

Table 10C–4
Potential Treatment-Related Skin Changes

Treatment	Erythema	Hyper-pigmentation	Dry/Moist desquamation	Urticaria	Telangi-ectasia	Photo-sensitivity	Rash/Pruritus	Nail Changes	Acral Erythema	Alopecia	Radiation Recall/Enhancement
Radiation Therapy	X	X	X		X					X	X
Alkylating agents											
• busulfan		X									
• carmustine	X										
• chlorambucil		X		X			X				
• cyclophosphamide	X							X	X	X	
• dacarbazine				X						X	
• estramustine				X							
• ifosfamide		X					X	X		X	
• lomustine							X			X	
• melphalan				X			X			X	
• mechlorethamine				X			X				
• thiotepa							X				
Antimetabolites											
• cytarabine							X		X	X	
• floxuridine	X						X	X	X		
• fluorouracil		X				X	X	X	X	X	X
• gemcitabine	X						X				
• hydroxyurea	X						X			X	X
• mercaptopurine							X		X		
• methotrexate				X		X	X		X	X	X
• thioguanine											
Antibiotics											
• bleomycin		X		X			X	X	X	X	X
• dactinomycin			X				X			X	X
• daunorubicin		X					X	X		X	X
• doxorubicin		X		X				X	X	X	X
• idarubicin		X					X	X		X	X
• plicamycin		X						X		X	
• mitomycin		X						X		X	

Plant alkaloids

- etoposide
- teniposide
- vinblastine
- vincristine
- vinorelbine

Hormones/Antihormone

- mitotane
- tamoxifen

Miscellaneous agents

- mitoxantrone
- procarbazine
- paclitaxel
- docetaxel

Biotherapy

Interferons
Interleukin-2
Hemopoietic growth factors (G-CSF, GM-CSF)
Monoclonal antibodies
Tumor necrosis factor (injection site)

Drug							
etoposide			x			x	
teniposide			x	x		x	
vinblastine	x		x			x	
vincristine	x		x			x	
vinorelbine			x			x	
mitotane	x		x				
tamoxifen	x		x			x	x
mitoxantrone		x	x			x	
procarbazine	x	x	x			x	
paclitaxel	x	x	x			x	
docetaxel	x		x			x	x
Interferons	x		x				
Interleukin-2	x	x	x			x	
Hemopoietic growth factors (G-CSF, GM-CSF)			x				
Monoclonal antibodies	x		x				
Tumor necrosis factor (injection site)	x						

Alopecia is loss of hair, partial or total. Hair loss can occur in any area of body hair, including scalp, eyebrows, eye lashes, facial hair, axillary hair, pubic hair, and fine body hair. Both radiation and chemotherapy cause injury to the rapidly dividing epithelial cells of the hair follicles, resulting in hair loss. Chemotherapy results in temporary hair loss beginning at one to two weeks after chemotherapy, with maximum loss at one to two months. Hair regrowth begins after completion of therapy when the treatment no longer affects hair growth. As with radiation new hair might have a different texture and slightly different color. Categories of drugs causing alopecia include alkylating agents, antimetabolites, and antibiotics.

Chemotherapeutic agents, such as cisplatin, carboplatin, vincristine, vinorelbine, and paclitaxel, can cause neuropathies that alter the sense of touch. Sensory alterations such as tingling and numbness increase risk of skin injury. Hypersensitivity to touch can also occur.

Cutaneous manifestations of hypersensitivity reactions are uncommon. Signs and symptoms range from urticaria to anaphylaxis. L-asparginase and cisplatin are the most common drugs associated with these reactions. Other drugs that can cause hypersensitivity reactions are paclitaxel, docetaxel, bleomycin, plicamycin, cytarabine, methotrexate, thiotepa, mechlorethamine, teniposide, and etoposide. Additional drugs that can cause rash, urticaria, or angioedema are procarbazine, levamisole, and melphalan.

Biotherapy

Skin rashes with biotherapy are common. Immunoreactive cells in the skin can be affected, resulting in redness, swelling, and itching. Rashes and dry desquamation can occur. Interleukin-2 (IL-2) can cause erythema followed by severe dryness, desquamation, and intense pruritus. More severe reactions can occur, resulting in skin ulcerations and sloughing of the nails and skin of the palms and soles. Hair might become thinner, but total alopecia rarely occurs. Skin gradually heals after completion of biotherapy. Sites of injection of biotherapy agents (e.g., interferon, colony stimulating factors) might exhibit inflammatory reactions with pain and edema for several days.

Hyperthermia

Hyperthermia (heat treatment) is used in the treatment of cancer usually in combination with radiation therapy or chemotherapy. Temperatures higher than 42.5°C (108°F) are toxic to cells. The effect of radiation therapy and some chemotherapeutic drugs is enhanced when combined with hyperthermia. Skin erythema and thermal blisters are affected by prior radiation therapy, dose of radiation therapy, dose during hyperthermia, and number of heat treatments. Skin reactions are more often observed in patients receiving higher doses of radiation with hyperthermia and more hyperthermia treatments. Patients who received previous radiation with relatively high doses are less likely to have skin reactions.

Protective mechanisms of the skin are compromised by surgical incisions, sutures, and drain sites. Cutaneous impairment can also occur secondary to surgical disruption of lymph node drainage and blood flow. Postoperative edema and fluid accumulation contribute to risk of infection after surgery.

Surgery

Manifestations of graft-versus-host disease (GVHD) after autologous or allogeneic bone marrow transplantation (BMT) are related to immunocompetent leukocytes attacking various organs, most commonly the skin, in the immunocompromised patient (see Table 10C–5). Acute cutaneous GVHD occurs up to several months after BMT, and signs range from erythematous macules and papules covering less than 25 percent of skin to the

Bone Marrow Transplantation (Graft-versus-Host Disease)

Table 10C–5
Potential Graft Versus Host Disease Skin Manifestations

	Factors	Manifestations
Acute GVHD	Occurs in 50%–80% of allogeneic BMT. GVHD after autologous BMT is generally mild and confined to skin. Can occur up to several months after BMT. Related to preparation for BMT, prophylaxis and treatment of GVHD, and donor and recipient characteristics.	Erythematous macules, particularly on palms, soles, and ears. Rash might cause edema and tenderness. Possible progression to wide distribution of macules involving trunk and extremities possible with erythroderma. Possible progression to edematous plaques. Possible progression to subepidermal bullae formation. Desquamation after rash subsides. Exacerbation of cutaneous disease can occur. Severe rupture, increasing risk of infection and electrolyte imbalance. Postinflammatory hyperpigmentation is frequent in sites of GVHD reaction.
Chronic GVHD	Rare after autologous BMT. Occurs months to years after BMT.	Lichenoid: violaceous or erythematous papules. Healed lesions leave hypo- or hyperpigmented areas of skin. Sclerodermoid: progressive; thickened lesions, hairless, hypo- or hyperpigmented. Ulceration and infection not uncommon.

GVHD—Graft-versus-host disease; BMT—bone marrow transplantation.

formation of severe vesicles and bullae. Treatment of acute GVHD begins with prophylaxis (cyclosporine, methotrexate, or both) on the day of infusion of bone marrow. Symptomatic GVHD is treated with systemic corticosteroids and additional immunomodulating agents (see Chapter 3A).

Cutaneous manifestations of chronic GVHD appear months to years after allogeneic BMT. Chronic lesions might be lichenoid or sclerodermoid, and both types can occur in the same person. Lichenoid lesions appear as violaceous or erythematous papules initially on the palms and soles. These can increase in number and spread to other regions of the body. Resolution of lesions leaves hypo- or hyperpigmented lesions. Sclerodermoid lesions are characterized by limited patches of progressively thickening skin, which could be erythematous and become hairless, hypo- or hyperpigmented, and sclerotic in appearance. Extension of disease can lead to generalized involvement of skin. The primary treatment for chronic GVHD is immunosuppressive agents, including systemic corticosteroids, cyclosporine, and azathioprine. Thalidomide has recently been found useful in chronic GVHD as an immunomodulating agent.

Other Treatment and Disease-Related Factors Affecting Skin

Adequate dietary intake and hydration are essential for wound healing, maintaining intact skin, and preventing infection.

Nutrition

The normal epidermis, hair follicles, and nail matrices receive their nutrition from the dermal vasculature. Protein, vitamins, and minerals facilitate wound repair and assist in maintaining skin integrity (see Table 10C–6). Protein promotes collagen synthesis and epidermal proliferation, and maintains immunocompetence to prevent infection. Calories provide energy for tissue defense and wound repair. The nutritional consequences of impaired skin integrity include loss of fluid and electrolytes, loss of cel-

Table 10C–6
Vitamin and Mineral Effects on Wound Repair

Vitamin or Mineral	Action
Vitamin C	Cofactor for collagen synthesis, capillary wall integrity
Vitamin A	Support wound healing
Vitamin B	Collagen cross-linking in maturation phase
Iron	Oxygen transport and cofactor for collagen synthesis
Zinc	Collagen and protein synthesis

lular components and nutrients, and increased energy requirements. Related signs of nutritional deficiency are albumin less than 3.4 g/dl; acute or chronic anemia; total lymphocyte count less than 200 cells/mm^3; inadequate intake of calories, vitamins, and minerals; and dehydration.

Edema includes ascites, lymphedema, or peripheral edema. Patients at risk for the development of edema are those who have had recent surgery (e.g., prostatectomy, mastectomy, lymphatic dissection), primary or metastatic lymphatic disease; primary or metastatic liver disease; concomitant cardiopulmonary deficiency; malnutrition (e.g., hypoalbuminemia, hypoproteinemia); and/or fluid and electrolyte imbalance (e.g., nausea/vomiting, diarrhea, hormonal impairment).

Edema

Normally the lymph system returns fluids and plasma from the interstitial spaces into the circulation. Both edema and lymphedema can occur when proteins cannot move freely out of the tissues and fluid accumulates in a body space or extremity. Ascites usually results from obstruction of the main thoracic and subdiaphragmatic lymphatic channels directly by tumor, or by tumor metastases to the liver; both conditions result in decreased clearance of fluid from the peritoneal cavity and increased peritoneal fluid accumulation. The goal of therapy is to treat the underlying condition, remove excess fluid when possible, control associated symptoms, and support and enhance comfort and quality of life.

A break in the skin's integrity at the site of edema is followed by bacterial colonization called cellulitis. Cellulitis is infection of the dermis and subcutaneous tissues characterized by redness, warmth, pain, and swelling. The most common pathogens are staphylococcal or streptococcal bacteria.

Bacterial infections can develop quickly in neutropenic patients, accounting for 85 percent to 90 percent of pathogens associated with febrile episodes. Invading organisms usually arise from endogenous flora colonizing the skin, respiratory system, and genitourinary and gastrointestinal systems. Breaks in the skin allow the organisms to invade. The most serious infections are gram-negative *enterobactoriaceae* and *pseudomonous aeruginosa*. Vascular access devices are commonly infected with gram-positive organisms: staphylococcus, streptococcus, corynebacteria, or clostridia.

Bacterial, Viral, and Fungal Infections
Bacterial Infections

Impaired skin can become colonized or infected with bacteria. Colonization of a wound refers to the loose attachment of a large number of bacterial organisms to devitalized tissue where there is no movement of bacterial cells into vital tissue and no host immune response. Infection results when bacteria invades vital tissue and stimulates an immune response. An infected wound is defined as having a bacterial count of more than 10^5 colonies. The infected wound has a prolonged inflammatory phase, and delayed collagen synthesis and epithelialization.

Bacterial infections are treated with systemic and topical antibiotics. The antibiotic chosen is based on the infecting organism. Topical antibiotics most commonly used are triple antibiotic ointment such as Neosporin,® and silver sulfadiazine. The wound is cleansed prior to each application of antibiotic, and the appropriate dressing applied. Meticulous hand washing is essential. Topical antiseptics such as povidone iodine, iodophor, sodium hypochlorite (Dakin's Solution), hydrogen peroxide, and acetic acid should not be used, as these agents have not been shown to clean an infected wound, but rather to destroy fibroblasts and new granulation tissue.

Viral Infections

Cancer patients are at high risk for the development of viral infections. At greatest risk are patients who are immunocompromised, have hematological malignancies, or are undergoing bone marrow transplantation. The virus enters the peripheral nerve root and rests dormant in the dorsal root ganglia. Recurrent herpes infection occurs when the latent virus becomes reactivated. Most cancer patients will experience recurrence of the virus three to four times per year during periods of stress, immunosuppression, fatigue, trauma, or surgical intervention.

Herpes virus is transmitted by direct contact with the lesions or respiratory droplets. Viral infections occurring most often in cancer patients are herpes simplex 1 and 2, varicella-zoster virus, cytomegalovirus, and Epstein-Barr virus. Herpes simplex 1 and 2 are usually localized, vesicular lesions in the oral or genital regions. The patient with herpes zoster virus is infectious to any person who has not had chicken pox or is immunocompromised.

Varicella-zoster virus's primary infection occurs in the nasopharynx via the respiratory tract and disseminates to the skin. Skin lesions begin approximately two weeks after exposure and are characterized as fluid-filled vesicles on an erythematous base. These lesions progress to pustules that erupt and crust over, signifying the end of viral shedding and infectivity. The lesions appear on the head and trunk and extend to the extremities. The reactivated varicella-zoster virus is called herpes zoster or shingles (see Table 10C–7).

Table 10C–7
Four Phases of Herpes Zoster Infection

Phase	Characteristics
Prodromal	Fever, malaise, pain, pruritus, change in sensation of affected body area; no lesions
Eruption	Fever, headache, malaise, chills, lymphadenopathy; erythematous patches progress to vesicles, then crust; located along dermatome
Dissemination	Lesions scattered over entire body and frequently visceral involvement; coalescence of bullae, can be hemorrhagic and gangrenous
Postherpetic	Pain at site after lesions have disappeared; increased incidence with age, neuralgia

Acyclovir is the treatment of choice for varicella-zoster virus and herpes simplex virus. This antiviral agent has been shown to decrease the number and healing time of the lesions, the duration of fevers and pain associated with the lesions, and viral shedding and new lesion formation. Systemic chemotherapy is discontinued until treatment of the infection is complete. The use of corticosteriods to decrease inflammation and pain at the lesion site is controversial.

Other nursing management considerations include minimizing discomfort from pain and pruritus, preventing or minimizing complications, preventing the spread of varicella-zoster virus to others, and supporting the patient and family. Complications arise from secondary bacterial infection of lesions and inadequate fluid and nutritional support.

Cytomegalovirus (CMV) causes a primary infection, becomes latent probably in peripheral monocytes, and can become reactivated in the immunocompromised individual. Petechiae or purpura can result due to thrombocytopenia, and jaundice can occur as a result of hyperbilirubinemia. Cutaneous manifestations are rare. The immunocompromised patient might exhibit lesions associated with disseminated disease, which need to be biopsied, or as a result of nonspecific antibiotic therapy. Lesions most commonly appear in the perineal area. The treatment of CMV in the immunocompromised person is with an antiviral agent, either ganciclovir or foscarnet.

Epstein-Barr virus (EBV) invades B-lymphocytes and nasopharyngeal and salivary gland epithelial cells. Recent reports state that EBV shedding has been found on cervical epithelium. Primary infections are most commonly found in young children and young adults. EBV is secreted in saliva and is transmitted through oral contact of a susceptible host. It remains in its latent state in B-lymphocytes and can be reactivated in the immunocompromised person. Within the B-lymphocyte, the EBV synthesizes viral proteins that promote cellular proliferation and transformation of cells. Epstein-Barr virus in children manifests itself on the skin as large papular lesions, which may be erythematous and are nonpruritic. Children are generally afebrile, with generalized lymphadenopathy. In young adults EBV is clinically present as infectious mononucleosis with pharyngitis, fever, cervical lymphadenopathy, macular erythema (3 percent), and upper eyelid edema (50 percent). Epstein-Barr virus has been associated with Burkitt's lymphoma and large-cell lymphoma in HIV-infected patients.

Epstein-Barr virus in an immunocompetent person is self-limiting and lasts approximately three weeks. Corticosteroids have been used in cases of extreme pharyngitis with airway edema and in the immunocompromised patient. Acyclovir has been shown to decrease viral replication but does not affect symptoms associated with the viral infection.

Fungal Infections

Fungal infections most commonly occur in persons who are immunosuppressed as a result of cancer or treatments such as chemotherapy, radiation therapy, and multiple antibiotic therapy. The most common fungal infection complicating the immunosuppressed person is candidiasis. Lesions most often appear as oral, vaginal, or intertriginous (inframammary, axillary, groin, perianal, interdigital). Oral or vaginal lesions appear as white plaques with underlying bright red mucosa; intertriginous lesions are red with scaling borders and macerated skin folds.

Treatment of fungal infections includes the imidiazoles (i.e. Lotrimin® topical, Mycelex® troche PO, or Mycelex® intravaginal) or polyenes (amphotericin B or nystatin PO, topically as a cream, ointment, or powder). Optimal treatment of a fungal infection is correction of cause of immunosuppression and local and/or systemic therapy.

Jaundice might indicate metastatic cancer or a hepatic or pancreatic primary cancer. Increased red blood cell (RBC) lysis in cancer patients could be a prehepatic cause of jaundice. Intrahepatic causes, other than carcinoma, include hepatitis, cirrhosis, or drug uptake impairment. Extrahepatic causes include biliary obstruction or primary carcinoma of the pancreas, gall bladder, or biliary tree.

Incontinence alters the resilience of the epidermis to external forces such as friction and shearing and increases the level of bacteria and moisture in a wound (Table 10C–8).

Pressure Ulcers

Cancer and the effects of treatment increase risk for pressure ulcer development. Radiation can result in tissue necrosis and fibrosis. Chemotherapeutic agents that cause cardiomyopathy, such as doxorubicin, can result in decreased tissue perfusion, and agents that cause nausea and vomiting can result in decreased nutritional status and fatigue.

Many factors contribute to the development of pressure ulcers, the most common being excessive pressure on soft tissue of prolonged duration and intensity. Factors that influence skin tolerance of pressure include

Table 10C–8
Nursing Protocol for the Management of Skin Care Related to Incontinence

Factor	Intervention
Incontinence	• Prevent skin breakdown • Maintain clean, dry skin and environment • Cleanse skin using periwash bottle with tap water or incontinent cleanser, and pat area dry (do not rub) after each elimination • Apply barrier ointments or creams • Use cloth absorbent pad instead of diaper or disposable pad • Offer assistance to bathroom or provide urinal or bedpan q 2 hours and PRN, and allow for adequate toileting time • Allow adequate toileting time • Promote patient/family time • Identify and correct causes of odor • Educate regarding skin care measures to patient and caregiver

decreased mobility, activity, and sensory perception, and increase in skin moisture and friction and shear, advancing age, poor dietary intake of protein and other nutrients, and hypotension.

ASSESSMENT

The major focus of assessment is the patient's current skin condition and the history of impairments. General observations include color; vascularity; evidence of bleeding or bruising (e.g., petechiae, hematoma); lesions (color, grouping, type, size, distribution); areas of edema or moisture; configurations, texture, mobility, and turgor; nails; and hair (see Table 10C–9). A complete history should be obtained with special emphasis on allergies, use of medication, past and present skin disorders, recent exposure to infection, and associated symptoms.

Assessment of any existing pressure ulcer is necessary to determine the status of the wound and identify appropriate treatments (see Table 10C–10). Reassessment of the site should take place at each dressing change. When there is no measurable improvement in wound healing after

Table 10C–9
Skin Terminology

Type of Lesion	Characteristic	Definition
Primary skin lesions	Macule	Circumscribed flat, colored (brown, red, or hypopigmented), <1.0 cm
	Plaque	Circumscribed, superficial, elevated, solid, >0.5 cm
	Pustule	Circumscribed collection of leukocytes and free fluid, vary in size
	Papule	Elevated solid lesion up to 0.5 cm, various colors
	Nodule	A papule >0.5 cm
	Vesicle	Circumscribed collection of free fluid, <0.5 cm
	Bulla	Circumscribed collection of free fluid, >0.5 cm
	Cyst	Semisolid or liquid area >1.0 cm
	Wheal	Edematous plaque
	Uticaria	Eruption of itchy wheals, usually systemic origin
Secondary skin lesions	Atrophy	Depression in skin as a result of epidermal or dermal thinning
	Crusts	Collection of dry serum and cellular debris
	Erosions	Loss of epidermis
	Ulcers	Loss of epidermis and dermis
Risk for pressure ulcer development	Friction	Epidermal surface damage caused by skin rubbing against skin
	Pressure	Force created between a bony prominence and support surface
	Shear	Trauma caused by tissue layers sliding against one another
Periwound skin changes	Erythema	Skin redness due to vasodilation, inflammation
	Induration	Abnormal tissue firmness with a definite margin
	Maceration	Tissue softened due to soaking in fluids
	Telangiectasia	Dilation of capillaries or terminal arteries; destruction of capillary bed

Table 10C–10
Pressure Ulcer Staging

Stage	Characteristics	Treatment
I	Non-blanchable erythema of intact skin	• Transparent film dressing (change dressing q 72 hrs) or application of lotion or ointment
II	Partial thickness skin loss involving the epidermis and/or dermis	• Cleanse wound • Apply hydrocolloid dressing, change dressing q 72 hrs
III	Full thickness skin loss involving damage or necrosis to underlying subcutaneous tissue, extending down to but not through the underlying fascia	• Irrigate wound with normal saline or in a shower • Apply appropriate wound dressing, i.e., moistened gauze with normal saline covered with dry gauze, or aliginate for highly draining wounds. • Change saturated dressing BID and PRN • Debride necrotic tissue: autolytic, surgical, or whirlpool
IV	Full thickness skin loss with destruction of tissues through and below the deep fascia, i.e., tendon, muscle, and bone	• Cleanse wound • Apply and change appropriate dressings according to physician orders

a period of two to four weeks, the patient should be reevaluated for the presence of inhibiting factors such as unrelieved pressure, friction, shear, excessive moisture, or malnutrition.

Factors included in the assessment of pressure ulcers include the following:

1. Size (length x width x depth in centimeters): include wound and affected surrounding skin;
2. Location;
3. Stage;
4. Skin color surrounding wound;
5. Presence or absence of necrotic tissue;
6. Presence, quantity, and type of exudate;
7. Presence or absence of peripheral tissue edema;
8. Presence or absence of peripheral tissue induration;
9. Presence or absence of odor;
10. Presence or absence of undermining;
11. Presence or absence of granulation tissue;
12. Presence or absence of epithelialization.

MANAGEMENT OF DISEASE AND TREATMENT-RELATED SKIN MANIFESTATIONS

Products

Many products have been developed to manage skin impairments (see Table 10C–11).

Symptom Management

Treatment for cutaneous metastases includes surgical excision, chemotherapy, or radiation therapy and depends on the location of the disease, signs and symptoms from the lesions, and total body tumor burden. Cutaneous metastases might have intact skin, or lesions might ulcerate, leaving an open wound (see Table 10C–12).

Alopecia (Table 10C–13) ranges from partial thinning to total body hair loss and can have a major impact on body image and feelings about sexuality. Cancer treatments interfere with the growth of rapidly proliferating epithelial cells of hair follicles. Alopecia due to radiation therapy is localized to the treatment field, whereas hair loss due to chemotherapy can occur anywhere that hair is found. The scalp is the most common site of hair loss due to chemotherapy and biotherapy.

Techniques such as peripheral scalp hypothermia and scalp tourniquet to prevent or minimize alopecia with chemotherapy have been investigated. The purpose is to decrease the amount of chemotherapy reaching the hair follicles by decreasing blood flow to the area. Use of these techniques is controversial because of concern regarding reduction of drug dose to the scalp, which creates the potential for creating sanctuary sites for metastatic disease. These techniques are contraindicated in patients with disease that is known to metastasize to the scalp.

Pruritus, or itching, associated with cancer and cancer treatment can be localized or generalized. Localized pruritus might be associated with tumor invasion of the skin or localized treatment such as radiation therapy. Generalized pruritus might be associated with systemic treatment (e.g., chemotherapy, biotherapy), GVHD, and malignancies such as Hodgkin's disease, non-Hodgkin's lymphoma, cutaneous T cell lymphoma, small cell carcinoma of the bronchus, leukemia, Kaposi's sarcoma, and multiple myeloma. The precise cause of pruritus is unknown. Disease-related generalized pruritus can be caused by toxic substances circulating in the blood. Biliary or hepatic obstruction from cancer results in pruritus related to increased blood levels of bile acids. Discomfort from pruritus ranges from mild to severe and can significantly affect quality of life.

Cutaneous Metastases

Table 10C-11
Wound Care Products

Category	Examples	Functions
Gauze Impregnated gauze	Kling®, Nu-Gauze®, Petrolatum Gauze, Xeroform®, Aquaphor Gauze, Iodoform	Absorb wound exudate and physically remove surface necrotic tissue. May remove viable tissue if allowed to dry in the wound, delaying wound healing.
Non-adherent dressings	Adaptic™, Telfa®	Provide a cover for wounds or incisions with minimal drainage. Will not adhere to wound, so new tissue protected during dressing change.
Film dressings	Bioclusive*, OpSite*, Tegaderm™	Help maintain a moist wound environment to enhance wound resurfacing, provide a bacterial barrier, conform to wound. Consider other products if wound has moderate amount of exudate as dressing may leak.
Hydrogel sheets Hydrogels	ElastoGel, Vigilon® IntraSite* Gel, Carrasyn™ Hydrogel	Provide cooling effect that relieves pain. Maintain a moist wound environment. Absorb small amounts of exudate. Hydrogels useful in conforming to entire wound bed in undermining wounds. Hydrogels require a secondary dressing.
Hydrocolloid dressings	Duoderm®, Tegasorb™, Ultec™ Comfeel®	Adhere to dry and moist skin surfaces. Absorb mild to moderate amounts of exudate. Soften over wound, and easy to remove, but can remove newly formed skin. Maintain a moist wound environment, provide a bacterial barrier. Should remain in place for several days; more difficult to remove if changed too soon.
Alginate dressings	Sorbsan™, Algiderm™, Kaltostat®, Kalginate	Highly absorptive, convert to gel after contact with wound exudate. Maintain a moist wound environment. Require a secondary dressing. Useful in covering wound bed in undermining wounds.
Wound fillers	Debrisan® Beads, Bard Absorption Dressing™	Absorb exudate, maintain a moist environment, facilitate debridement. Useful in filling small cavities. Require a secondary dressing.
Debriding agents	Elase®, Panafil®, Santyl	Promote elimination of necrotic tissue in wound bed.
Wound cleansers	Biolex™, Constant Clens™, Sea-Clens®	Reduce debris and slough in wound. May not need to be rinsed out.
Topical antimicrobial agents	Dakin's, acetic acid, povidone-iodine	Interfere with normal wound healing; for short-term use only except when wound healing unlikely.
Barrier creams	Carrington Moisture Barrier Cream™, Proshield™ Plus	Provide a barrier to moisture. Useful in resolving or preventing redness due to moisture, incontinence.

This table is not comprehensive. Many other wound care products are available. Consult an enterostomal therapist or wound care specialist for assistance in choosing the most appropriate dressing materials for specific clinical situations.

Table 10C–12
Nursing Protocol for the Management of Cutaneous Metastases

Related Factors	Management
Intact skin lesions	Skin Care • Wash lesions with tepid water, mild soap. • Prevent irritation: avoid rubbing (pat dry), avoid friction and pressure (nonbinding, soft clothing); avoid tape in area. • Apply topical medication or moisturizer as prescribed. • Apply dressing (dry if topical medication; possibly use hydrocolloid dressing).
Ulcerated skin lesions	Skin care • Cleanse lesions with tepid water using irrigating syringe, shower, or hand spray. • Irrigate with wound cleansing agent or dilute hydrogen peroxide, dilute Dakins, or povidine-iodine (toxic to fibroblasts) to facilitate debridement if wound unlikely to heal, and rinse with normal saline. • Prevent irritation: avoid rubbing (pat dry), avoid friction and pressure (nonbinding, soft clothing); avoid tape in area. • Do not use wet-to-dry dressings. • Surgically debride PRN. • Apply dressings: hydrogel or hydrocolloid dressing over ulcerations; change PRN for odor or saturation. • Control pain: PRN and prior to painful wound care. Odor control • Shallow lesions: apply plain, fresh yogurt (room temperature) to lesions and surrounding skin for 5–10 minutes q 6–8 hours; apply thin layer of petroleum jelly; apply absorbent dressing; odor control occurs in 2–4 days. • Deep lesions: apply plain, fresh buttermilk (room temperature) to lesions and surrounding skin for 5–10 minutes q 6–8 hours; apply absorbent dressing (consider hydrogel or hydrocolloid dressing or activated charcoal dressing); apply occlusive dressing, such as transparent dressing or wrap with saran wrap, to cover absorbent dressing and protect clothing. • Deodorize room: activated charcoal; frequent dressing changes; seal or remove used dressings from room; commercial deodorizers. Prevent infection • Culture lesions weekly and PRN. • Use aseptic technique to change dressings. • Apply topical antibacterial agents and irrigations. • Administer systemic antibiotics PRN.
Bleeding lesions	Skin care • Irrigate gently with sterile water or normal saline. • Apply hydrogel or hydrogel sheet and cover with nonadherent dressing. • Apply gentle direct pressure with dressing to decrease bleeding (e.g., elastic bandage). • Change dressing q day and as needed for odor control and drainage. • Apply local hemostatic agent to small areas of bleeding. • Do not debride. • Consider cautery (silver nitrate, electrocautery, laser cautery).

Table 10C–13
Nursing Protocol for the Management of Alopecia

Factors	Management
Radiation therapy (localized alopecia to area treated)	Assess:
	• Assess risk of alopecia prior to treatment
	• Assess body image and/or self concept disturbance (hair loss could adversely affect self-esteem, perception of sexual attractiveness, social activities; alopecia might be the only visible sign of cancer or cancer treatment)
Chemotherapy	
Biotherapy	• Assess patient's self perception and coping prior to hair loss and provide emotional support
	• Assess and educate patient with regard to potential impact
	• Assist patient/family in adapting to alopecia
	• Encourage verbalization of feelings and concerns about hair loss
	Educate the patient/family regarding:
	• Timing of expected alopecia
	• Resources to help restore self-image and self-esteem: wigs, head coverings (turbans, hats, scarves), American Cancer Society Look Good, Feel Better program, support groups
	• Temporary nature of alopecia
	• Possible changes in color and texture of hair with regrowth
	• Reimbursement (prosthetic coverage; tax deduction as medical expense)
	Maintain skin integrity
	• Minimize scalp irritation (avoid excessive brushing, harsh shampoos, hot dryers, hair dyes, sun exposure; use soft brush, mild shampoos)
	Protect eyes related to loss of eyelashes and eyebrows
	• Use sunglasses, wide-brimmed hat, false eyelashes

Severe pruritus causes an overwhelming urge to scratch. The goals of nursing management for pruritus are to minimize or reduce injury to the skin and to promote comfort (Table 10C–14). Antipruritic drugs can be prescribed for itching (e.g., hydroxyzine, diphenhydramine), and lorazepam can be used for severe itching.

Xerosis

Xerosis, or dry skin, can occur from the underlying disease and from treatment-related conditions such as edema and GVHD. (Table 10C–15).

Table 10C–14
Nursing Protocol for the Management of Pruritus

Factor	Intervention
Assessment	• Obtain patient description of onset, duration, intensity, sensation, pattern, location • Observe skin color, temperature, turgor, lesions, integrity, infection • Determine factors that reduce or aggravate pruritus
Need for systemic medications	Consider: • Steroids • Antihistamines • Cholestyramine (renal or hepatic pruritus) • Cimetidine + antihistamine • Tricyclic antidepressants (doxepin)
Need for topical medications	Consider: • Corticosteroids • Diphenhydramine • Astringents for inflamed lesions or vesicles • Moisturizing agents (lubricants, bath oils, lotions, creams, ointments) • Tepid or cool wet compresses/soaks
Protection of skin integrity	• Prevent skin trauma (shorten fingernails, use cotton gloves, soft cotton clothing and bedding, non-binding clothing) • Avoid scratching; use gentle, firm pressure or gentle rubbing around area of itch with open palm or soft cloth • Pat skin gently to dry • Rotate IM or SC injection sites when appropriate
Promotion of comfort	• Prevent dry skin • Humidify environment • Maintain cool room temperature • Encourage tepid baths for 10 to 20 minutes • Use mild soap, colloidal oatmeal baths • Provide adequate systemic hydration and nutrition • Reduce anxiety • Employ techniques of diversion, distraction, guided imagery, relaxation • Avoid activities that cause perspiration
Prevent further irritation	• Use hypo-allergenic soap/detergents • Avoid chemicals (perfume, deodorant) • Prevent vasodilation
Educate patient/family	• Focus on self care techniques to relieve/minimize pruritus • Instruct regarding reportable signs and symptoms (worsening of pruritus, pain, bleeding, infection, fever)

Table 10C-15
Nursing Protocol for the Management of Xerosis

Factor	Intervention
Assessment	• Assess previous or current treatment
Protect skin integrity	• Avoid scratching • Avoid use of tape on dry skin • Encourage diet with adequate iron, zinc, and protein to promote skin integrity
Prevent dry skin	• Bathe no more often than every 1 to 2 days using tepid water • Wash with mild soaps (e.g., Dove®, Basis®, Neutrogena®, Aveeno®) • Use medicated baths (Aveeno® Colloidal Oatmeal Bath) • Use bath oils • Apply topical anesthetic creams, emollients (Lubriderm®, Alpha Keri®, Nivea®, Aquaphor®) • Use topical corticosteroids when there are eczematous changes • Use topical preparations on wet skin for increased absorption • Use mild shampoo (e.g., baby shampoo) • Avoid heating pads, hot-water bottles, ice bags • Wear non-binding, soft cotton clothing • Avoid chemicals on dry skin (perfume, deodorant) • Ensure adequate hydration (2 to 3 quarts of fluid per day) • Humidify room to 30% to 40% • Maintain cool room temperature

Radiation Therapy-Induced Skin Changes

Possible skin side effects in the radiation treatment field include early changes (erythema, dry desquamation, moist desquamation, and alopecia) and late effects such as fibrosis, atrophy, pigmentation, and telangiectasia (see Chapter 2B and Table 10C–16). Dry desquamation can begin after approximately two weeks of treatment. Moist desquamation can begin after approximately four weeks of treatment, or could be due to radiation recall or enhancement from prior chemotherapy. Aims of care include minimizing symptoms by avoiding actions and substances that will increase side effects, educating patients and families, promoting healing, and providing comfort.

Edema, Lymphedema and Ascites

The therapeutic treatment of ascites is paracentesis, intraperitoneal therapy, and peritoneovenous shunting to remove accumulated fluid, providing relief of symptoms and discomfort (Table 10C–17). However, paracentesis causes disruption to skin integrity due to the introduction of a paracentesis

Table 10C–16
Nursing Protocol for the Management of Radiation Induced Skin Changes

Factor	Intervention
Dry desquamation	Assess • Assess for changes in radiated skin during and after treatment course • Assess recent or concurrent chemotherapy or hyperthemia Educate patient/family: • Teach self-care as follows Provide skin care for radiated skin • Avoid sun exposure to radiated skin • Wash radiated area with mild soap (e.g., Dove®, Neutrogena®) and tepid water and gently pat dry • Use mild shampoo (e.g., baby shampoo) • Avoid heating pads, hot-water bottles, ice bags in radiated sites • Use electric shaver • Moisturize skin: apply thin layer and use only recommended water-soluble lotions and creams to relieve dryness 2–3 times per day (e.g., Aquaphor®, Eucerin®, Sween Cream®, aloe lotions and creams, non-perfumed substances) • Avoid application of lotions and creams for 2–3 hours prior to daily radiation treatment • Avoid chemicals in radiated area (e.g., perfumes, harsh deodorants)
Hyperpigmentation	Educate patient/family: • Some degree of hyperpigmentation could be permanent
Moist desquamation	Assess: • Assess for infection • Assess skin folds in treatment field for breakdown (e.g., inframammary area, axilla, groin) Education patient/family: • Teach self-care • Teach that adequate nutrition is required for optimal wound healing Minimize pain Provide skin care for radiated skin: • Avoid irritation and trauma to the area • Teach that wound healing is better in a clean, moist wound bed that is free of debris, eschar, and infection • Cleanse area to keep free of crusts; consider use of autolytic debriding hydrogels • Mild astringent soaks: Domeboro® solution soak for 10–15 minutes 3–4 times per day for gentle debridement of dead cells and exudate • Provide moist wound environment to promote healing (e.g., hydrogels, hydrocolloids, moisture vapor permeable dressings) • Avoid maceration of area

Table 10C–17
Nursing Protocol for the Management of Edema, Lymphedema, and Ascites

Factors	Intervention

Promote circulation	• Palpate peripheral pulses
	• Assess skin temperature, color, and capillary refill
	• Measure girth and extremity circumference comparing with opposite extremity
	• Weigh patient daily
	• Position patient for maximum drainage:
	  Elevate extremity
	  Use of supportive devices: scrotal support
	  Use high Fowler's position for ascites
	  Use compression therapy: pneumatic pump, jobst stocking
	• Provide physical therapy: ROM, ambulation
	• Avoid blood pressure in affected extremity

Maintain skin integrity	• Provide meticulous skin care: keep skin clean, dry • Assist in mobility and position changes q 1–2 hours to relieve pressure points • Apply lotions and creams to relieve pruritus and dry skin • Encourage adequate nutritional intake (refer to Chapter 9) • Use of absorbent dressing in skin folds • Avoid IV therapies and venipunctures • Assess respiratory distress from ascites
Provide medical treatment	• Administer colloids (albumin), diuretics, and antibiotics as ordered • Monitor need for and provide supportive care related to paracentesis, intraperitoneal therapy, and peritoneovenous shunting
Educate patient/family	• Inform that lymphedema is normal in the first 6 weeks following surgery • Instruct medication regimen • Instruct dietary considerations, related restriction of sodium and water, and the addition of protein • Instruct self-care techniques and treatment plan

needle through the abdominal wall into the peritoneal cavity. This becomes a potential site of ascitic fluid leakage when the ascitic fluid reaccumulates rapidly. Attention to this site is necessary by placement of an absorbent dressing or drainage bag (if more than 100cc of drainage over 24 hours) over the needle site to collect the fluid and protect the skin.

Pressure Ulcers

The goal in the management of pressure ulcers is to reduce or eliminate pressure, optimize the environment, and support and educate the patient (see Table 10C–18). Reducing or eliminating pressure can be accom-

Table 10C-18
Nursing Protocol for the Management of Pressure Ulcers

Factor	Intervention
Skin integrity	Prevent friction and shear • Use draw sheet on bed to raise patient in bed • Elevate head of bed to a maximum of 30 degrees except at meals • Have trapeze on bed to assist patient in movement • Lift (do not pull or slide) to help patient change position, use powder on surface contacting patient's skin • Apply protective dressing, such as a hydrocolloid or transparent film, or lotion to high risk areas • Utilize specialty bed as needed, i.e., low air-loss mattress • Interrupt duration and intensity of pressure by changing position q 1–2 hours; have a planned schedule • Elevate heels off of bed, position pillows to prevent direct contact between bony prominence and to maintain side lying position • Do not use donuts • Practice meticulous hygiene, maintain clean, dry skin, pay special attention to skin folds and moist areas
Ameliorate cachexia	• Use a low air-loss mattress • Provide nutritional support (see Chapter 9) • Assess high-risk areas daily including bony sacrum, coccyx, heels, elbows, trochanters, and ischial tuberosities
Immobility	• Perform range of motion exercises; assist with ambulation and transfers; referral to physical therapy if indicated
Other high-risk factors	• Utilize a pressure assessment tool, such as the Braden scale, to assess risk factors • Consider other risk factors such as sensory perception, advancing age, poor dietary intake of protein, incontinence, and hypotension
Education	• Collaborate with health care team members in determining prevention and treatment plan • Instruct patient and caregiver on prevention, treatment plan and goals

plished by choosing the appropriate support surfaces such as high or low air-loss specialty bed, and foam or gel pads for wheelchairs, and assisting the patient in position changes at least every two hours utilizing pillows to maintain side lying positions. Optimizing the wound environment includes minimizing or eliminating risk factors such as shear and friction, choosing the appropriate topical treatment and dressing, assessing and documenting wound repair, and changing therapy as needed.

To support the patient, attention is focused on nutritional status and prevention of infection. Protein, calories, vitamins, and minerals are important elements for supporting wound repair and maintaining intact skin. Dietary supplements, tube feedings, or parenteral nutrition might be necessary to meet nutritional requirements. Preventing infection can be accomplished by meticulous skin and wound care such as cleansing perineal skin after each elimination, removal of necrotic tissue by debridement, and providing systemic and/or topical antibiotics when indicated. Wounds are cultured by needle aspiration of tissue and fluid, and indicated when the wound does not respond to two to four weeks of treatment. Educating the patient and caregiver is essential for the prevention and treatment of pressure ulcers. The patient and caregiver need to understand the significant

Table 10C–19
Nursing Protocol for the Management of Surgical Wounds

Factor	Management/Description
Ensure wound closure	• Use Steri-strips™: Place over wound incision at time of wound closure or after staples have been removed • Monitor staples or sutures for inflammatory reactions, tissue ischemia
Provide primary dressing	• Use nonadherent, absorptive dressing with sterile technique
Monitor healing	• Palpate indurated ridge over incisional line 5–9 days after primary wound closure (if no ridge palpated, evaluate for wound dehiscence) • Reduce straining forces on incisional site
Monitor wound site	• Assess drainage: color, odor, quantity • Document changes in periwound skin: color, induration, temperature, pain
Promote healing by secondary intention	• Irrigate wound with normal saline or in a shower • Apply appropriate wound dressing, i.e., moistened gauze with normal saline covered with dry gauze, or alginate for highly draining wounds. • Change dressing BID and PRN for saturated dressing • Debride necrotic tissue: autolytic, surgical, or whirlpool
Educate patient/family	• Teach deep-breathing exercises • Encourage activity and rest • Instruct importance of adequate hydration • Teach patient to refrain from straining: use stool softeners or laxatives • Teach patient signs and symptoms of infection: wound site changes, and fever • Teach patient wound care

factors that contribute to pressure ulcer development, prevention measures, the significance of nutritional requirements for wound repair, and the indicators of wound healing.

The surgical wound will progress through the phases of wound healing. Surgical wounds are most often closed by primary intention (see Table 10C–19). It is necessary for the clinician to assess and evaluate the incision carefully and support the healing process. Assessment of the surgical wound includes primary dressing, presence of epithelial resurfacing, type of wound closure, presence of a healing ridge, and local changes at the wound site.

Surgical Wound Management

Table 10C–20
Nursing Protocol for the Management of Herpes Virus

Factor	Intervention
Prevent spread	• Assess for prodromal signs and appearance of lesions in high-risk populations • Practice strict isolation of suspected or confirmed patients • Ensure adequate varicella titers for staff and restrict pregnant staff from contact
Minimize discomfort	• Assess involved areas and characteristics of the discomfort • Administer analgesics, antihistamines, and corticosteroids as necessary • Relieve discomfort locally using cool compresses • Cover lesions with a nonadherent dressing to protect from mechanical trauma (friction and shear) and to absorb drainage from erupted lesions. • Provide a quiet environment to promote relaxation; distraction activities, or biofeedback
Prevent secondary infection	• Assess for signs and symptoms of infection, i.e., fever, purulent drainage • Culture indicated areas • Administer antipyretics as needed • Avoid introduction of pathogens by meticulous handwashing, skin care, and perineal hygiene; avoid use of Foley catheter if possible • Avoid breaking lesions from scratching (shorten finger nails or provide mitten) • Gently clean broken lesions daily either by showering or using spray cleanser, pat dry, do not rub.
Detect systemic involvement	• Seek immediate attention of ophthalmologist for any lesions of the head or face. • Be alert for signs of widespread dissemination including evaluation of neurological and pulmonary status. • Administer antiviral agents.
Maintain adequate fluid and food intake	• If oral lesions are present: use saline mouthwashes and analgesics (see Chapter 10B) • Assess swallowing ability and adjust diet accordingly, i.e., soft diet, nutrition shakes • Set fluid intake goals and monitor.
Promote mobility	• Perform range-of-motion exercises to all affected extremities and joints; assist with ambulating.
Educate patient/family	• Teach disease characteristics and sequelae of disease and treatment. • Teach self-care techniques for lesion care, pain control, and prevention of infection.

Viral Infection

For nursing management of the patient with herpes virus see Table 10C–20.

SUMMARY

The skin is the largest organ of the body and serves as a major protective mechanism. Cancer and its treatment modalities often affect the skin. Skin lesions have both physiological and psychological consequences that can affect quality of life. Goals of nursing care include aiding healing, promoting comfort, and preventing infection. Collaborating with patients to manage side effects of treatment can help alleviate distress caused by these symptoms, minimize symptoms, and improve the patient's quality of life during and following treatment.

BIBLIOGRAPHY

1. Alexander, L., C. Kononenko, and C. Hess. The 1997 Ostomy/Wound Management Buyers Guide. *Ostomy* 43(6). 1997.

   This volume provides a complete overview of current products on the market utilized for wound management, including an explanation of major classes of wound products.

2. Archambeau, J. O., R. Pezner, and T. Wasserman. Pathophysiology of irradiated skin and breast. *International Journal of Radiation Oncology, Biology, and Physics* 31(5): 1171–1185. 1995.

   This article provides information regarding effects of radiation on the skin.

3. Boyton, P., and C. Paustian. Wound assessment and decision making options. *Critical Care Nursing Clinics of North America* 8(2): 125–139. 1996.

   This article describes wound characteristics and treatment criteria.

4. Bryant, R. *Acute and Chronic Wounds: Nursing Management.* Mosby Yearbook, St. Louis. 1992.

   This comprehensive book describes the nursing management of acute and chronic wounds associated with diseases and treatments.

5. Burke, M. B., G. M. Wilkes, and K. Ingwersen, eds. *Cancer Chemotherapy: A Nursing Process Approach.* Jones and Bartlett Publishers, Sudbury, MA. 1996.

   This comprehensive book reviews information about chemotherapy with standardized nursing care plans for toxicities as well as detailed information on specific agents.

6. Braden, B. J., and N. Bergstrom. Clinical utility of the Braden Scale for Predicting Pressure Sore Risk. *Decubitus* 2: 44–51. 1989.

   This article describes the Braden Scale, a widely used and reliable tool for assessing pressure ulcer risk.

7. Byers, J. Local and systemic effects of major traumatic wounds. *Critical Care Nursing Clinics of North America* 8(2): 107–113. 1996.

   This article presents effects of a traumatic wound locally and systemically.

8. Engin, K., L. Tupchong, F. M. Waterman, J. D. McFarlane, L. L. Hoh, and D. B. Leeper. Predictive factors for skin reactions in patients treated with thermoradiotherapy. *International Journal of Hyperthermia* 11(5): 357–364. 1995.

This article presents factors related to skin effects of combined radiation therapy and chemotherapy.

9. Flynn, M. Wound healing and critical illness. *Critical Care Nursing Clinics of North America* 8(2): 115–123. 1996.

This article describes the phases of wound healing.

10. Gallagher, J. Management of cutaneous symptoms. *Seminars in Oncology Nursing* 11(4): 239–247. 1995.

This article presents management of cancerous cutaneous lesions related to disease and treatment.

11. Goodman, M., L. Hilderley, and S. Purl. Integumentery and mucous membrane alterations. In Groenwald, S. L., M. Goodman, M. H. Frogge, and C. H. Yarbro. *Cancer Nursing: Principles and Practice.* 768–822. Jones and Bartlett Publishers, Boston. 1997.

This is a comprehensive chapter describing the normal anatomy and physiology of the skin and the alterations in skin integrity–related cancer and the treatment of cancer.

12. Krieg, T. Collagen in the healing wound. *Wounds: A Compendium of Clinical Research and Practice* 7(Supplement A): 5A–9A. 1995.

This article provides a thorough description of the wound healing process.

13. Leshin, B. and W. L. White. Malignant neoplasms of keratinocytes. In Arndt, K. A., P. E. LeBoit, J. K. Robinson, and B. U. Wintroub. *Cutaneous Medicine and Surgery: An Integrated Program in Dermatology.* 1378–1440. W. B. Saunders Company, Philadelphia. 1996.

This chapter presents a thorough review of cancers arising from keratinocytes and treatment of these lesions.

14. Longman, A. Skin cancers. In Mc Corkle, R., M. Grant, M. Frank-Stromborg, and S. Baird, eds. *Cancer Nursing: A Comprehensive Textbook.* WB Saunders Co., Philadelphia. 1996.

This comprehensive chapter provides a description of the skin's structure and carcinogenic changes.

15. Maklebust, J. Using wound care products to promote a healing environment. *Critical Care Nursing Clinics of North America* 8(2): 141–158. 1996.

This article describes how wound care products can be utilized to promote a healing environment.

16. McDonald, A. Skin ulceration. *In* Groenwald, S. L., M. Goodman, M. H. Frogge, and C. H. Yarbro. *Cancer Symptom Management.* Jones and Bartlett Publishers, Sudbury, MA. 364–381. 1996.

This chapter describes the development and treatment of skin ulcerations in cancer patients.

17. McLean, D. I. and H. Lui. Paraneoplastic syndromes. *In* Arndt, K. A., P. E. LeBoit, J. K. Robinson, and B. U. Wintroub. *Cutaneous Medicine and Surgery: An Integrated Program in Dermatology.* 1843–1852. WB Saunders Company, Philadelphia. 1996.

This chapter describes multiple paraneoplastic syndromes with cutaneous manifestations.

18. Oncology Nursing Society. *Cancer Chemotherapy Guidelines and Recommendations for Practice.* Oncology Nursing Press, Inc., Pittsburgh. 1996.

    These excellent guidelines and recommendations for practice provide referenced information regarding nursing practice for patients receiving chemotherapy, including tables regarding symptom management for these patients.

19. Pickard-Holley, S. The symptom experience of alopecia. *Seminars in Oncology Nursing* 11(4): 235–238. 1995.

    This article presents management of alopecia, including patient education, resources, support, and impact on body image and quality of life.

20. Seiz, A. M. and C. H. Yarbro. Pruritus. *In* Groenwald, S. L., M. Goodman, M. H. Frogge, and C. H. Yarbro. *Cancer Symptom Management.* 137–149. Jones and Bartlett Publishers, Sudbury, MA. 1996.

    This comprehensive chapter provides information on etiology of pruritus, in addition to pathophysiology, assessment, symptom management, and patient education.

21. Sitton, E. Managing side effects of skin changes and fatigue. *In* Dow, K. H., J. D. Bucholtz, R. R. Iwamoto, V. K. Fieler, and L. J. Hilderley. *Nursing Care in Radiation Oncology,* 2d Ed. 79–100. WB Saunders Company, Philadelphia. 1997.

    This chapter provides a comprehensive review of what is currently known about management of skin side effects from radiation therapy.

22. ———— Early and late radiation-induced skin alterations, part I: Mechanisms of skin changes. *Oncology Nursing Forum* 19(5): 801–807. 1992.

23. ———— Early and late radiation-induced skin alterations, part II: Nursing care of irradiated skin. *Oncology Nursing Forum* 19(5): 907–912. 1992.

    These articles provide an overview of the mechanisms of skin changes and management of these changes related to radiation.

24. Department of Health and Human Services. *Clinical Practice Guideline Number 15: Treatment of Pressure Ulcers.* AHCPR Publication # 95-0652. Washington, DC. 1994.

    These guidelines are written to assist practitioner and patient decisions about treatment of pressure ulcers.

25. Walczak, J., and C. Heckman. Ascities. *In* Groenwald, S. L., M. Goodman, M. H. Frogge, and C. H. Yarbro. *Cancer Symptom Management.* 385–398. Jones and Bartlett Publishers, Sudbury, MA. 1996.

    This chapter provides a comprehensive review of the assessment and management of ascites, a symptom of advanced cancer.

26. Zimmerman, G. C., J. H. Keeling, H. A. Burris, G. Cook, R. Irvin, J. Kuhn, M. L. McCollough, and D. D. vonHoff. Acute cutaneous reactions to docetaxel, a new chemotherapeutic agent. *Archives of Dermatology* 131: 202–206. 1995.

    This article describes the cutaneous side effects of docetaxel found in phase I and II studies of the drug.

Neurologic Complications

Johanna LaRoss Meehan

INTRODUCTION

Neurologic complications of systemic cancer represent an important challenge to oncology nurses because of the complexity of neurologic dysfunction resulting from either primary or secondary effects of cancer. The incidence and scope of neurologic involvement has increased in recent years due to the increase in survival among cancer patients, allowing the development of central nervous system (CNS) metastases as a late effect of cancer, as well as the development of latent toxicities of therapy. The continuing emergence of novel neurotoxic cancer drugs and use of dose-intensive chemotherapy strategies have also contributed to an increase in neurologic complications. These complications often produce frightening and disabling symptoms that require careful management by the oncology nurse, in collaboration with other medical disciplines, in order to avoid, control, or eliminate functional disabilities. Early identification of the signs and symptoms of neurologic deficits is crucial, because the impairment can progress or become permanent if not addressed in its earliest stage. Physical disability reduces a person's quality of life by limiting career options, housing, social interactions, and general well-being. Prompt intervention can ameliorate disabilities and improve quality of life for many patients.

PATHOPHYSIOLOGY

The scope of neurologic complications is broad (see Table 11–1), and etiology is often difficult to determine. Dysfunction can result from a combination of interactions involving drugs, tumor, or host factors. Up to 20 percent of patients with systemic cancer can develop neurologic symptoms during the course of their illness. Autopsy reports indicate that up to 25 percent of patients have CNS metastases. Neurological damage can result from primary CNS tumors, systemic metastases to the brain and spinal cord, complications resulting from therapy or procedures, or secondary effects of malignancy. Primary or secondary effects of unrelated chronic illness or conditions also produce neurologic complications. It is important for the physician and nurse to differentiate among the effects of the malignancy, the treatment, and other possible alterations in the nervous system.

11

Table 11-1
Etiology of Neurologic Complications of Cancer

Malignant Causes	
Primary brain tumors	Metastases to spinal cord
Metastases to brain	Leptomeningeal carcinomatosis
Primary spinal cord tumors	

Nonmalignant Causes	
Treatment-related effects	Vascular disease
Systemic chemotherapy	Hyperviscosity syndrome
Intrathecal chemotherapy	Thromboembolic disease
Biotherapy	
Radiation therapy	Paraneoplastic syndromes
Leukoencephalopathy	Cerebellar degeneration
	Sensory and motor neuropathies
	Opsoclonus/myoclonus
Support medications	Retinopathy
Antiemetics	Dermatomyositis
Sedatives	Eaton Lambert syndrome
Corticosteroids	Giullian-Barre syndrome
Antimicrobials	Polymyositis
Cyclosporin	
Analgesics	Underlying chronic illness
	Addison's disease
Secondary complications	Alcoholism
Metabolic encephalopathy	Alzheimer's disease
Infection of CNS	Diabetes
Meningitis	Thyroid disorders
Abscess	Malnutrition
Systemic infection	Multiple sclerosis
Encephalomyelitis	AIDS

MALIGNANT CAUSES OF NEUROLOGIC DYSFUNCTION

Brain Tumors

Tumors arising in the brain or spinal cord represent only 2 percent of all cancers. The majority of brain tumors occur in two age peaks: childhood (3–12 years), and later life (55–70 years). The incidence of primary brain tumors in the United States is increasing, especially in the older population.

Primary brain tumors are the second most common tumor in children, exceeded only by leukemia, and the fourth leading cause of cancer death in middle-aged adult males.

Primary tumors of the brain spread locally and through CNS seeding; they rarely metastasize to distant locations. The enclosed cranium restricts expansion of tumor, producing profound neurologic defects and death in a relatively short time span. The inability of the brain to regenerate after damage has occurred also contributes to a high degree of permanent disability. The presenting signs and symptoms of brain tumors depend on the area of the brain involved (focal symptoms) and the effects of increased intracranial pressure (generalized symptoms). Symptoms can appear gradually or develop rapidly. Knowledge of the tumor site enables the nurse to plan care based on predicted problems and behaviors.

In most patients with brain tumors, the initial presenting symptoms include headaches, seizures, and alterations in consciousness. The headaches are described as deep and dull, and are characteristically worse in the morning, improving as the day proceeds. Weakness; sensory loss; deficits in vision, hearing, or smell; personality changes; vomiting; and papilledema also occur in adults with brain tumors. Symptoms of increased intracranial pressure (ICP) include lethargy, drowsiness, irritability, and difficulty with ambulation (see Chapter 15A).

Surgical resection is the initial therapy for brain tumors. Corticosteroids and radiation therapy are also critical to the treatment plan. Chemotherapy is used as an adjunctive treatment with modest success. When the patient has seizures, anticonvulsant therapy must be instituted and followed carefully.

Metastases to the brain represent a common neurologic complication of systemic cancer, occurring in 20 percent to 40 percent of cancer patients. The incidence of brain metastases is highest in the 50- to 70-year-old group. Lung cancer is the most common malignancy found to metastasize to the brain. Other common sources include breast, melanoma, renal, and gastrointestinal malignancies. Most metastases reach the brain via hematogenous spread. Distribution of metastases parallels the blood supply to the brain, with the cerebrum the most common site (80 percent), followed by the cerebellum (17 percent), and the brainstem (3 percent). Although patients with metastatic brain lesions might be asymptomatic, the progression and type of symptoms are determined by the site of the lesion (see Tables 11–2 and 3), the growth rate, and type of underlying tumor. Generalized signs and symptoms of brain metastases mimic those of primary brain tumors: headache, seizures, loss of motor function, impaired mentation, lethargy, sensory loss, and increased intracranial pressure.

Radiation therapy is standard treatment for brain metastases. Supportive therapy also includes the use of corticosteroids and anticonvulsant management for patients with suspected seizures or in whom surgical resection is planned. Brachytherapy and stereotactic radiation therapy deliver high-dose radiation to focal lesions with few acute toxicities. Surgical excision is rarely an option, and chemotherapy is generally not helpful.

Table 11-2
Neurologic Symptoms Associated with Specific Areas of Brain Involvement

Focal Symptoms	
Frontal Lobe	*Occipital Lobe*
Personality changes	Seizures
Altered mental status	Decreased visual fields
Decreased sphincter control	Hallucinations
Hemiparesis	Headache
Emotional lability	Nausea/vomiting
Memory deficits	Vertigo
Flat affect	Aphasia
Seizures	
Expressive aphasia	*Brainstem*
Papilledema, diplopia	Cranial nerve palsy (IV–XII)
Decreased visual fields	Papilledema
Gait disturbances	Cerebellar dysfunction
	Vomiting
Parietal Lobe	Dysphagia
Focal seizures	Motor & sensory deficits
Visual field change	Ataxia
Dyslexia	
Nystagmus	*Cerebellum*
Agnosia, agraphia	Ataxia
Receptive aphasia	Impaired coordination
Altered body image	Nystagmus
Perceptual changes	Cranial nerve dysfunction (VIII–XII)
Impaired cognition	
Paresthesia	*Pituitary and Hypothalamus*
Hypesthesia	Sleep disturbance
Hemianopsia (contralateral or homonymous)	Headache
	Nausea/vomiting
Altered emotions	Hormonal imbalance
Sensory deficits	Optic atrophy
	Paralysis of extraocular muscles
Temporal Lobe	Fat and carbohydrate metabolic imbalance
Psychomotor or generalized seizures	Water and temperature control imbalance
Visual field changes	Cushing's Syndrome
Memory impairment	
Aphasia	
Dysphagia	
Papilledema	

Adapted with permission from McDonnell, K. K. Increased intracranial pressure. In Johnson, B. L., and J. Gross, *Handbook of Oncology Nursing*. 1st ed. John Wiley & Sons. New York. 1985. 403.

Table 11-3
Neurologic Symptoms Associated
with Generalized Brain Involvement

Generalized Symptoms
Headache
Vomiting
Papilledema
Pituitary dysfunction
Seizure activity
Mental changes
Deterioration in level of consciousness
Visual disturbances
Motor deficits
Personality changes

Spinal Cord Tumors

Primary spinal cord tumors present much less frequently than intracranial tumors. Just as the brain is contained in the skull, the spinal cord is contained in the vertebral column, eliminating room for tumor expansion and displacement.

These tumors can be classified by cellular origin, anatomic location, tumor type, or location in relation to vertebral column. Anatomic classification distinguishes extramedullary tumors (occuring outside the spinal cord) from intramedullary tumors (occuring within the spinal cord). Extramedullary tumors, which account for 90 percent of all primary spinal cord tumors, are further defined as extradural (outside the dura; within epidural area) or intradural (within or under the spinal dura, not within the spinal cord).

Spinal cord tumors present with a combination of pain and alterations in sensory, motor, and autonomic function. Extramedullary tumors tend to produce symptoms by compression or destruction of nerve roots or bone before the cord itself is involved. Intramedullary tumors are manifested by symptoms of spinal cord compression. The most common and earliest presenting symptom is back pain. Weakness, loss of sensation, and difficulty with bowel and bladder control can follow. Weakness tends to appear in distal extremities and progress proximally. Reflexes are initially hyperactive and later become hypotonic, with flaccid paralysis. Temperature, proprioception, and touch can all be affected. Sensory testing determines the dermatome affected by the lesion. Many tumors can be identified through detailed history and neurologic examination.

Radiation therapy, or surgical decompression followed by radiation therapy, is the principal therapy for all primary intraspinal tumors. Corticosteroids are also an important part of the treatment plan.

Metastases to the spinal cord occur in 5 percent to 10 percent of patients with cancer and can be either a late effect of advanced disease or an early sign of underlying malignancy. Spinal cord metastases are presenting symptoms of malignancy in one-third of childhood tumors. The most common adult tumors to metastasize to the spine are carcinomas of the lung, breast and prostate, and myelomas.

Clinical presentation depends on the level of spinal involvement. Back pain is the most common presenting symptom (95 percent), with the thoracic region the most common site (70 percent), followed by lumbarsacral (20 percent) and cervical (10 percent) spine. Spinal cord compression is a neuro-oncologic emergency (see Chapter 15B). Preservation of neurologic function through early diagnosis is mandatory to prevent the catastrophic consequences of paraplegia and bowel and bladder incontinence. When neurologic symptoms other than pain develop, progression is often quite rapid, with possible paraplegia in a matter of hours or days. The site of the lesion determines the character of the symptoms, which can range from paresthesia to death.

Treatment is aimed at pain relief and preservation and restoration of neurologic function. Radiation therapy is the treatment of choice for spinal metastases with or without surgical decompression. High-dose steroids are also employed.

Leptomeningeal Carcinomatosis

Leptomeningeal carcinomatosis is the diffuse multifocal seeding of the surface layers of the brain (pia mater and arachnoid membranes) with tumor deposits. Seeding could block cerebrospinal fluid (CSF) pathways, producing increased intracranial pressure and hydrocephalus. It occurs in approximately 8 percent of patients with systemic cancer and is frequently associated with carcinomas of the breast and lung, lymphomas, malignant melanomas, and adult acute leukemias. Multiple cerebrospinal fluid exams (up to four lumbar punctures) are often required to confirm the diagnosis in suspicious cases. Leptomeningeal metastases typically present with symptoms of transient neurologic dysfunction. Signs and symptoms of leptomeningeal carcinomatosis include headache and altered mental status, cranial nerve dysfunction (exhibited as diplopia and visual changes), spinal root symptoms (with neck, back, and radicular pain), paresthesia, and focal weakness.

Optimal treatment has not been established, but radiation of clinically involved areas combined with intrathecal administration of chemotherapeutic agents such as methotrexate, cytarabine, or thiotepa is generally used. The drug can be administered by lumbar puncture or by intraventricular reservoir. Surgical placement of an Ommaya intraventricular reservoir facilitates delivery of chemotherapy agents directly into the ventricle for circulation throughout the CSF (see Chapter 3B).

NONMALIGNANT CAUSES
OF NEUROLOGIC DYSFUNCTION

Complications Caused by
Cancer Treatment

The use of new investigational drugs, as well as standard drugs used in new combinations or in higher doses, has contributed to an increased occurrence of neurotoxicity. The incidence of neurotoxicity related to antineoplastic agents has been estimated at 60 percent in patients receiving standard therapy and as high as 70 percent in the bone marrow transplantation population. Many risk factors contribute to the occurrence of neurotoxicities associated with antineoplastic agents, including advanced age, hepatic or renal insufficiencies, dose-intensive chemotherapy, combined modality therapy, and new schedules or routes of drug delivery. Chemotherapy agents can produce a broad spectrum of neurologic deficits, resulting in peripheral, cerebral, or cerebellar deficits. It is of utmost importance to attempt to differentiate the effects of therapy from the effects of the disease in order to adjust or discontinue treatment. Anti-tumor agents with high potential for neurologic toxicities include L-asparaginase, carboplatin, cisplatin, cytarabine, docetaxel, fludarabine, fluorouracil, ifosfamide, high-dose interferons, methotrexate, paclitaxel, procarbazine, suramin, tretinoin and the vinca alkaloids. (See Table 11–4 for chemotherapy agents and associated neurotoxicities.)

Systemic Chemotherapy

Intrathecal (IT) administration of antineoplastic agents to treat or prevent CNS metastases can result in several types of neurologic dysfunction, such as alterations in mental status and signs of subacute meningeal irritation (headache, nausea, vomiting, fever, stiff neck). The most frequently used intrathecal drugs are methotrexate (MTX), cytarabine, and thiotepa. Five to ten percent of patients treated with MTX will exhibit signs of acute meningeal irritation. Arachnoiditis is the most common type of MTX neurotoxicity, occurring in 5 percent to 40 percent of prophylactic intrathecal MTX courses. Combined modality therapies, such as those used in the treatment of acute lymphocytic leukemia, potentiate the CNS effects of MTX. The patient's age, total dose of drug, concurrent radiation therapy, preexisting neurologic deficit, or presence of active leukemia will also place the patient at risk for CNS toxicity.

Intrathecal Chemotherapy

CNS toxicities are common and distressing side effects seen with the use of biological response modifiers (see Chapter 2D). The toxicities appear to be dose dependent and cumulative. Symptoms include memory loss, confusion, attention deficits, depression, fatigue, somnolence, leth-

Biotherapy

Table 11–4
Neurotoxic Signs Caused by Agents Commonly Used in Patients with Cancer

Acute Encephalopathy (Delirium)

Corticosteroids
Methotrexate (high-dose IV, IT)
Cis-platinum
Vincristine
Asparaginase
Procarbazine
5-Fluorouracil (± levamisole)
Ara-C
Nitrosoureas (high-dose or arterial)
Cyclosporine
Interleukin-2
Ifosfamide/mesna
Interferons
Tamoxifen
VP-16 (high-dose)
PALA

Chronic Encephalopathy (Dementia)

Methotrexate
BCNU
Ara-C
Carmofur
Fludarabine

Visual Loss

Tamoxifen
Gallium nitrate
Nitrosoureas (intra-arterial)
Cis-platinum

Cerebellar Dysfunction/Ataxia

5-Fluorouracil (± levamisole)
Ara-C
Phenytoin
Procarbazine
Hexamethylmelamine
Vincristine
Cyclosporine

Aseptic Meningitis

Trimethoprim-sulfamethoxazole (Co-trimoxazole)
IVIg
NSAIDs
Levamisole
Monoclonal antibodies
Metrizamide
OKT3
Ara-C
Carbamazepine
Methotrexate (IT)

Headaches without Meningitis

Retinoic acid
Trimethoprim-sulfamethoxazole
Cimetidine
Corticosteroids
Tamoxifen

Seizures

Methotrexate
VP-16 (high-dose)
Cis-platinum
Vincristine
Asparaginase
Nitrogen mustard
BCNU
Dacarbazine (intra-arterial or high-dose)
PALA
mAmsa
Busulfan (high-dose)
Cyclosporine
Mitronidazole
Misonidazole
Beta-lactam antibiotics
Iodinated contrast material (IV or IT)

Myelopathy (Intrathecal Drugs)

Methotrexate
Ara-C
Thiotepa

Peripheral Neuropathy

Vinca alkaloids
Cis-platinum
Hexamethylmelamine
Procarbazine
5-Azacytidine
VP-16
VM-26
Misonidazole
Methyl-G
Ara-C
Taxol
Suramin
Mitotane

Ara-C = cytosine arabinoside or cytarabine: BCNU = carmustine; IV = intravenous; IVIg = intravenous gamma globulin; IT = intrathecal; mAmsa = acridinvlaniside or AMSA; NSAIDs = nonsteroidal anti-inflammatory drugs; OKT3 = orthoclone; PALA = N-phosphonoacetyl-L-aspartate; VM-26 = teniposide; VP-16 = etoposide, Taxol = paclitaxel.

Reprinted with permission from Posner, J. B. *Neurologic Complications of Cancer*. F.A. Davis Company, Philadelphia. 1995.

argy, and loss of cognitive function. Interferon can also cause encephalopathies and mild peripheral neuropathies. Interleukin-2 has been noted to produce ophthalmic alterations, and the vascular leak syndrome associated with intravenous IL-2 administration has been observed to induce encephalopathy and/or coma.

Radiation Therapy

CNS radiation damage can occur acutely, subacutely, or several years after treatment, producing damage to the brain, spinal cord, or peripheral nerves (see Chapter 2B). Although neurological damage from radiation therapy is rare, the incidence of neurological disability is related to the dose, area radiated, vascularity of tissue, and patient's age and sensitivity to radiation. Headache, nausea and vomiting are common signs and symptoms of acute radiation toxicity to the brain. Somnolence syndrome with drowsiness, nausea, and malaise typically occurs approximately six weeks after radiation. Chronic CNS damage is usually manifested as cognitive impairment.

Recent data suggest that children who receive cranial radiation experience long-term functional problems and significant intellectual decrements. These late effects generally occur 24 to 36 months after treatment. Children under 5 years of age and adults over 60 are at greatest risk for the deleterious effects of CNS radiation.

Radiation myelopathy due to CNS radiation therapy can result in reversible Lhermittes' syndrome 1 to 4 months after treatment to the spinal cord. A more serious, progressive transverse myelitis produces weakness, radicular pain, and loss of pain and temperature sensation in the 6 to 12 months following spinal radiation treatment. The major risk factor is the dose. Steroid therapy sometimes delays progression, but prevention is the only successful therapy.

Chronic radiation encephalopathy, due to brain necrosis and occlusion of small vessels, is manifested by increased intracranial pressure and focal neurological dysfunction. This is irreversible and can be fatal.

Radiation necrosis occurs in 4 percent to 9 percent of patients. Although uncommon, it is an irreversible and devastating neurologic complication of radiation therapy. It is dose dependent and can be difficult to diagnose because an area of edema seen on CT scan might be either metastatic disease or changes caused by radiation therapy. Rarely seen in radiation therapy doses less than 5,000 cGy, it is seen more frequently at doses in the 6,000–7,000 cGy range used for intracranial and head and neck tumors. Vascular changes to the brain appear to be responsible for damage. Radiation necrosis is usually treated by surgical resection, as steroids offer only temporary relief. Therapy is primarily palliative, and nursing care focuses on safety measures for the demented, sensory-impaired, or somnolent patient. The patient with cerebral edema will benefit from measures to decrease increased cranial pressure.

New techniques such as stereotactic radiation therapy and radio-surgery, interstitial brachytherapy, and proton beam delivery spare normal tissue, thereby decreasing radiation induced toxicities.

Leukoencephalopathy, destruction of the white matter of the brain, can result from the use of MTX. It has been observed in patients receiving MTX intrathecally over a long period of time, in patients whose brains have been radiated and who are receiving intravenous MTX in standard doses, and in patients receiving high doses of MTX (8–20 grams) without radiation therapy. A 45 percent incidence is reported when CNS radiation, IT MTX, and high-dose systemic MTX are combined. MTX given before radiation therapy is less neurotoxic than MTX given after or concurrently with radiation. Leukoencephalopathy has also been associated with IT cytarabine, thiotepa, and high-dose cytarabine, as well as intra-arterial carmustine or cisplatin. Signs and symptoms include lethargy, somnolence, dementia, coma, seizures, and personality changes.

Support Medications

Antiemetic agents such as metoclopramide, prochlorperazine, and haloperidol can cause extrapyramidal reactions due to dopamine blocking activity. Extrapyramidal signs generally occur in the young and are characterized by dystonic posturing, akathisia, and severe agitation. Ondansetron, a serotonin antagonist, also can cause extrapyramidal reactions.

Sedatives are a common cause of altered mental status in cancer patients, who are more susceptible to pharmacologic side effects due to compromised metabolism, cachexia, depression, and the use of multiple drug regimens. Tricyclic antidepressants, anxiolytic antidepressants (such as alprazolam and fluoxetine), and psychotropic drugs are all frequently used for cancer patients and can have neurotoxic effects.

Steroids are the most widely used drugs in neurooncology and are the key therapy for edema and ICP. They commonly cause muscle weakness (often incapacitating), infection, hyperglycemia, gastrointestinal disturbances, insomnia, and mental status changes ranging from mood swings and anxiety to steroid psychosis. Symptoms arising from the use of these agents also include headache, confusion, seizures, and coma. Steroid doses should be tapered immediately upon detection of neurologic changes, because rapid withdrawal from steroids also causes neurologic disability.

Antimicrobials can cause neurologic dysfunctions. Penicillin-like agents, for example, can cause multifocal myoclonus, seizures, and aseptic meningitis. Bactrim™ has also been reported to cause aseptic meningitis as well as painful sensory and autonomic neuropathies. Amphotericin B causes brain white matter damage following bone marrow transplantation. Acyclovir can cause tremor, myoclonus, or delirium with or without focal symptoms. Metronidazole, an antimicrobial agent sometimes used as a radiosensitizer, can produce neuropathies, seizures, cerebellar dysfunction, and encephalopathy.

Cyclosporine, an immunosuppressive agent used to prevent and treat graft-versus-host disease in BMT recipients, causes neurologic complications in 8 percent to 29 percent of patients. Tremors and seizures are most commonly seen, followed by visual changes, musculomotor changes, peripheral neuropathies, and encephalopathies.

Analgesics are frequently used in the oncology patient population due to the high incidence of pain in patients with end-stage disease. Opioid analgesics often add to existing neurologic dysfunction. Side effects of analgesics include sedation, visual disturbances, hallucinations, myoclonus, and seizures.

Secondary Neurologic Complications

Metabolic encephalopathy occurs when the brain is unable to regulate or detoxify substances due to interference by extracerebral factors. This common neurologic complication results in behavioral changes such as delirium or an acute confusional state. The etiology of metabolic encephalopathy includes hypoxia, organ failure, fluid, acid/base and electrolyte imbalance, sepsis, drug effects, and alteration of nutritional status. Any change in mental status is an early sign, followed by more severe behavior change, disturbance in cognition, and perceptual errors. Motor dysfunction, myoclonus, respiratory changes, and coma can ensue if not addressed and reversed in early stages. Hepatic encephalopathy and hypercalcemia are the most frequent neurologic syndromes seen in cancer patients.

Infection is common in immunosuppressed patients and can cause neurologic deficits. CNS infections occur most commonly in patients with lymphoma and leukemia, and in the bone marrow transplant population due to abnormal host defense mechanisms. The CNS can be invaded by an infectious agent through the blood stream (septicemia) or by direct extension from nearby structures such as the ears or sinuses, resulting in abscess formation, arachnoiditis, or meningitis. Symptoms of CNS infection include fever, stiff neck, headache, mental status changes, seizures, and focal neurologic signs. Bacterial, fungal, viral, and protozoan infections can all result in neurologic complications. If diagnosed early, most infections of the CNS respond to systemic antibiotic therapy. Third-generation cephalosporins cross the blood brain barrier well, particularly in the presence of inflammation, and yield therapeutic CNS levels of drug. In patients who do not respond to systemic treatment, direct intraventricular injection of antimicrobial agents via an Ommaya reservoir (see Chapter 3B) may be indicated.

A frequent example is herpes zoster, the most common viral infection of the nervous system in cancer patients (see Chapter 10C). Shingles is caused by reactivation of the varicella-zoster virus. The virus remains latent in neurons following a primary case of chicken pox until reactivated by a breakdown in immune surveillance. It is transported to the skin via axons, causing a vesicular eruption within a dermatome. It affects the thoracic dermatome in more than 50 percent of cases. The trigeminal nerve is the next most frequently involved site. Pain, described as constant, deep, and burning, can occur prior to, during, or after eruption. Postherpetic neuralgia is pain that persists for weeks or months after the clearing of skin lesions. Disseminated herpes zoster can result in encephalopathy, Guillain-Barre syndrome, transverse myelitis and myositis, as well as pneumonia, thrombocytopenia, hepatitis, and arthritis.

Vascular Disorders

Cerebrovascular disease in cancer patients can be caused by either thrombocytopenia-induced hemorrhage or excessive coagulopathy. Intracranial or spinal hemorrhages can occur when patients are thrombocytopenic. Vessel occlusion due to a hypercoagulable state can result in infarction. More than 90 percent of patients develop a coagulation abnormality during the course of cancer or its treatment. Cerebrovascular lesions are found in 15 percent of autopsied cancer patients. Cerebrovascular pathology is the second most common neuropathological finding in autopsies of patients with systemic cancer. Disseminated intravascular coagulation, nonbacterial thrombotic endocarditis, septic or tumor embolism, atherosclerosis, and cerebral vein occlusion can cause cerebral infarction. Cerebral hemorrhage and hematomas are usually associated with metastatic brain tumors, thrombocytopenia, and hypercoagulable states. Tumors most likely to hemorrhage into a brain tumor include lung cancer, melanoma, and germ cell tumors.

Paraneoplastic syndromes are rare clinical abnormalities caused by cancer but not resulting from direct invasion by tumor or metastases. Although uncommon, their effects are sometimes more disabling than the tumor itself. The patient with no known malignancy who develops a paraneoplastic syndrome should be evaluated for occult malignancy, as about 50 percent of these syndromes precede the discovery of cancer. The four most common involved organ systems are endocrine, nervous, haematologic, and dermatologic.

The "remote" effects of cancer on the nervous system produce various clinical syndromes, such as subacute cerebellar degeneration, encephalomyelitis, subacute motor or sensory neuropathy, polymyositis, opsoclonus-myoclonus, Gullian-Barre syndrome, retinopathy, or Eaton-Lambert syndrome. Symptoms such as dementia, gait disturbance, dysarthria, adiadochokinesis, past-pointing, abnormal heel-shin test, nystagmus, loss of proprioception, motor weakness, or abnormalities of speech and vision may precede the malignancy or become evident after development of the neoplasm. Severity of symptoms can remit or progress over time, without regard to the course of the tumor or its treatment.

Patients with small cell lung cancer, breast, stomach, bowel and ovarian carcinomas, and Hodgkin's lymphoma are most likely to experience paraneoplastic syndromes.

Assessment

Nurses participate in monitoring the functional status of cancer patients at the time of diagnosis and throughout their course of therapy. A thorough nursing assessment is the foundation for identification of neurologic dysfunction, evaluation of the effects of the dysfunction on activities of daily living, and the prevention of progressive or permanent neurologic disabilities. Various scales, including the Karnofsky Performance Scale (see Table 11–5), have proven reliable, valid, and easy to use to assess the physical functioning of patients. The scales measure the patient's ability to perform normal activities of daily living or the degree of dependency on others for assistance.

A complete medical history should be taken for every patient, regardless of diagnosis. If a patient is unreliable, the history should be obtained from a qualified party, such as a family member. The physical exam provides objective information to verify the absence or presence of reported abnormalities. Table 11–6 provides a model for standard neurologic assessment. The neurologic examination encompasses a review of the cerebellar system (balance and coordination), cerebral system (cognition), and the sensory, motor, cranial, and autonomic systems. An overview of the patient can be gained by observing the patient as he or she enters the area. General posture, gait, skin integrity, willingness to move and cooperate, and overall disposition should be noted. Speech patterns can be evaluated during the interview.

CEREBELLAR NERVOUS SYSTEM

Assessment

The major function of the cerebellum is to regulate the coordination of movement. Cerebellar lesions manifest in lack of balance and coordination. This functional deficit is different from that due to spinal cord compression, in which a peripheral nerve injury causes weakness and loss of reflexes. Loss of cerebellar function results in problems with planning the movement (ideation, motivation, programming), initiating the movement, and maintaining rhythmic activity such as speech and gait. Common signs

Table 11-5
Karnofsky Performance Scale

Description: Karnofsky Scale	Karnofsky Scale	Zubrod Scale (ECOG)	TNM Scale (AJC)	Description: AJC and ECOG Scales
No complaints, no evidence of disease	100	0		Normal activity
Able to carry on normal activity, minor signs or symptoms of disease	90		H0	
Some signs or symptoms of disease	80			Symptoms of disease, but ambulatory and able to carry out activities of daily living
Cares for self with effort, unable to carry on normal activity or to do active work	70	1	H1	
Requires occasional assistance but is able to care for most personal needs	60			Out of bed more than 50% of time; occasionally needs assistance
		2	H2	
Requires considerable assistance and frequent medical care	50			
Disabled: Requires special care and assistance	40			In bed more than 50% of time; needs nursing care
		3	H3	
Severely disabled: Hospitalization indicated, although death not imminent	30			
Very sick, hospitalization necessary, requires active supportive treatment	20			Bedridden, may need hospitalization
		4	H4	
Moribund, fatal processes progressing rapidly	10			
Dead	0			

NOTE: ECOG = Eastern Cooperative Oncology Group; AJC = American Joint Commission for Cancer Staging and End Results Reporting

Table 11–6
Standard Neurological Assessment

Factor	Assessment
Consciousness	
Arousal	Observe for:
	Spontaneous eye opening
	Response to auditory environmental stimuli
	Ability to follow verbal directions
Self-Awareness	Determine orientation:
	What is your name?
	What is the year, season, month?
	Where are we now (state, town, institution)?
Motor Function	
Seeing	Observe for:
	Spontaneous eye movements
	Ability to follow objects with eyes
	Pupillary response to light, accommodation
	Voluntary eye movements
Speaking	Assess spontaneous speech for:
	Clarity of articulation
	Phonation (speech volume, sounds)
Moving	Observe for:
	Rapid initiation of movement
	Large muscle, small muscle coordination
	Strength, muscle mass
	Symmetry of movement
Walking	Observe for:
	Erect posture
	Feet together
	Steps approximately a single line
	Normal associated arm swing
	Ability to turn at a normal pace
	Brisk gait
	Maintenance of gait
Sensation	
Special Senses	Assess:
Sight	Visual acuity (newsprint, Snellen)
	Visual fields
Smell	Ability to detect odor
Hearing	Ability to detect voice, tuning fork

Continued

Table 11–6 *(Continued)*
Standard Neurological Assessment

Factor	Assessment
Somatic Senses	
Feeling	Assess:
	Perception of touch
	Perception of pain
	Perception of temperature
	Perception of limb position
Cortical sensation	Perception of form, shape, texture, and point localization
Regulation	Assess:
Breathing	Rate, rhythm, pattern, breath sounds
Circulation	Heart rate, blood pressure, postural change in blood pressure, heart sounds, color and blanching of extremities
Temperature	Temperature

and symptoms of cerebellar dysfunction are described in Table 11–7. The patient's balance and coordination are evaluated while the patient performs skilled acts such as the following:

1. Upper extremities: With arm extended to side and index finger pointing, touch nose by moving arm while looking straight ahead; repeat with other arm. If the finger-to-nose test is smooth and accurate, further evaluation of the upper extremities is not necessary.

   While sitting, the patient is asked to supinate and pronate the hands alternately, or to tap up and down rhythmically on the knee or a flat surface.

2. Lower extremities: While lying on back, place heel of dorsiflexed foot on knee of other leg and move the heel along the shin to the toe; repeat with other leg.

   Stand erect with arms at side, first with eyes open, then with eyes closed. Inability to maintain balance is a positive Romberg's sign and indicates a cerebellar lesion on the side to which he or she leans.

   Hop or stand on each leg.

3. Eye coordination: Abnormal nystagmus is an early sign of cerebellar dysfunction and consists of sustained eye jerks that occur when the patient is asked to direct the gaze from one side to the other (horizontal), then up and down (vertical). This can be done by asking the patient to follow your finger or pencil as you move in the six fields of gaze (see Table 11–6).

Table 11–7
Signs/Symptoms of Cerebellar Dysfunction

Sign/Symptom	Description
Asthenia	Generalized weakness; sense of "heaviness." Excessive effort required for simple tasks with early onset of fatigue.
Dysmetria	Disturbance of posture and balance; lack of coordination in tandem walking. Rapid, brisk movements made with more force than necessary.
Gait disturbance	Staggering gait resembling one who is intoxicated. Arm swing absent.
Movement decomposition	Performance of a movement with distinct sequence rather than smooth pattern.
Dysdiadochokinesia	Performs rapidly alternating movements slowly with loss of rate and rhythm.
Speech aphasia	Inability to process or produce language.
Speech dysarthria	Weakness, slowness, or incoordination of speech.
Scanning speech	Words or syllables pronounced slowly, accents misplaced, inappropriate pauses.
Eye movement (lateral or vertical nystagmus)	At edge of peripheral vision, eye movements are jerky, with involuntary drift back to neutral position.
Dyssynergia	Inability of body to make a coordinated muscle contraction in proper sequence.

Management of Cerebellar Dysfunction

Cerebellar dysfunction can result in decreased mobility due to loss of balance and coordination. Although the signs and symptoms can vary considerably, the goal is to overcome the resulting muscle weakness and to prevent and correct deformity such as flexion contracture. Physical therapists should be enlisted to work with patients in programs for postural stability, gait training, and accuracy of limb movements. Resistive exercises, with or without weights, are used to enhance muscle tone and can improve a patient's posture and endurance in ambulation. Proprioceptive neuromuscular facilitation (PNF), or slow-reversal-hold for the lower extremities, allows patients to ambulate with better control. Frenkel exercises (see Table 11–8) can also be used to modify dysmetria in the lower extremities. These exercises can be modified for use with upper extremities; the greater the movement error, the heavier the weight needed. Energy conservation tech-

Table 11-8
Frenkel Exercises

Supine

1. Flex and extend one leg, heel sliding down a straight line on table.
2. Abduct and adduct hip smoothly with knee bent, heel on table.
3. Abduct and adduct leg with knee and hip extended, leg sliding on table.
4. Flex and extend hip and knee with heel off table.
5. Place one heel on knee of opposite leg and slide heel slowly down shin toward ankle and back to knee.
6. Flex and extend both legs together, heels sliding on table.
7. Flex one leg while extending other leg.
8. Flex and extend one leg while abducting and adducting other leg.

Sitting

1. Place foot in therapist's hand, which will change position on each trial.
2. Raise leg and put foot on traced footprint on floor.
3. Sit steady for a few minutes.
4. Rise and sit with knees together.

Standing

1. Place foot forward and backward on a straight line.
2. Walk along a winding strip.
3. Walk between two parallel lines.
4. Walk, placing each foot in a tracing on floor.

niques maximize and prolong strength and endurance. As mobility deteriorates, whether due to weakness, pain, or lack of coordination, simple walking aids such as canes, crutches, or walkers can help considerably. The patient should be protected from injury.

CEREBRAL FUNCTION

Assessment

Assessment of mental status gives an indication of how the patient is functioning. Higher-level functions of the cerebrum include cognitive and integrative functions, personality, and affect, as well as level of consciousness. Alterations can vary from one exam to the next due to fatigue, stress, or pathophysiology.

Many parts of the mental status exam are incorporated into the history-taking section of the assessment. The actual assessment process follows a systematic plan of data collection, but a large part of the assessment can be accomplished as part of a routine neurological assessment or an informal conversation, while administering nursing care, or through a formal structured interview. The nurse must consider the patient's age, occupation, socioeconomic and educational background, and baseline data, when available.

Many standardized tools are currently available (e.g., Wechsler Adult Intelligence Scale, Galveston Orientation and Amnesia Test) but may be either too lengthy, too limited, or inappropriate for simple screening at the bedside or in the outpatient setting.

The patient's status should be determined by a brief assessment of his or her affect; behavior; orientation to person, place, and time; recent and remote memory; concentration; arithmetic and abstract reasoning; and auditory comprehension.

The ability to respond to commands involving multiple functions (e.g., "Take the paper in your right hand, fold it in half, and put it on the table.") is a good general measure of mental status. Serial subtraction from 100 allows evaluation of arithmetic function and concentration. Repetition of phrases, content, and appropriateness help assess whether aphasia or dysphasia is present. The mood of the patient can be discerned by listening and observing general movements, facial expressions, and reactions.

Mood changes, such as euphoria, apathy, irritability, and lability, occur in some individuals with cerebral dysfunction. Distinguishing between reactive and endogenous depression might be difficult but has important implications for treatment.

Dyspraxia (impairment of learned movements in the absence of weakness, sensory loss, or paralysis) can occur in frontal or parietal lobe disease. Cerebral lesions affecting motor function tend to produce spastic paralysis and often affect distal extremities first (fine motor function).

Delirium is an acute confusional state associated with septic states or drug intoxication. It has been reported to be present in 25–40 percent of patients with cancer at various stages and up to 85 percent of cancer patients who are terminally ill. It is often difficult to differentiate the initial stages of delirium from anxiety or depression. The delirious patient experiences a sudden change in mental status, resulting in an altered level of consciousness and inability to make judgments, to understand and maintain thought processes, or to make decisions. Confusion, agitation, hallucinations, or disturbance of the sleep-wake cycle are also associated with delirium.

Dementia is the impairment of higher intellectual function without a reduction in arousal. The demented patient is unable to process incoming sensory information into the highly complex cerebral neuronal system that integrates past and present experiences and allows appropriate behavioral responses. The nurse should note evidence of aphasia, agnosia (response to a common environmental stimulus as though it had never been encountered before), or apraxia (impairment of learned movements in the absence of weakness or sensory loss). The diagnosis of dementia requires the demonstration of decline in cognitive function. The demented patient almost always has problems with perception and is prone to agitation and confusion. Dementia, usually an irreversible disorder, severely impairs the person's ability to function independently.

Management of Cerebral Dysfunction

The primary goals of nursing management are patient safety and optimal function. Specific problems such as communication disorders, disorientation, memory loss, and inability to perform activities of daily living will vary from patient to patient. It is important that the patient be able to maintain a sense of control over his or her life to the greatest extent possible.

The nurse can acknowledge behavior changes (e.g., lability, anxiety) and then try to put the patient at ease and work through the behavior change. Distractions can also be used for the patient experiencing loss of behavior control—for example, having the patient raise his hand or turn his head or simply changing the topic of conversation.

Patients are often devastated and depressed when they sense that their intellectual function is failing. Appropriate consultations with a medical psychiatric team might be warranted. The oncology nurse should counsel the family and significant others to place fewer demands on the patient, to maintain stability, and to decrease excess stimuli or noise in the environment in order to promote function and independence. The patients's eyeglasses or hearing aid should be provided. Use of a nightlight can often prevent fear and control confusion. Recruiting a family member to sit with the patient can be dramatically effective in restoring function. The nurse should assist with self-care as needed; provide information in clear, simple terms; orient the patient as needed; and provide reassurance to the patient and family frequently. As the level of confusion deteriorates, the nurse must assume responsibility for protecting the patient from injury.

PERIPHERAL NERVOUS SYSTEM

The peripheral nervous system (PNS) includes all the nerve structures that lie outside the CNS. It consists of cranial, sensory, and motor nerves and portions of the autonomic nervous system. The peripheral nerves serve as a conduit for flow of information from the CNS to the periphery and from the periphery back to the CNS. Most peripheral nerves have mixed functions and carry motor, sensory, and autonomic fibers.

Assessment of Sensory Dysfunction

A common sign of peripheral neuropathy is symmetric, distal sensory and motor loss with absent or decreased reflexes, though variation can occur. Progressive peripheral neuropathy commonly results in loss of motor function; however, it can also present with irritative effects, such as pain, paresthesia, dysesthia, and continuous motor activity.

Sensory loss is commonly detected in distal extremities first. Testing with pin prick, temperature, vibration, and tactile discrimination is important, as sensory dysfunction can be diagnosed prior to the onset of motor loss. Frequency of assessment depends on the patient's acuity and stability.

Peripheral nerve injury, caused by such agents as vincristine, typically produces a decrease or loss of sensation and a decrease in perception of touch, proprioception, and stereognosis. The most common presenting symptom is numbness in the feet. Hands are affected later. Less frequently, temperature and pain sensation are involved. Contact dysesthia, hyperalgesia, burning, and "pins and needles" sensations, or proprioceptive losses, are common symptoms.

The patient interview should include questions related to subjective feelings of numbness and changes in sensation. It is helpful for the patient to keep eyes closed during the sensory exam to avoid visual clues. Sensation is tested as follows:

- Light touch: Stroke a cotton wisp over each of the four extremities and ask the patient to report feeling the stimulus.
- Pain: Touch the skin with the sharp end of a safety pin, irregularly alternating with the dull end of the pin to determine if the patient can distinguish between the two stimuli.
- Temperature: Apply test tubes filled with warm and cold water to skin and ask the patient to identify the sensation. A cool tuning fork can also be used to compare temperature perception. If reaction to pain stimuli is intact, assessment of temperature can be omitted, as both are carried by the same ascending pathways.
- Vibration: Apply a vibrating C-128 tuning fork to fingernails and/or bony prominence of thumb and great toe. If vibration sense is impaired, move to the next proximal prominence and repeat until vibration is sensed.
- Proprioception: Place the thumb and forefinger on either side of the patient's great toe or forefinger and gently move the digit up and down. Ask the patient to indicate the direction of movement.
- Stereognosis: Have the patient identify the size and shape of easily recognized objects (e.g., coin, key) placed in his hands.
- Graphesthesia: Have the patient identify numbers traced on the palm of his hand.

Management of Sensory Dysfunction

Treatment is aimed at preventing disuse syndrome, compensating for loss, maximizing safety using visual feedback, and increasing awareness of the extent of the sensory impairment. Coordination exercises for the extremities, in combination with sensory stimulation, can enhance sensory awareness. Inability to perceive temperature or pain must be addressed by teaching safety techniques.

Serious threats to skin integrity should be identified and avoided, because pressure on any area for more than two hours can lead to ischemia and tissue damage. Skin breakdown or pressure sores can be prevented by turning the patient at least every two hours, reducing shearing forces, avoiding wrinkles in clothing and bedding, and using cushions or air mattresses when indicated (see Chapter 10C).

The wish to appear normal is of paramount importance to some patients. Simple measures such as the substitution of Velcro for zippers and buttons can be helpful. Long-handled combs, makeup appliances to hold cosmetics, and electric toothbrushes are all readily available and not obvious symbols of disability. If standard crockery proves too heavy, a lightweight mug or cup with a large, conveniently shaped handle can be grasped more easily. Straws can facilitate drinking.

Fluctuation in neurologic dysfunction can occur (e.g., drug-induced neuropathy), or it may be progressive (e.g., leukoencephalopathy). Knowledge of the likely course prepares the patient and family for potential problems, teaching needs, and ancillary service needs. The patient and family should be informed of anticipated changes to the degree that they want to know about or can accept them.

Assessment of Motor Dysfunction

Voluntary motor function is primarily controlled by the pyramidal system (the corticospinal and corticobulbar tracts). These tracts originate in the posterior frontal lobe of the brain and descend through the brain stem to the point of decussation. Thus, voluntary motor function on one side of the body is controlled by the opposite side of the brain. The cerebellum controls much of the coordination of the extrapyramidal system.

Deficits in motor function can be due to a lesion in the center of the brain, tracts, or peripheral nerves. Tumor infiltration, compression, infection, and the secondary effects of cancer therapies are all potential causes of peripheral nerve dysfunction. Dysfunction can be characterized by changes not only in muscle strength but also in muscle tone; the ability to initiate, organize, and coordinate movement; the presence of abnormal movements; and reflex changes. Symptoms of pain, anesthesia, motor weakness, or paralysis can also appear.

A major complication of the neurotoxicity of chemotherapy is the loss of deep tendon reflexes (DTRs), with ensuing weakness and possible impairment of mobility. Ataxic gait from proprioceptive loss resulting from peripheral neuropathy should be differentiated from cerebellar ataxia. Motor weakness and sensory loss suggest the possibility of a spinal cord tumor. The motor exam assesses bulk, tone, and strength of major muscle groups of the body as well as gait, posture, and deep tendon reflexes:

- Strength: Put muscles of the major joints through full range of motion, first against gravity and then against the examiner's resistance. Compare muscles on each side of the body to note strength or weakness on a scale of 0 (no muscle contraction) to 5 (active movement against resistance).
- Tone: Assess at rest and during passive range of motion, comparing alternate sides of the body. Involuntary movements (tremors, rigidity, spasticity, or uncoordinated movements) should be noted. Flaccid muscles (hypotonia) are weak, flabby and fatigue easily. Spasticity refers to increased resistance to passive movement followed by release of resistance.
- Size: Observe for atrophy or wasting; inspect and compare for symmetry, size and contour. Note atrophy or hypertrophy.
- Romberg test: Have patient stand with feet together and eyes open. With eyes closed, balance should be maintained with minimal swaying.
- Babinski reflex: Stroke the lateral aspect of the sole from the heel to the ball of the foot with a moderately sharp object. Fanning of the toes with dorsiflexion of the big toe is an abnormal response, or positive Babinski.
- DTRs: Tap a relaxed tendon or bony prominence with a reflex hammer; skeletal muscles contract when tendons are stretched. Reflexes to be tested include biceps, triceps, radial, patellar, and Achilles. The response is measured as follows: 0 = absent, 1 = weak, 2 = normal, 3 = exaggerated, 4 = hyperreflexia. Abnormal responses include hyperreflexia, an exaggerated reflex response usually seen in upper motor neuron disease, and hyporeflexia, diminished reflex response to stimuli usually seen with lower motor neuron disease.
- Pronator drift: Ask the patient to close eyes and stretch out the arms parallel to the floor with palms up for 20–30 seconds. Downward drifting of an arm or pronation of the palm on one side suggests mild paresis of the involved extremity.

Management of Motor Dysfunction

The goals of nursing management for the patient with disturbed motor function are to preserve normal physiologic function and to prevent the complications of immobility. If a patient has generalized weakness, rest periods should be encouraged and supportive devices might be appropriate. A physical therapist should be consulted for gait training when appropriate and for supportive devices such as braces, crutches, and other ambulatory aids, as necessary.

When paralyzed limbs and joints are allowed to remain in the same position for prolonged periods, contractures can develop. The tendency to form a contracture is most pronounced in the early weeks after the onset of paralysis; during that time a full passive range of motion (ROM) must be given to every joint at least twice a day. Applications of heat to stretch tendons also act as an analgesic when pain is present. Splinting can be helpful to provide support and prevent deformity. Strengthening exercises for improving function and coordination must be practiced frequently if they are to be effective. Energy-conserving techniques must become habitual to maximize and prolong strength and endurance.

Ankle-foot orthoses are used to stabilize the ankle and compensate for foot drop. Clog-style rocker shoes can be helpful in improving ambulation in persons with specific patterns of lower extremity weakness. Well-fitting boots or high-top sneakers often obviate the necessity for orthosis. A wrist splint can be invaluable in supporting the wrist in dorsiflexion with wrist drop resulting from peripheral neuropathy. In patients with permanent weakness, adaptations to the environment such as ramps and lifts can reduce disabilities and allow patients to retain independence.

AUTONOMIC NERVOUS SYSTEM

The autonomic nervous system regulates, adjusts, and coordinates visceral activities including all smooth (involuntary) muscles, cardiac muscles, and glands. Bowel and bladder functions involve both motor and sensory pathways and are assessed by determining whether the client has normal elimination patterns. Bowel and bladder dysfunction was found in 50 percent of patients at the time of spinal cord compression. Impotence, ortho-static hypotension, and Horner's syndrome are other autonomic dysfunctions. Evidence of autonomic dysfunctions is elicited from the patient history or from clinical observation. Autonomic functions, with the ability to maintain continence of the bowel and bladder, have a profound impact on the patient and command high priority for independence and social acceptance. (Refer to Chapter 12 for management of bowel and bladder function.)

CRANIAL NERVES

There are 12 pairs of cranial nerves that provide sensory and/or motor function (Table 11–9). There are three pure sensory nerves (I, II, VIII), five pure motor nerves (III,IV, VI, XI, XII), and four mixed cranial nerves (V, VII, IX, X). Cranial nerve and visual field deficits provide important information to assist in the diagnosis of CNS dysfunction. Deficits can be detected with close attention to the patient's face, eye movements, speech, and swallowing. Early diagnosis of cranial nerve dysfunction is critical because tumors can directly infiltrate or compress the nerves, and because continued antineoplastic treatment could contribute to progressive neurotoxicity.

Dysfunction of motor nerves can present as facial weakness, dysarthria, diminished or lost gag reflex, dysphagia, ptosis, diplopia, visual field limitations, jaw weakness or paralysis, or neck and shoulder weakness.

Table 11-9
Cranial Nerves

	Nerve	Function	Dysfunction	Assessment
I	Olfactory	Smell	Disturbance in smell	Ask patient to identify distinctive odors (e.g., coffee, spices)
II	Optic	Vision Pupil Response	Visual field defect Papilledema, optic neuritis Blurred vision Blindness Retrobulbar neuritis	Fundoscopic exam Check visual acuity—Snellen Chart Check Rosenbaum Chart Check peripheral vision Confrontation
III	Oculomotor	Elevation of upper eyelid Inward eye movement Pupil constriction	Outward strabismus Nystagmus Dilated pupil Diplopia Ptosis	Check convergence & accommodation Check eyelid position Check light reflex, and pupillary reaction to light
IV	Trochlear	Downward eye movement Outward eye movement	Nystagmus Inward strabismus	Check eye movements in six fields of gaze
V	Trigeminal	Jaw movement Corneal reflex Pain, temperature Light touch Facial sensation Chewing	Loss of pain & temperature sensation Jaw pain, weakness, or paralysis Difficulty chewing Corneal reflex absent or missing Trigeminal Neuralgia	Assess for jaw pain, difficulty with mastication Assess pain and light touch Palpate mandible strength
VI	Abducens	Lateral eye movement	Strabismus Diplopia Ptosis	Check extraocular movements Check eyelid position
VII	Facial	Taste in anterior two-thirds of tongue Close, blink eyes Corneal reflex Facial expression	Salt, sugar not discriminated Facial palsy weakness Increased/decreased saliva or tears Bell's Palsy	Check symmetry of expressions (ask patient to smile, frown, show teeth, and raise eyebrows) Assess taste changes Assess changes in saliva, tears
VIII	Auditory	Hearing acuity Equilibrium	Tinnitus Nausea Loss of balance Deafness Nystagmus Meniere's Disease	Rinne and Weber tests Whisper test Assess for history of ringing in ears, dizziness Observe eye movements

Continued

Table 11–9 (Continued)
Cranial Nerves

	Nerve	Function	Dysfunction	Assessment
IX	Glossopharyngeal	Taste in posterior one-third of tongue Gag reflex Swallowing	Dysphagia Diminished gag reflex Taste changes Deviation of uvula Glossopharyngeal neuralgia	Touch either side of palate with tongue blade Assess dysphagia, taste changes Check uvula
X	Vagus	Swallowing Gag reflex Vocal quality	Dysphonia, dysphagia Difficulty swallowing Diminished gag reflex Hoarseness	Monitor hoarseness, dysphagia Check gag reflex Check rise of palate
XI	Spinal accessory	Shrug shoulders Rotate head	Inability to shrug shoulders or rotate head Weakness	Check bulk and strength of sternocleidomastoid and trapezius muscles Check asymmetry of muscles
XII	Hypoglossal	Tongue movement Articulation	Tongue deviates or atrophies	Observe protruded tongue for asymmetry or atrophy

Sensory symptoms that can occur with cranial nerve dysfunction include pain, alteration in taste, smell, or hearing, visual loss or deficits, visual perceptual problems, and dysphonia.

Management of Cranial Nerve Dysfunction

Visual pathways involve all the lobes of the cerebral hemisphere, and visual defects are a common symptom of intracranial lesions. The ability to function independently is severely compromised, and the patient requires protective and supportive measures. Optic and oculomotor nerve involvement can cause blurred or double vision. Eye patches can be useful. The environment should be made safe to prevent falls or other injuries. Large-print or talking books, volunteer readers, or diversional activities can enhance the independence of the visually impaired. Adequate lighting should be employed, and the patient should be informed of any necessary changes in the physical environment. An ophthalmologist should be consulted, since prescription glasses may be warranted.

Speech might become slurred when the tongue and throat muscles are involved. Speech therapists should be consulted to increase fluency and rhythm. The patient should be allowed adequate time to express thoughts.

Cisplatin, an antineoplastic alkylating agent, is known to be ototoxic in 24 percent of patients. Manifested by tinnitus and hearing loss, impairment is related to age, dose, and schedule of administration. The nurse should face the patient and speak slowly, repeating as necessary. An alternate method of communication should be developed if the patient is severely disabled. To encourage nonverbal communication, pencil and paper should be available at all times. Touch can convey a great deal to the patient and should be used whenever appropriate.

PREVENTION

Neurotoxicity can remain the major dose-limiting toxicity of cancer therapy. Several types of interventions have been investigated in hopes of ameliorating neurotoxicity. Early clinical data suggest that several agents have shown promise in reducing the incidence and severity of neurotoxicities without adversely affecting anti-tumor efficacy.

Nucleophilic sulfur thiols, neurotrophic factors, phosophonic acid antibiotics, and free oxygen radical scavengers have been tested as chemoprotectants. Amifostine, a radioprotective agent released for neuroprotection, is an organic thiophosphate compound that prevents cellular damage through free-radical scavenging, hydrogen donation, and inhibition of DNA damage. In some studies, amifostine has protected against cisplatin-induced neuropathy without reducing anti-tumor effect. In preliminary trials, the neuropeptide Org 2766, an ACTH analog, has restored nerve function over a period of several months. Nerve growth factor is the only agent reported to prevent, rather than partially protect against cisplatin-induced neuropathy in an experimental model.

Summary

Neurologic dysfunction constitutes a significant oncologic nursing challenge because of the overwhelming emotional and physical consequences and their relatively high incidence in the total cancer population. The cancer patient might experience various emotional and psychological reactions to neurologic dysfunctions, including changes in body image, self-esteem and lifestyle, sensory deprivation, social isolation, powerlessness, frustration, anger, hostility, depression, loss, grief, and bereavement. It is extremely important that the oncology nurse provide psychological and emotional support along with expert technical nursing skills.

As improved antitumor therapy prolongs the life of patients with cancer, it is critical that oncology nurses address neurologic dysfunction before it becomes permanent or disabling. Nurses can organize and coordinate the comprehensive care of the cancer patient with neurologic complications through knowledge of the nervous system, identification of patient needs, provision of appropriate nursing care, and applicable referrals for multidisciplinary care (Table 11–10). The overall objective of nursing management should be to restore and maintain the cancer patient's fullest physical, psychological, and social capability. This can be achieved

Table 11–10
Nursing Management of Common Neurologic Dysfunctions

Factor	Intervention
Alteration in Mobility	
General	Identify and discuss limitations and strengths
	Teach safety awareness for prevention of injury
	Promote energy conservation to prolong endurance; schedule adequate rest periods
	Encourage patient participation in ADLs
	Initiate and coordinate appropriate referrals
	Collaborate with multidisciplinary caregivers
	Provide positive reinforcement to patient
Ataxia, dysmetria, aesthenia, and hypotonicity	Refer to physical therapy/occupational therapy for exercise programs to:
	Enhance muscle tone
	Practice precise posturing of trunk and extremities
	Teach and practice coordination exercises for extremities (Frenkel's exercises)
	Teach gait training
	Instruct in active and passive exercises to maintain functional ROM and prevent contractures
	Position patient in proper alignment, reposition frequently
	Examine immobilized patient for signs of thrombophlebitis (tenderness, erythema, warmth)
	Supply support hose when appropriate
	Preserve skin integrity and prevent decubitus ulcers
	Promote optimal nutrition for strength and healing with supplements as needed
	Remove splints regularly to monitor skin
	Discuss individual needs for use of adaptive equipment
	Apply devices to prevent foot drop and hand, leg, and arm deformities (pillows, cushions, and commercial devices may be used)
	Provide assistive devices for eating and dressing
	Apply braces and supports for ambulation
	Teach patient how to perform ADLs with use of devices and how to modify them according to functional impairment
	Safely anchor beds, chairs for patient transfers
Alteration in Level of Consciousness	
General	Document onset, duration, and intensity of impairment
	Enlist family assistance
	Instruct family to report all changes
	Provide appropriate information to patient and family
	Identify and address underlying medical disorder when possible
	Initiate appropriate referrals when indicated

Table 11–10 *(Continued)*
Nursing Management of Common Neurologic Dysfunctions

Factor	Intervention
Decreased memory	Assess memory function
	Identify self and wear name tag
	Explain all procedures
	Repeat information only as necesary
	Simplify and organize environment
	Provide paper and pencil for patient to record information
	Place items patient needs to use where he can easily see them
Decreased orientation	Assess disorientation frequently
	Orient patient frequently to person, place, and time
	Identify self to patient on each encounter
	Promote safe environment and protect from injury
	Provide environmental and sensory stimulation (e.g., family photographs)
	Place clock and calendar near patient
	Schedule daily routines
	Encourage visits from significant others
Decreased concentration and attention	Assess degree of cognitive alteration
	Assist with self-care as necessary
	Modify educational procedures and provide information in a clear, concise way
	Reinforce information
	Teach patient and family regarding avoidance of unnecessary contributing items (e.g., alcohol, OTC drugs, toxins)
Increased anxiety	Address patient by familiar nickname
	Provide information in simple, concise form
	Focus on one health concern at a time
	Reorient patient at regular intervals
	Introduce self and maintain open communication
	Reassure patient
	Explain all procedures and medications
	Use calm, supportive, nonthreatening approach with active listening to encourage verbalization
	Ensure safety through controlled environment

Peripheral Neuropathies

Teach safety measures:
  Set water temperature at safe level—110 degrees F
  Pretest bath water and dishwater
  Avoid steam and hot utensils when cooking (use pot holders, pots with wooden or plastic handles)
  Protect against contact with sources of extreme heat or cold (radiators, oven, light bulbs)
Dress warmly in cold weather, wear gloves and well-fitting footwear

Continued

Table 11-10 *(Continued)*
Nursing Management of Common Neurologic Dysfunctions

Factor	Intervention
Peripheral Neuropathies	
	Examine skin daily for signs of irritation, breakdown
	Teach hand and foot care (e.g., use of massage, lotions)
	Encourage patient to ambulate as much as possible
	Provide heel protectors, footboard, high-top sneakers, or support shoes as required
	Use functional aids such as triangular pencils, adaptive crockery, Velcro, button hook, or zipper ring-pull when appropriate
	Instruct patient to become mentally aware of where extremities are when performing activities
	Refer to PT/OT for exercise and sensory stimulation, gait, training, ROM
	Instruct patient to stretch muscles before getting out of bed
Visual Disturbance	
General	Assess visual acuity, eye mechanics
	Assist with ADLs as necessary
	Structure environment to increase stability, decrease meaningless stimuli, and promote safety
	Provide good lighting
	Ambulate patient with assistance as necessary
	Explain all procedures to patient and allow patient to verbalize fears
	Provide referrals to ophthalmology service or occupational therapy as necessary
Diplopia	Encourage use of adaptive materials such as large print books, talking books, volunteer readers
	Alternate eye patches every four hours while awake, warn patient of alteration in depth perception. Tear solutions when necessary
Hemianopsia	Approach patient from unimpaired visual field side. Place objects in range of vision. Instruct patient to visually scan environment
Hearing Deficit	
	Assess hearing loss, acuity
	Refer to specialist for audiometric testing, hearing aids when appropriate
	Assist with hearing aid placement/fitting if necessary
	Face patient when speaking to him and talk to unaffected side
	Provide safety measures
	Decrease extraneous noise
	Provide pencil and paper at all times
	Increase awareness of nonverbal communication

by preventing further complications, promoting recovery to the greatest extent possible, teaching adaptive strategies, and facilitating the highest quality of life for the patient.

BIBLIOGRAPHY

1. Abeloff, M. *Clinical Oncology.* Churchill Livingstone, New York. 1995.

   This comprehensive oncologic textbook includes chapters on CNS tumors, brain metastases and carcinomatous meningitis, and neurologic complications of cancer and cancer treatment. The authors address incidence, presenting signs and symptoms, diagnosis, and treatment options in detail.

2. Armstrong, T., D. Rust, and J. R. Kohtz. Neurologic, pulmonary, and cutaneous toxicities of high-dose chemotherapy. Oncol Nurs 24(1)(suppl. Jan–Feb): 23–33. 1997.

   Dose-intensive chemotherapy and their asssociated toxicities are discussed. Interventions and goals are detailed.

3. Bates, B. *A Guide to Physical Examination and History Taking,* 6th Ed. J. B. Lippincott Co., Philadelphia. 1995.

   This is an invaluable resource for detailed physical assessment and identification of common or important pathophysiologic abnormalities.

4. Bender, C. M. Cognitive dysfunction associated with biological response modifier therapy. *Oncol Nurs Forum* 21(3): 515–523. 1994.

   This is a review of current knowledge regarding cognitive dysfunction related to administration of biological response modifiers. It includes a review of studies performed in this area as well as assessment and nursing intervention.

5. Dietz, J. H., Jr. *Rehabilitation Oncology.* John Wiley & Sons, Inc., New York. 1981.

   Organized by anatomic region, which facilitates use, this text focuses on rehabilitation of cancer patients and includes selection and use of adaptive equipment.

6. Furlong, T. G. Neurologic complications of immunosuppressive cancer therapy. *Oncol Nurs Forum* 20(9): 1337–1354. 1993.

   This article presents an overview of neurologic complications specific to common immunosuppressive agents associated with cancer therapy. Risk factors, nursing assessment, and clinical management are discussed.

7. Hickey, J. V. *The Clinical Practice of Neurological and Neurosurgical Nursing,* 4th Ed. J. B. Lippincott Co., Philadelphia. 1997.

   This is a comprehensive text on neurologic nursing, encompassing anatomy and physiology, neurologic assessment, and nursing management of patients with neurologic complications of disease.

8. Meehan, J. L., and B. L. Johnson. The neurotoxicity of antineoplastic agents. In Hubbard, S. M., P. E. Greene, and M. T. Knobf, eds. *Current Issues in Cancer Nursing Practice.* J. B. Lippincott Co., Philadelphia. 1992.

   This article describes the neurotoxic sequelae of chemotherapeutic agents and includes neurologic assessment, symptom management, and an overview of drug-specific neurologic effects.

9. Murphy, G. P., ed. Brain tumors. *Ca—A Cancer Journal for Clinicians* 43(5) (September/October).

   This issue contains articles that review the classification, symptoms, diagnosis, and treatment of adult brain tumors, pediatric brain tumors, and the pathology and treatment of peripheral nerve tumors and tumor-like conditions.

10. Murphy, G. P., W. Lawrence, and R. E. Lenhard, Jr. *American Cancer Society Textbook of Clinical Oncology*, 2d Ed. American Cancer Society, Inc., Atlanta. 1995.

    This is a comprehensive resource for clinicians who tend to cancer patients with timely, in-depth discussions of pathology, etiology, and nature of cancer. It includes chapters on CNS malignancies, quality of life, rehabilitation, and supportive care of cancer patients.

11. Newton, H. B. Primary brain tumors: Review of etiology, diagnosis, and treatment. *American Family Physician* 49(4): 787–797. 1994.

    Epidemiology, etiology, presentation, exam, diagnostics, and treatment are covered.

12. Posner, J. B. *Neurologic Complications of Cancer*. F.A. Davis Co., Philadelphia. 1995.

    This text presents an overview and integration of neurologic and oncologic complications of cancer. Guidance on appropriate clinical assessment, diagnosis, and treatment is detailed.

13. Raney, D. J. Malignant spinal cord tumors: A review and case presentation. *Journal of Neuroscience Nursing* 23(1): 44–49. 1991.

    This journal article discusses the pathophysiology, signs and symptoms, medical management, and nursing implications of malignant spinal cord tumors. A case study is presented with nursing diagnoses and interventions.

14. Sims, L. B. Neurologic involvement of systemic cancer. *Critical Care Nursing Clinics of North America* 7(1): 171–177. 1995.

    Selected neurologic complications of systemic cancer are discussed, including tumor involvement, paraneoplastic syndromes, and non-neoplastic and treatment-related complications.

15. Tuxen, M. K. and S. W. Hansen. Neurotoxicity secondary to antineoplastic drugs. *Cancer Treatment Reviews* 20(2): 191–214. 1994.

    This review focuses on antineoplastic agents that commonly cause neurotoxic manifestations. The author briefly discusses new drugs in which neurotoxicities have been clinically noted.

16. Umphred, D. A. *Neurological Rehabilitation*, 2d Ed. C. V. Mosby Co., Philadelphia. 1990.

    This presents an interdisciplinary approach to management of persons with neurologic disabilities, including physical, occupational, and speech therapy, as well as nursing care plans for selected diagnoses.

17. Zimberg, M., and S. Berenson. Delirium in patients with cancer: Nursing assessment and intervention. *Oncol Nurs Forum* 17(4): 529–538. 1990.

    This article includes standards of care and nursing diagnoses associated with delirium. Assessment criteria, interventions, and expected patient outcomes are included.

12

Elimination

A. Anatomical Alterations

Alice Basch

FECAL DIVERSION

Pathophysiology

The surgical alteration of the gastrointestinal (GI) tract is commonly undertaken when a tumor invades the system or a mechanical blockage occurs. After the initial physiologic recovery from the surgical procedure and anesthesia, the remaining alimentary system returns to what was previously normal functioning for the person. Fecal consistency depends on the site of intervention, the amount of intestine removed, and whether additional treatments or medications are needed for symptom management or control of disease.

Most frequently the stoma, or opening, will be matured (i.e., the inner lining of the intestinal tract is turned over onto itself, as one would turn up a cuff on a sleeve) at time of surgery. This creates a surface that is moist pinkish-red in color and closely resembles other healthy mucosal tissue. The color is due to the high number of blood vessels found in the mucosa, which account for the occasional drops of blood seen when wiping with a cloth or tissue. The stoma is unaffected by digestive materials found in the stool and will move slightly, consistent with peristalsis.

The descending, or sigmoid, colon, located in the lower left quadrant, is the most common site for colostomy placement. Stomas located at this site are usually one to two inches in diameter and protrude slightly from the skin surface. Effluent from the sigmoid colostomy will return to the stool consistency normal to the person prior to disease.

The higher in the colon the surgical intervention is performed, the softer the fecal output and the higher the concentration of enzymatic material. A left transverse colostomy might produce stool of peanut-butter to semiliquid consistency and be mildly irritating to skin surfaces. Transverse colostomies, usually placed at waist level, are 2 to $3\frac{1}{2}$ inches in diameter and are often unmatured at the time of surgery, creating a moist light-red to pink cauliflower-shaped structure. Because of positioning, effluent consistency, and size, these colostomies are the most difficult to manage in terms of maintaining a seal and protecting peristomal skin.

12A

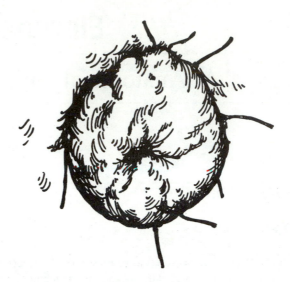

Figure 12A-1. Healthy ileostomy, protruding one inch from abdominal wall.

The ascending colostomy, an intervention higher in the colon, is located on the right side of the abdomen. Effluent produced at this stoma will be primarily liquid and highly enzymatic to surrounding skin; that is, the effluent digests the skin and is therefore a potential source of skin breakdown.

Small-bowel ostomy output occurring with an ileostomy or jejunostomy is primarily liquid in nature and extremely enzymatic. Skin breakdown from fecal contact can occur within several hours when ostomies are located in the small bowel. Stoma diameter is usually small, 1 to $1\frac{1}{2}$ inches, and is placed in the right lower quadrant. For improved pouch seal, the stoma will protrude $\frac{1}{2}$ to 1 inch (Figure 12A–1).

Management

During the first several days after a stoma is created, all types of ostomies should be managed in a similar manner. Appropriate pouching systems should include an open-ended, odor-proof pouch and some type of skin barrier to be used between the pouch and the skin. Each institution may choose a particular manufacturer according to availability of products and the facility's ability to maintain a varied inventory. The general management of the new colostomy should include procedures and equipment that protect the skin from the fecal material; provide an odor-proof material for patient, staff, and visitor comfort; and provide an opening in the bottom of the bag to empty waste material.

Pouching procedures should be demonstrated to the new ostomate and/or the primary caregiver. Following are two sample procedures. The first is for changing the drainable appliance with precut washer. Necessary supplies are as follows:

1. The correct appliance with an opening of $\frac{1}{8}$ to $\frac{1}{4}$ inches larger than stoma diameter (e.g., Hollister, Convatec, Coloplast).
2. Skin sealant (e.g., United Skin-Prep™ wipes #4204 or Skin-Prep™ spray, Hollister skin gel, Bard Protective barrier film).
3. Warm water, washcloth, and towel.

Procedure

1. Remove old appliance. Be careful to support the skin as the adhesive area is gently removed.
2. Wash area around the stoma with warm water. Do not use soap, which can leave a film on the skin, causing irritation or poor appliance adherence. Do not rub. Do not be concerned if small amounts of skin barrier do not come off the skin. It will not interfere with the new appliance. If difficulty is experienced removing a large amount of the skin barrier, soak a tissue with water and hold it on the area. The material will soften and can be removed more easily.
3. Pat area dry; do not rub.
4. Measure stoma, using a measuring guide, to identify the correct opening in the appliance.
5. Wipe area to be covered by appliance adhesive with skin sealant or spray with skin sealant spray.
6. Allow skin sealant to dry thoroughly (20–30 seconds).
7. Remove clear and/or paper covering from adhesive backing.
8. Center opening in appliance around stoma.
9. Apply gentle pressure over skin barrier to ensure that it seals to the skin.
10. Smooth adhesive backing carefully to eliminate wrinkles.
11. Insert pouch deodorant if it is being used.
12. Apply clamp to end of pouch.

Next are instructions for use of a two-piece, open-ended appliance. Necessary supplies are as follows:

1. Two-piece, open-ended appliance (Hollister two-piece or Convatec Sur-Fit®).
2. Skin sealant (Skin-prep™).
3. Stomahesive™ or Hollihesive™ paste (optional).
4. Warm water, washcloth, and towel.

Procedure

1. Remove old appliance.
2. Cleanse gently with warm water and pat dry.
3. Cut opening in adhesive to fit stoma.
4. Apply skin sealant to peristomal area and allow to dry well. Apply paste around stoma or at inner opening of adhesive backing (optional).
5. Remove paper backing from wafer.
6. Center appliance opening around stoma. Press gently around opening to ensure seal.
7. Snap bag onto flange. You will hear a snap or click when it is secured. It might be helpful to start at the bottom and evenly press as you move toward the top. You can also attach bag to flange before securing the appliance over the stoma.
8. Insert pouch deodorant if it is being used.
9. Apply clamp to end of pouch.

After several days of bowel functioning and regular dietary intake, the patient with a sigmoid colostomy who fits the criteria listed in Table 12A-1

Table 12A-1
Considerations for Irrigation in Patients with Sigmoid Colostomy

Positive	Negative
Regular bowel movements prior to current disease and surgery	History of irregular bowel movements
Motivation	Lack of motivation
Full mental and emotional capacities	Poor orientation or depression
Full dexterity	Severe arthritis, amputation, or other factors affecting dexterity
Appropriate bathroom facilities, including running water	Lack of appropriate bathroom facilities, including lack of running water
	Blindness
	Frequent travel
	Frequent changes in daily schedule
	Diarrhea
	Terminal status
	Temporary colostomy

can be instructed in irrigation. To obtain a thorough irrigation and fluid return, proper height of the irrigation fluid is important. A bag held too high can cause water to flow high in the colon, causing a more liquid return lasting over several hours. If the patient is standing or sitting, the bag should hang between shoulder and nipple level. If the patient is supine, the bottom of the irrigation bag should hang 18 inches above the stoma. An irrigation that takes longer than $1\frac{1}{2}$ hours from time of start to fluid return should be evaluated for proper technique. Instructions for an appropriate colostomy irrigation are as follows:

1. Choose a convenient time for irrigation.
2. Fill irrigation bag with 1,000 ml (1 quart) lukewarm tap water.
3. Let water run through the tubing to clear it of air.
4. Hang irrigating bag so that the bottom of the bag will be between breast and shoulder level. (If patient is supine, nurse or caregiver will perform the procedure. Bag will hang 18 inches above stoma.)
5. Remove old appliance carefully, supporting skin as the adhesive is pulled off. If using two-piece system, remove drainage pouch and attach irrigation sleeve to flange.
6. Place faceplate of irrigating sleeve over stoma and secure with belt. The patient should sit on the toilet or place a chair adjacent to the toilet.
7. Direct open end of irrigating sleeve into the toilet or other receptacle. Irrigating sleeve will be open at the top for insertion of cone into stoma.
8. Identify opening in stoma from which stool is being discharged. With a double-barrel colostomy, a second opening might be present. Solution can be inserted into this opening, but the water will probably be eliminated from the rectum.
9. Lubricate the cone with water-soluble lubricant (K-Y Jelly®, Lubafax®).
10. When the cone is in front of the stoma, in position to insert, begin slow water flow as you insert the cone.
11. Insert cone until there is no backflow of water. It is not necessary to insert all the way to the flat edge. Never force the cone into the stoma.
12. Allow water to flow in quickly. If cramps develop, slow the flow of the solution; also, check to see if the water is too hot or too cold.
13. When most of the water has gone in or if a full feeling occurs, stop the water flow.
14. Remove the cone from the stoma and the irrigating sleeve.
15. Clip the top of the irrigating sleeve closed, so that fluid return will not escape.
16. Allow irrigation to return. Results can take from 20 to 45 minutes. While waiting for the return, you can continue with regular

morning routine by cleaning the bottom of the irrigation sleeve and folding or clipping the end of the sleeve. A slight cramping might be felt with the return or a feeling of warmth as the water and stool is eliminated. If the return takes longer than 45 minutes, contact the enterostomal therapist.

17. When the return is complete, remove the faceplate and the irrigating sleeve.
18. Cleanse area around the stoma with warm water (no soap).
19. Apply new appliance.

The first irrigation should be done with not more than 500 ml warm water to evaluate the patient's tolerance of the procedure. To determine the direction of the colon, dilate the stoma gently before beginning the procedure. With few exceptions, a cone tip or shield should always be used for irrigations. A cone tip will prevent too high a water infusion or possible bowel perforation if the catheter is forced. Because the colon lacks nerve endings and the patient cannot feel the catheter against the wall of the bowel, caution must be used to avoid perforation. An experienced nurse or enterostomal therapist can be consulted to determine when a catheter can be used.

When a person with a sigmoid colostomy achieves bowel regulation (no stool leakage during 24- to 48-hour period between irrigations), he or she might feel comfortable pouching the stoma with a small closed-ended pouch or gauze covering. The patient should be reminded to keep a supply of open-ended pouches for use during travel or with changes in medication, treatment for disease, and viral illness that could cause diarrhea resulting in unsuccessful irrigations.

Regularity cannot be achieved for stomas not located in the sigmoid colon. If a patient is not regulated within six weeks of initiating proper irrigations, the likelihood of future bowel regulation is minimal.

COMMON PROBLEMS

Stoma Complications

Most stoma complications occur within the first year of surgery. Stoma viability and functioning should be assessed with each appliance change and recorded for future reference.

The first assessment for any stoma is a determination of viability. A healthy stoma is deep pink to red in color. A compromise in blood flow to the stoma from trauma, edema, or other causes will appear as a purplish-to-black stoma. If not reversed or surgically altered, the stoma will become necrotic and slough off, leaving an opening that may be difficult to pouch.

Stricturing, or narrowing, of the stoma opening is another frequently seen complication. Unless the condition causes obstruction, intervention is

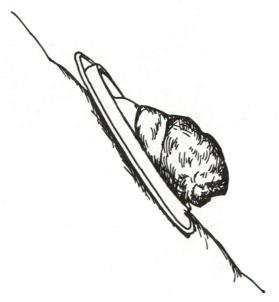

Figure 12A-2. Prolapsed colostomy.

not required. Occasionally dilation of the stoma is recommended, but it seems to have little effect on the stricturing and may cause formation of additional scar tissue if performed too rigorously.

Stoma retraction, which creates an opening below skin level, will cause effluent to undermine the appliance, creating skin breakdown and leakage. An appliance with a flexible faceplate or increased convexity can aid in adherence.

Visually, stoma prolapse (Figure 12A–2) can be one of the most distressing of complications to the patient. Stomas matured and not having internal fixation of the mesentery seem to prolapse more frequently, but the causes of prolapse are not clear. Occasionally a stoma will prolapse and spontaneously retract with no further problems. If the prolapse recurs or remains extended over long periods of time, a feeling of pressure and abdominal discomfort can occur. A mild support, such as pantyhose or a manufactured prolapse belt, and avoidance of injury can help relieve symptoms. Surgical revision can be made if the prolapse compromises blood flow or if abdominal discomfort occurs.

Alteration in Consistency, Volume, Odor

The nature and volume of colostomy and ileostomy effluent is determined by normal physiology and location of the stoma. A change in the individual's normal output can result from a variety of causes (Table 12A–2).

Diarrhea in the regulated or sigmoid colostomy presents as frequent soft to liquid stools. The colostomate should switch to an open-ended ap-

Table 12A-2
Potential Sources of Alteration in Consistency/Volume/Odor of Effluent

Cause	Constipation	Diarrhea	Odor	Gas
Food	Apple juice and sauce Carrot juice Celery Corn Bananas Chinese food Mushrooms Nuts Popcorn Milk products	Beer Fried and greasy foods Excessive fruit Milk products Nutritional supplement Rich sauces Spicy foods	Asparagus Beans Broccoli Cabbage Cheese Fish Eggs Garlic and spices Onions Antibiotics Vitamins	Beer Carbonated beverages Cabbage family Dairy products Legumes Onions
Drugs	Chemotherapy: Vincristine Iron Antibiotics Aluminum hydroxide B-adrenergic blockers Codeine and opioids Tricyclic antidepressants	Chemotherapy: Busulfan Doxorubicin Fluorouracil Methotrexate Plicamycin Mitotane Antibiotics Antihypertensives Sulfasalazine (Azulfidine) Digitalis Lithium Vitamin D	Antibiotics Vitamins	
Other	Decreased fluid intake Inactivity Tumor blockage	Emotional upset Infection Virus	Bacterial colonization Poor hygiene Stricture, dysfunction, or obstruction of intestine	Chewing gum Improper colostomy irrigation Talking or swallowing air while chewing

pliance, if not already using one, and empty fecal material PRN. If the colostomate is to begin therapy that could result in diarrhea, such as abdominal radiation or chemotherapy, he or she should stop irrigation until treatment is concluded and bowel functioning returns to previous condition. On occasion, after radiation treatment, a formerly regulated ostomate will be unable to achieve beneficial results from irrigation. He or she should then be encouraged to stop the procedure and manage the colostomy like a higher colonic stoma.

When transverse colostomy, ascending colostomy, or ileostomy patients develop diarrhea, severe complications can result from dehydration and changes in electrolytes. Fluids, electrolytes, and skin integrity should be carefully monitored and any alterations treated. A bland, low-roughage diet, including rice, toast, applesauce, bananas, yogurt, and other foods that can help create bulk, will aid in controlling the high–liquid-volume output. Fluids containing sodium and potassium should be provided. Examples include tea, coffee, strained orange juice, bouillon, manufactured sport drinks, cola, and other sodas.

With severe or chronic diarrhea, oral medication may be of benefit in treating symptoms. Nonprescription oral agents may include Kaopectate®, Pepto-Bismol®, and agents containing aluminum hydroxide. Prescription medications include diphenoxylate with atropine (Lomotil®), loperamide (Imodium®), tincture of opium, and codeine derivatives.

Continued diarrhea may indicate changes in the mucosal lining, stricture, mechanical blockage, or viral disease, and a physician's examination is indicated to rule out pathologic causes. Cases of severe fluid-and-electrolyte depletion can require IV therapy for replacement of lost nutrients.

Constipation after bowel diversion often has the same causes as with the intact bowel (see Chapter 12B). Fluid loss, inactivity, diet, and medication can all contribute to constipation. As with the intact bowel, diet changes, stool softeners, mild laxatives, and retention enemas or irrigation can be used to treat bowel problems. Paralytic ileus, bowel stricture, adhesions, tumor, and kinks in the colon are other causes of constipation and should be treated medically.

Minimal fecal output over 24 hours or forceful liquid spurts, associated with nausea, vomiting, and abdominal discomfort could indicate a blockage in the ileostomate. Foods such as corn, mushrooms, popcorn, coconut, and Chinese foods are common offenders. If blockage occurs and is unrelieved with gentle stomal dilation and oral fluids after 24 hours, an ileostomy irrigation can be performed by a qualified professional. IV fluids, discontinuation of oral intake, and pain medication may also be necessary.

The newly formed stoma will produce large amounts of flatulence and strong odors, a result of increased bacterial colonization during the first days after surgery, when anesthesia and mechanical manipulation have decreased peristalsis of the colon. With increased activity and normalization of diet, gas and odor will decrease. Continued problems with gas and odor could result from diet, medication, treatment, or disease (see Table 12A–2). Odor can be effectively controlled with a variety of commercially prepared pouch deodorants, odor-proof bags, and oral agents, such as parsley, charcoal, and bismuth subgallate, in moderation.

Alterations In Skin Integrity

The peristomal skin, although often exposed to a variety of irritations, will maintain integrity if properly protected. Irritated and even severely excoriated skin will heal rapidly when promptly and properly treated. Basic principles to follow in skin care of the ostomate include protecting the skin from irritating fluids and chemicals, maintaining a clean and moisture-free environment, and treating irritations early. If the skin under the appliance becomes irritated from fecal discharge, the following procedure should be used as soon as possible. Necessary supplies are as follows: Karaya or Stomahesive powder and skin sealant (e.g., United Skin-Prep™ spray/Skin-Prep™ Wipes #4204/Convatec AllKare™ Protective Barrier Wipe #37444).

Procedure

1. Remove old appliance, clean and dry peristomal skin, and sprinkle irritated area with powder (it might sting slightly).
2. Brush off excess powder, using a tissue.
3. Spray or wipe with skin sealant to seal powder to irritated area.
4. Allow sealant to dry completely. (It will go through three stages: wet, sticky, and completely dry.)
5. Apply appliance in usual manner.
6. If irritation does not improve, assess skin or consult with enterostomal therapist to determine if skin allergy or Monilia infection is present, or whether a change in application procedure is necessary.

The patient with an ileostomy or a transverse colostomy is highly susceptible to skin breakdown from a variety of causes. A skin barrier (e.g., Hollister Premium Skin Barrier, Squibb Stomahesive™, Eakin Cohesive Seals, karaya washers) should always be used to keep problems from developing. Choice of barrier will be determined by availability, cost, and effectiveness. A skin sealant (e.g., United Skin Prep™, Sween Prep™, Hollister skin gel, and Bard Protective barrier film, Convatec AllKare™ Protective Barrier Wipes) will provide added protection from mechanical irritation when adhesives are removed and from irritating fluids and chemicals.

Assessment of skin irritation requires consideration of location of irritation in relation to barriers and appliance, skin exposure to effluent, description of irritation, and the patient's subjective complaints (Table 12A–3). Examining a recently used appliance and barrier for patterns of erosion is another useful way to determine the etiology of irritation. A patient history of allergic reactions and sensitivity will also assist in documenting and eliminating irritants. A final assessment can be made by observing the patient's pouching procedures, which could indicate a need to modify the application process, perhaps by providing a longer drying period for skin sealants or adhesives.

When the cause of the irritation is identified, a remedy can be easily determined, and the skin will usually heal within several days. In most cases, simply eliminating the irritant or adding a sealant or barrier to the pouching procedure will reverse the skin damage. Severe excoriation or infection might require additional treatment or prescription medication, such as systemic antibiotics or topical antifungal agents (Table 12A–4). Re-

Table 12A–3
Assessment of Alteration in Skin Integrity

Irritant	Signs	Symptoms
Fecal	Irritation will be seen in areas of skin that have contact with fecal effluent. There may be slight erythema to denuded, bleeding, or weeping skin. Most commonly seen in ileostomy, ascending, or right transverse colostomies.	Itching, burning, or stinging. Mild to severe pain intermittently or continually. Stinging with application of alcohol- or acid-containing products.
Urine	Irritation seen on stoma or peristomal area in contact with urine. Skin may be erythemic, lacerated, or bleeding, and encrustations may be seen on the skin, stoma, or old appliance (white sandpaper-textured particles). Excessive skin growth (hyperplasia) may develop on stoma or skin.	Itching or burning. Patient will complain of poor appliance adherence and urine leakage. Also may complain of strong urine odor.
Chemical Soap detergents skin cement or solvents	The peristomal area on which the barrier or appliance adheres may or may not follow pattern of adhesive. Irritated areas may be erythemic or edematous.	Itching or burning.
Mechanical	Irritation will be seen in areas of adhesives and under belt tabs or edges of faceplates. Irritated areas will be erythemic, eroded, or abraded.	Mild to severe pain will be felt on skin. Cuts or abrasions of the stoma will have no associated pain because of lack of nerve endings.
Infection/fungus *Candida albicans Staphylococcus aureus*	Irritation does not follow pattern. It may extend beyond the pouch or barrier and frequently will be seen in skin folds. Lesions will show up as patchy dry or scaly areas. They may also present as moist erythema or white papular lesions.	Severe itching will be the major complaint. A few individuals will complain of stinging.
Allergy	Irritation will follow a distinct pattern, corresponding to the suspected allergen. Skin area will appear erythemic, edematous, and may have a rash.	Itching.

peated excoriation because of a poorly placed or constructed stoma might require evaluation for surgical reconstruction.

   The person with a regulated colostomy will have very few skin problems associated with his or her diversion. Effluent from a sigmoid colostomy is usually firm, with little remainder of digestive enzymes. Because the person might often use only a gauze pad to protect clothing from mucus discharge, allergic reactions are minimal. When skin irritation does occur, it should be assessed and treated in the same manner as for other fecal diversions.

Table 12A–4
Management of Alteration in Skin Integrity

Irritant	Medical Intervention	Nursing Intervention
Fecal	Chronic severe fecal excoriation may be caused by poor stoma placement. Surgical revision may be required if pouching procedures are inadequate for skin protection.	Add or change type of skin barrier to protect the skin from fecal contact. A seal of >3 will aid in skin healing. Follow procedure for treatment of mild to severe excoriation.
Urine	See above.	Maintain a urine pH of 5.5–5.6. Use vinegar-and-water soaks 1:2 for 15–30 min daily to treat skin. If irritation chronic, use disposable appliance to prevent crystal buildup, antireflux valve, and night-drainage hookup. Maintaining a leak-proof appliance seal will prevent further skin damage.
Chemical	Not applicable.	Discourage use of soaps. If using soap, rinse thoroughly and use only oil- and fragrance-free soaps (Ivory®). Allow cements or solvents to dry completely. If irritant isolated, eliminate, or use barrier or skin sealant between irritant and skin.
Mechanical	Severe lacerations to the stoma may require assessment for reconstruction.	Maintain pouch seal for 3–5d to decrease abrasions from tape removal. Use push/pull method to remove the old pouch. Use skin sealants for friable skin and gauze padding under belt tabs. Measure opening in appliance for proper fit and center appliance over stoma.
Infection/ fungus	Prescription of nystatin powder for *Candida,* topical or systemic antibiotics for *Staphylococcus.*	Areas not covered by an appliance will heal spontaneously if kept clean and dry. Lesions will need to be cultured if etiology unknown.
Allergy	Antihistamines if severe.	Remove or substitute for the source of irritation. Include a skin sealant or barrier between the skin and irritant. Skin may be tested if source of irritation is uncertain: 1. Place a 3–5 cm patch of the suspected item on the forearm or abdomen. 2. Cover with a clear adhesive film (Op-Site®). 3. Observe in 24 and 48 hr for reaction.

Alterations In Appliance Adherence

An appliance is expected to maintain a seal for three to seven days. A decrease in adherence should alert the ostomate to the need for reassessment of application procedure or equipment. Aging, changes in hormones, weight, activity, or environment can affect ostomy management.

Aging, pregnancy, and other hormonal alterations can affect the texture of the skin and oil production of skin pores. Oily skin will interfere with adhesive adherence. Dry skin promotes adherence. A particularly oily skin might benefit from a denaturing agent (e.g., UniSolve® Adhesive Remover) after the old appliance is removed and prior to application of any powders, sealants, barriers, or adhesives. A change of weight of more than ten pounds will likely alter stoma size. Significant weight changes can also change abdominal contours, thus affecting adherence. A convex faceplate could increase wearing time on protruding bellies. Changes in abdominal contours may also occur after additional surgery for other causes, and a change in appliance or procedure may then be beneficial.

Other considerations include weather and activity. Humidity and hot weather will often affect the normal wearing time of an appliance, and appliances might require more frequent changes. Hot moisture, as found in saunas and steam rooms, can also loosen adhesive and melt skin barriers.

Increased activity could affect adherence of the appliance if the person perspires heavily. In most cases, an acceptable wearing time of three days can be achieved by adding adhesive or by substituting barriers that disintegrate less rapidly on that person (e.g., Convatec Stomahesive™, Hollister Premium Skin Barrier, Colly-Seel, Eakin Cohesive Seals).

The formation of abdominal hernias also alters adherence. Hernias develop when the muscle wall weakens, and this often occurs in the peristomal area. A portion of the intestine will slide through a weak area during the day and recede when lying down. A girdle with an opening cut for the stoma or a hernia belt manufactured for the ostomate can be used for patient comfort. A faceplate with a flexible adhesive area is usually adequate. A surgical repair of the hernia might be required or elected for some persons. Hernias often recur after surgery if the stoma location remains unchanged.

All stoma, skin, or contour changes should be assessed by a qualified enterostomal therapist, nurse, or physician to determine comfort, safety, appropriateness of the pouching procedure, and need for surgical revision.

Another type of drainage pouch is the continent ileostomy or continent reservoir (Figure 12A–3). This type of ostomy has a stoma located low in the right quadrant, and fecal material is drained three to four times a day with a 28 French catheter. A surgically created nipple valve is designed to prevent gas, odor, or stool leakage between intubations. This nipple valve remains closed by the pressure of the contents of the ileal pouch and is opened by insertion of the catheter. Construction of the reservoir is limited to a select group of patients and medical centers because of the complexity of the surgery. Specific information on care of the continent ileostomy should be obtained from an enterostomal therapist or a surgeon experienced in caring for this type of ostomy.

In recent years, the ileal-anal pull-through or J-Pouch has been performed on selected candidates who might otherwise have a conventional ileostomy. In this procedure, the rectum and anus are stripped of the inner

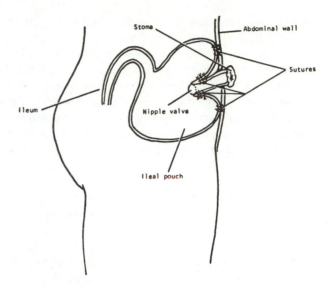

Figure 12A–3. Schematic drawing of a continent ileostomy.

lining, leaving the muscle wall intact. The diseased portion of the small intestine is removed and the healthy proximal end of the intestine is anastamosed to the remaining rectum. Bowel movements, although of more liquid content and more frequent, are achieved in a normal manner via the rectum. The person is provided specific instructions on diet, perineal muscle strengthening, and care of the peri-rectal skin.

URINARY DIVERSION

Pathophysiology

The construction of a urinary diversion bypasses the bladder, the storage area of the urinary tract. After bypass, urine drains continually, requiring a collection pouch in place at all times. Normal urine is clear yellow, has no odor, and averages 1,500 ml per day.

The most common type of diversion created is the ileal or colon conduit, which is usually located in the right lower quadrant. Figure 12A–4 illustrates the construction of the ileal conduit, in which the surgeon takes a six- to eight-centimeter segment of the ileum (or the colon if it is a colon conduit) to use as a conduit between the ureters and the skin surface. With the peristalsis moving toward the outside, backflow of urine to the kidneys is decreased.

Other common diversions are the ureterostomy, in which one or both ureters are brought directly to the skin surface; the vesicostomy, in which

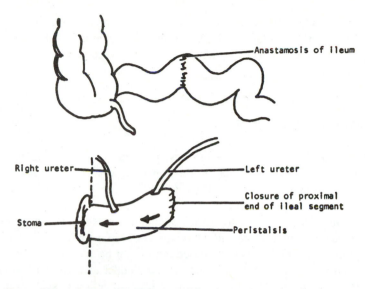

Figure 12A-4. Schematic drawing of the formation of an ileal conduit.

the bladder is brought to the abdominal wall and an opening is constructed in the suprapubic region; and the nephrostomy, in which an opening is made directly in the kidney on one or both sides in the lower flank area. Continent ileal bladders are also constructed in select persons at some medical centers. This surgery creates an internal urine reservoir that can be emptied by intermittent catheterization during the day.

A surgical procedure for males exists in which the urinary sphincter is salvaged. An ileal bladder is constructed from a segment of the small intestine and attached to the urethra in the pelvic region, allowing for intermittent catheterization via the penis. As with the previous procedure, candidates for this surgery are carefully selected due to the complexity of the procedure.

Management

Proper management of urinary output includes pouching of the stoma for three days without leakage (see procedures for changing appliances outlined previously). A pouch containing an antireflux valve will prevent backflow of urine and decrease skin or urinary problems. The opening in the pouch or barrier should be $\frac{1}{16}$ to $\frac{1}{8}$ inch larger than the stoma in order to avoid skin problems associated with urine contact on skin. Skin barriers (e.g., Bard Coloplast ReliaSeal® and Convatec Stomahesive™ or Convatec Durahesive®) will aid in adherence and not melt as quickly as karaya in the urinary diversion. Many urinary ostomates can also achieve excellent seals without the use of a skin barrier.

Use of a leg bag during the day and straight drainage at night will prevent urine buildup in the pouch. A bag more than one-third full of urine is more likely to leak and create skin problems or provide a medium for bacterial growth.

Common Problems

Dysfunction In Consistency/Volume/ Odor

A change in volume, consistency, or odor of urine could indicate problems. A decrease in urine production will be seen when inadequate quantities of fluid are consumed. Urine will appear darker, more concentrated, and have a stronger odor.

Odor in urine can be the result of dietary intake, bacteria, or urine pH. Asparagus is known to cause a distinct odor in ostomate and nonostomate alike. Infection and an increased number of bacteria will change the odor and appearance of urine. Because the bladder and its nerve endings are lacking, the usual signs of urinary tract infections—such as pain, burning, and frequency—will not be present, so the ostomate needs to assess urine periodically for change in odor and appearance. Sterile cultures should be performed to prevent misdiagnosis of infection. As in the case of the nonostomate, if infection is determined, medications will be prescribed.

The following is the procedure for the collection of a sterile urine specimen using the ileal conduit single-lumen method. Necessary supplies are as follows:

1. A standard catheterization kit (14 or 16 French straight catheter);
2. Water soluble lubricant (K-Y® Jelly) and antiseptic solution if not found in kit;
3. Warm water, soap, washcloth, and towel;
4. Clean urinary diversion (urostomy) appliance.

Procedure

1. Gently remove urostomy appliance. (If appliance is a two-piece system, it is not necessary to remove the faceplate.)
2. Wash stoma and area around it to remove mucus and traces of adhesive.
3. Rinse well with clear water.
4. Open catheterization kit. Proceed to clean stoma with antiseptic solution and skin using sterile technique.
5. Wait for peristalsis of ileal conduit to force urine out of the stoma. This will wash the antiseptic from the stoma.
6. Lubricate catheter.

7. Gently advance catheter $1\frac{1}{2}$ to 2 inches into the stoma and collect urine into a sterile container. (Note: Wait for the stoma and conduit to relax before advancing catheter to desired distance.)
8. Adhere clean urostomy appliance or pouch according to procedure outlined previously or other preferred procedure.

Alkaline urine is a common cause of urine odor and can create a host environment for bacterial growth. Urine pH should be tested periodically and should measure 5.5 to 6.5. Phenaphthazine paper (Nitrazine paper) is used to measure the pH of urine as it falls on the skin, not while on the stoma or in the pouch. Methods for acidifying urine include ingestion of cranberry juice and administration of 2–10 grams ascorbic acid (vitamin C) in divided doses during the day, providing an acid-ash diet and increasing fluids.

Skin problems are often associated with alkaline urine and can show up as encrustations or hyperplasia (an overgrowth of skin). Along with acidification of the urine and treatment of infection if present, skin should be treated with daily vinegar-and-water 1:2 soaks for 15 to 30 minutes. A similar solution can be instilled through the bottom of the pouch to decrease bacterial count in the pouch.

Alterations In Skin Integrity

Other skin problems seen in the urinary ostomate are caused by factors similar to those affecting the fecal ostomate, and assessment is made (see Table 12A–3) and management is performed (see Table 12A–4) in a similar manner.

Urinary appliances should maintain a leak-free seal for more than three days. When applying a urinary pouch, the skin should be thoroughly dry or the seal will not hold. Other considerations involve skin barrier breakdown caused by urine and a poorly fitting appliance. Alterations in adherence also can result from the same causes, described previously, as for fecal diversions.

In recent years, surgical techniques have been developed to construct a neo-bladder or continent bladder. The goal is to provide a continent bladder substitute, at low intravesical pressure, and that provides an antireflux valve to prevent upper urinary tract infection. A pouch is created using a portion of the small intestine in a similar manner as that used with the continent ileostomy. An antireflux valve is created utilizing a segment of ileum at the ureteroileal anastomoses. The reservoir is attached to the urethra and patients are instructed in voiding techniques to increase neo-bladder capacity. As with other complicated procedures, patient selection is important in success of the neo-bladder. In women, it might be difficult to achieve adequate anastomosis at the urethra, and a nipple valve could be created that is located at the lower right quadrant of the abdomen. Catheterization of the neo-bladder is performed at regular intervals.

MANAGEMENT OF OTHER DRAINING WOUNDS

Draining wounds other than those described previously are managed according to the same concepts. As with fecal diversions, skin protection, odor containment, and drainage collection are the expected outcome of all wound management.

Small drainage openings, such as fistulas or Penrose drain sites, can be managed using the technique described previously. As with other fecal diversions, skin should be protected from irritating discharge or chemicals.

Large draining wounds, such as wound dehiscence or abscess, that are not contained with conventional pouches might require specialized care and creative management from an experienced nurse or enterostomal therapist. Several products for wound containment are available; these provide access to wounds for irrigation or connection to active or passive draining techniques.

Drainage sites located in skin folds or creases, such as suprapubic catheters, can become management problems. The use of additional pastes (e.g., karaya, Stomahesive™) and skin cements can increase adherence and protect surrounding skin.

BIBLIOGRAPHY

1. Abrams, J. *Abdominal Stomas: Indications, Operative Technique and Patient Care*. John Wright. PSG Inc., Littleton. 1984. Grune & Stratton, New York. 1984.

   This monograph on abdominal stomas presents indications for surgery, stoma construction, postoperative care, complications, and management.

2. Bradley, M., and M. Pupiales. Essential elements of ostomy care. *AJN*. 97(7): 38–46. 1997.

   This article describes anatomy and physiology of ostomy surgery, techniques for pouching ostomies, stoma assessment, complications, basic instructions and tips on patient teaching, and psychosocial concerns.

3. Fischer, J., M. Nussbaum, L. Martin, B. Warner, L. Flesch, J. Staneck, E. Niemer, S. Bjornson, R. Thompson, K. McFadden, L. James. The pull-through procedure: Technical factors in influencing outcome, with emphasis on pouchitis. *Surgery,* 114 (October): 828–35. 1993.

   This article provides excellent information on a wide range of factors related to ileal-anal pull-through surgery.

4. Hampton, B. *Ostomies and Continent Diversion: Nursing Management*. C. V. Mosby Co., St. Louis. 1992.

   This book provides a complete guide to ostomy and wound care. Contributing authors cover areas related to the role of enterostomal therapy, pathology, and medical management of ostomy-related disease, anatomy and physiology, nursing management, psychosocial issues, age-related issues, and future trends.

5. Heneghan, G., N. Clark, B. Hensley, and Yang. The Indiana pouch: A continent urinary diversion. *Journal of Enterostomal Therapy* 17(6): 231–236. 1990.

    This article describes a continent urinary diversion. Pros and cons are presented, as well as care of the reservoir and psychosocial aspects of the procedure.

6. Jeter, K. F. Hyperplasia or what? *Journal of Enterostomal Therapy* 10(5): 181–184. 1983.

    This article presents and defines common urinary ostomy skin conditions. Using case study methods, two classic situations are presented and appropriate therapy discussed.

7. Krasner, D. Managing draining wounds: Fistulas, leaking tubes and drains. *Ostomy/Wound Management* (Summer): 79–85. 1988.

    Concepts in the management of draining wounds are discussed. In selecting approaches to management, the author considers factors such as amount of drainage, type of drainage, consistency, and configurations. Case studies are provided that incorporate these factors.

8. Thielman, D. E. Patient teaching guidelines. *Journal of Enterostomal Therapy* 10(5): 166–168. 1983.

    The author provides four concise, one-page guidelines for patient teaching after ostomy surgery. Included are colostomy, ileostomy, urinary diversion, and a general guideline for all types of ostomies.

9. Watt, R. Colostomy irrigation: Yes or no? *AJN* 74(10): 1806–1811. 1974.

    This complete article on irrigation includes the pros and cons of colostomy irrigation.

10. Watt, R. Ostomies; why, how and where: An overview. *Nurs Clin North Am* 11(3): 427–444. 1976.

    This classic article provides a general overview of ostomy management.

B. Functional Alterations: Bowel

Jody Gross

12B

Constipation and diarrhea are alterations in bowel function that frequently occur in cancer patients. As diarrhea most commonly has an adverse effect on the nutritional status of the patient, it is discussed in detail in Chapter 9; this section focuses on constipation. Interventions to resolve constipation are often inconsistently implemented and geared to episodic rather than prophylactic management. Constipation is an expected side effect of numerous treatments for cancer, but measures to treat constipation are often not instituted until after constipation has developed. No standard accepted regimen or protocol is used in practice, with the result that many patients suffer discomfort, take numerous laxative doses, and require enemas or other invasive procedures to reestablish normal bowel habits. Patients prone to constipation are easily identified, and measures should be instituted to *prevent* changes in bowel habits, because resolution of constipation is a more difficult and time-consuming task for both the patient and the nurse.

PATHOPHYSIOLOGY

Defecation is a complex process that involves several intrinsic and extrinsic reflex mechanisms and the action of both voluntary and involuntary muscles. Activities such as food ingestion initiate, via the myenteric plexus, the *gastrocolic reflex*. This reflex, and others at various gastrointestinal (GI) tract junctures intrinsic to the GI tract, such as the duodenocolic and jejunocolic reflexes, result in mass movements that propel fecal matter into the rectum. *Mass movements*, propulsive peristaltic waves that arise in the colon, occur three or four times a day and are strongest during the first hour after breakfast. When enough stool has collected in the rectum to exceed the threshold of stimulation, receptors in the rectum initiate the *defecation reflex* by transmitting afferent impulses through the myenteric plexus to the spinal cord and the brain. The myenteric plexus initiates further peristaltic waves, and spinal cord reflexes intensify these peristaltic motions, which are weak without central nervous system (CNS) augmentation, causing contraction of rectal musculature and relaxation of the internal anal sphincter. The impulses to the brain arouse awareness of the urge to stool and lead to voluntary contraction of the external anal sphincter. If the person does not allow defecation to proceed, the intensity of the urge decreases and the reflex dies out; it will usually not return until more feces have entered the rectum. Continually ignoring the call to stool will result in diminished sensitivity of the rectum, so the arrival of more feces or further peristaltic mass movements fail to initiate defecation. As feces remain in the colon and rectum, water is continually absorbed across the wall of the gut, so that the stool is further compacted and hardened. Though more stool is required to initiate defecation, the stool already present in the rectum has become hard, dry, and small.

When defecation is allowed to proceed, the most physiologically comfortable position is squatting, with hamstring muscles in the posterior thigh contracted. The glottis is closed, and the diaphragm and abdominal muscles contracted. These actions serve to increase intra-abdominal and intrathoracic pressures to aid in expelling stool. Voluntary cortical inhibition of the external anal sphincter ceases, and the sphincter relaxes, allowing stool to pass. This process normally occurs between three times a day and three times a week in 98 percent of the population.

ASSESSMENT

Constipation is defined as the passage of hard, dry stools, associated with an undue amount of straining, that is decreased in frequency from normal and leave the patient with a sensation of incomplete evacuation. Consistency of stool and the degree of difficulty in defecation are objective signs of constipation, as is the presence of a firm abdomen or decreased bowel sounds. Occasionally, liquid stool can be passed around constipated or impacted stool and might be mistaken for diarrhea. The diagnosis of constipation in this case can be made by the person's complaints of rectal fullness and decreased frequency of bowel movements, and by the presence of increased bowel sounds and stool in the rectum on digital examination. X-rays might be required to distinguish a fecal impaction higher in the colon from bowel obstruction or other pathology.

Even if objective signs are not in evidence, the diagnosis of constipation should be based on the subjective report of the patient, as with pain. If the patient complains of a change in bowel habits that he or she considers constipation, the problem should be treated. Frequency and feelings of rectal fullness are issues of great concern to patients and should be dealt with as part of treatment. Rectal fullness could also indicate underlying disease—such as hemorrhoids, prolapsed rectal mucosa, or tumor—and should be investigated.

Constipation can be classified by physiologic and pathologic causes. Appropriate assessment of the patient includes identification of risk factors for the development of constipation.

Primary Constipation

This condition exists without any underlying organic disease. It can be self-induced by a decreased intake of food or dietary fiber, lack of exercise, or ignoring the call to stool. Decreased stool bulk from decreased intake can contribute to constipation by two mechanisms: by decreasing GI motility and peristalsis associated with a full gut, contributing to the production of small, dry stool; and by lack of stimulation of sensory receptors in the rectum and therefore initiation of the defecation reflex. Lack of exercise leads to a decrease in GI tract motility and in the muscle tone needed to generate adequate intra-abdominal pressure for defecation. Environmental factors can also cause the person to ignore the urge to defecate; these factors include poor or inaccessible toilet facilities or conditions that prevent answering the call to stool, such as hospitalization, which interrupts normal routines and affects activity and food and fluid intake.

Lack of physical activity because of illness or hospitalization, and surgical trauma, which can halt peristalsis, also interfere with maintenance of normal bowel function. Bedpan use can contribute to constipation because the patient might suppress the urge to defecate if a bedpan is not readily available. Evacuation on a bedpan is a difficult and uncomfortable process, because the patient cannot assume the normal squatting position. Attempting the passage of a normal bowel movement on a bedpan is often unsuccessful, increasing the tendency toward constipation as well as exhausting the patient and endangering his or her cardiovascular status. Oxygen consumption increases when a bedpan is used rather than a commode or toilet, and intrathoracic pressure can be raised enough to be classified as a Valsalva maneuver (greater than 40 mm Hg for greater than 8 sec). If a patient is already constipated, attempts to defecate using a bedpan can result in Valsalva maneuvers in more than 50 percent of straining episodes.

Motility Disorders

Diverticular disease, irritable bowel syndrome, idiopathic slow transit, and other conditions that cause hypomotility can cause constipation.

Psychiatric Conditions

Emotional states can have a profound effect on the GI tract. Disorders in which constipation is a common symptom include anorexia nervosa and depression, because these conditions are associated with decreased mobility, food intake, and muscle tone.

Known Organic Disease

Known organic disease is less often the source of constipation in cancer patients than the factors that cause primary constipation. Constipation can be a presenting symptom of bowel carcinoma, as a result of internal or external compression of the colon by tumor. Hemorrhoids, anal fissures, and perianal abscesses cause pain or difficulty with defecation, so the person suppresses the call to stool. Other GI or pelvic diseases can interfere with defecation reflexes. Neurologic conditions—such as spinal cord or cerebral injuries, tumors, or metastases—can give rise to severe constipation by interfering with the extrinsic innervation of the gut. Hypercalcemia, by disturbing the electrophysiology of colon muscle; dehydration, by causing hardened feces and decreased fecal mass in the rectum; fluid and electrolyte imbalances, which interfere with absorptive processes and gut musculature; and debility associated with impaired metabolism and nutrition, and generalized weakness can all contribute to constipation.

Medical and Surgical Treatment

Constipation can be related to drugs, including aluminum- and calcium-containing antacids, because these ions are constipating; opioids, which bind to receptors in the myenteric plexus as well as in the CNS and prevent peristaltic waves; and anticonvulsants, antidepressants, anesthetics, and other drugs that act on the CNS or affect transmission of nerve impulses. Patients receiving cytotoxic therapy with vinca alkaloids, particularly vincristine, might experience constipation or obstipation as a result of autonomic neuropathy.

Opioids are the most common cause of constipation in cancer patients because they decrease propulsive peristalsis and thus prolong the transit time of fecal matter. Unlike other side effects of opioids, little if any tolerance is developed to the constipating effects with prolonged administration of these drugs. In addition to the direct effect of opioids on the gut, use of these medications also contributes to constipation via indirect effects, as opioids can cause decreased appetite secondary to nausea and decreased mobility secondary to sedation. Patients are infrequently started on a laxative program at the same time they begin taking opioids, so the opportunity for prevention is often missed.

Other iatrogenic causes include fluid depletion and decreased food intake resulting from treatment for disease, such as chemotherapy, radiation therapy, and diagnostic procedures. Less acute effects of treatment include adhesion formation and radiation colitis, which can result in constipation due to a decrease in the size of the lumen of the colon, interference with motility, or pain.

Complicating Conditions

Thrombocytopenia and granulocytopenia enhance the dangers of constipation for the patient. In the patient prone to bleeding, Valsalva maneuvers performed while straining at stool can increase intracranial pressure, which can cause a retinal or potentially fatal cerebral hemorrhage (see Chapter 15A). Perirectal abscesses account for approximately 25 percent of infections in patients with acute leukemia and can occur in patients who are leukopenic as a result of cytotoxic therapy. The presence of any abnormality of bowel function, whether diarrhea or constipation, that increases the likelihood of rectal mucosal tears or irritation increases the risk of infection at this site. These risks are compounded for the patient suffering from mucositis as a result of cytotoxic therapy.

Patients experiencing anemia or fatigue might lack the energy or muscle tone required to pass a constipated stool. If dietary intake has changed, with a reduction in fiber intake, stool may become soft and unformed. Lack of energy and muscle tone make it difficult to pass these stools, so that the stool remaining in the rectum will become harder and dryer. Defecation on the toilet or bedside commode requires less energy expenditure than the use of a bedpan, but some patients do not have the energy required to get to the bathroom or commode.

MEDICAL MANAGEMENT

There are many agents to treat constipation. Currently more than 700 different over-the-counter laxative preparations are available in the United States. The majority can be divided into five categories. Table 12B–1 lists common agents, doses, and onset of action.

Table 12B–1
Laxative Dosages and Onset of Action

Agent	Usual Daily Dose	Onset of Action (Hours)
Bulk producers		
Bran	10 g/1 tbsp	
Psyllium/cellulose derivatives	1–3 tbsp, 1–3	12–24
Calcium polycarbophil	1–4 tab, 1–4	
Saline laxatives		
Milk of magnesia	15 ml	
Magnesium citrate	200 ml	3–6
Epsom salt	15 g	
Osmotic laxatives		
Lactulose	15–60 ml	24–48
Sorbitol	30–60 ml	
Stimulant laxatives		
Bisacodyl	10–15 mg	6–10
Phenolpthalein	30–200 mg	6–10
Senna (standardized senna concentrate)		
Granules	326 mg/1 tsp, 1–4 tsp/d	6–10
Tablets	187 mg/tab, 2–8 tabs/d	6–10
Syrup	218 mg/5 ml, 10–30 ml/d	6–10
Cascara sagrada	325 mg/tab	6–10
Bisacodyl suppository	10 mg	$\frac{1}{4}$–1
Surfactant laxatives		
Docusate	50–500 mg	6–10

Bulk Producers

Bulk producers are hydrophilic agents that absorb significant quantities of water in the gut, consequently softening as well as increasing the size of the stool. Peristaltic waves, though initiated by intrinsic reflexes, are also stimulated by adequate quantities of fecal matter in the bowel lumen. The best source of bulk is dietary fiber, most commonly bran, a substance often lacking in the diet of many Americans, and especially in the elderly, who might have decreased their food intake because of debility. Decreased intake of dietary fiber can also occur in cancer patients who move to softer diets in response to stomatitis from chemotherapy or radiation therapy, ill-fitting dentures after weight loss, or a need for bland, easily digested food.

Among geriatric patients on regular diets, a decrease to approximately half the former number of laxative doses has been noted after an increase in dietary fiber. The inclusion of 10 to 20 grams of bran in the daily diet can have a positive effect on evacuation, though it remains difficult to establish the minimum amount of dietary fiber required to treat constipation. The fiber content of foods is determined as either crude or dietary. Crude fiber content in food is determined by measuring the cellulose and lignin content that remains after the food is boiled in acid and alkaline solutions. Dietary fiber consists of the cellulose, lignin, and other polysaccharides that are not digested by the small intestine; 20 grams of crude fiber equals approximately 60 grams of dietary fiber. A multitude of high-fiber foods are available from many sources, including whole wheat bread (9.5 g dietary fiber/100 g of food), all-bran cereals (26.7), peanuts (9.3) and peanut butter (7.5), unpeeled pears (8.6), peas (7.9) and carrots (3.7).

Polysaccharides and cellulose derivatives, such as psyllium (Metamucil®) and methylcellulose (Citrucil®), or calcium polycarbophil (FiberCon®), can be utilized in place of dietary sources. The dosage range of these agents is flexible, allowing adjustment to the individual person's needs. Psyllium preparations often contain dextrose as a dispersing agent, so there is little danger of bolus formation in the gut if they are taken with enough fluid. Fluid intake must be sufficient to deal with the increase in bulk, or water will be pulled across the colonic mucosa from the extracellular fluid. Each dose of bulk laxative should be taken with at least one glass (eight ounces) of fluid. Intake of fluids in all forms should be two to three liters per day. Occasionally, bulk producers can cause flatulence or abdominal cramping. These side effects can be decreased or avoided by gradually introducing these agents into the diet and by using divided doses. If possible, dietary fiber should be ingested at every meal, other bulking agents should be given therapeutically one to four times a day. Increasing dietary fiber is preferred to using other types of bulking agents, because high-fiber foods provide nutrients and calories as well as normalizing bowel function.

As constipation in cancer patients most frequently occurs in persons who are experiencing decreased functional capacity, the usefulness of bulk producers to treat constipation is limited. Many patients will be unable to ingest a therapeutic amount of bulk, either dietary or from over the counter products, or the volume of fluid needed for these agents to be effective.

Lubricants

Lubricants, the most common of which is mineral oil, lubricate and soften the stool. Mineral oil is infrequently used, because it results in unpleasant seepage from the rectum and can cause lipid pneumonia, especially in a debilitated and bedridden patient. If mineral oil is used—for example, in the resolution of fecal impaction—the patient should be instructed to sit up for several hours after taking the oil orally. A lubricant does not increase GI motility, and bulk producers are probably as effective in softening stool. Mineral oil is useful when given as an enema, where it remains in the rectum, and can soften constipated stool more effectively than a similar volume of water. It also lubricates the outside of the stool when given rectally, allowing easier passage.

Saline and Osmotic Laxatives

Epsom salt, milk of magnesia, and other sodium, magnesium, and potassium salts are unabsorbed solutes that retain water in the small bowel and increase the flow of fluid into the colon. The cathartic effect of these saline laxatives is unpleasant, can be associated with cramping and bloating, and can lead to excessive absorption of cations by the bowel. The sodium salts must be used with caution in patients with congestive heart failure; magnesium and phosphate salts might be contraindicated in those with renal insufficiency. These agents do not encourage a return to normal bowel function but are useful as preparative agents for diagnostic tests and in rapid resolution of existing constipation.

Osmotic laxatives include lactulose (Chronulac®, Cephulac®), sorbitol, and glycerin. Lactulose and sorbitol are synthetic disaccharides for which no corresponding disaccharidase exists in the small bowel, so they enter the colon unmetabolized. Action of colonic bacteria may enhance the osmotic catharsis. These agents are effective in the treatment of vincristine- or opioid-induced constipation, where bulking agents might not work, because increasing the size of the fecal mass without the necessary peristaltic stimulation will produce more discomfort rather than resolve the constipation. Sorbitol is inexpensive compared with lactulose. Dosages can be titrated to produce bowel movements with a frequency and consistency acceptable to the patient. Excessive dosages can cause cramping, bloating, and nausea.

Stimulant Laxatives

Stimulant laxatives include castor oil, whose violent cathartic action should preclude its use, and the anthraquinone and polyphenolic compounds. The most common anthraquinones are senna (Senokot®) and cascara. The polyphenolics are usually represented by bisacodyl (Dulcolax®) and phenolpthalein (Ex-Lax®). These agents are effective for management of opioid-induced constipation. Caution should be exercised with chronic use, because these agents are habit forming, can lead to electrolyte disturbances and histologic changes in the bowel, and cause myenteric plexus degeneration after prolonged use.

Senna and cascara are also active only in the colon after interaction with colonic bacteria. These laxatives work by inducing peristalsis through intrinsic stimulation of the colon. Approximately one-half of a senna tablet can be effective in treating or preventing constipation caused by 60 mg of codeine or 5 mg of morphine. At higher opioid doses, less senna per mg of opioid is needed to cause a laxative effect or prevent constipation.

Phenolpthaleins are active only in the colon, where they increase peristalsis by stimulating sensory nerves. Effective doses of phenolpthaleins vary widely among patients; dosages should be adjusted to the person to maintain bowel function with minimal side effects. Bisacodyl should not be administered with alkali, such as antacids, which causes activation of the agent in the small intestine. These medications can color the urine.

Because of their specific site of action, these agents are recommended for general use as a temporary measure, in the minimal effective dose. They are available as oral and rectal agents. Senna and cascara, which are plant derivatives, can also be found in products such as teas and cookies. Prunes contain a phenolic substance as well as fiber and should be considered as therapeutic agents for their laxative effect. It should be noted that prune juice contains no fiber.

Surfactant Laxatives

Dioctyl sulfosuccinate, or docusate, is a surface-active agent with detergent properties that allows water to penetrate the feces and increases the permeability of the gut mucosa. Docusate sodium (Colace®), calcium (Surfak®), and potassium (Dialose®) are ineffective in altering the incidence of constipation among elderly medical patients. However, for patients who have difficulty drinking adequate amounts of fluid, these agents are useful to soften the stool, when used in combination with another type of laxative.

Suppositories and Enemas

Suppositories act mechanically by stimulating sensory receptors in the rectum. If indicated, glycerine suppositories are a useful stimulus to defecation when no further laxative action is warranted, and they also draw fluid into the rectum. Other suppository preparations contain an active agent, usually a stimulant laxative, and exert the same effect as when taken orally; in addition, the anorectal reflex is stimulated by placement of the suppository. Because they are administered rectally, the onset of their therapeutic effect is rapid. Patients might experience mild burning sensations in the rectum. Suppositories might not be effective if hard, dry stool is present in the rectum and sigmoid colon, as this stool must be moistened in order to be evacuated.

Enemas are useful in the resolution of constipation related to diagnostic procedures, management of fecal impaction, or as a first step in reestablishing normal bowel habits after medication-induced constipation develops. Enemas evacuate only the distal colon. Tap water enemas add water to constipated stool; soap suds enemas add water and have an irritant effect. Sodium phosphate/biphosphate (Fleet®) exerts an osmotic effect; an oil-retention enema softens and lubricates hard, dry stool.

Agents that are administered per rectum should be used with caution in cancer patients who are receiving chemotherapy or radiation therapy or are otherwise at risk for granulocytopenia, thrombocytopenia, or mucositis, because of the hazards of perirectal infection or hemorrhage.

NURSING MANAGEMENT

A comprehensive bowel program for cancer patients susceptible to constipation is presented in Table 12B–2. This program advocates a preventive approach as the best method of treating constipation, which can be a long-term problem.

The protocol should be applied with caution to patients who have GI disease or bowel obstruction. Program modifications can be made for patients unable to tolerate a significant amount of bulk-producing agents or with disease involving the spinal cord. Patients with a history of constipation should first embark upon a retraining program that includes the judicious use of enemas and suppositories and that can be based on the format presented in Table 12B–2. When the patient is retrained, the prophylactic approach of the program should prevent recurrence of constipation. Cancer patients previously identified as being at risk for constipation or whose condition is threatened by granulocytopenia or thrombocytopenia and who are not in the excluded categories listed previously can use this program.

The intake of adequate dietary fiber and fluid should be the first step in any bowel regimen. Pharmacological agents should not be used in place

Table 12B–2
Nursing Protocol for Prophylactic Bowel Management

Problem	Intervention
Maintain adequate bulk and softness of stool	Provide a high fiber diet, approximately 10 g dietary fiber daily. Ensure adequate fluid intake, approximately 2–3 L daily. Provides psyllium or other bulk producers as needed, in recommended dosages. Avoid caffeine-containing beverages. Provide stool softener (surfactant) if fluid intake inadequate.

Encourage normal bowel function	Ensure adequate physical activity to maintain abdominal and other muscle tone and promote GI motility.
	Use toilet or bedside commode for all bowel movements:
	    If patient only OOB once/d, use this time for toileting.
	    Place commode near weakened patients; when hospitalized, place patient in bed nearest bathroom.
	Provide privacy to lessen suppression of call to stool.
	Provide footstool if raised toilet seat is used.
	Plan bowel movements for same time each day.
	Provide hot drink approximately $\frac{1}{2}$ hr before planned defecation to stimulate gastrocolic reflex.
	Insert glycerine suppository 15 min to $\frac{1}{2}$ hr prior to planned defecation to stimulate anorectal reflex.

Ensure bowel movement at least once every 3 days	Add prunes to diet; give in PM for laxative effect in AM, in AM for laxative effect in PM. Provide senna, cascara, or bisacodyl for patients receiving opioids or vincristine therapy, or who do not establish or maintain routine habits. Provide lactulose or sorbitol for patients who do not achieve regularity with senna, cascara, or bisacodyl.

GI—gastrointestinal; OOB—out of bed.

of these two easy, cost-effective, and normal methods of maintaining bowel regularity. Patients at risk for constipation should avoid excessive quantities of coffee, tea, or other beverages containing caffeine, because these act as diuretics, decreasing available body fluids. It might be helpful to exclude these beverages from tabulations of daily fluid intake.

Monitoring patients on a prophylactic bowel program includes assessing daily dietary fiber, calorie, and fluid intake; medications; performance status; frequency and consistency of stools; and the number of laxative doses given.

Successful implementation of the program should result in decreased need for laxatives and other interventions; easy passage of a soft, formed stool approximately once every two to three days; and fewer complaints of discomfort or constipation.

This protocol is easily instituted for all patients, whether they are receiving care in an inpatient setting, an ambulatory care setting, or at home. All therapeutic agents used, with the exception of sorbitol and lactulose, are available without a prescription. As an aspect of preventive self-care, this program presents an excellent opportunity for nurses to engage in patient teaching.

BIBLIOGRAPHY

1. Basch, A. Changes in elimination. *Seminars in Oncology Nursing* 3(4): 287–292. 1987.

   This article provides a good review of the causes and treatments of diarrhea and constipation in cancer patients.

2. Benton, J. , H. Brown, and H. Rusk. Energy expended by patients on the bedpan and bedside commode. *Journal of the American Medical Association* 144 (December 23): 1443–1447. 1950.

   This interesting study documents increased energy consumption during bedpan usage.

3. Bisanz, A. Managing bowel elimination problems in patients with cancer. *Oncology Nursing Forum* 24(4): 679–686. 1997.

   This article presents information on management of elimination problems in cancer patients, including constipation and diarrhea. It also offers continuing education credits for the reader.

4. Canty, S. L. Constipation as a side effect of opioids. *Oncology Nursing Forum* 21(4): 739–745. 1994.

   This review article presents the causes, complications, and treatment of constipation in cancer patients and presents a decision tree for management of this patient problem.

5. Cimprich, B. Symptom management: Constipation. *Cancer Nursing* 8(3): 9–43. 1985 (suppl. 1).

   This reviews the assessment, causes and prevention, and management of constipation.

6. Halpern, A., N. Shafter, D. Selman, et al. The straining forces of bowel function. *Angiology* 11 (October): 426–436. 1960.

   This is another study that documents the physiological effects of constipation, specifically the increase in intrathoracic pressure during straining.

7. McMillan, S. C., and F. A. Williams. Validity and reliability of the Constipation Assessment Scale. *Cancer Nursing* 12(3): 183–188. 1989.

   This article reports on the development of an assessment tool for constipation, which utilizes the patients' subjective report to appropriately identify the problem of constipation.

8. Portenoy, R. K. Constipation in the cancer patient: Causes and management. *Medical Clinics of North America* 71(2): 303–311. 1987.

This article reviews the subject of constipation in cancer patients, with the goal of allowing the clinician to prevent or manage this common problem so that therapeutic regimens for pain and other problems will be adequate.

9. Sykes, N. P. Current approaches to the management of constipation. *Cancer Surveys* 21: 137–145. 1994.

This article reviews the management of constipation in cancer patients, including those in the terminal phases of illness.

10. Twycross, R. G. Managing constipation: A not-so-easy problem in cancer patients. *Primary Care and Cancer* 9(8): 23–30. 1989.

This article discusses the management of opioid-induced constipation, with a review of available agents.

11. Wald, A. Constipation and fecal incontinence in the elderly. *Gastroenterology Clinics North America* 19(2): 405–418. 1990.

This review covers the incidence of constipation and fecal incontinence in the elderly, physiological changes associated with aging, and etiology and management of these problems in a geriatric population.

12. Yakabowich, M. Prescribe with care: The role of laxatives in the treatment of constipation. *Journal of Gerontological Nursing* 16(7): 4–11. 1990.

This review article focuses on the management of constipation, especially the pharmacological agents used in treatment of this problem.

C. Functional Alterations: Bladder

Mikel Gray

INTRODUCTION

Voiding dysfunction exists when the filling/storage or elimination functions of the lower urinary tract are compromised. Several symptoms can indicate dysfunctional voiding. *Urinary incontinence* is a symptom that might represent a simple mechanical disorder of the urinary system or the direct or indirect result of a serious underlying disorder such as a malignant process.

Urinary retention occurs when the bladder fails to empty itself by the process of micturition. *Painful disorders of the bladder* occur when the sensations of bladder filling are altered. Inflammation of the bladder wall

12c

or a specific inflammatory lesion can cause increased urgency or pain during bladder filling, resulting in a voiding dysfunction characterized by frequency, urgency to urinate, and significant lower urinary tract discomfort.

Urinary system distress occurs when lower urinary tract physiology becomes so compromised that renal function is threatened. Common presenting symptoms of urinary system distress are voiding dysfunction with recurrent urinary tract infection (usually febrile) or signs of uremia. Urinary system distress can coexist with symptoms of incontinence, retention, or a painful bladder disorder. Regardless of its presentation and relative threat to physiological well-being, voiding dysfunction represents a serious threat to a person's psychological and social well-being.

PHYSIOLOGY

The lower urinary tract (vesicourethral unit) comprises the bladder, urethra, pelvic floor muscles, and endopelvic fascia. The function of the lower urinary system is to receive and store urine manufactured by the renal parenchyma until a socially appropriate time for elimination.

Urinary continence is the term applied to the control of bladder functions. In most cultures, control of urinary continence is expected by the time a child reaches the fourth year of life. The characteristics of urinary continence are the ability to (1) store urine for at least two hours while awake; (2) hold urine without leaking despite physical exertion or the desire (urge) to urinate; and (3) completely empty the bladder using voluntary command.

Urinary continence relies on three factors: an anatomically intact lower urinary system, a functioning central nervous system, and a competent urinary sphincter mechanism. Failure of any one of these mechanisms will compromise urinary function and predispose the person to voiding dysfunction.

A continuous, anatomically intact urinary tract begins at the level of the kidney where blood is filtered in large quantities, resulting in the production of urine (1,000–2,500 cc/day) containing water and the metabolic waste products of the body. When filtration, secretion, and excretion is completed by the nephron, urine collects in the renal pelvis for transport to the urinary bladder via the ureters. The urinary bladder, in turn, stores urine before it is expelled from the body by micturition. Loss of anatomic integrity of the urinary system, by ectopia (an abnormal opening of the urinary system caused by a birth defect) or a fistulous tract (an abnormal, epithelialized passage caused by a malignancy, trauma, or iatrogenic lesion), produces extraurethral urinary leakage, bypassing the normal route for urinary elimination.

An intact nervous system is essential for urinary continence because it regulates detrusor stability and urinary sphincter control. *Detrusor stability* is the term used to describe normal continence. The stable detrusor produces a contraction of sufficient magnitude to empty the bladder of urine only when its owner gives permission. The brain contains multiple centers that modulate detrusor control. Although the exact mechanism remains unclear, the net effect of the brain's influence on the bladder is to inhibit detrusor contractions until an appropriate time and place for urination. The detrusor motor area, located in the prefrontal cortex, contributes to detrusor stability by an unknown mechanism. In addition, the thalamus, cerebellum, and basal ganglia interact with the detrusor motor area to provide voluntary modulation of bladder contractions. The hypothalamus and limbic system also influence autonomic system function and are presumed to exert an influence on detrusor function, although dysfunction of the limbic system fails to produce clinically apparent detrusor instability.

The brain stem influences both detrusor and urethral sphincter function. Within the pons are two neural centers crucial to lower urinary tract function. The "M" center of the pons is a group of neurons that act under direction from higher brain centers to initiate the micturition reflex. The adjacent "L" center also contains a group of neurons that coordinate detrusor contraction with sphincter mechanism relaxation. While the brain controls the social aspects of continence (the timing of bladder contractions), the pons is the origin of the detrusor reflex. After the brain releases its inhibitory influence over the lower urinary tract (gives "permission" to urinate), the "M" center of the pons is activated, initiating a detrusor contraction. Stimulation of the adjacent "L" center of the pons causes the sphincter mechanism to relax, allowing complete evacuation of the bladder. Following urination, the brain restores its inhibitory influence over the bladder and the "M" center remains quiet, allowing the detrusor to relax for bladder filling while the "L" center causes contraction of the muscular elements of the urinary sphincter, preventing stress urinary incontinence.

The spinal cord contains two centers that directly affect bladder function; both act under the influence of modulatory centers in the brain and pons. Sympathetic output to the bladder originates at spinal levels T12 to L2. The sympathetic nervous system promotes bladder filling and storage, causing the detrusor muscle to relax and the sphincter mechanism to remain closed. Parasympathetic output to the bladder favors micturition, producing detrusor contraction and (indirectly) sphincter mechanism relaxation. The parasympathetic neurons originate at sacral spinal levels 2–4. Somatic input from spinal levels S1–3 also affects bladder function. These nerve roots provide segmental and volitional control of the pelvic floor muscles.

Three peripheral nerves join the spinal central nervous system to innervate the lower urinary tract. The inferior hypogastric plexus carries sympathetic nerve fibers to the detrusor muscle and sphincter mechanism, and the pelvic plexus carries parasympathetic fibers to the bladder and urethra. In addition, the pudendal nerve carries somatic fibers to the pelvic floor muscles.

Direct nervous control of the detrusor muscle is achieved through the actions of specific neurotransmitters that affect the smooth and skeletal muscle of the lower urinary tract. Acetylcholine, the primary excitatory neurotransmitter of the parasympathetic nervous system, is primarily responsible for detrusor muscle contraction. Cholinergic receptors in the detrusor muscle are subdivided into muscarinic and nicotinic, according to specific pharmacologic properties. The cholinergic receptors of the detrusor muscle are muscarinic, and anticholinergic drugs are frequently administered to diminish the frequency and magnitude of hyperactive or unstable contractions that occur when the control of the detrusor muscle is compromised. The muscarinic receptors have been further subdivided, and it is now known that the cholinergic receptors of the detrusor muscle are predominantly M3. This subdivision is significant, because it could allow the development of anticholinergic medications that are more specific to bladder function and less likely to produce the unpleasant side effects (e.g., dry mouth, blurred vision, and intolerance to heat) that limit the efficacy of current agents.

Relaxation of the detrusor muscle probably represents a combination of inhibition of cholinergic action and the inhibitory influence of adrenergic receptors. Adrenergic receptors rely on the neurotransmitter noradrenaline (norepinephrine), and the detrusor muscle primarily contains beta-adrenergic receptors. The significance of these receptors remains unclear, and beta-adrenergic agonists are not suitable for the control of unstable detrusor contractions because of the side effects produced by these drugs.

The normal urethral sphincter also prevents urinary incontinence; it is best conceptualized as a single mechanism containing elements of compression and tension, rather than a combination of internal and external muscles. These produce a watertight seal against urinary leakage. The elements of compression are the soft urethral lining, the mucus produced by specific cells with the urethral epithelium, and the submucosal vascular cushion. The soft lining of the urethra easily folds on itself while mucosal secretions fill the microscopic grooves to prevent urinary leakage. Finally, the rich vascular bed that lies between the epithelium and muscular elements of the sphincter promotes the transmission of tension (closure pressure) from the intrinsic urethral and pelvic floor muscles, ensuring continence in the presence of physical stress.

Compression and tension are necessary for urethral competence (closure) when physical stress is present. Smooth muscle bundles at the bladder neck and proximal urethra are arranged in circular and longitudinal configurations, providing active tension that opposes leakage. In addition, a specialized group of skeletal muscle fibers, in the middle third of the female's urethra and in the membranous urethra of the male, are arranged in a semicircular fashion, contributing to urethral closure. These muscle fibers are collectively referred to as the *rhabdosphincter*. Innervated by sympathetic, parasympathetic, and somatic nerve endings, the rhabdosphincter is particularly suited for the prolonged periods of tension required to maintain urinary continence.

Like the detrusor muscle, the muscles of the urethral sphincter mechanism are under the direct control of specific neurotransmitters. The smooth muscle of the bladder neck and proximal urethra (including the prostatic urethra of the male) contain primarily adrenergic receptors. Unlike the detrusor, these receptors are primarily alpha adrenergic, and stimulation causes muscle contraction rather than relaxation. The rhabdosphincter also contains alpha adrenergic receptors; alpha adrenergic antagonists (blockers) can be used to treat detrusor sphincter dyssynergia, and alpha adrenergic agonists can be used to treat stress urinary incontinence caused by intrinsic sphincter deficiency.

The pelvic floor also contributes to urethral tension, especially when bursts of intense physical intensity occur. Contraction of the pelvic floor muscles in response to coughing, lifting a heavy object, walking, or running provides the additional urethral closure needed for short bursts of intense physical stress.

The competence of the ureteral sphincter mechanism also relies on support outside the urethra. The pelvic floor muscles are the primary supportive structure, but the endopelvic fascia and adjacent organs, including the rectum, prostate, and vagina, provide additional support for the bladder base and urethral sphincter mechanism. Failure of these support mechanisms compromises the anatomic position of the urethra, often leading to urinary incontinence in the presence of physical stress.

PATHOPHYSIOLOGY

Urinary Incontinence

According to the International Continence Society, urinary incontinence is the uncontrolled loss of urine that produces a social or hygienic problem perceived by the patient, family, or caregivers. Urinary incontinence can occur as the direct or indirect result of a malignant disease. Incontinence is best conceptualized by its various types. Multiple classification schema for incontinence exist; for the purposes of this discussion, the schema described by Gray and Dougherty will be used. Table 12C–1 correlates this schema with the nursing diagnoses proposed by the North American Nursing Diagnosis Association.

Detrusor instability is the occurrence of bladder contractions during vesicle filling/storage that produce urinary leakage or compromise bladder capacity. Detrusor instability produces urge incontinence when contractions are accompanied by the sudden urge to urinate and reflex incontinence when contractions occur without sensations. Detrusor instability is caused by neuropathic disorders (e.g., cerebrovascular accident, brain tumors, spinal injury, and multiple sclerosis), obstruction of the bladder outlet, or irritative bladder disorders; or it can be idiopathic. Detrusor instability is associated with stress urinary incontinence, but no causative relationship has been found.

When malignant tumors affect the neurological modulation of the detrusor muscle, produce irritation of the bladder wall, or obstruct the vesical

Table 12C-1
Comparative Classifications for Urinary Dysfunction

Gray/Dougherty Schema	NANDA* Diagnosis
Stress incontinence	Stress incontinence Total incontinence**
Instability incontinence	Urge incontinence Reflex incontinence
Overflow incontinence	Urinary retention
Extraurethral incontinence	Total incontinence**

*North American Nursing Diagnosis Association

**Total incontinence is used to refer to extraurethral leakage and to severe cases of stress incontinence produced by sphincter incompetence.

For further information, refer to Gray, M. L., and M. C. Dougherty. Urinary incontinence: Pathophysiology and treatment. *Journal of Enterostomal Therapy* 14: 152–62. 1987, *and* Kim, M. J., E. H. McFarlane, and A. M. McLane. *Pocket guide to nursing diagnoses.* Mosby-Yearbook, St. Louis. 1991.

outlet, they predispose the person to instability incontinence. Primary intracerebral tumors, extracerebral tumors, and metastatic brain lesions produce urge incontinence when, by direct invasion or compression, they compromise one or more of the modulatory centers for the urinary bladder. Detrusor instability and urge incontinence also can occur when obstruction of the flow of cerebrospinal fluid increases intracranial pressure.

Urge incontinence can also result from a specific inflammatory lesion of the bladder. Primary urothelial tumors, including transitional cell carcinoma and particularly carcinoma *in situ,* produce irritative voiding symptoms and urge incontinence in addition to grossly visible hematuria.

Detrusor instability can result from obstruction of the bladder outlet. In this case, unstable detrusor contractions coexist with urinary retention, causing a prolonged or intermittent urinary stream, frequent urination, feelings of incomplete bladder emptying and nocturia. Prostatic tumors that encroach upon the proximal urethra, primary urothelial tumors located near the bladder base, and urethral tumors produce obstruction that often leads to detrusor instability. Because urge incontinence in the presence of bladder outlet obstruction produces urinary stasis while increasing detrusor contraction pressures, urinary system distress also might exist.

Reflex incontinence occurs when a primary spinal tumor, meningeal tumor, or metastatic lesion compromises spinal segmental function below the pons and above the sacral micturition center. Reflex incontinence is distinguished from urge incontinence by two factors. Because the lesion lies below the brain, sensations of bladder filling are compromised or absent. In addition, because communication between the bladder and pontine micturition center is disrupted, detrusor–sphincter coordination is lost and detrusor–sphincter (vesicosphincter) dyssynergia occurs. *Dyssynergia* is a loss of muscle coordination between the bladder muscle and sphincter mechanism, causing a functional obstruction of the vesical outlet. Dyssynergia often leads to urinary system distress.

Stress incontinence is the leakage of urine in response to physical exertion in the absence of a detrusor contraction. It is produced by two mechanisms, pelvic descent and intrinsic sphincter deficiency. Pelvic descent occurs when the structures of the pelvic floor are weakened, resulting in a change in anatomic relationships of the lower urinary tract. Pelvic descent is rarely the direct result of a malignant process. The predisposition toward pelvic descent and urethral hypermobility is probably familial, and the condition is exacerbated by changes in circulating estrogens, multiple vaginal deliveries, a chronic cough, or prolonged high-impact activities such as long-distance running or weightlifting. In certain cases, pelvic descent could be related to radical hysterectomy or pelvic exenteration with oophorectomy and subsequent loss of muscle tone.

In contrast, intrinsic sphincter deficiency is more commonly related to cancer and its treatment. Primary or metastatic tumors that affect spinal segments S2–4 produce weakness of the detrusor muscle and incompetence of the sphincter mechanism. Surgical excision of tumors of the bladder base also can damage the sphincter mechanism. Radical prostatectomy, by its very nature, interrupts the sphincter mechanism, often resulting in incontinence when extensive resection is required. The risk of stress urinary incontinence following radical prostatectomy can be affected by multiple factors, including the surgical approach used to remove the malignancy.

Extraurethral incontinence occurs when the normal sphincter mechanism is bypassed, causing a continuous urinary leakage unaffected by physical exertion or detrusor contractions. Urinary fistulae can be caused by an invasive tumor or radiation therapy near the bladder and urethra. Fistulae are a rare complication of extensive abdomino-pelvic surgery.

Functional incontinence occurs when alterations in mobility, dexterity, or cognition prevent the person from reaching the bathroom, manipulating clothing, and moving onto the toilet before voiding occurs. Functional incontinence might exist in a person with otherwise normal bladder control, or it can complicate stress, urge, or extraurethral incontinence. The person with a malignant process is particularly prone to functional incontinence during periods of acute debilitation or during a terminal disease stage when mobility, dexterity, and/or cognition are compromised.

Urinary Retention

Urinary retention occurs when the bladder is unable to completely evacuate itself by spontaneous micturition. It is caused by two factors: bladder outlet obstruction and deficient detrusor contraction strength. Malignant tumors that encroach upon the bladder base, enlarge the prostatic stroma, or invade the urethra will obstruct the bladder outlet. Lower spinal tumors or malignancies that compress the pelvic plexus produce urinary retention related to deficient detrusor contraction strength. Extensive abdomino-pelvic surgery could compromise detrusor contractility even though there is no obvious interruption of the neural supply of the bladder. In addition, bladder contractions can be compromised by acute debilitation or prolonged immobility related to a malignant process.

The construction of a neobladder also can produce urinary retention. A neobladder is created when a patient with bladder cancer undergoes a radical cystectomy with preservation of the bladder outlet and urethra. Detubularized bowel is isolated from the fecal stream and reconstructed into a reservoir for urine. Urinary evacuation requires strain voiding, and urinary residual volumes can be significant.

Painful Bladder Disorders

Painful bladder disorders occur when a specific inflammatory lesion or inflammatory process compromises the person's ability to store urine in the lower urinary tract. Primary urothelial tumors can produce irritative voiding symptoms that provide important clues to early detection. Carcinoma *in situ,* in particular, produces irritative voiding symptoms and bladder discomfort; papillary tumors can produce mild inflammation.

Chemotherapeutic agents, particularly cyclophosphamide and ifosfamide, can produce a painful bladder syndrome characterized by urinary frequency, urgency, dysuria, and nocturia. Urine cultures will be negative; cystoscopic examination will reveal hemorrhagic lesions of the bladder epithelium. Gross or microscopic hematuria is often noted on urinalysis. The risk of cystitis is related to the total dosage of the chemotherapeutic agent and the rapidity of administration, which increase the person's risk of accumulating the toxic metabolic waste products of these agents in the bladder. External beam radiation therapy or radioactive seeds implanted near the bladder can also produce a painful bladder syndrome, similar to that caused by the alkylating agents. Most patients note that inflammatory symptoms cease 12 to 18 months after treatment, but a few continue to experience symptoms for months or years.

Irritative voiding symptoms often result from intravesical chemotherapy for primary bladder tumors. Antineoplastic agents mitomycin, thiotepa, or doxorubicin are often administered intravesically for superficial bladder tumors, causing transient symptoms of cystitis, possibly associated with hematuria. These symptoms rapidly subside following completion of therapy. Bacillus Calmette-Guerin (BCG) therapy uses an immunological approach to the management of superficial bladder tumors. The irritative voiding symptoms produced by BCG are often severe, although they rarely persist after therapy is discontinued.

External beam radiation of the pelvis structures can lead to radiation-induced cystitis, affecting approximately 30 percent to 40 percent of those treated by this modality. These effects are typically transient, although they might occasionally persist following the end of treatment. Urethral stricture and bladder outlet obstruction can complicate external beam radiation therapy of the pelvis, particularly when therapy follows surgery of the bladder outlet. Because of improvements in technique, brachytherapy (interstitial therapy using I-125 seeds) has regained popularity in the management of localized prostate cancer. Brachytherapy has been historically associated with a significant risk of debilitating cystitis or proctitis. Using updated techniques, however, the risk of irritative bladder disorders has been greatly reduced, and the risk of subsequent urinary incontinence is less than that associated with radical prostatectomy.

Urinary System Distress

Urinary system distress occurs when voiding dysfunction produces elevated pressures in the urinary tract, compromising the production, transport, or elimination of urine. The presenting symptoms of urinary system distress vary among persons; they include voiding dysfunction coexisting with recurrent urinary tract infection (usually with febrile infections) and signs of renal insufficiency. Diagnosis relies on radiographic imaging, urodynamic evaluation, and laboratory tests. Bladder trabeculation, hydronephrosis, vesicoureteral reflux, low (poor) bladder wall compliance, elevated voiding pressures, and elevated creatinine and blood urea nitrogen might be noted when urinary system distress is present.

Cancer can directly or indirectly produce urinary system distress. Primary tumors of the prostate, bladder, or ureters can compromise renal and urinary function when they obstruct the renal pelvis, ureteral course, or bladder outlet. Tumors of the retroperitoneum or pelvis can cause extrinsic obstruction of the urinary system by compressing the ureters.

Radiation therapy or systemic chemotherapy occasionally causes fibrosis of the bladder wall, resulting in poor compliance, or accommodation, of the bladder to filling with urine. Poor bladder wall compliance produces chronic elevation of intravesical (bladder) pressure, which adversely affects ureteral drainage and, in later stages, filtration of blood within Bowman's capsule.

Spinal tumors can indirectly produce urinary system distress by causing reflex incontinence and vesicosphincter dyssynergia. In this case, functional obstruction of the bladder outlet causes high voiding pressures and residual urine that predispose a patient to infection, hydronephrosis, and vesicoureteral reflux.

ASSESSMENT

The Agency for Health Care Policy and Research's Clinical Guideline Panel on Urinary Incontinence in Adults recommends that all basic evaluations for incontinence confirm the condition in some objective manner, identify contributing, causative, or complicating factors associated with urinary leakage, and distinguish patients who require further evaluation from those who are ready to receive treatment without additional testing. The basic nursing assessment of incontinence comprises a history, focused physical examination, functional and environmental evaluation, voiding (bladder) diary, and limited laboratory testing. Further laboratory tests, urodynamic evaluation, and imaging procedures are indicated when

---

Urologic History/Voiding Patterns:

    Spontaneous Voiding: Diurnal Frequency _____ (hrs)

                            Nocturia ___ (episodes per noc)

    Containment Devices: Pads _____ (number per day)

                            Type of Pad _____

                            Diapers _____ (number per day)

    Intermittent Catheterization Program: _____ (hrs)

    Indwelling Catheter: Urethral _____   Suprapubic _____

Sensations of Urinary Filling:

    Irritative Bladder Symptoms (frequency, urgency, dysuria):

    Cystitis (recurrent infections, current infection, febrile infections):

    Predisposing Factors (systemic chemotherapy with alkylating agents, pelvic radiotherapy, implantation of radioactive seeds):

Incontinence Type:

    Stress   Urge   Reflex   Functional   Continuous (extraurethral)

Urinary Retention:

    Acute _____ (number of episodes, precipitating factors)

    Chronic _____ (catheterization required?)

    Feelings of incomplete bladder evacuation _____

LIMITED SYSTEMS REVIEW

Neurologic:

    Brain Tumor (type, location, treatment):

    Spinal Tumor: (type, location, treatment)

    Other: _____

Figure 12C-1. Voiding history.

Adapted from Gray, M. L. Genitourinary Disorders. Mosby-Yearbook, St. Louis, 1992.

more complex cases of incontinence, painful bladder syndromes, or urinary distress exist.

The history (Figure 12C–1) includes a review of the type and duration of voiding symptoms, focusing on the bladder management program, patterns of urinary elimination, and patterns of incontinence. The person is asked to describe the conditions that create, exacerbate, and alleviate uri-

---

Related Medical Conditions:

   Related Malignant Tumors (type, location, treatment):

   Other:_____

Reproductive System (Male):

   Prostate Disorders (benign prostatic hyperplasia, prostatitis, prostatic cancer):

   Erectile dysfunction _____   Ejaculatory dysfunction _____

   Other: _____

Reproductive System (Female):

   Number of Vaginal Deliveries: _____   (forceps assistance, breech deliveries)

   Reproductive System Tumors (type, location, treatment):

   Other:_____

Bowel Habits:

   Frequency/Pattern: _____   Usual Consistency: _____

   Constipation: _____   Fecal Incontinence: _____

   Bowel Program (laxatives, suppository, digital stimulation):

Surgical History:

Current Medications:

Figure 12C–1. *(Continued)*

nary leakage. A limited review of systems focuses on urinary, reproductive, neurological, and related medical disorders. The type of tumor and treatment, including surgery, chemotherapy, biotherapy, or radiation therapies, are explored to determine their potential impact on bladder function.

The physical examination begins with a general examination of the body habitus, including mobility and dexterity. Any assistive devices needed to ambulate are noted, as is the patient's ability to remove clothing and the general choice of garments (e.g., zippers versus buttons, layers of clothing). The clothing or containment device is assessed for evidence of urinary leakage. An abdominal examination can detect obvious masses produced by a distended bladder, hydronephrotic kidney, or impacted colon. The pelvic skin is inspected for evidence of impaired integrity such as monilial rash or ammonia contact dermatitis, indicating significant urinary leakage. Pelvic examination will determine the presence and extent of pelvic descent, the status of the vaginal and urethral mucosa, and evidence of local infection. In males, the penis and scrotum are inspected for impaired skin integrity, presence and consistency of the testes, and evidence of local infection. A digital rectal examination in males is used to determine the size and consistency of the prostate and the presence of asymmetry, nodules, or induration. A rectal examination in both males and females is used to determine the presence of the bulbocavernosus response, anal sphincter tone, and the presence of sensations in the genitourinary area.

Reproduction of an episode of urinary leakage and measurement of the post-void residual (obtained by catheterization or ultrasonic estimation of urine remaining in the bladder immediately after micturition) complete the physical examination. Stress urinary incontinence is reproduced with a comfortably full bladder. The patient is asked to cough, strain, or physically exert, and any leakage is noted. A dribbling of urine with exertion in the absence of a precipitous desire to urinate indicates stress incontinence. Urge incontinence can be reproduced by one of several provocative maneuvers. Bladder filling with a catheter attached to a syringe can be used to provoke detrusor instability. Other maneuvers, including walking, washing the hands, or exposure to cool air, can also produce unstable contractions. Extraurethral leakage occurs in the absence of physical exertion or a precipitous urge to urinate. By filling the bladder with methylene blue and observing the vagina or perineum, the examiner can track the dye through a fistulous tract.

A voiding diary is another tool to evaluate urinary incontinence (Figure 12C–2). The voiding diary is a record or log of episodes of micturition and urinary leakage. The document can be extended to include the volume voided and patterns of fluid intake. Stress urinary incontinence typically occurs as leakage related to physical exertion; the voided volume is typically normal and micturition patterns are normal. The patient with urge incontinence will experience frequent episodes of urination (greater than every two hours during waking hours) and nocturia. Episodes of inconti-

Time	Amount Voided	Leakage	Amount Drank

Instructions for Completing Voiding Diary

1. Measure all amounts using the plastic cup provided or another measuring container marked with "ccs" or "ounces."
2. Record the amount you urinated under the column marked "Amount Voided."
3. Record the amount you drink under the column marked "Amount Drank." Approximate volumes are fine.
   - A cup of coffee or tea is 4 ounces; a mug of coffee or tea is 8 ounces.
   - A glass of tea or water is 8 ounces.
   - A larger tumbler is 12 ounces.
   - A can of soda is 12 ounces.
4. If you experience leakage, place a check beside the approximate time it occurred. Do not try to estimate amounts.

Keep this diary for two days only and we will evaluate whether further recordings are necessary.

For questions call:

Figure 12C-2. Voiding diary.

nence are associated with a precipitous desire to urinate. Extraurethral incontinence will present as a continuous dribbling leakage not affected by physical exertion or the urge to urinate or as a continuous discharge of urine with insufficient bladder storage for urination.

Urinary retention is assessed by measuring the post-voiding residual (PVR) volume within five to ten minutes of voiding. Ideally, the voided volume is measured and the bladder is catheterized, allowing assessment of the bladder's total capacity: the portions eliminated by micturition added to the remaining or residual volume. Because catheterization is an invasive procedure carrying some risk of subsequent infection, ultrasonic evaluation of the lower urinary tract can be substituted for catheterization.

Limited laboratory tests are helpful for the basic evaluation of urinary incontinence. A dipstick urinalysis is used to screen for urinary infection, which could produce transient incontinence. Urinalysis also provides an assessment of certain metabolic conditions causing polyuria (such as diabetes insipidus or mellitus) or signs of significant renal insufficiency. The presence of hematuria and pyuria also can be used to indicate the presence of a previously unsuspected tumor or inflammatory mass in the urinary system. When signs of urinary tract infection (bacteriuria and pyuria) are found, a urine culture and sensitivity testing are completed.

Further evaluation of the urinary system is indicated when urinary incontinence cannot be adequately assessed by basic measures, when dysfunction is complicated by a painful bladder condition of undetermined origin, or when there is evidence of urinary retention with or without urinary system distress. Table 12C–2 summarizes the imaging and other diagnostic tests used to evaluate voiding dysfunction.

MEDICAL MANAGEMENT

The medical management of voiding dysfunction depends on the type of dysfunction and the presence of complicating factors. Instability (urge) incontinence is often managed by antispasmodic medications. Oxybutynin or propantheline are commonly used; alternate agents include dicyclomine, hyoscyamine, or flavoxate. Electrostimulation using a transcutaneous, transvaginal, or transrectal approach is an alternative to pharmacotherapy. Bladder retraining techniques or bladder drill therapy are occasionally employed, although these modalities are more commonly managed by nurses. Surgical interventions play a limited role in the management of urge incontinence. Surgical repair of stress incontinence related to pelvic descent often ablates symptoms of urge incontinence as well. Resection of an inflammatory or obstructive lesion can also relieve urge incontinence caused by bladder wall irritation or obstruction. Surgical denervation of the bladder is seldom used because of the risk of unacceptable complications such as rectal or urethral sphincter incompetence or erectile dysfunction in the male.

Table 12C-2
Diagnostic Tests for Urinary Dysfunction

Test	Brief Description	Indications
Cystourethroscopy	Endoscopic inspection of the urethra, bladder neck, bladder vesicle, and ureterovesical junction.	Incontinence caused by sphincter incompetence or fistulae, inflammatory lesions of the bladder, tumors, or bladder calculi.
Intravenous pyelogram/urogram (IVP, IVU)	Intravenous injection of contrast material with serial images of the urinary system; provides views of urinary system anatomy and limited information concerning renal function.	Urinary system distress causing urinary system dilation (hydronephrosis, ureteral dilation) or impaired renal function (delayed or absent concentration and excretion of contrast material).
DTPA renal scan	Intravenous injection of a radionuclide for evaluation of renal plasma flow; injection of furosemide provides evaluation of renal excretion.	Urinary system distress with obstruction of the upper urinary tracts.
DMSA renal scan	Intravenous injection of a radionuclide for evaluation of differential renal function.	Compromised function related to obstruction or poor compliance, focal scarring of reflux nephropathy.
MAG3 renal scan	Intravenous injection of a radionuclide that combines advantages of the DTPA and DMSA scans.	Upper urinary tract obstruction, compromised renal function, or focal scarring related to vesicoureteral reflux.
Voiding cystourethrogram (VCUG)	Retrograde injection of contrast material via urethral catheter to visualize the bladder and urethra.	Incontinence related to intrinsic sphincter incompetence; or pelvic descent and urethral hypermobility; large inflammatory or malignant mass; or bladder calculi, trabeculation, or vesicoureteral reflux with urinary system distress.
Radionuclide cystogram	Retrograde injection of radionuclide material to visualize the bladder and urinary tract.	Vesicoureteral reflux with urinary system distress.
Retrograde urethrogram (RUG)	Retrograde injection of contrast material into the penis via urethra.	Urethral obstruction related to a tumor or mass.
Urodynamics	Collection of diagnostic tests used to evaluate the function of the lower urinary tract: the cystometrogram (CMG) is the graphic representation of bladder pressure as a function of volume, the sphincter electromyogram (EMG) is a graphic or audio representation of the movements of the pelvic muscles, and the urinary flow studies evaluate micturition via urinary flow alone or with voiding.	Complex cases of incontinence that are not diagnosed or successfully managed by simpler tests; urinary retention caused by deficient contractility or obstruction.
Videourodynamics	Combines urodynamic data with fluoroscopic monitoring of the lower urinary tract during bladder filling and micturition.	Complex voiding dysfunction not amenable to water urodynamics or simpler tests, urinary system distress, or sphincter incompetence.

The medical management of instability (reflex) incontinence requires the prevention of high-pressure, potentially harmful detrusor contractions or the alleviation of obstruction produced by a dyssynergic sphincter. Anticholinergic agents are administered in an attempt to pharmacologically "paralyze" the detrusor, and the bladder is drained via intermittent catheterization. Initially, an anticholinergic agent such as oxybutynin or propantheline is administered. A second drug, usually imipramine, can be administered to supplement the action of the anticholinergic drug. Occasionally, a calcium channel blocker, such as nifedipine, is given to supplement the action of anticholinergic agents at an intracellular level. If pharmacotherapy fails to relieve unstable detrusor contractions, augmentation enterocystoplasty is considered to improve bladder capacity and alleviate instability permanently.

Because a number of acceptable condom devices are available, male reflex incontinence can also be managed by condom containment rather than intermittent catheterization. This alternative is usually reserved for those patients who are unable to self-catheterize (because of cervical spinal lesions producing quadriplegia) or unwilling to catheterize. In some instances, they can be managed with condom containment only; more often, they will require relief from the obstructive effects of vesicosphincter dyssynergia. An alpha adrenergic antagonist such as doxazosin or terazosin can be administered to reduce tone at the smooth muscle of the bladder outlet and the rhabdosphincter. A transurethral sphincterotomy, the surgical incision of the membranous urethra, can reduce bladder outlet resistance and avoid urinary system distress. The success of transurethral sphincterotomy is limited by the subsequent development of deficient detrusor contractility. Implantation of prosthetic urethral stents, designed to place the urethra in a slightly open position, provides an attractive alternative to traditional sphincterotomy, because these devices can be removed if detrusor contractility causes a recurrence of urinary retention.

Under certain circumstances, an indwelling Foley catheter can be used to manage instability incontinence. Because these catheters ultimately lead to chronic bacteriuria and increase the risk of urinary system distress, they are limited to persons unable to take advantage of alternative bladder management programs or those with guarded prognosis for whom alternative techniques are not realistic. Figure 12C–3 provides guidelines for the choice of an indwelling catheter and its management.

Stress urinary incontinence (SUI) caused by pelvic descent can be managed by drugs, surgical repair, or placement of a urethral barrier device. More than 100 procedures to repair the anatomic defects contributing to SUI have been described in the medical literature. The majority use an abdominal approach, a vaginal approach, or a needle technique. Although these devices produce excellent initial results, their long-term (five- and ten-year) efficacy is considerably less. Alpha sympathomimetics also provide relief for mild to moderate cases of SUI. Alpha adrenergic agents are available in many over-the-counter preparations, including decongestants and certain diet pills.

Size	Smaller is generally better; 14–16 French with a 5 cc balloon is adequate for most adults. Remember to increase catheter size *only* when sphincter incompetence is proven.
Material	Silastic catheters with Teflon are appropriate for short-term use only; a silicone catheter is better for catheters expected to remain in place for more than 7 days. Catheters constructed with relatively biocompatible, hydrophilic materials with low friction coefficients are preferred.
Leg bag	A leg bag should hold at least 500 ml of urine, the valve between catheter and leg bag should prevent reflux, and the drainage valve should be relatively easy to manipulate (preferably with one hand); the bag should be constructed so that it is easy to conceal under clothing with a baffling system preventing a single bulge when filled with urine; the straps of the leg bag should be constructed of a stretch material other than rubber for greater comfort and minimal skin irritation; the leg bag may be concealed in a cloth sleeve next to the skin, or its posterior aspect (facing the skin of the leg) should be constructed of material that allows the skin to receive air.
Bedside bag	The bedside bag should contain approximately 2,000–3,000 ml, the valve between bag and catheter should prevent reflux, and the tubing of the bedside bag must be long enough to allow the patient to move while in bed. A bedside stand may be needed to enhance drainage.

Figure 12C-3. Selecting an indwelling catheter.

Urethral barrier devices constitute a relatively new class of products used to manage stress urinary incontinence. The urethral insert is similar to a catheter and is effective for mild to severe stress urinary incontinence, including SUI caused by intrinsic sphincter deficiency. This device is inserted into the urethra of a woman, and a small balloon is used to secure placement. The urethral insert can be worn for up to six hours, or until urination is again completed. The patient then deflates the balloon, the device is removed, and urination can proceed. A urethral patch can be applied over the urethral meatus. The woman is taught to apply this device herself, and it is removed and discarded prior to urination. The patient also can be taught to use a bladder neck support prosthesis. This device is similar to a pessary, and it is used to temporarily occlude the urethra in order to prevent SUI.

Men with SUI can be taught to apply one of several devices used to constrict the penile urethra and prevent urinary leakage. The Cunningham clamp has been available for many years, but its efficacy is limited by the relative discomfort associated with wearing the device and by the risk of distal ischemia if the clamp is applied too tightly. Several alternative devices have been developed that provide similar results without the discomfort or risk of ischemia.

Stress urinary incontinence related to intrinsic sphincter deficiency can be managed by surgical repair, implantation of an artificial urinary sphincter, or injection of a periurethral bulking agent. The pubovaginal sling can be used to treat sphincter incompetence in the female. The surgeon suspends the proximal third of the bladder using a sling fashioned from fascia or a synthetic material. Care is exercised during the procedure to avoid placing excessive tension on the urethra, causing bladder outlet obstruction. Males and females are appropriate candidates for implantation of an artificial sphincter device. A cuff implanted around the urethra is connected to an abdominal reservoir, and a pump mechanism is placed in the scrotum or under the skin of the labia majora. A periurethral bulking agent, GAX collagen, has been approved for the treatment of SUI related to intrinsic sphincter deficiency.

Extraurethral incontinence can be managed by surgical repair. Surgical repair of a fistulous tract can be complicated by the lack of healthy, well-vascularized tissues needed to close the tract. An alternative management technique is to inject a sclerosing agent designed to seal the tract by promoting the formation of scar tissue. A suspension of tetracycline is a potent sclerosing agent that is injected into the fistulous tract; nonetheless, repeat treatments are often required to completely seal the tract and eradicate urinary leakage.

Urinary retention caused by obstruction is managed by surgical or transurethral ablation of the obstructive lesion. Retention related to deficient detrusor contraction is typically managed by pharmacotherapy, intermittent catheterization, or indwelling catheter. Cholinergic agents, primarily bethanechol, can be administered in an attempt to maximize detrusor contraction strength, but they are rarely effective. More commonly, retention produced by poor bladder contractility is managed by intermittent catheterization or an indwelling catheter. Because it is associated with fewer urinary system complications, intermittent catheterization is preferred (see Table 12C–3).

The medical management of painful bladder disorders varies according to the underlying etiology of the lesion. Specific inflammatory lesions, such as urothelial tumors, are managed by surgical or laser resection, chemotherapy, radiation therapy, or biotherapy. The discomfort produced by radiation- or chemotherapy-induced cystitis is eased by a urinary analgesic medication or an anticholinergic agent, or by transvaginal or transrectal electrical simulation. Protracted cases might require more aggressive therapy such as reconstructive surgery, particularly when bladder inflammation coexists with urinary system distress.

Urinary system distress often requires aggressive medical intervention. Bladder outlet obstruction can be relieved by surgical resection or dilation of an anatomic lesion or pharmacologic relaxation of a hypertonic sphincter mechanism. Poor bladder wall compliance produced by radiation

Table 12C-3
Procedure for Clean Catheterization

Female	Male
1. If possible, wash your hands. Catheterization should *not* be postponed because you cannot wash your hands or your perineum; the risk of infection from retained urine is too great.	1. If possible, wash your hands. Catheterization should *not* be postponed because you cannot wash your hands or your penis; the risk of infection from retained urine is too great.
2. Sit on a table, with your feet on the table and your knees flexed apart. With a well-lighted mirror, identify your vagina, clitoris, and urethral meatus.	2. Sit on a chair or toilet with your feet on the floor. If you are uncircumcised, retract your foreskin for the rest of the procedure.
3. Separate your vaginal folds. Using a washcloth, soap, and water, thoroughly wash the exposed area with downward strokes.	3. Using a washcloth, soap, and water, thoroughly wash the end of your penis.
4. Place some lubricant on a paper towel and use this to lubricate the first 3 inches of the catheter.	4. Place some lubricant on a paper towel and use this to lubricate the first 7–10 inches of the catheter.
5. With the hand you normally use for skilled tasks, hold the catheter as you would a pencil or a dart. Hold the catheter on the unlubricated part.	5. With the hand you normally use for skilled tasks, hold the catheter as you would a pencil or a dart. Hold the catheter on the unlubricated part.
6. While using the index and ring fingers of your other hand to separate your labia, press (locate) your urethral meatus with the middle finger.	6. Hold your penis at a right angle to your body and slowly insert the catheter 7–10 inches, until urine begins to flow steadily.
7. Raise your middle finger and insert the catheter about 3 inches into your urethra until urine begins to flow steadily.	7. After all urine has drained, carefully and slowly remove the catheter.
8. After all urine has drained, carefully and slowly remove the catheter.	8. Wash and soak the used catheter in warm, soapy water. Then rinse it inside and outside, dry it, and place it in a clean plastic bag for future use.
9. Wash and soak the used catheter in warm, soapy water. Then rinse it inside and outside, dry it, and place it in a clean plastic bag for future use.	

NOTES:

This table is intended to assist the nurse with teaching the patient clean catheterization. It is suggested that the nurse (1) perform the procedure, explaining the various steps to the patient; (2) have the patient perform the procedure, in the nurse's presence, explaining the various steps to the nurse; and (3) once the patient demonstrates competence, allow the patient to perform the procedure in private.

This procedure should be performed in a well-lighted area. Necessary equipment includes rubber catheter, water-soluble lubricant, paper towel, plastic bag for used catheter, and receptacle (e.g., toilet) for urine collection. Optional equipment includes washcloth, soap, and water.

If the female patient lacks perineal sensation, she should probably always perform this procedure with a mirror reflecting her perineum. If perineal sensation is present, and if the patient is proficient at self-catheterization, she can use the touch technique, which provides more freedom and flexibility because mirrors and lights are not necessary.

Adapted from Wahlquist, G. Bladder: functional alterations. In Johnson, B. L., and J. Gross, eds. *Handbook of oncology nursing.* 1st ed. 360–362. John Wiley & Sons, New York. 1985.

therapy or chemotherapy cystitis or chronic obstruction might respond to anticholinergic therapy; more often, these conditions represent significant fibrous or collagenous elements of the bladder wall that require surgical reconstruction. Reconstruction could be an augmentation enterocystoplasty, continent urinary diversion, or incontinent urinary diversion. An indwelling Foley catheter can be used for drainage when these other options are not feasible.

NURSING MANAGEMENT

The nursing management of urinary incontinence has undergone significant transition and expansion, thanks to efforts to explore nonsurgical and nonpharmacologic management of common forms of leakage. Factors leading to selection of a management program for urge incontinence include patient choice, the availability of alternative treatment modalities, and the presence of complicating factors such as inflammatory lesions of the lower urinary tract or urinary system distress. Table 12C–4 outlines a nursing care protocol for patients with urinary dysfunction.

The nursing management of urge incontinence often combines pharmacologic or other measures with behavioral therapy. Pharmacologic management using anticholinergic medications is inadequate unless the patient is taught to control fluid intake and to time voiding. A voiding schedule is derived from a voiding diary. The person who urinates every $\frac{1}{2}$ hour will initially postpone micturition to every hour with gradual progression to every $2\frac{1}{2}$ to 3 hours. The patient is informed that no antispasmodic medication will allow indefinite postponement of urination, although the medication will increase the length of time between voiding. The nurse teaches the patient the dosage, schedule, and common side effects of all anticholinergic medications.

Patient teaching also includes specific strategies to manage the immediate urge to urinate. For example, the patient might respond to a sudden urge to urinate with a rush to the toilet; instead, the nurse could teach the patient to respond by stopping and forcefully contracting the pelvic and periurethral muscles while relaxing the abdominal muscles to prevent precipitous leakage. This maneuver is followed by a prompt but more deliberate trip to the toilet.

Bladder retraining or habit retraining is another alternative for the patient with urge incontinence. Patients undergoing bladder retraining are taught to urinate during waking hours on a highly structured schedule, beginning with urination every $\frac{1}{2}$ to 1 hour and progressing to every $2\frac{1}{2}$ to 3 hours. Therapy stresses cognitive control of bladder function.

Transvaginal or transrectal electrostimulation has been used in the management of urge incontinence. Therapy requires the use of a 5–20 Hertz frequency current that is applied during daily sessions to increase bladder capacity and reduce the frequency and amplitude of unstable de-

Table 12C-4
Nursing Protocol for the Management of Patients with Voiding Dysfunction

Urge Incontinence

- Institute timed voiding program based on results of voiding diary.
- Teach technique of urge suppression.
- Teach fluid management program ensuring adequate fluid intake ($\frac{1}{2}$ ounce per pound of body weight or approximately 1,500ml/d) while avoiding intake of large volumes within a short period of time.
- Eliminate or reduce bladder irritants, including caffeinated beverages, alcoholic drinks, and beverages with aspartane.
- Begin bladder retraining (habit retraining) program in consultation with patient and physician.
- Institute transvaginal or transrectal electrical stimulation program in consultation with patient and physician.

Reflex Incontinence

- Teach intermittent catheterization program as indicated using a clean technique (see Table 12C-3). Include family members and significant others whenever possible.
- Teach the patient and family to apply a condom catheter and leg bag when reflex voiding with containment is indicated. Emphasize routine care and assessment of penile skin.

Stress Incontinence (related to pelvic descent)

- Begin a pelvic muscle exercise program using principles of physiotherapy and biofeedback techniques in consultation with the patient and physician.
- Teach the patient to apply, remove, and care for urethral barrier devices as indicated.
- Assist the patient to synchronize administration of pharmacologic agents with periods of physical activity.
- Begin transvaginal or transrectal electrical stimulation in consultation with patient and physician.

Stress Incontinence (related to intrinsic sphincter deficiency)

- Teach the patient to apply, remove and care for urethral barrier devices as indicated.
- Teach the patient undergoing implantation of an artificial urinary sphincter device to manipulate the device prior to implantation. Repeat instruction following implantation to ensure proper use and to promote wound healing such that the device remains in an accessible location.
- Provide the patient with a Medi-Alert® bracelet whenever a prosthesis device is placed.

Functional Incontinence

- Identify and assist the patient and family to minimize or remove environmental barriers to toileting.
- Provide the patient with a referral to an appropriate health care professional for physical therapy, fitting with an assistive cane, wheelchair, or other device as indicated.
- Provide non-scuff shoes to enhance balance and ambulation.
- Assist the patient to alter clothing to maximize ease of removal for toileting.
- Teach the patient's caregivers to maximize opportunities for toileting and to begin a prompted voiding regimen when indicated.

Extraurethral Incontinence

- Teach the patient and family to apply an absorptive device to contain urinary leakage, protect the skin, and minimize or eliminate odor.
- Teach preventive skin care and provide specific instructions for odor control as indicated.

Urinary Retention

- Teach a double voiding technique for mild urinary retention.
- Teach the patient with a neobladder to urinate using a Valsalva voiding technique. Begin intermittent catheterization if the patient is unable to effectively evacuate the bladder by Valsalva voiding.
- Teach intermittent catheterization as indicated using a clean technique (see Table 12C-3).

Continued

Table 12C-4 *(Continued)*
Nursing Protocol for the Management of Patients with Voiding Dysfunction

Urinary Retention

- Place an indwelling catheter as directed. Choose a catheter constructed of an inert material or one that is hydrophilic with a low friction coefficient.
- Teach the patient and family to care for the catheter. Emphasize adequate fluid intake and the treatment of only symptomatic urinary tract infections.
- Assist the patient to choose appropriate leg and bedside drainage bags.

Painful Bladder Disorders

- Instruct the patient to reduce his/her intake or avoid foods or beverages that contain bladder irritants, including caffeine, alcohol and aspartame.
- Advise the patient to avoid dehydration because this maneuver exacerbates rather than reduces bladder discomfort while increasing the risk of bacterial urinary tract infection.
- Administer transvaginal or transrectal electrical simulation for pain control in consultation with the physician and patient.
- Assist the patient to obtain a referral to investigate the cause of a painful bladder disorder as indicated.

Urinary System Distress

- Teach the patient to recognize the signs and symptoms of a urinary tract infection and to differentiate a febrile episode from a lower urinary tract infection.
- Encourage the patient with low bladder wall compliance to adhere to a rigid schedule of catheterization.
- Teach intermittent catheterization to the patient who undergoes augmentation enterocystoplasty, neobladder procedure, or a continent urinary diversion.
- Reinforce the significance of strict compliance with long-term suppressive antibiotic therapy when vesicoureteral reflux is present

trusor contractions. The patient is taught to self-regulate the voltage to just below the threshold of discomfort.

The nursing management of reflex incontinence balances the need for continence with the potential for urinary system distress caused by vesicosphincter dyssynergia. Pharmacologic paralysis of the detrusor muscle is accompanied by instruction in intermittent catheterization for the patient and family. When reflex voiding is the management program of choice, the nurse teaches the patient and family to apply and care for a condom catheter. Because of the risk of urinary system distress, the patient is also taught to recognize signs of symptomatic urinary infection and to seek treatment promptly should they occur. When the male patient is managed by condom catheter drainage and an alpha blocking agent, he is taught the care of the catheter, drainage bag, and the dosage, administration, and potential side effects of the specific drug.

Stress urinary incontinence produced by pelvic descent can be managed by pelvic muscle exercises. The nurse instructs the patient to isolate and contract the correct muscles, using biofeedback techniques. The patient is then taught an exercise program applying principles of physiotherapy. Initially 5–10 repetitions of exercises that stress improvements in maximal strength and endurance are performed every day or every other day. The repetitions are gradually increased to 35 to 50 repetitions in a graded manner. Improving pelvic muscle tone requires three to six months of vigorous exercise. A program consisting of exercises three times a week is used to maintain results.

Patients who manage stress urinary incontinence with drug therapy are taught the dosage, administration, and potential side effects of their medications. Specifically, the scheduling of the medication is discussed with the patient. Administration of medications for SUI should be limited to those periods of physical stress likely to induce leakage. Thus, long-acting drugs—such as Sudafed® L.A., Entex® L.A., or Dexatrim®—are administered in the morning only; short-acting drugs can be given prior to periods of intensive physical exertion, e.g., exercise class, jogging, or walking for a prolonged distance.

The patient who chooses barrier therapy is taught to apply and remove the specific barrier device. The woman who chooses to use a urethral insert must be taught the location of her urethra and the technique of inserting the device. She is then taught to inflate the balloon and test the device for placement. She also is instructed on the technique for device removal and to monitor herself for potential complications, including mild hematuria or urinary tract infection. The nurse also teaches the patient to apply the urethral patch or male constriction device. These devices are relatively easy to apply, and patients typically grasp their application in one session. In contrast, the bladder neck support prosthesis must be carefully fitted; teaching the woman to correctly place this device might require more than one session.

Stress incontinence related to sphincter incompetence might respond to pelvic muscle exercises, although improvement in the volume and frequency of leakage is more likely than cure. The patient who undergoes implantation of an artificial sphincter is taught to use the device prior to implantation. Following surgery, the device is left in an open (nonactivated) position. The patient is taught to place gentle, downward traction upon the device for the next several weeks to promote formation of a fibrous capsule around the implant. Following activation of the device, use of the implant is again reviewed with the patient and family. The patient is also instructed about the potential long-term complications associated with implantation of an artificial urinary sphincter, including infection and mechanical complications. The patient is advised to ask his or her urologist prior to invasive procedures whether prophylactic anti-infective medications are needed. A Medi-Alert® bracelet is provided to advise health care professionals of the presence of the prosthetic device.

Whenever possible, the patient with functional incontinence is given assistance to limit or eliminate environmental barriers to toileting. A portable toilet could be placed near the bed, or the patient's bed might be moved nearer to the bathroom. The toilet seat is equipped with adequate supports, and door frames are widened to accommodate a wheelchair or walker as indicated. The patient is given a cane, walker, or other assistive devices to maximize mobility and dexterity. Patients with altered cognition could be encouraged and helped to the toilet or in using a prompted, urge-response toileting program in which the patient's normal voiding patterns are ascertained and caregivers are taught to prompt a toileting response using verbal and visual cues, with physical assistance as indicated.

The patient with extraurethral incontinence might require a prolonged period of urinary containment with protection of the perineal skin. The nurse also assists the patient undergoing sclerosing agent therapy to protect the skin around a fistula both during and following the procedure.

The patient who experiences urinary retention can be taught to void on a specific schedule or to double void (urinate, rest on the toilet for three to five minutes, and urinate again). Other patients will be placed on intermittent clean catheterization (Table 12C–3). When spontaneous voiding or intermittent catheterization is not feasible, the bladder is drained via an indwelling Foley catheter. The choice to place the catheter is typically made by the physician, and the type of catheter is often chosen by the nurse. The ideal indwelling catheter is made of an inert or hydrophilic material that minimizes bacterial adherence and urethral irritation. It should have a maximal internal versus external (French) diameter. The patient is advised that regular catheter changes (approximately every month) will be necessary. A leg bag is chosen to contain urinary output during waking hours. The ideal bag has tubing of adequate length to provide good drainage between catheter and bag. It should be backed by a cloth or breathable material to minimize skin irritation and discomfort. The bag can be attached to the leg using a cloth pocket or nonrubberized straps. The leg bag should hold at least 500 cc and baffle urine in a way that avoids creating a bulge clearly visible under clothing. A bedside bag is used for urinary drainage overnight. The overnight bag should be relatively large (2,000–3,000 cc) and attached to the catheter with a tube long enough to allow the patient to turn over in the bed. The bag should be vented to prevent backflow of urine, and it should be hung from a stand or bed rail lower than the urinary bladder.

The patient is taught to maintain an adequate intake of fluids to ensure adequate drainage from the indwelling catheter. Typically, 1,500 cc of fluid is considered adequate, although the patient might need 2,000–2,500 cc per day to promote adequate drainage and to prevent symptomatic bacteriuria. The patient is taught to recognize the signs and symptoms of symptomatic bacteriuria. He or she is further advised that asymptomatic bacteriuria is inevitable with an indwelling catheter and that asymptomatic bacteria in the urine should not be treated. The patient is taught to drain and regularly clean the overnight (bedside) and leg bags to prevent bacterial overgrowth and odor. The importance of regular follow-up care of the Foley catheter is emphasized.

The patient who experiences a painful bladder disorder is taught to self-administer urinary analgesic, anticholinergic, or anti-infective medications as indicated. The patient is advised against limiting fluids, because this strategy only intensifies discomfort by concentrating the urine and enhancing bladder irritability. The patient is also taught that certain foods and beverages can increase bladder irritability. Beverages that contain caffeine, carbonation, or alcohol are eliminated or limited, although the volume of fluid intake (at least 1,500 ml/day) is maintained. Spicy or greasy foods and chocolate also can irritate the bladder. The patient is advised to eliminate these foods from the diet one at a time to determine any effects on bladder irritability.

The patient who experiences urinary system distress is taught to recognize the signs of urinary infection (dysuria; urinary frequency; hematuria; cloudy, foul-smelling urine; fever) and to seek treatment promptly should these symptoms occur. The patient managed by anticholinergic medications for poor bladder wall compliance is taught to adhere to a rigid schedule of spontaneous voiding or intermittent catheterization to prevent dangerously high filling pressures. The patient who undergoes reconstructive urologic surgery using the bowel is managed by intermittent catheterization. The nurse teaches the patient to manage mucus produced by the detubularized bowel by increased intake of cranberry juice (a mucolytic agent), adequate fluid intake, and irrigation of the augmented bladder or continent bowel with normal saline when needed.

The patient with urinary system distress and vesicoureteral reflux will benefit from suppressive anti-infective medications. The patient is taught to administer the medicine in the evening before going to sleep, because the night is the longest period of urinary stasis. The patient is informed that signs and symptoms of urinary infection require immediate medical intervention, because untreated bacteriuria can rapidly lead to pyelonephritis and sepsis unless promptly managed.

SUMMARY

Altered bladder function can occur as the direct or indirect result of a malignant process. Voiding dysfunction can produce symptoms of urinary incontinence, painful bladder conditions, or urinary system distress. With proper management, these conditions can be alleviated or ablated, avoiding or reversing the psychological, social, and physiological complications of a dysfunctional voiding condition.

BIBLIOGRAPHY

1. Agency for Health Care Policy and Research, Urinary Incontinence Clinical Guideline Panel. Urinary Incontinence in Adults: *Acute and Chronic Management.* U.S. Department of Health and Human Services, Rockville, Maryland. 1996.

   Clinical practice guidelines based on a review of specific literature in the area of urinary incontinence are provided.

2. Bradley, W. B. The physiology of the urinary bladder. In Walsh, P. C., R. F. Gittes, A. D. Perlmutter, and T. A. Stamey, eds. *Campbell's Urology* 5th Ed. W. B. Saunders, Philadelphia. 1986.

   This chapter reviews the neurophysiological aspects of the lower urinary tract.

3. Burgio, K. Biofeedback assisted behavioral training for elderly men and women. *NIH Consensus Development Conference: Urinary Incontinence in Adults* (proceedings book). 87–90. NIH, Bethesda, MD. 1988.

A detailed description of biofeedback techniques, including specific strategies to treat episodes of urge incontinence, is provided.

4. Colling, J., J. Ouslander, B. J. Hadley, E. J. Campbell, and J. Eisch. Patterned urge-response toileting for urinary incontinence. In S. G. Funk, E. M. Tornquist, M. T. Champagne and R. A. Wiese, ed. *Key Aspects of Elder Care*. Springer Pub. Co. New York. 169–186. 1992.

A description of the patterned urge response toileting program is provided.

5. Dougherty, M. C., et al. The effect of exercise on the circumvaginal muscles in postpartum women. *Journal of Nurse-Midwifery* 34(1): 8–14. 1989.

This paper describes the effects of pelvic floor muscle exercises on postpartum females; the paper emphasizes principles of exercise physiology.

6. Fantl, J. A., J. F. Wyman, D. K. McClish, S. W. Harkins, R. K. Elswick, J. K. Taylor, and E. C. Hadley. Efficacy of bladder training in older women with urinary incontinence. *JAMA* 265: 609–613. 1991.

This article describes a bladder drill (retraining) program among elderly women living in the community.

7. Gallo, M. Clinical experience with a balloon tipped urethral insert for stress urinary incontinence. *Journal of Wound, Ostomy and Continence Nursing* 24 (1): 51. 1997.

This article reviews the nursing management of the urethral insert used for urinary incontinence in women.

8. Gray, M. L. Assessment of patients with urinary incontinence. In D. Doughty, ed. *Nursing Management of Urinary and Fecal Incontinence*. Mosby-Yearbook, St. Louis. 1991.

This offers a detailed discussion of the nursing evaluation of urinary leakage; interpretation of urodynamic and imaging studies is included.

9. Gray, M. L. *Genitourinary Disease*. Mosby-Yearbook, St. Louis. 1992.

This book contains detailed discussions of the nursing assessment and management of urinary incontinence, painful bladder disorders, and disorders that produce urinary system distress.

10. Gray, M. L. Electrostimulation in the management of voiding dysfunction. *Urologic Nursing* 12(2): 73–74. 1992.

An overview is provided of the indications and techniques of electrostimulation in the management of urinary incontinence.

11. Gray, M. L. *Urology Nursing Drug Reference*. Mosby-Wolfe, Philadelphia. 1996.

This handbook summarizes the dosage, indications, side effects and nursing implications of medications used to manage altered urinary elimination and common antineoplastic agents used to manage genitourinary malignancies.

12. Griffiths, D. J., G. Holstege, H. Dewall, and E. Dalm. Anatomic and physiologic observations on suprasacral control of bladder and urethral muscle contractions in the cat. *Neuro-urology and Urodynamics* 9(1): 63–82. 1990.

The effects of specific neural clusters in the pons on bladder function are described.

13. International Continence Society. *The Standardization of Terminology of Lower Urinary Tract Function.* Glasgow, Scotland. 1984.

    This reports the system of nomenclature commonly used to describe urodynamics and incontinence by investigators in this field.

14. Long, J.P. Is there a role for cryoablation of the prostate in the management of localized prostate cancer? *Hematology—Oncology Clinics of North America* 10 (3): 675. 1996.

    This article summarizes the place of modern brachytherapy techniques in the management of localized prostate cancer, including the risk of subsequent genitourinary complications.

15. Mitchell, M. E. and M. W. Burns. Surgical treatment of urinary incontinence. In Kelasis, P. P., L. R. King, and A. B. Belman, eds. *Clinical Pediatric Urology* 3d Ed. W. B. Saunders, Philadelphia. 1992.

    This chapter describes surgical techniques of augmentation enterocystoplasty and related procedures.

16. M'Liss, A. and W. J. Catalona, Bladder cancer. In Gillenwater, J. Y., J. T. Grayhack, S. S. Howards, and J. W. Duckett, eds. *Adult and Pediatric Urology.* 3d Ed. Mosby-Yearbook, Chicago. 1996.

    The chapter discusses the management of bladder cancer, including the potential complications of chemotherapy and radiation therapy on bladder function.

17. Sant, G. R. Inflammatory diseases of the bladder. In Gillenwater, J. Y., J. T. Grayhack, S. S. Howards, and J. W. Duckett, eds. *Adult and Pediatric Urology* 3d Ed. Mosby-Yearbook, Chicago. 1996.

    This provides a detailed discussion of painful bladder disorders caused by specific inflammatory lesions.

18. Staskin, D. R., et al. Pathophysiology of stress incontinence. *Clinics in Obstetrics and Gynecology* 12(3): 357. 1985.

    This paper describes the pathophysiology of SUI.

19. Steers, W. D., D. M. Barrett, and A. J. Wein. Voiding dysfunction: diagnosis, classification and management. In Gillenwater, J. Y., J. T. Grayhack, S. S. Howards, and J. W. Duckett, eds. *Adult and Pediatric Urology* 3d Ed. Mosby-Yearbook, Chicago. 1996.

    This chapter reviews the pathophysiology, diagnosis and management of voiding dysfunction from a urological (surgical) perspective.

20. Torrens, M., and J. F. B. Morrison. *The Physiology of the Lower Urinary Tract.* Springer-Verlag, London. 1987.

    This book remains the definitive source that describes in detail the physiology of the lower urinary tract.

21. Wallner, K., J. Roy, and L. Harrison. Dosimetry guides to minimize urethral and rectal morbidity following transperineal I-125 prostate brachytherapy. *International Journal of Radiation Oncology, Biology, Physics.* 32 (2): 465. 1995.

    This paper reviews modern methods used to minimize radiation cystitis and radiation proctitis among men undergoing brachytherapy for localized prostate cancer.

Sexuality

Dorothy B. Smith

INTRODUCTION

Sexuality as a health care issue has slowly but increasingly emerged in the literature of various professions over the past five decades, motivated in large part by the Kinsey reports of 1948 and 1953 and Masters and Johnson's classic text on human sexual response in 1966. Among nursing publications, texts devoted to geriatrics were the first to incorporate sexuality as a concern, followed by texts on the care of patients with spinal cord trauma and those on ostomy care. An outcome for oncology nursing care is to enable the patient and his or her sexual partner to identify aspects of sexuality that would be impaired by the disease and decide on methods of maintaining their sexual identity. The role of the oncology nurse in this process is as follows:

1. To become aware of potential sexual concerns specific to the population under his or her care;
2. To demonstrate sensitivity to the private nature of sexuality and the vulnerability of the patient;
3. To develop a professional attitude toward sexual health promotion that eliminates personal biases;
4. To attain the knowledge necessary for identifying patients' sexual concerns and for responding with correct information; and
5. To keep informed of resources available to address patient concerns.

Many nurses still experience difficulty implementing discussions of sexuality in their clinical practice. The reasons are varied (Table 13–1), but most can be categorized under lack of information, embarrassment with the subject, or a belief that the subject is not of concern to the patient.

PATHOPHYSIOLOGY

To detect the patient's concerns regarding sexual activity and to respond appropriately, the nurse needs to know about the physiological cycle of sexual response and about sexuality during the course of life. Sexuality is in part biological, encompassing the genetic makeup of the chromosomes, the phenotype of the individual person, and hormonal dominance

13

Table 13–1
Reasons Nurses Give for Not Discussing Sexuality with Their Patients

1. I don't feel comfortable.
2. I don't have the knowledge.
3. The patient is not married.
4. I am not married.
5. He is as old as my father.
6. This is the Bible Belt, so the subject is taboo.
7. The patient has not brought it up.
8. It is the physician's job.
9. I don't have time.
10. There is no privacy.

and development of secondary sex characteristics. However, sexuality is also cultural and inseparable from social mores and the person's past experiences. Sexuality is multifaceted and highly individual, much more than the act of sexual intercourse; it is a form of communication, which can be conscious or unconscious, with varying degrees of intimacy. Although cancer or its treatments can alter forms of sexual expression, sexuality cannot be destroyed.

The phases of the physiological cycle of sexual response are described in Table 13–2. To teach patients accurately, nurses must be aware that sexuality does not begin and end with procreative capabilities and appreciate that humans are sexual beings throughout their lives. For instance, infants and young children can respond to stimulation with erections, vaginal lubrication, and orgasm, although Western cultures generally recognize active sexuality as beginning with the burst of hormones during puberty and the development of secondary sex characteristics. Even active, procreative sexuality, however, is not simply a biological function but rather occurs in a cultural context and is affected by social attitudes. Couples in their twenties and thirties, for instance, often are simultaneously involved in family life and career work. Time and energy for intimacy must frequently be negotiated because of the multitude of demands on the husband and wife. For these reasons, many couples find that middle age is a time of renewed interest in sexual activities; by this time, they often have met their career goals and their children might have left the home. Finally, although aging might bring a decrease in sexual function and response time, couples can remain active if they have maintained good health and are cooperative with each other as sexual partners.

A person who has a diagnosis of cancer might have problems related to the sexual and psychosocial impact of the disease and therapy. In addition to the disease itself, therapies such as surgery, radiation therapy, chemotherapy, and biotherapy can affect a patient's self-image and general quality of life as much as they affect sexual functioning. Disease-related causes of disruption to the sexual response cycle are discussed in Table

Table 13–2
Sexual Response Cycle

Phase	Physiologic Factors	Response
Desire	*Male* Requires testosterone, prolactin at normal levels.*	Interest in sex.
	Female Requires androgens, prolactin at normal levels.*	
	Both male and female Central nervous system process: dopamine (a neurotransmitter) is involved.	
Arousal	*Male* Innervation: prostatic plexus (parasympathetic and sympathetic fibers), sensory (pudendal nerve) messages to brain.	Corpus cavernosum, surrounded by tunica albuginea, fills with blood and stiffens the penis.
	Vascularization: arteries of the penis dilate and fill the cavernous venous sinusoids and occlude venous outflow. Amount of blood flow increases 25–60 times above normal during erection.	Corpus spongiosum fills with blood and widens to become the glans of the penis. It does not grow rigid and serves to cushion the penis during intercourse.
	Female Innervation: adrenergic nerves, sensory (pudendal nerve) messages to brain.	Blood pools in the labia majora and minora and clitoris.
	Vascularization.	The vagina deepens and widens, and the mucosa lining secretes drops of lubrication.
	Both male and female	Changes in heart rate, blood pressure, respiration rate, and overall muscle tension.
Orgasm	*Male* Sympathetic nervous system activates smooth muscles of genital area.	Emission: vas deferens, prostate, and seminal vesicles contract.
	Pudendal nerve activates the striated muscles at the base of the penis.	Mature sperm cells combine with rest of semen, are deposited in the prostatic urethra and ejaculated.
	Female Pudendal nerve stimulation (clitoris, perineum, anus, vagina).	Striated muscles contract, ejaculation of a fluid (disagreement exists as to whether this is from the urethra or distinct from urine).
	Both male and female	Sensation of pleasure centered in genital area, often described as inevitable or "point of no return."
Resolution	Central nervous system (has not been as fully researched as the other phases of the cycle and mechanisms are not defined).	Physiologic measures (blood pressure, pulse, respiration, muscle tension) return to their baseline levels; genital vasocongestion decreases, and a sense of relaxation and satisfaction results.

*High levels of the pituitary hormone prolactin decrease sexual desire.

Table 13–3
Disease-related Causes of Disruptions to the Sexual Response Cycle

Phase	Disease Factors Affecting Responses
Desire	Fatigue Pain Anxiety (patient and partner) Changes in body image Alteration in hormones (adrenal and testicular malignancies can produce ectopic hormones) Depression Neurocognitive problems Immobility Myths about cancer and sexuality
Arousal	Tumor invasion of genital structures Innervation or vascular involvement by the tumor Hormonal influences Tumors of the central nervous system
Orgasm	None

13–3. However, most problems affecting the sexual response cycle result from the treatments for the disease; these are presented in Table 13–4.

Fertility problems can be a major concern to cancer patients treated either before or during the years of procreation. Children or adolescents with cancer might have therapies that will retard their sexual development or create problems with fertility later. Infertility can be caused by surgical treatments that affect the genitals, including penectomy, vaginectomy, oophorectomy, hysterectomy, orchiectomy, and prostatectomy. Erection dysfunction can result from surgery that disrupts the prostatic nerve plexus, radiation that damages the arteries that supply blood to the penis, or drugs that disrupt peripheral neurotransmission. Ejaculation dysfunction from emission failure or retrograde ejaculation can occur if sympathetic nerves that control the prostate seminal vesicles or bladder neck are damaged. Ovarian failure and premature menopause can result from radiation treatments, chemotherapy, and hormonal treatments.

MEDICAL MANAGEMENT

The physical examination should include routine blood chemistry, assessment of the peripheral vascular system, a brief neurologic exam, and a pelvic examination. Specific studies for the male include exams for penile erectile function such as monitoring nocturnal penile tumescence by a sleep lab evaluation, a stamp test, or a snap-gauge test; measuring penile blood pressures by a Doppler ultrasound probe; and assessing vascular function by Papaverine tests and venography. Blood tests are done to measure levels

Table 13–4
Treatment-related Causes of Disruption
to the Sexual Response Cycle

Phase	Treatment Factors Affecting Responses
Desire	Effects of chemotherapy
	This therapy can cause nausea, vomiting, fatigue, ovarian failure, weakness, and altered body image from loss of facial and body hair and weight changes.
	Effects of drugs
	Opioids, sedatives, and antiemetics can lower desire. Hormonal therapy for metastatic prostate cancer decreases serum testosterone levels. Endocrine therapy can alter mood, pleasure and desire.
	Effects of surgery
	Alterations may affect hormones, e.g., orchiectomy, removal of the pituitary.
	Alterations to areas of the body may affect sexual image, e.g., mastectomy, head and neck, surgery, ostomies, penectomy, orchiectomy.
	Effects of radiation therapy
	Radiation to the pelvis can cause dry and less pliable skin, altering body image.
	Myths about radiation.
Arousal	Effects of chemotherapy
	Fatigue.
	Peripheral neuropathy.
	Infusion of chemotherapeutic agents through pelvic arteries.
	Effects of drugs
	Some antidepressants prevent erection.
	Effects of surgery—Male
	Damage to the prostatic plexus preventing erection can occur in the following:
	Radical prostatectomy
	Radical cystoprostatectomy
	Abdominoperineal resection
	Total pelvic exenteration
	Effects of surgery—Female
	Capacity for vaginal lubrication and expansion can be reduced by radical cystectomy and total pelvic exenteration. Ligation of blood vessels can occur in pelvic surgery.
	Effects of radiation therapy—Male
	Pelvic radiation for prostate, bladder, and colon cancers can cause vascular erection problems.

Continued

Table 13–4 *(Continued)*
**Treatment-related Causes of Disruption
to the Sexual Response Cycle**

Phase	Treatment Factors Affecting Responses
	Effects of radiation therapy—Female Radiation for cervical, vaginal, or colon cancers can result in vaginal dryness and stenosis.
Orgasm	Sensations of orgasm are reportedly unchanged or slightly less intense for patients treated with chemotherapy, radiation, or surgery in combination or alone. Patients with arousal impairments (erection dysfunction or vaginal alterations) report orgasms from touch or friction to the genital areas.

Orgasm—ejaculation	Effects of drugs
	  Tranquilizers, antihypertensives, long-term opioid use, cocaine or excessive alcohol can inhibit ejaculation; neurotoxic chemotherapy agents, e.g., vincristine, can impair ejaculation.
	
	Effects of surgery
	  Radical prostatectomy—dry orgasm.
	  Radical cystoprostatectomy—dry orgasm.
	  Abdominoperineal resection—possibility of dry orgasm if presacral sympathetic nerves are damaged.
	  Total pelvic exenteration—dry orgasm.
	  Retroperitoneal lymph node dissection—possible retrograde ejaculation or emission dysfunction.

of FSH (follicle-stimulating hormone), LH (luteinizing hormone), and testosterone. A semen analysis of sperm volume, count, motility, pH, and morphology is essential. A testicular biopsy might be indicated. Some of these tests might be done to get baseline information before a treatment that could affect erectile function or fertility is begun or to provide diagnostic information when assessing a problem in either. Assessment of fertility in the female might include an assessment of the menstrual cycle, basal body temperature, and blood levels of FSH, LH, estradiol, prolactin, and serum progesterone. An endometrial biopsy might be indicated and an in vitro sperm, cervical mucous interaction to detect an antigen-antibody response between the ovum, vagina, and sperm could be performed.

The medical management of sexual problems related to cancer or its treatment includes surgical procedures that can be either preventive or supportive (Table 13–5). Preventive approaches can be very effective with psychosocial problems; for example, giving the patient and partner correct information can help relieve anxiety, increase awareness of options for renewing sexual relations, and prevent the development of anger and resentment. In addition, helping the couple communicate with each other regard-

Table 13–5
Medical Management of Sexual Problems

Medical interventions	Hormones
	Oral medications
	Change medications
	Pharmacological erection (oral, topical, intraurethral, or intracavernous)
	Stop smoking, alcohol intake
	Vacuum erection device
	Electroejaculation therapy
	Psychosexual therapy
	Alternative techniques
Surgical interventions	Penile arterial reconstructive techniques
	Penile venous procedures
	Penile prosthesis
	Malleable rods
	Hinged prosthesis
	Inflatable prosthesis
	Testicular prosthesis
	Breast reconstruction
	Implants
	Tissue expanders
	Flaps
	Vaginal reconstruction
	Skin grafts
	Myocutaneous flaps
	Head and neck reconstructive techniques

ing their sexual needs, desires, and concerns can prevent misunderstanding and imagined feelings of rejection.

Prevention techniques are also useful for physical dysfunction. For example, shielding the gonads during radiation therapy can reduce levels of radiation to the ovaries or testicles. Sperm or embryo (fertilized eggs) cryopreservation might be offered for selected patients at risk for infertility. Still another effort entails employing surgical nerve-sparing techniques for patients with testicular cancer following retroperitoneal lymph node dissection, in order to prevent postoperative failure of ejaculation. These techniques have also been used to prevent postoperative erection dysfunction in patients who have had a radical prostatectomy, radical cystoprostatectomy, or abdominoperineal resection. Continent urinary diversion might be used to spare selected persons the psychological adjustment to an ostomy and external appliance (see Chapter 12A). For some women, breast or vaginal reconstruction at the time of the initial radical surgery is an attempt to avoid the feeling that they have lost an organ. Similarly, a penile prosthesis could be implanted in men at the time of cystectomy or a testicular prosthesis after orchiectomy. Post-therapy medical treatments for men include hormonal therapy; pharmacologically induced erections by oral

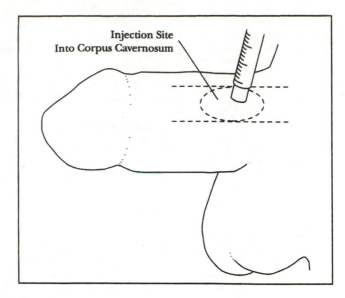

Figure 13–1. Injection site.

Reprinted with permission from Bruner, D. W. and R. R. Awamoto. Altered Sexual Health, in Cancer Symptom Management, *Groenwald, S. L., Frogge, M. H., Goodman, M., & Yarbro, C. H., eds, Jones & Bartlett, Sudbury, MA. p. 540. 1996.*

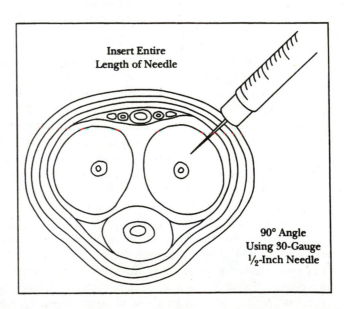

Figure 13–2. Insert the needle at a 90-degree angle (cross-section view).

Reprinted with permission from Bruner, D. W. and R. R. Awamoto. Altered Sexual Health, in Cancer Symptom Management, *Groenwald, S. L., Frogge, M. H., Goodman, M., & Yarbro, C. H., eds, Jones & Bartlett, Sudbury, MA. p. 540. 1996.*

topical or intraurethral (suppository) drugs, or intracavernous self-injections of vasoactive drugs into the cavernous bodies at the base of the penis for erectile dysfunction (see Figures 13–1 and 13–2); and electroejaculation for emission dysfunction. Post-therapy medical treatments for women include addressing postmenopausal symptoms if necessary via systemic or topical estrogen/testosterone replacement, vaginal lubrication, and/or dilatation if needed. For fertility issues, there are assisted reproductive techniques such as husband or donor insemination, in vitro fertilization, donor eggs, and surrogate carriers. Adoption might also be an option for cancer survivors with fertility issues.

NURSING MANAGEMENT

Nursing management is based on four components: assessment, education, counseling, and referral. Patients' sexual concerns can be further categorized as preventive, with an emphasis on education and communication skills, or supportive, including the use of counseling methods and referrals as needed. In 1976, Jack Annon proposed a model (PLISSIT) for sexual rehabilitation that includes these four components (Table 13–6). Specific nursing actions for each component of the nursing model appear in Table 13–7.

ASSESSMENT

Just as nursing assessment of the patient's medical status is a continuous component of the nursing process for the duration of the illness, so is sexual assessment. During the course of sexual assessment, the nurse becomes the patient's counselor and educator, helping the patient and sexual partner discover what sexuality means to them and what adjustments might be required because of the diagnosis and treatment of cancer. Sexual assessment involves a series of discussions about the specific effects of treatment on sexual function and the options for adaptation or resumption of sexual activity. The nurse must consider the psychosocial and physical characteristics of the couple prior to the diagnosis, along with problems presented by the cancer, in order to ascertain preexisting problems or factors affecting the couple's sexuality.

Table 13–6

Corresponding Models for Care of the Patient with Sexual Concerns

Jack Annon Model	Nursing Model
P = Permission	Assessment
LI = Limited information	Education
SS = Specific suggestion	Counseling
IT = Intensive therapy	Referral

Table 13–7
Components of Nursing Management of Patients' Sexual Concerns

Phase	Interventions
Assessment	Give the patient permission to express sexual concerns. Let the patient know you are concerned about him or her as a whole. Make assessment an ongoing component of nursing care throughout the illness and follow-up care. Be aware of your own attitudes and beliefs about sexuality and do not impose biases on the patient. Do not make light of the sensitivity of the subject or the patient's vulnerability. Use open-ended questions when asking the patient and partner about sex. Privacy and confidentiality are essential.
Education	Prepare yourself with proper information regarding sexual implications for your patient population (through literature, conferences, physician rounds, questions). Include sexual education as a component of care for all of your patients. Develop a relationship with the patient by becoming informed about the patient and showing concern. Talk to the patient and partner as a couple so they hear the same information. Know what information and patient education materials the patient has been given by the physician. Start with basic educational facts using drawings or models to show normal anatomy and physiology. Never assume the patient knows normal sexual physiology. Show how the disease or treatment may affect sexual function. Help the patient and partner see sexuality as a whole and not just a single act of intercourse. Allow time and opportunity for questions to be asked. Correct myths and misinformation. Provide written patient education as a follow-up if appropriate.
Counseling	Help the couple to communicate regarding sexual concerns. Provide specific suggestions related to population served, e.g., vaginal lubrication for RT patients, pouch covers for ostomy patients, alternative positions, elastic underwear for semirigid penile prosthesis, touch techniques for foreplay, birth control measures, safe sex guidelines, sperm banking.
Referral	Be aware of possible medical and surgical interventions. Provide available resource personnel for the patient. Be alert to patient clues and requests for referral. Continually assess the patient in regard to his need for further intervention. Serve in a supportive educational role when the patient is involved in a referral service.

A sexual assessment to identify problems could rely upon medical questionnaires designed to indicate the patient's ability to cope with illness and his or her need for psychological intervention. Medical evaluation, including a history and examination, is important in order to create a record of major illnesses, surgical procedures, medications, and use of alcohol and recreational drugs.

As previously noted, nurses often feel uncomfortable when assessing patients' sexual concerns. Nurses, like all people, have their own sexual experiences and values. Objectivity and empathy are necessary for the nurse to effectively and accurately assess a patient's sexual concerns or needs. Ver Steeg, a nurse and sex therapist, suggests that because nurses provide all kinds of bodily care during birth, disease, and death, a nurse's sense of intimacy with a patient can alternate between or conflict with a sense of intrusion. This conflict is usually not acknowledged or addressed in nursing education. Yet, the nurse must constantly be aware of personal struggles with sexuality and be able to separate personal from professional concerns. Although part of the nursing assessment can come from the health care records, test results, and the nurse's clinical observations and knowledge, much of the psychosexual assessment must come from communication with the patient and partner during the period of illness and follow-up care. Suggestions for discussing sex are included in Table 13–8.

Table 13–8
Guidelines in Discussing Sexuality

1. Clearly establish your professional identity. A patient wants to know with whom he is talking (e.g., you might say, "Hello, Mr. Brendom, I am Mrs. Smith, an enterostomal therapy nurse. I am one of the nurses here who works with patients who have their bladder removed.")
2. Be sensitive to timing and the patient's most immediate concerns. If the patient is in shock or tears over a new diagnosis, let him or her absorb some of this pain before attempting to discuss emotionally charged issues.
3. Let the patient know you are interested in him or her as a person. Establish rapport in the beginning by asking the patient questions about home and work (e.g., "Tell me about some of the things you do at home, at work.").
4. Use open-ended questions; if the patient can answer simply yes or no, he or she may not reveal much information. (E.g., do ask, "What kinds of touching or sexual activities do you use to reach a climax?" Do not ask, "Do you have orgasms?")
5. Start with the least threatening material. Begin with educational facts, advance to fears and concerns. (E.g., do not ask, "What kind of foreplay do you use?" Do ask, "Tell me a little about the importance of sex in your relationship.")
6. Do not impose your own values on the patient.
7. Let the patient know that his or her behavior is normal and common.
8. Correct any myths or misinformation the patient may have.
9. Know basic information about genital anatomy, sexual functioning, and the effects of illness on sexuality.
10. Give the patient permission to express feelings.

It might be helpful to realize that communication skills are learned; discussing sexual information does not come naturally but requires practice. Role-playing and discussing sexual information with peers is one way to build confidence with the subject.

EDUCATION

Education might be the nurse's single most effective method of managing the patient's sexual concerns. The goal of education is to help the patient and partner understand the physiology of their own sexual function and the impact that cancer and its treatment will have on their sexuality. Education is best provided to the couple to ensure that they both hear the same information. Nurses should start by providing factual information, using models or drawings to explain the normal anatomy and function, and subsequently to show how disease or therapy is affecting sexual performance. Nurses should not assume that patients understand basic sexual functioning. For example, they do not necessarily know that the penis has three compartments, or where the prostate is and what it does. Women might not know the location of the cervix or that the vagina expands during foreplay. Using models or drawings keeps the information factual and allows the patient to look initially at something other than the nurse. This reduces tension and discomfort about the discussion. Nurses should use simple but medically correct language, encouraging and allowing time for the couple to ask questions. In this way, nurses can help dispel misinformation, explore the couple's fears, and assess attitudes toward sex, including changes in sexual practices.

COUNSELING

As described by Annon, counseling entails giving the patient and the partner specific suggestions related to their needs. Nurses, for instance, should be prepared to suggest to couples how to communicate fears, needs, and desires about sexuality. For example, couples might schedule sexual activity when pain and nausea are controlled, when energy is not depleted, and when anxieties are reduced. Nurses might also need to suggest medical procedures; e.g., breast prosthesis, reconstructive surgery, or a pouch cover to conceal an ostomy pouch. Further, nurses could suggest vaginal lubrication, positions to reduce pressure on the vagina or conserve energy, or other hints in resuming intercourse after recovery from vaginal surgery or pelvic irradiation. Clearly, the possible suggestions are numerous and depend upon the individual patient's circumstances and needs.

REFERRAL

Sexual rehabilitation is best provided through a team approach. The physician, the social worker, the chaplain, and the sex therapist are all resources available to the patient, but frequently, the nurse is the team member most closely involved with the patient. The nurse must be aware of each team member's personal and professional contributions in order to help make appropriate resources available to the patient. When the patient is under referral care, whether for psychosexual therapy pertaining to the emotional aspects of sexuality or surgical reconstruction or prosthesis, the nurse fills a supportive and educational role.

SUMMARY

Sexual rehabilitation need not be as difficult as many nurses and patients fear. The nurse who gives the patient permission to express concerns about sexuality and responds with sensitivity will open communication to assess and solve problems. A commitment to approaching the problem with a professional demeanor and an emphasis on education can assist the nurse in including the promotion of sexual health as a component of clinical nursing care in oncology.

BIBLIOGRAPHY

1. Annon, Jack S. *Behavioral Treatment of Sexual Problems: Brief Therapy.* Harper and Row, Hagerstown, MD. 1976.

   This book presents a model of a behavioral approach to the treatment of sexual problems.

2. Averette, H. E., G. M. Boike, and M. A. Jarrell. Effects of cancer chemotherapy on gonadal function and reproduction capacity. *CA—A Cancer Journal for Clinicians* 40(4): 199–209. 1990.

   This article deals with the impact of various chemotherapeutic agents on testicular and ovarian function and reproductive capacity.

3. Fogel, C. I., and D. Lauver, eds. *Sexual Health Promotion.* W. B. Saunders, Philadelphia. 1990.

   This comprehensive text covers human sexuality and health care, including the life cycle of sexuality and potential disturbances.

4. Hughes, M. Sexuality issues: keeping your cool. *Oncol Nurs Forum* 23(10): 1597–1600. 1996.

   This article describes the psychosexual effects of cancer treatment for patients and how nurses can help the patient and partner cope.

5. Lamb, Margaret A. Effects of cancer on the sexuality and fertility of women. *Seminars in Oncology Nursing.* 11: 120–127. 1995.

A thorough review of the impact cancer and therapies have on women with regard to both sexual expression and fertility is provided.

6. Nishimoto, Patricia W. Sex and sexuality in the cancer patient. *Nurse Practitioner Forum.* 6(4): 221–227. 1995.

   This article presents a brief yet thorough overview of specific sexual issues in the cancer patient.

7. Schover, L. R., and S. B. Jensen. *Sexuality and Chronic Illness: A Comprehensive Approach.* The Guilford Press, New York. 1988.

   This book provides an excellent model for integrating sexuality and illness. It includes assessment and therapy approaches, and it is highlighted with case studies to demonstrate approaches.

8. Shell, J. A., and C. K. Smith. Sexuality and the older person with cancer. *Oncol Nurs Forum.* 21: 553–558. 1994.

   This article presents the physiological changes of aging that can affect sexual functioning in relationship to a diagnosis of cancer.

9. Smith, D. B., and R. J. Babaian. The effects of treatment for cancer on male fertility and sexuality. *Cancer Nursing* 15(4): 271–275. 1994.

   A brief overview of the impact on sexuality of various types of cancer therapies for men and possible treatment interventions is presented.

10. Ver Steeg, M. A. Developing a sexual assessment. In von Eschenbach, A. C., and D. B. Rodriguez, eds. *Sexual Rehabilitation of the Urologic Cancer Patient.* G. K. Hall, Boston. 1981.

    This chapter focuses on the philosophy of a sexual assessment and cautions the nurse to provide sensitivity for the patient. Clinical scenarios with guidelines provide approaches for the nurse.

11. Young-McCaughan, Stacey. Sexual functioning in women with breast cancer after treatment with adjuvant therapy. *Cancer Nursing* 19(4): 308–319. 1996.

    This article is a research-designed paper that has a good review of the literature and an extensive bibliography.

Pulmonary Function

Rebecca Stockdale-Wooley
Linda Celentano Norton

INTRODUCTION

The prevention, diagnosis, and management of pulmonary problems is one of the most challenging aspects of caring for cancer patients. Most cancer patients are at risk for pulmonary problems because of their disease or its treatment. Cancer of the lung, pleural effusions, pneumonia, effects of radiation therapy (RT) and drugs, and respiratory failure are the most common pulmonary problems in cancer patients.

Pathophysiology and Presentation

Primary carcinoma of the lung accounts for 29 percent of all cancer deaths. In the United States, lung cancer is the leading cause of cancer death in both men and women. Furthermore, the lung parenchyma is the most common site for tumor metastases, particularly from cancers of the breast and prostate. Tumors of the pleura, chest wall, diaphragm, and mediastinum often present with respiratory symptoms.

Malignant pleural effusions are among the most common symptomatic complications of cancer. Ten percent of patients with cancer and 50 percent of patients with disseminated cancer develop a pleural effusion. It is most often caused by lung cancer, breast cancer, ovarian cancer, or lymphoma. The severity of the symptoms is related to how rapidly the effusion develops rather than the amount of fluid present. The common presenting complaints of malignant effusion include dyspnea, nonproductive cough, and chest pain; they are due to pulmonary compression and pleural irritation and inflammation.

The lung is the most common site of serious infection in the cancer patient, and pneumonia is a frequent cause of fatal infection. The patient with cancer is at significant risk for developing pneumonia, because of both altered systemic immune function and local defense mechanisms in the lung; this is due to disease progression and related therapies, as well as such factors as malnutrition and decreased mobility. For these reasons, clinicians seek prompt diagnosis and treatment for new pulmonary infiltrates, particularly those accompanied by fever. Table 14–1 lists some infectious causes of new pulmonary infiltrates. Some of the noninfectious

Table 14-1
Pathogens that Cause Pneumonia in Cancer Patients

Classification	Organism
Bacteria	Actinomyces
	Chlamydia
	Escherichia coli
	Hemophilus influenzae
	Klebsiella
	Legionella
	Moraxella catarrhalis
	Mycobacterium tuberculosis
	Mycoplasma pneumoniae
	Nocardia
	Pseudomonas aeruginosa
	Streptococcus pneumoniae
Fungi	Aspergillis
	Candida
	Coccidioides
	Cryptococcus
	Histoplasma
	Mucor
	Zygomycetes
Virus	Adenovirus
	Cytomegalovirus
	Herpes simplex
	Influenza
	Respiratory syncytial
	Varicella-zoster
Protozoa	Pneumocystis carinii
	Strongyloides stercoralis
	Toxoplasma gondii

causes are tumor, pneumonitis, intrapulmonary hemorrhage or edema, radiation- or drug-induced lung disease, and pulmonary embolism.

The incidence and severity of radiation damage to the normal lungs are related to the volume radiated, the total dose, rate of its delivery, and the quality of the radiation (see Chapter 2B). Other contributing factors include concomitant chemotherapy, previous radiation therapy, and withdrawal of steroids. Early radiation damage consists of pulmonary capillary damage with pulmonary vascular congestion and edema. During the intermediate phase, alveolar walls are infiltrated with fibroblasts. Radiation toxicity could subside if the injury is mild. If the injury is severe, a chronic phase of pulmonary fibrosis develops.

Five to 15 percent of radiated patients develop radiation pneumonitis, usually developing symptoms two to three months after completing radiation therapy. The primary complaint is usually dyspnea. Patients might also complain of a cough—either nonproductive or producing small amounts of pink sputum. Pulmonary function tests reveal decreased lung volumes, diffusing capacity and compliance, and the presence of hypoxia. Although some patients' symptoms resolve, most patients develop gradual progressive fibrosis with varying degrees of dyspnea.

The number of chemotherapeutic drugs implicated as causes of drug-induced lung disease (DILD) is increasing as pulmonary toxicity is recognized more frequently. The subacute pattern of DILD affects the interstitium, the alveolar wall, its lining cells, and occasionally the bronchiolar and arteriolar walls. Late in the course of the disease, a fibrotic process becomes evident. Factors that contribute to the risk of drug toxicity are prior or concomitant RT, prior treatment with chemotherapy, the use of high fractions of inspired oxygen (35 percent or greater), preexisting lung disease, and high total dosage of antineoplastic agents. A dose-related risk has been identified for bleomycin and carmustine. Age, specific disease (e.g., lymphoma), route of administration of the drug, and renal dysfunction are other factors that could predispose the patient to DILD.

The most common symptom of DILD is dyspnea. Commonly associated complaints include nonproductive cough, fatigue, and malaise. Decreased diffusing capacity and a restrictive ventilatory defect are seen in pulmonary function tests (PFTs). With improvements in diagnosis and better description of the variables contributing to DILD, the incidence of lethal and nonlethal disease should decrease.

Respiratory failure in patients with cancer has been associated with mortality rates of 75–90 percent. Some causes, also seen in the general patient population, are adult respiratory distress syndrome, pulmonary emboli, and bacterial pneumonia. Other causes are disease or treatment related. Pulmonary fibrosis secondary to RT or chemotherapy can lead to respiratory failure. It can also be caused by metastatic lung disease, sepsis during neutropenia, intrapulmonary hemorrhage in association with thrombocytopenia, pneumonitis, and pulmonary opportunistic infections.

Nursing care for cancer patients with pulmonary problems focuses on measures to support the patient until lung function improves, symptom relief, and prevention of common respiratory problems. An understanding of the complications arising from lung tumors and treatment reveals four major nursing care problems encountered with cancer patients. **Airflow obstruction** can be acute or chronic; it results from tumor or infection. Symptoms of dyspnea and breathlessness and a laboratory pattern of restrictive lung disease are present in patients with **hypoxia** and **hypoventilation.** Problems with **secretion clearance** can be caused by a tumor impeding the airway or an alteration in normal defense mechanisms. The prevention and early detection of **respiratory failure** must be an important consideration in the care of cancer patients. Table 14–2, which illustrates the correlation between these nursing care problems and the medical diagnosis, can be used as a problem identification tool when designing care for the cancer patient.

Table 14-2
Problem Identification for Nursing Care

Medical Diagnosis	Airflow Obstruction	Hypoxia and Hypoventilation	Inadequate Secretion Clearance	Respiratory Failure
Cancer of the lung	Secondary to tumor obstruction of airflow	Secondary to gas exchange impairment	Secondary to obstruction of airflow	Secondary to gas exchange impairment
Neoplasms of the pleura, chest wall, mediastinum	Secondary to bronchial obstruction or mediastinal shift	Secondary to decreased chest wall or diaphragm motion	Secondary to loss of adequate cough or gag reflex	Secondary to gas exchange impairment
Tracheal obstruction secondary to tumor or metastasis	Secondary to tumor	Secondary to decreased ventilation from obstruction or pulmonary infiltrates	Secondary to loss of adequate cough and/or altered defense mechanisms	Secondary to obstruction of airflow and gas exchange impairment
Pleural effusions	Secondary to fluid impeding chest expansion	Secondary to restriction of lung expansion and ventilation–perfusion mismatch		Secondary to gas exchange impairment
Pulmonary infections and infiltrates	Secondary to consolidation or secretions	Secondary to decreased lung volumes; decreased surface area for O_2 diffusion	Secondary to postobstructive pneumonia	Secondary to gas exchange impairment
Radiation fibrosis	Secondary to bronchial epithelial injury (cough, bronchospasm [asthmatic reaction])	Secondary to radiation pneumonitis (hypoxemia and restrictive pattern on PFTs)	Secondary to obstruction or increased secretions	Secondary to fibrosis and gas exchange impairment
Drug-induced lung disease	Secondary to impaired cough; increased secretions	Secondary to fibrosis (restrictive pattern on PFTs)	Secondary to altered defense mechanisms	Secondary to fibrosis and gas exchange impairment

PFT—pulmonary function test

Assessment

Evaluation of lung function is dependent on a history, physical examination, and laboratory data. Table 14–3 lists the clinical findings of these three assessment areas for the patient with airflow obstruction, hypoxia/hypoventilation, inadequate secretion clearance, and respiratory failure. Although a complete history and physical examination are necessary for evaluating these patients, Table 14–3 is intended to focus on the pulmonary database and move the reader from a specific assessment to interpretation of the data based on the four common nursing care problem areas.

Management

Improving the quality of life is the aim of managing pulmonary problems in cancer patients. The overall goals of therapy are to (1) optimize oxygenation and ventilation, (2) decrease the work of breathing, and (3) prevent infection. Tables 14–4 to 14–6 provide management protocols for three of the common nursing care problem areas.

Airflow obstruction can be characterized by its location along the tracheobronchial tree and by whether it is acute or chronic. Obstructions, which are central or peripheral, originate in the airway lumen itself, the airway wall, or outside the tracheobronchial tree. The more central the location, the more severe the disturbance to airflow. Examples of intraluminal obstruction include secretions (mucus plug), pneumonia, neoplasms, and foreign bodies. Obstructions arising in the wall of the airway can be caused by tumors or more diffuse processes such as chronic obstructive pulmonary disease, fibrosis, or asthma. Finally, obstructions outside the tracheobronchial tree are caused by tumors (e.g., head/neck region, thorax, abdomen) that impede air and secretion movement. The management of acute airflow obstruction differs from that of chronic airflow obstruction in that the focus is immediate removal of the obstruction and/or provision of an artificial airway.

The nursing protocol for management of airflow obstruction is detailed in Table 14–4. Because cancer patients face a high risk for pneumonia, a preventive protocol is presented. Breathing exercises and relaxation techniques are aimed at increasing expiratory flow and decreasing anxiety. Physical conditioning should be geared toward achieving maximal tolerance for the activities of daily living. The treatment of reversible bronchospasm can include the use of methylxanthines, sympathomimetics, anticholinergics, steroids, and mediator blockers. The concomitant use of oxygen and mechanical assistance devices improves exercise tolerance,

Airflow Obstruction

Table 14–3
Clinical Findings According to Nursing Care Problems

Assessment	Airflow Obstruction	Hypoxia and Hypoventilation	Inadequate Secretion Clearance	Respiratory Failure
History	Dyspnea and/or shortness of breath, cough, hemoptysis, recurrent upper respiratory infections.	Dyspnea, tachypnea, lethargy, fatigue, restlessness, headache, irritability, confusion.	Cough, with or without sputum; inadequate cough; sputum: change in color, odor, consistency, and amount; fever; dyspnea; tachypnea; generalized weakness; postoperative patient; history of smoking and/or COPD.	Rapidly progressive air hunger; restlessness, confusion, diaphoresis, headache. Refer to history data under Airflow Obstruction, Hypoxia and Hypoventilation, Inadequate Secretion Clearance.
Physical examination	Cyanosis; tripod posture; $\uparrow$ RR, $\downarrow$ chest excursion, prolonged expiration; accessory muscle use; pursed lip breathing; $\uparrow$ A-P diameter (if COPD); retractions, stridor; tracheal shift; $\downarrow$ fremitus; flat or hyperresonant percussion; rhonchi, rales, wheezing; signs of consolidation if acute obstruction: snoring—partial, complete, marked; inspiratory effort without air movement.	Coma; cyanosis; tachycardia, hypertension, and then hypotension; $\downarrow$ respiratory excursion, $\downarrow$ diaphragm excursion; $\downarrow$ breath sounds, rhonchi, rales, wheezing; signs of consolidation.	Cyanosis; increased work of breathing—$\uparrow$ RR, accessory muscle use; rhonchi, rales, wheezing; signs of consolidation; systemic signs of dehydration.	Tachycardia; hypotension; cyanosis; confusion, coma, tremors, asterixis; $\downarrow$ respiratory excursion, $\uparrow$ RR with progression to $\downarrow$ RR; papilledema.
Laboratory data	ABGs: $\downarrow$ PO_2; may have $\uparrow$ or $\downarrow$ PCO_2. CXR: may show tumor, pleural effusion, pneumonia. COPD pattern. PFTs: obstructive defect.	ABGs: $\downarrow$ PO_2; may have $\uparrow$ PCO_2. CXR: may show tumor, pleural effusion, pneumonia, fibrosis, pulmonary edema. PFTs: obstructive or restrictive defect.	ABGs: normal or $\downarrow$ PO_2; may have $\uparrow$ PCO_2. CXR: may show tumor, pleural effusion, pneumonia, fibrosis, pulmonary edema. PFTs: obstructive or restrictive defect.	ABGs: $\downarrow$ PO_2; may have $\uparrow$ or $\downarrow$ PCO_2. CXR: may show tumor, pleural effusion, pneumonia, fibrosis, pulmonary edema. PFTs: obstructive or restrictive defect.

A-P diameter, anterior-posterior diameter; COPD, chronic obstructive pulmonary disease; PCO_2, partial pressure of carbon dioxide; PO_2, partial pressure of oxygen; RR, respiratory rate; ABG, arterial blood gas; CXR, chest x-ray; PFT, pulmonary function test.

Table 14–4
Nursing Protocol for the Management of Airflow Obstruction

Factor	Intervention
Prevention of pneumonia	Wash hands thoroughly. Practice aseptic technique, e.g., during suctioning. Use laminar air flow when available. Monitor for signs and symptoms of infection. Obtain surveillance cultures. Provide adequate nutrition. Decrease hospital stay. Avoid contact with people with respiratory infections. Perform tuberculin screening prior to immunosuppression. Hydrate adequately. Encourage deep breathing, coughing, and ambulation. Instruct and practice prior to surgery. If necessary, institute chest physical therapy. Instruct patient and family in signs of respiratory infection to monitor and report for early treatment: fever; change in color, consistency, amount, viscosity, or odor of sputum; or increased cough, shortness of breath, chest tightness, or wheezing. Encourage/maintain smoking cessation. If risk of aspiration pneumonia, refer below to Management of tracheostomy tube.
Position needs	Turn head laterally with neck extended and inspect mouth for cause of acute (short-term) obstruction. Prepare for insertion of an artificial airway to relieve the obstruction, protect the airway, provide a route for secretion removal, and provide a port for supporting ventilation.
Chronic (long-term)	Reposition q 2 hr. Get patient out of bed to maximize thoracic excursion and improve oxygenation and secretion removal. Position for best alveolar ventilation: Check ABGs and lung sounds after position change and after the patient is stable (allow approximately 30 min). Patient will likely report being most comfortable in position with best alveolar ventilation. Have patient use tripod position (leaning forward on elbows) while sitting. While in bed use the position that provides the least obstruction to airflow. The patient should be less symptomatic, the lung sounds clearer and ABGs improved in this position. Educate patient and family as to rationale for management and patient care.
Breathing exercises and relaxation techniques	To slow respiratory rate and prolong expiration, use pursed-lip expiration: Inhale through nose and exhale slowly and steadily through pursed lips. Use diaphragmatic breathing: Place one hand (yours or patient's) on abdomen and one on thorax; inhale deeply through nose and let abdomen expand; exhale through pursed lips while pushing abdomen in and up. Hand on chest should not be moving with respirations.

Continued

Table 14–4 *(Continued)*
Nursing Protocol for the Management of Airflow Obstruction

Factor	Intervention
	Count during inhalation and exhalation. Check that exhalation is longer (roughly twice as long). Counting also serves as a distraction and decreases anxiety when trying to get shortness of breath under control.
	For retraining of chronic patients, pursed lip and diaphragm exercises should progress from the supine position to sitting to walking, and to stair climbing. Mechanical assistance can be used to strengthen the diaphragm further; e.g., place a weight (book, sandbag) on the abdomen when practicing in the supine position.
	Patients with pulmonary fibrosis normally breathe or pant more shallowly and at a faster rate due to the changes in the lungs. With exertion it is normal for them to pant even faster. This increased rate facilitates gas exchange and is not to be discouraged.
	Thoracic expansion exercises for patients with chronic obstructive or restrictive pulmonary disease and for post-thoracic surgery patients:
	Place hands over the lateral bases of thorax. Push ribs/hands out during inhalation.
	Lie on right side with left arm overhead and right hand on left lateral chest. Concentrate on expanding left lateral thorax. Reverse and repeat lying on left side.
	Use slow deep breathing with diaphragmatic pursed lip breathing as a relaxation technique. Imagery (guided or nonguided) and progressive muscle relaxation can also be used.
	Allow patient and family adequate time to learn exercises, particularly those that will be continued at home. Assist in identifying causes/signs of shortness of breath. Teach family to coach with breathing exercises and when to call for help.
Physical conditioning	Collaborate with physical therapy department in designing program.
	Provide adequate pain relief.
	Proceed from starting point to maximum tolerance: range of motion, to sitting, to walking with assistance, to level walking, to treadmill exercise, to bicycling, to stair climbing.
	Encourage daily exercise with gradual increase in activity. Keep a daily log to document progress and provide encouragement.
	Assist in energy conservation. Teach patient to lift, push, pull, and go up a step on exhalation; pace activities, rest, sit when possible, eliminate unnecessary steps; plan activities after breathing medications and treatments; set priorities: simplify, postpone, eliminate certain activities, spread activities out over day/week; use assistive devices, e.g., oxygen, a chair in the shower, devices to help put on socks.
	Provide low-flow O_2, if necessary, for continuous use or with activities.
	Involve family in activities, because they will be continued at home.
	Refer patient to agencies that provide assistance at home.

Table 14-4 *(Continued)*
Nursing Protocol for the Management of Airflow Obstruction

Factor	Intervention
Bronchodilators	Administer according to individual patient needs: Evaluate effects, side effects, optimum timing, and sequencing of drugs and activities, e.g., bronchodilator inhaler before steroid inhaler; ensure proper administration of inhaled drugs and proper dosage based on duration of action; encourage use before breathing exercises, postural drainage and coughing exercises, conditioning exercises, and strenuous activities. Optimize MDI technique: Shake MDI, hold mouthpiece 1½ inches in front of mouth or between teeth with mouth open, exhale completely, depress canister and inhale slowly and maximally, hold breath to count of ten or as long as able, exhale, and wait two minutes before taking next puff. Spacer devices are helpful for patients who are unable to use the MDI correctly. Collaborate with patient and family on how to avoid allergens, dust, fumes, and cigarette smoking at home or at work. Teach patient and family about bronchodilators.
Oxygen and mechanical assistance	Assess factors determining mode of delivery: Presence of an artificial airway, e.g., T-piece, tracheostomy mask. Fraction of inspired oxygen required: Low-flow systems (e.g., nasal cannulas) are less sensitive to changes in ventilatory pattern. High-flow systems (e.g., Venturi) provide a specific FIO_2 and bag reservoirs provide higher FIO_2. Assess patient comfort and tolerance, particularly if candidate for home oxygen. Provide home oxygen. Delivery options: compressed O_2, liquid systems, concentrators, devices to conserve oxygen. Factors determining type of delivery: oxygen requirement (e.g., FIO_2 and number of daily hours needed), portability (patient's lifestyle), cost of oxygen and financial status of patient and family. Patient and family education: machinery operation, cleaning and assembly, signs and symptoms of hypoxia and hypercapnia, home safety precautions. Provide other devices: Nebulizer to administer medications. To increase humidity: Wick or drum humidifier—cleaning unit and changing water and filter regularly are imperative. Incentive inspiratory devices to encourage maximal inspiration. Nasal BI PAP device to deliver nasal pressure support ventilation in obstructive and restrictive lung disease, upper airway obstruction, respiratory insufficiency, and chest wall disorders. Pneumobelt—for severe diaphragm weakness (corset cuff intermittently inflates and deflates at preset rate).

Continued

Table 14-4 *(Continued)*
Nursing Protocol for the Management of Airflow Obstruction

Factor	Intervention

Management of tube tracheostomy	Maintain airway patency:
	  Provide a humidification source because the normal warming and humidifying mechanism, the nose, is bypassed. Remove secretions: hydrate and provide humidity; institute deep breathing and huff coughing (see Table 14–5); suction as necessary; reposition patient and get patient out of bed.
	Provide tube care:
	  Suction as necessary: wash hands and wear sterile gloves; instill 2–3 cc sterile NS if secretions are very thick; hyperoxygenate and hyperventilate before suctioning; use 10, 12, or 14 French catheter and 120 mm Hg pressure; introduce catheter and apply suction for maximum of 15 seconds; then withdraw catheter; reoxygenate and hyperventilate.
	  Clean inner and outer cannula q 2–4 hr and PRN: prepare equipment and suction patient; release lock, remove inner cannula, and place in a solution of 1:1 NS and hydrogen peroxide; clean inner cannula; then rinse in NS; clean outer cannula; suction outer cannula if necessary; dry inner cannula and reinsert.
	  Change tracheostomy dressing and ties: Remove dressing and ties and clean tracheostomy stoma with 1:1 solution of NS and hydrogen peroxide; wipe stoma area with NS and apply antimicrobial ointment; replace precut tracheostomy dressing; replace ties.
	Change tube one or two times per week, frequency according to local standards:
	  Thread outer cannula with neck tapes. If a cuffed tube, test for leaks by inflating and observing for deflation or immerse in NS and check for air bubbles; deflate prior to insertion. Place obturator in outer cannula; lubricate end with water-soluble lubricant. If a cuffed tube is in place, deflate before removing. Cut neck tapes, grasp neck plate and remove entire tube in a straight downward motion. Insert new tube using gentle inward pressure; remove obturator. Secure neck tapes with square knot with tension, allowing one finger between tape and neck. Insert inner cannula; lock into place.
	Prevent complications:
	  Pneumonia and mucus plugging: Humidify and hydrate, mobilize secretions, suction, and maintain asepsis.
	  Aspiration pneumonia: inflate tracheostomy cuff, if appropriate, for duration of feeding and one hour afterward; allow rest for one hour before and after meals; place in semi-Fowler's position for duration of meals and for one hour afterward.
	  Inadvertent extubation: Have an extra tube available.
	Promote communication and comfort with:
	  Assistive devices: trach talk, artificial larynx, esophageal speech.

Table 14-4 *(Continued)*
Nursing Protocol for the Management of Airflow Obstruction

Factor	Intervention
	Short-term solutions: letter board, writing tablet. Comfort measures: mouth care, involving patient and family in care and care decisions, explanation of all aspects of care. Extubate: Gradually decrease tube size and/or tracheostomy plugs. Use fenestrated tracheostomy tube. Use tracheal button.

FIO_2, fraction of inspired oxygen; IPPB, intermittent positive pressure breathing; ABG, arterial blood gas; MDI, metered dose inhaler; BI PAP, bilevel positive airway pressure; NS, normal saline.

Table 14-5
Nursing Protocol for the Management of Secretion Clearance

Factor	Intervention
Prevention of pneumonia	See Table 14–4.
Positioning	Position q 2 hr; include supine, prone, lateral, and sitting positions. Modify if post-lung surgery. Get patient out of bed to maximize thoracic excursion and improve oxygenation and secretion removal. Ambulate, if possible.
Coughing exercises	Hydrate patient adequately; humidify supplemental O_2, if receiving more than 2 liters per minute; increase room humidity; inhale shower steam. Liquefy secretions by nebulization treatment, if necessary. Administer bronchodilators first, if prescribed. Provide adequate pain relief, assist with splinting of abdominal or thoracic incisions. Cascade cough: Instruct patient to take a deep breath followed by three to four coughs until the air has been emptied out of the lungs. Repeat. Huff cough: Instruct patient to take a deep breath then forcefully exhale with mouth open, without closing the glottis, resulting in a "huff" sound. Effective for postoperative patients and patients with airway collapse due to compliant airways. Manually assist coughing for patients with extremely weak abdominal muscles: Apply manual pressure over the abdominal wall during coughing.
Chest physical therapy and drainage (Fig. 14–1)	Provide adequate pain relief. Liquefy secretions: Maximize fluid intake, humidify, and/or nebulize. Define affected lung regions and therapy positions. Auscultate lungs before, during, and after treatment. Provide O_2 if hypoxemic during chest therapy. Position for drainage of first lobe(s). If possible, use Trendelenburg's position for lower and middle lobes.

Continued

Table 14-5 (Continued)
Nursing Protocol for the Management of Secretion Clearance

Factor	Intervention
	Percuss defined area with cupped hands in a rhythmic fashion for a given time, e.g., three to five minutes, or use mechanical percussor. Follow with vibration. Instruct patient to deep-breathe. Place flat hand over area and vibrate on exhalation while gently compressing chest wall. Follow with coughing exercises. Proceed to next position, percuss, vibrate, assist with coughing exercises. Perform two to four times daily.
Suctioning (if unable to cough effectively)	If intubated: Refer to Table 14–4, Management of tracheostomy tube. If not intubated: Use aseptic technique; preoxygenate and ask patient to take a few deep breaths; lubricate 10, 12, or 14 French catheter tip and insert through a naris to the back of the throat; ask the patient to inhale and pass catheter into the tracheobronchial tree to the level of the carina; apply intermittent suction, no greater than 120 mmHg for a maximum of 15 seconds; rotate the catheter while removing it; reoxygenate and have the patient take a few deep breaths.

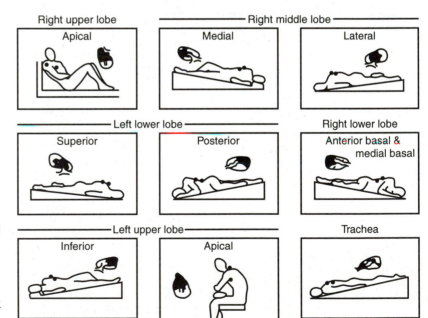

Figure 14-1. Basic postural drainage positions. Each position is used to drain the segment of the lung indicated by the shaded areas. • indicates the points where percussion and vibration are to be applied.

Adapted with permission from Haas, A., H. Pineda, F. Haas, and K. Axen. Pulmonary Therapy and Rehabilitation Principles and Practice. Williams & Wilkins Co., Baltimore. p. 127. 1979.

Table 14–6
Nursing Protocol for the Management of Respiratory Failure

Factor	Intervention
Prevention of infection	Prevent pneumonia (see Table 14–4), remove secretions by coughing or suctioning, and perform chest physical therapy and postural drainage (see Table 14–5). Change ventilator tubing regularly. Secure the endotracheal tube. Use aseptic suctioning technique. Humidify inhaled air. Provide frequent mouth care for intubated patients.
Oxygen and mechanical ventilation	Administer supplemental oxygen to bring PO_2 and PCO_2 to normal. Monitor vital signs, level of consciousness, lung sounds, and use of accessory muscles. Monitor ventilator settings and alarm systems.
Positioning	See Table 14–4.
Hemodynamic and fluid balance	Hydrate adequately. Monitor cardiac output. Minimize the effects of positive pressure breathing: use intermittent mechanical ventilation; minimize peak airway pressure; restrict fluids if water retention secondary to vasopressin release; control pain, stress, and increases in CO_2; use diuretics.
Prevention of complications of mechanical ventilation	Maintain airway patency: humidify inhaled air and hydrate patient; remove secretions (see Table 14–4, Management of tracheostomy tube, suctioning); secure endotracheal tube; sedate patient as necessary; have Ambu bag and mask on hand. Prevent laryngeal and tracheal complications: secure endotracheal tube; use low-pressure cuffs; use minimal occluding volume in inflating cuff; measure cuff pressures. Prevent barotrauma: Identify population at risk (patients with high peak airway pressures). Minimize peak airway pressure: Use intermittent mechanical ventilation; prolong expiratory time or decrease respiratory rate. Provide for mechanical emergencies: Have Ambu bag at bedside.
Communication and comfort	See Table 14–4, Management of tracheostomy tube.

PCO_2, partial pressure of carbon dioxide; PO_2, partial pressure of oxygen.

decreases symptoms of hypoxia, and prevents the development of cor pulmonale. A tracheostomy tube might be necessary to relieve obstruction on a temporary or permanent basis. Tracheostomy tubes also facilitate secretion removal and, when necessary, provide a medium for administering positive pressure ventilation. Other non-nursing aspects of managing airflow obstruction include surgical removal of a tumor, radiation, and chemotherapy.

Hypoxia and Hypoventilation

Adequate tissue oxygenation is dependent upon an intact cardiovascular–respiratory–hematopoietic transport system.

Hypoventilation is the inability of the respiratory apparatus to maintain alveolar ventilation adequate for the metabolic needs of the body. Cancer patients, because of functional or structural impairments, have a propensity to hypoventilate. Fatigue and malnutrition are the common examples of *functional* limitations that cause a patient to hypoventilate. Tumors obstructing air movement, surgery involving the thorax or lungs, treatment effects such as radiation pneumonitis or DILD, and pneumonia are all examples of *structural* causes of hypoventilation. Hypoventilation places a patient at risk for hypoxia, hypercapnia, and pneumonia. If air movement is diminished, so too is the oxygen available for transport across the alveolar-capillary membrane.

Hypoxia, a decrease in oxygen tension, can result from hypoventilation or can occur in isolation. Problems of oxygen transport occur (1) at the alveolar-capillary membrane, as in interstitial fibrosis or lymphangitic metastases; (2) as a result of hemodynamic dysfunction, as in pericardial effusion or doxorubicin cardiomyopathy; or (3) because of an alteration in the chemical composition of the blood, as in anemia.

Prevention of hypoxia and hypoventilation and optimizing oxygen transport in irreversible lung disease are essential aspects in the care of the cancer patient. Factors for the nurse to consider include the prevention of pneumonia, oxygen administration, patient positioning, physical conditioning, and bronchodilator administration (all of these factors are discussed in Table 14–4). In addition, breathing exercises (Table 14–4) are essential for the patient, particularly thoracic expansion exercises (e.g., periodic deep breathing, segmental breathing), as are incentive inspiratory devices and coughing exercises (Table 14–5). Other aspects of management include transfusions, drugs to improve cardiac output, drainage of effusions or pleurectomy, and the administration of steroids, chemotherapy, or RT.

Secretion Clearance

Hypoventilation or airway obstruction hampers secretion removal and predisposes the patient to pneumonia. Immunosuppression secondary to chemotherapy, RT, malnutrition, disease, or advanced age add to the risk of pneumonia. Prevention is the hallmark of nursing management of this potential patient care problem (see Table 14–5). Other aspects of management include antibiotics or antiviral drugs, judicious use of chemotherapy, bronchoscopy (e.g., to remove mucus plugs), endotracheal intubation, and removal of airway obstruction.

Respiratory Failure

Respiratory failure is the inability of the respiratory system to maintain adequate oxygenation and carbon dioxide elimination. Identification of the oncology patient at risk and the early clinical manifestations of respiratory failure is the basis for decreasing patient morbidity and mortality.

Critically ill cancer patients are those with sepsis, for example, or fulminant pneumonia, interstitial fibrosis, intrapulmonary hemorrhage, and large-airway obstruction. A more common cause of respiratory failure is narcotic suppression of respiration in an already compromised patient. Diagnosis and treatment of the cause of respiratory failure is of paramount importance. During the treatment phase, however, symptomatic management prevails (see Table 14–6). Additional treatment might include drugs to treat the cause of respiratory failure (e.g., antibiotics), bronchoscopy to aid in secretion removal, and chemotherapy or RT to treat tumor growth.

BIBLIOGRAPHY

1. Advances in oncology nursing. *Nurs Clin North Am* 25(2) (June, 1990).

   This issue includes articles on nursing management of patients with lung cancer, effects of chemotherapy, and advances in radiation therapy.

2. American Cancer Society. *Cancer Facts & Figures—1997*. American Cancer Society, Inc. Atlanta, GA. 1997.

   This is a compilation of the latest facts and figures on cancer cases, mortality, incidence, and survival rates in the United States.

3. Armstrong, T., D. Rust, and J. R. Kohtz. Neurologic, pulmonary, and cutaneous toxicities of high-dose chemotherapy. *Oncology Nursing Forum* 24(1) supplement: 23–33. 1997.

   This article discusses the pulmonary toxicities associated with chemotherapy including signs and symptoms, diagnosis, medical treatment, and nursing interventions, and includes excellent tables.

4. DeVita, Jr., V. T., S. Hellman, and S. A. Rosenberg. *Cancer: Principles and Practice of Oncology*. Lippincott-Raven Publishers, Philadelphia. 1997.

   This includes concise explanations of pulmonary toxicity (radiation and drug induced), malignant pleural effusions, and comprehensive information on lung cancer and respiratory tract infections. Pathophysiology, symptoms, and management are presented.

5. Drings, P., and I. Günther. Relief from respiratory distress in advanced cancer patients. *Recent Results in Cancer Research* 121: 366–377. 1991.

   This features good coverage of cause, diagnosis and management of respiratory problems in cancer patients.

6. Fishman, A. P. *Pulmonary Rehabilitation*. Marcel Dekker, New York. 1996.

   The art and science of pulmonary rehabilitation is presented, with good coverage of breathing exercises, mobilization, and physical therapy for obstructive and restrictive lung disease and respiratory failure.

7. Groeger, J. S. *Critical Care of the Cancer Patient*. Mosby Year-Book, St. Louis. 1991.

   This book contains comprehensive chapters on respiratory failure and the infectious complications of neoplastic diseases.

8. Luce, J. M., D. J. Pierson, and M. L. Tyler. *Intensive Respiratory Care*. W.B. Saunders Company, Philadelphia. 1993.

   The presentations of pulmonary anatomy and physiology, respiratory failure, and respiratory care techniques (including airway clearance, oxygen therapy, artificial airways) are excellent and comprehensive.

9. Sexton, D. L. *Nursing Care of the Respiratory Patient*. Appleton & Lange, Norwalk, CT. 1990.

   This features excellent review chapters on respiratory failure and lung cancer.

10. Stover, D. E., and R. J. Kaner. Pulmonary complications in cancer patients. *CA Cancer J Clin* 46(5): 303–320. 1996.

    This article provides an excellent review of the presentation, diagnosis, and treatment of common pulmonary complications in cancer patients.

ONCOLOGIC EMERGENCIES

Chapter 15 Obstructive Emergencies — 15

    A. Increased Intracranial Pressure — 15A

    B. Spinal Cord Compression — 15B

    C. Superior Vena Cava Syndrome — 15C

    D. Tracheal Obstruction — 15D

    E. Bowel Obstruction — 15E

    F. Cardiac Tamponade — 15F

Chapter 16 Metabolic Emergencies — 16

    A. Hypercalcemia — 16A

    B. Tumor Lysis Syndrome — 16B

    C. Syndrome of Inappropriate Antidiuretic Hormone Secretion — 16C

    D. Anaphylaxis — 16D

    E. Septic Shock — 16E

    F. Coagulopathies — 16F

Chapter 17 Infiltrative Emergencies — 17

    A. Carotid Artery Erosion and Rupture — 17A

    B. Leukostasis — 17B

Obstructive Emergencies

A. Increased Intracranial Pressure

Diahann Kazierad

Increased intracranial pressure (ICP) is defined as change in intracranial volume, either increased brain tissue volume, cerebral spinal fluid (CSF), or blood. This is supported by the Monro-Kellie doctrine, which states that the expansion of one of these volumes requires adjustment of the other two volumes to maintain a steady state within the rigid skull. Adjustment of the volumes keeps ICP constant. If compensatory mechanisms fail, increased ICP with neurological deterioration occurs.

PATHOPHYSIOLOGY

Brain Volume

Brain volume can be increased by a number of mechanisms: space occupying lesions such as primary or metastatic tumors of the brain, hematomas, intracerebral hemorrhages, abscesses, and aneurysms. Edema of the cerebral tissue caused by an accumulation of fluid in the intracellular space, extracellular space, or both is also associated with increased brain volume. There are three types of cerebral edema that have been identified and will be discussed in more detail: vasogenic, intracelluar, and interstitial edema. Regardless of the type of cerebral edema or space occupying lesion, uninterrupted increased ICP will lead to herniation of the brain and death.

Vasogenic cerebral edema, the most common form of brain edema, is characterized by an alteration in the permeability of the specialized capillary network called the blood-brain barrier (BBB). The permeability of the capillary walls is increased, causing fluid to leak into the extracellular space (ECF). Cerebral edema is the result of this fluid shift. In the oncology patient population, vasogenic edema can be precipitated by primary or metastatic tumors of the brain, intracranial surgery, local or total cranial radiation, intracerebral bleeds, hematomas, and central nervous system (CNS) infections.

Intracellular edema is characterized by movement of fluid into the cellular space. In this situation, sodium is unable to leave the cell. Fluid is drawn into the cell causing it to swell and increase intracranial pressure. Intracellular edema is caused by hypoxia or hypercapnea, such as occurs during a cardiac arrest, respiratory arrest, cerebral ischemia and infarction, or severe, prolonged hypotension. Intracellular edema can also occur in the syndrome of inappropriate antidiuretic hormone (SIADH), hyponatremia, and exudative CNS infections. Vasogenic and intracellular edema can occur together.

Interstitial edema occurs when pressure within the ventricular system forces the cerebral spinal fluid out of the ventricles and into the tissues surrounding the ventricles. This situation is seen with acute and subacute hydrocephalus (see the section "Cerebrospinal Fluid").

Blood Volume

An increase in cerebral blood volume can occur either through increased arterial blood flow or because of a decrease in the venous outflow. Normally, arterial cerebral blood flow is maintained at a relatively constant pressure by *autoregulation,* a process that allows both small and large cerebral arterioles to change their diameter in response to variations in arterial pressure. Autoregulation operates within the limits of a mean arterial pressure (MAP) of 60 to 150 mm Hg; at a MAP less than 60 mm Hg cerebral blood flow is reduced, and at a MAP greater than 150 mm Hg cerebral blood flow is increased. The arterioles consist of smooth muscle fibers that respond to an increase in volume by constricting and to a decrease in volume by dilating. These arterioles are also responsive to chemical and metabolic influences. Carbon dioxide (CO_2), the end product of cellular metabolism, is the most potent chemical to influence cerebral blood flow. Increased CO_2 causes vasodilation, whereas decreased CO_2 causes vasoconstriction. Oxygen and pH also influence cerebral blood flow; decreases in either lead to vasodilatation and increases cause vasoconstriction. The venous system does not contain smooth muscle and is therefore a passive system. Distention of the venules occurs as a result of increased intraluminal volume. The venous system is not capable of vasoconstriction.

Increased cerebral blood volume due to increased arterial blood flow with loss of autoregulation can occur in hyperemia and malignant hypertension. Increased cerebral blood volume due to decreased venous outflow can occur with obstruction of the internal jugular (IJ) veins, which can complicate postsurgical resection of head and neck cancers, tumor compression, and superior vena cava syndrome.

Cerebrospinal Fluid

Alteration in CSF volume is the third mechanism by which ICP is increased. Most CSF is produced by the choroid plexus, a highly vascularized structure, which projects into the lateral, third, and fourth ventricles. The CSF is circulated through the ventricles and leaves the fourth ventricle at the foramen of Magendie and the foramen of Luschka, exiting either downward around the cord or upward over the surface of the brain to be reabsorbed by arachnoid villi and drained into the venous sinuses. Approximately 500 mls of CSF is produced per day or 25 mls per hour. Reabsorption of CSF is proportional to the CSF pressure.

Obstruction of CSF flow, reduced reabsorption of CSF by the arachnoid villi, or increased production of CSF results in increased ICP. Obstruction of CSF flow, termed noncommunicating hydrocephalus, can occur due to tumor compression within the ventricular system. Blood cells from subarachnoid hemorrhage and exudate from CNS infections can interfere with reabsorption of CSF by the arachnoid villi. Finally, rare tumors of the choroid plexus can increase CSF production.

Herniation

Intracranial pressure that continues to rise will result in herniation of the brain. Herniation is defined as the protrusion of an organ or part of an organ through a defect or natural opening that normally contains it. The cerebrum can shift laterally and/or downward against the tentorium cerebelli, a part of the dura matter that separates the cerebrum from the cerebellum; and through the foramen magnum, the opening in which the brain stem and spinal cord pass at the level of the first cervical vertebrae. Pressure exerted by a mass or cerebral edema, called the *mass effect,* will shift the brain tissue from an area of high pressure to an area of lower pressure. The brain will be compressed against these structures, and neurological dysfunction results.

Life-threatening herniation syndromes are caused by lesions that are either supratentorial or infratentorial, depending on their location in relationship to the tentorium cerebelli. Generally speaking, with supratentorial lesions, the structures above the tentorium press down on the brain stem, pushing it through the tentorial notch. This action will have detrimental effects on level of consciousness, cranial nerve function, and brain stem function. Most importantly, compression of the medulla within the brain stem can lead to loss of respiratory and cardiac function. Infratentorial lesions can directly press on the brain stem structures, forcing them up through the tentorial notch or down through the foramen magnum and resulting in dysfunction and death. Either herniation syndrome can cause vascular compression or hemorrhage leading to brain ischemia or CSF obstruction leading to hydrocephalus. Both complications can further exacerbate the ICP.

Within the oncology population, patients with the following are at risk for increased ICP:

1. Fast-growing primary and metastatic brain tumors;
2. Thrombocytopenia with or without concomitant head trauma or hypertension resulting in intracranial hemorrhage or hematoma;

3. Local or total cranial radiation;
4. CNS infection;
5. Cerebral hypercapnia, hypoxia;
6. SIADH or hyponatremia (see Chapter 16C);
7. Head and neck tumors followed by surgical resection;
8. Superior vena cava syndrome (see Chapter 15C);
9. Intracranial surgical manipulation;
10. Hyperleukocytosis associated with leukemia (see Chapter 17B);
11. Seizures.

CLINICAL MANIFESTATIONS

Early signs and symptoms of increased ICP indicate general impairment of cerebral function (see Table 15A–1). Changes in the level of consciousness can be subtle or overt and include behavior such as restlessness, drowsiness, loss of the perception of time, disorientation to surroundings, and memory and cognitive deficits. If headaches occur, they usually worsen upon awakening from REM sleep due to increased metabolism and production of CO_2, which cause intracranial vasodilation. Seizure activity can occur especially in a patient with brain metastasis. Pressure on the vomiting center causes sudden projectile vomiting not preceded by anticipatory nausea.

Late signs and symptoms are ominous. These include changes in vital signs, posturing, and loss of gag and corneal reflexes. They generally indicate pressure on the vital structures within the brain stem. Immediate intervention is required to decompress the brain.

ASSESSMENT

Ongoing serial assessment of neurologic status is necessary for early diagnosis and treatment of increased ICP. A baseline neurological exam is performed on admission, and subsequent exams are compared with base-

Table 15A-1
Signs and Symptoms of Increased Intracranial Pressure

Early Findings	Late Findings
Altered level of consciousness	Deterioration of level of consciousness
Cranial nerve dysfunction	Hemiplegia
Motor weakness	Decorticate, decerebrate posturing
Sensory deficits	Change in vital signs (Cushing's reflex, Cushing's triad)
Headache	Ipsilateral or bilateral dilated & fixed pupils
Seizures	Loss of brain stem reflexes
Projectile vomiting	Flaccidity mixed with occasional decerebration

line. A standard neurological examination includes assessment of level of consciousness, cranial nerves, motor function, and vital signs (see Chapter 11). The Glasgow Coma Scale (GCS) is widely used for neurological assessment (see Figure 15A–1). The scale evaluates the eye-opening, motor, and verbal responses. The range of possible scores is 3–15, with 15 indicating a fully alert and oriented person, and 3 indicating a deep coma. The GCS is a visual guide used to track trends in neurologic functioning.

Level of Consciousness

Level of consciousness can be defined as the state of wakefulness. The state of wakefulness is controlled by a diffuse network of neurons that includes the cerebral cortex, reticular activating system (RAS), thalamus, and hypothalamus. This network of neurons is sensitive to hypoxia, which occurs with increased ICP and responds with a change in the level of consciousness. Assessment of level of consciousness is one of the most reliable and sensitive predictors of early neurologic deterioration.

Level of consciousness is tested by applying a stimulus and observing the response. The stimuli include verbal sounds such as the normal and loud voice, tactile sensation such as light touch, and painful stimuli. The patient is either aroused spontaneously, to voice, to loud voice, to light touch, and to painful stimuli, or not at all. The patient's response to pain is either purposeful, nonpurposeful, or unresponsive. If the patient is arousable the nurse then tests for orientation to person, place, and time. Documentation of the response to the stimuli is more meaningful with the use of descriptive terminology. For example, "The patient opened her eyes when spoken to."

Cranial Nerves

The cranial nerve assessment provides information about brain stem functioning (see chapter 11, Table 11–9). The cranial nerves exit the brain stem in pairs. At the top of the brain stem, cranial nerves I and II exit from the cerebral cortex. The next structure in the stem, the midbrain, includes cranial nerves III and IV. Cranial nerves V, VI, and VII exit the pons. Lastly, cranial nerves VIII, IX, X, XI, and XII exit the most caudal structure, the medulla. Increasing ICP will exert pressure on the brain stem, starting at the midbrain and proceeding downward to the pons and medulla, causing predictable cranial nerve dysfunction.

It is of crucial importance to identify early signs and symptoms of increasing ICP (see Table 15A–2). Early symptoms of cranial nerve II dysfunction are subjective complaints of blurred vision, diplopia, decreased visual acuity, and field cuts. Also in the early stages, pressure on one nerve tract in the cranial nerve III pair results in ipsilateral pupil dilation and a

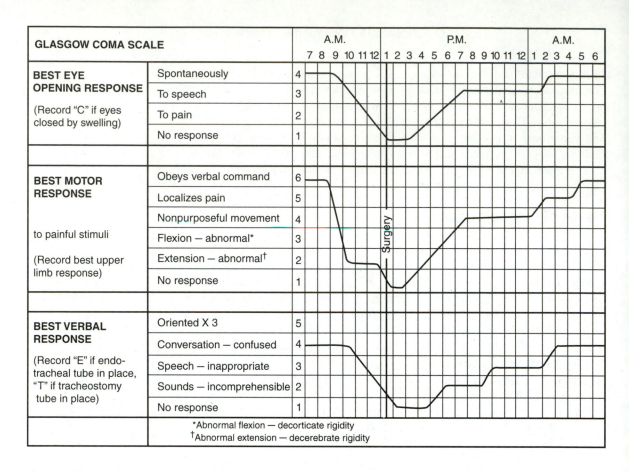

GLASGOW COMA SCALE			A.M. 7 8 9 10 11 12	P.M. 1 2 3 4 5 6 7 8 9 10 11 12	A.M. 1 2 3 4 5 6
BEST EYE OPENING RESPONSE (Record "C" if eyes closed by swelling)	Spontaneously	4			
	To speech	3			
	To pain	2			
	No response	1			
BEST MOTOR RESPONSE to painful stimuli (Record best upper limb response)	Obeys verbal command	6			
	Localizes pain	5			
	Nonpurposeful movement	4			
	Flexion — abnormal*	3			
	Extension — abnormal†	2			
	No response	1			
BEST VERBAL RESPONSE (Record "E" if endo-tracheal tube in place, "T" if tracheostomy tube in place)	Oriented X 3	5			
	Conversation — confused	4			
	Speech — inappropriate	3			
	Sounds — incomprehensible	2			
	No response	1			
	*Abnormal flexion — decorticate rigidity †Abnormal extension — decerebrate rigidity				

Scoring of Eye Opening

- 4   Opens eyes spontaneously when the nurse approaches
- 3   Opens eyes in response to speech (normal or shout)
- 2   Opens eyes only to painful stimuli (*e.g.*, squeezing of nail beds)
- 1   Does not open eyes to painful stimuli

Scoring of Best Motor Response

- 6   Can obey a simple command, such as "Lift your left hand off the bed"
- 5   Localizes to painful stimuli and attempts to remove source
- 4   Purposeless movement in response to pain
- 3   Flexes elbows and wrists while extending lower legs to pain
- 2   Extends upper and lower extremities to pain
- 1   No motor response to pain on any limb

Scoring of Best Verbal Response

- 5   Oriented to time, place, and person
- 4   Converses, although confused
- 3   Speaks only in words or phrases that make little or no sense
- 2   Responds with incomprehensible sounds (*e.g.*, groans)
- 1   No verbal response

Figure 15A–1. Example of completed Glascow Coma Scale.

Reprinted with permission from J. V. Hickey, The Clinical Practice of Neurological and Neurosurgical Nursing. *Lippencott-Raven, Philadelphia. p. 139. 1997.*

Table 15A–2
Cranial Nerve Assessment Related to Brainstem Location

Cranial Nerve	Brain Stem Structure	Test
II, III	Top of stem & midbrain	Inspect size & shape of pupil
III, IV, VI	Midbrain & pons	Pupillary reaction to light EOMs, "Doll-Eye" Movements
VII	Pons	Symmetry of facial movement
V, VII	Pons	Corneal reflex
IX, X	Medulla	Gag reflex

sluggish reaction to light. If the patient is able to follow commands, the nurse can instruct the patient to follow an object with his or her eyes to test extraocular movements (EOMs). In the unconscious patient, oculocephalic reflexes can be tested. This test, called "Doll-Eye Movements," requires the nurse to hold open the upper lids to observe the eyes. Next the patient's head is turned quickly to one side and then the other. The appropriate response is that the patient's eyes move in the opposite direction of head movement. An abnormal test of EOMs or loss of this reflex suggests pressure on the midbrain and pons.

In later stages of increased ICP, pontine and medullary dysfunction occurs. To test function of the pons, the nurse assesses cranial nerve VII by tickling each nostril with a cotton tip applicator. He or she should observe facial movements for symmetry and test the corneal reflex by dropping sterile saline into the corner of the open eye. Blinking is the appropriate response. Also in the later stage, the ipsilateral pupil becomes dilated and unresponsive to light. In the terminal stage, both pupils are dilated and fixed. Loss of the gag reflex suggests medullary dysfunction. Both these late signs indicate herniation and impending death.

Motor Capability

Motor and sensory nerve impulses travel throughout the cerebral cortex, cerebellum, and spinal cord. Both motor and sensory functions are altered due to compression on their respective descending and ascending tracts. The sensory assessment is deferred in patients with altered level of consciousness.

Assessment of the motor system in the patient with increased ICP consists of assessing for spontaneous movement, motor response, posturing, and muscle tone:

1. Observe the patient for spontaneous movement. In the absence of spontaneous movement, apply a noxious stimulus peripher-

ally. The motor response is either purposeful (the patient withdraws from the stimulus and the extremity crosses midline), nonpurposeful (the extremity moves slightly but does not withdraw or cross midline), or unresponsive (the patient does not react).

2. Observe the patient for abnormal posturing. Posturing can occur spontaneously or in response to a noxious stimulus. Decorticate rigidity is characterized by flexion of the arms at the elbows with the wrists and fingers flexed across the chest. The legs are extended, internally rotated and the feet are plantar flexed. In decerebrate rigidity, the jaws are clenched, the arms are adducted and extended to the patient's sides, wrists and fingers are flexed, legs are extended, and the feet are plantar flexed.

3. Assess muscle tone for spasticity, rigidity, or flaccidity by guiding the extremities through passive range of motion.

In general, an early sign of motor dysfunction is contralateral weakness as a result of pressure within the cortex motor tracts. As increased ICP progresses, contralateral hemiparesis to hemiplegia develops. Ipsilateral decorticate rigidity occurs with pressure on the uppermost structures of the brain stem. Continued pressure on the midbrain results in bilateral decerebration. In the later stages of compression on the medulla the patient becomes flaccid and decerebrate.

Vital Signs

Vital signs in the patient with increased ICP are relatively stable in the early stages. Respiration, pulse, blood pressure, and temperature are regulated by the structures within the brain stem. Changes in vital signs are indicative of direct compression and ischemia.

Blood Pressure

In an attempt to maintain blood pressure, a compensatory mechanism called Cushing's reflex occurs. Inadequate cerebral blood flow due to increased ICP stimulates the sympathetic "fight or flight" response in order to reestablish cerebral perfusion. As a result the systolic blood pressure rises (SBP), the diastolic falls (DBP), and pulse is bounding and slow. However, the resulting increased cerebral perfusion exacerbates the ICP, which further elevates the blood pressure. Cushing's triad refers to the loss of this compensatory mechanism and is characterized by hypertension, bradycardia with a thready pulse, and irregular breathing patterns. In the terminal phase, the patient can also become hypotensive. Therefore, it is critical to assess the patient for trends such as rising SBP, falling DBP, hypertension, and hypotension.

Pulse

In addition to the effects of Cushing's reflex, compression of the vagus nerve (cranial nerve X) within the brain stem causes bradycardia. Assess trends in the pulse rate, rhythm, and quality.

Table 15A–3
Respiratory Patterns in Patients with Altered Brainstem Function

Name	Brain Stem Structure	Pattern
Cheyne-Stokes	Bilateral, deep, cerebral lesion, diencephalon, basal ganglia	Rhythmic waxing and waning of depth and rate followed by apnea
Hyperventilation	Midbrain, upper pons	Increased rate and depth
Apneustic	Lower pons	Two- to three-second pauses after a full or prolonged inspiration alternating with an expiratory pause
Cluster	Lower pons, upper medulla	Clusters of irregular breaths along with periods of apnea at irregular intervals
Ataxic	Medulla	Irregular, unpredictable breaths, with deep and shallow random breaths and pauses

Respirations

Alterations in the respiratory pattern are associated with compression of specific brain stem structures (see Table 15A–3). Assessment must take into account the rate, rhythm, and characteristics of the inspiratory and expiratory phases.

Temperature

Hypothermia or hyperthermia can occur in the setting of increased ICP. A full evaluation for infectious and noninfectious etiologies should be initiated. See the section "Nursing Management" for more detail.

MEDICAL AND SURGICAL MANAGEMENT

The medical management of the patient with increased ICP consists of assisted hyperventilation, osmotic diuresis and fluid balance, CSF drainage, blood pressure control, and maintenance of normal body temperature. Surgical management for increased ICP is limited to resection or debulking of tumor, evacuation of hematomas, and drainage of an abscess.

Hyperventilation reduces $PaCO_2$, causing vasoconstriction within the brain, and reduces cerebral blood flow. Hyperventilation could be spontaneous, as in patients with meningitis, or mechanically induced via intubation. In an emergency, the patient can be hyperventilated (14–16 breaths per minute) by using an Ambu bag until mechanical ventilation is established.

Osmotic diuresis is a short-term treatment option that attempts to move water from brain tissue into the vascular bed. This is accomplished by creating a gradient between the plasma in the intravascular space and the fluid within the brain extra- and intra-cellular spaces. Mannitol, given intra-venous as a 0.75–1.0 gm/kg bolus dose, followed by 0.25–0.50 gm/kg every three to five hours, will draw the brain water into the vascular space, where it can be excreted in the urine. In addition, diuretics such as furosemide can be used in combination with mannitol. Osmotic diuresis can cause hypokalemia, hyperglycemia, dehydration, and hypovolemia. Frequent electrolyte and glucose analysis, accurate intake and output records, and daily weights are imperative. Intravenous medications and fluids should be infused using normal saline. Hypotonic solutions, such as D5W and Ringer's Lactate, should be avoided, as they can increase brain water.

Drainage of cerebral spinal fluid via ventriculostomy can help to reduce ICP. A *ventriculostomy* is the insertion of a catheter into a lateral ventricle. In this way, too, ICP can be directly measured and monitored. However, this procedure carries the risk of infection.

It is important to keep the systemic blood pressure within normal limits. Hypertension increases cerebral blood flow and ICP, whereas hypotension can directly cause cerebral ischemia. The SBP should be kept above 100mm Hg. Hypertension resulting from Cushing's response requires immediate intervention to reduce ICP, rather than antihypertensive medications.

Elevated body temperature increases cerebral metabolism, which increases $PaCO_2$ locally within the brain. Normothermia is essential to prevent a further increase in ICP. Fever must be worked up for possible infectious source, keeping in mind that higher than normal temperatures could also herald brain stem herniation.

In addition to these measures, sedation might be necessary. Agitation, restlessness, disorientation, and confusion can increase ICP and put the patient at greater risk for injury. Sedatives such as benzodiazepines (midazolam, lorazepam), opioids (morphine), and neuroleptics (haloperidol) can be used to keep the patient calm. In cases of extremely increased ICP, paralytic agents or barbiturate coma could be indicated, necessitating mechanical ventilation and intensive care nursing.

High-dose corticosteriods are useful in the setting of increased ICP related to edema associated with primary or metastatic tumors. Radiation therapy directed at the tumor can reduce tumor size, but it can cause cerebral edema. For this reason, corticosteroids are used concomitantly with radiation therapy to the brain.

NURSING MANAGEMENT

Nursing management of the patient with risk for increased ICP consists of frequent assessment, controlling factors known to increase ICP, and supporting homeostasis, with special attention to preventing complications. The goal of nursing management is to protect the patient from sudden increases in ICP.

Assessment of the patient at risk for increased ICP requires serial evaluation. Depending on the status of the patient, neurological assessment could be required every 15 minutes to every four hours. Included in the neurological nursing assessment is level of consciousness, cranial nerve function, motor function, brain stem reflexes, and vital signs (see the section "Assessment"). Quite frequently, changes in neurological function are subtle. Therefore, each assessment must be compared with the previous ones to make appropriate nursing decisions. Management of the patient with increased ICP might require admission to an intermediate care unit or the intensive care unit.

Many of the activities that increase ICP are related to the Valsalva maneuver. The Valsalva maneuver occurs when the patient attempts to forcibly exhale against a closed glottis, which increases intra-abdominal and intrathoracic pressures, impeding venous return from the brain. Changing body positioning, straining, coughing, vomiting, and crying are actions during which the Valsalva maneuver could occur (see Table 15A–4).

Positioning and turning of the patient should avoid stimulating the Valsava maneuver and focus on keeping the patient in proper body alignment. Proper body alignment includes avoiding angulation of body parts, such as lateral flexion of the neck, Trendelenberg position, prone position, or extreme flexion of the hips. The neck must be kept in a neutral position at all times to facilitate venous drainage. Soft collars, towel rolls or pillows can aid in keeping this position. The head of the bed should be kept at a 30 degree angle, if blood pressure allows, for optimum venous drainage. Passive range of motion is encouraged over isometric muscle contractions.

Bowel management to prevent constipation should be initiated (see Chapter 12B). Bowel function is negatively influenced by bedrest, decreased activity, and opioid use. Osmotic and saline laxatives can cause increased abdominal pressures and electrolyte abnormalities and should be used with caution. Enemas are contraindicated in this population.

External stimulation should be kept to a minimum. Emotionally upsetting conversations—such as those concerning legal proceedings, financial matters, marital conflict, prognosis, and the like—should not be discussed in the presence of the patient with increased ICP. Rather, they should be deferred until the patient is more stable. Noxious stimuli such as pain, nursing procedures, and invasive procedures should also be kept to a minimum. Soft stimuli such as a soothing voice, pleasant conversations, soft music, and voices of loved ones are encouraged. The external environment should be calming with limited visitors and activities.

Routine nursing care is known to increase ICP. Activities clustered together, such as bathing and turning, can put the patient at risk for increasing ICP as well. Therefore, nursing activities must be paced and planned in advance to limit the effect on ICP.

In addition to providing neurological care, the nurse must support homeostasis of the patient as a whole with special attention to preventing

Table 15A–4
Nursing Protocol for the Management of Increased Intracranial Pressure

Factor	Intervention
Airway/adequate ventilation maintenance	Auscultate chest sounds q 4–8 hr.
	Monitor the administration of oxygen. Use suctioning if necessary only after preoxygenating with 100% FIO_2 for 1 minute. Suction should be intermittent and brief (< 15 sec).
	Use opioids cautiously because they depress respirations. Monitor SaO_2 to keep saturation > 90%.
	Monitor blood gases.
	Keep PaO_2 > 60 mm Hg + $PaCO_2$ < 40 mmHg.
Body positioning	Maintain bed rest.
	Make use of pressure-distributing mattresses (egg-crate or alternating-pressure mattress), sheepskin paddings.
	Change position every 2 hrs.
	Offer gentle body massage.
	Encourage patient to keep head in neutral position. Avoid rotated head positions, flexion or extension of the neck, and extreme hip flexion.
	Keep head of bed elevated 30 degrees to promote venous drainage.
	Side lying position will decrease risk of aspiration in patients with an altered level of consciousness. Avoid prone position.
Physical stressors	
Isometric muscle contractions	Encourage patient to allow passive movement. Use pull sheet to turn and move patient. If the patient must move, encourage him to do so while exhaling. Avoid using restraints.
	Logroll patient.
Cough	Determine etiology of the cough. A cough suppressant may be indicated.
Vomiting	Assess etiology of vomiting. Administer antiemetics.
Constipation	Discourage straining. Maintain bowel regimen to prevent constipation (see Chapter 12B). Avoid the rectal route for medication administration and temperature assessment. No enemas.
Emotional stressors	Avoid emotional stress.
	Counsel family to maintain a calm atmosphere.
	Avoid disturbing conversations at the patient's bedside.
	Help to maintain open channels of communication between patient, family, and interdisciplinary team.
	Cautious use of benzodiazapines, opioids & neuroleptics for sedation.
Environmental factors	
Excess stimulation	Explain the unavoidable hallway and equipment noises. Make attempts to minimize excess stimulation. Provide a quiet, darkened room. Discourage the use of television or radio.
	Restrict visitors to close family and friends.
	Make other hospital personnel (e.g., housekeeping, venipuncture team) aware of the need to avoid excess stimulation. Place sign in doorway.

Table 15A–4 *(Continued)*
Nursing Protocol for the Management of Increased Intracranial Pressure

Factor	Intervention
Stability of surroundings	Provide consistent nursing personnel.
	Develop a predictable daily care routine. Provide periods of uninterrupted rest.
	Avoid clustering of nursing activities because of risk for increasing ICP.
Safety factors	Observe frequently.
	Create a mechanism for patient to call the nurse if unable to use call light/bell.
	Maintain all bed side rails in the elevated position.
	Supervise and/or assist with ambulation and ADL.
	Minimize hazards of immobility.
	Assess skin integrity. Institute measures to maintain skin integrity. Assess for signs/symptoms of deep vein thrombosis. (See Chapter 16F.)
	Apply pneumatic compression devices or elastic stockings as ordered.
	Institute seizure precautions if a history of seizures exists or if patient is at risk.
	Monitor for seizure activity. Administer anticonvulsant medications and monitor their blood level.
Treatment factors Steroids	Establish baseline mental status and monitor for changes. Minimize risk for GI disturbances. Steroids should be taken with meals, antacids, or milk. Avoid aspirin. Guaiac stool for occult blood. Minimize risk of infection. Avoid invasive procedures. Monitor CBC. Encourage all persons who come in contact with patient to wash hands. Maintain nutritional status. High-protein, high-calcium diet. Monitor for hyperglycemia and glucosuria. Monitor electrolytes, especially sodium and potassium. Weigh patient daily. Teach patient and family about visible changes (acne, abnormal fat distribution, facial changes, hirsutism). Advise them that these changes are reversible and will subside when steroid therapy is discontinued.
Diuretics	Monitor serum electrolytes glucose and chemistries. Keep an accurate record of intake and output. Monitor BP.

FIO_2—fraction of inspired oxygen; SaO_2—saturated arterial oxygen; PaO_2—partial pressure of arterial oxygen; $PaCO_2$—partial pressure of arterial carbon dioxide

complications. In supporting the respiratory system, the nurse must protect the patient's airway. Proper positioning of the neck, as previously mentioned, provides for an open airway, drainage of secretions, and prevention of aspiration, especially in the patient with altered level of consciousness. The nurse must auscultate the chest for breath sounds. Atelectasis can occur with prolonged bedrest. In this setting, deep breathing and coughing is contraindicated due to its effect on intrathoracic pressure. Monitoring oxygen saturation and blood gases will provide information on the oxygenation of the patient.

In addition to prolonged bedrest, a diagnosis of cancer and the presence of intravenous catheters puts the patient at an even higher risk for deep vein thrombosis. Pneumatic extremity compression devices and low-level anticoagulation therapy are indicated. Special attention must be given to the skin because of the medical necessity of bedrest (see Chapter 16F).

If the patient is unable to eat, intravenous or enteral nutrition should be provided. The patient should be monitored for electrolyte imbalances, hydration status, intake and output, and daily weights. Finally, the stress of the illness and the use of antibiotics and steroids put the patient at risk for gastric ulcerations. Gastrointestinal prophylaxis is indicated.

CONCLUSION

Patients with diagnosis of cancer can suffer from increased ICP due to a variety of etiologies. The nurse's role is to identify patients with changes in their neurological function, limit activities that could increase ICP, and provide support to the patient and family.

BIBLIOGRAPHY

1. Ackerman, L. L. Alteration in level of responsiveness: A proposed nursing diagnosis. *Neuroscience Nursing,* 28, 729–745. 1993.

   This article includes overview of neurological nursing assessment.

2. Bates, B. *A Guide to Physical Examination and History Taking.* J.B. Lippincott, Philadelphia. 1995.

   This classic reference includes a thorough neurological assessment.

3. Ganong, W. F. *Review of Medical Physiology.* Appleton & Lange. Norwalk, CT. 1995.

   This book reviews basic medical physiology, including a chapter on cerebral blood flow and circulation, CSF circulation, blood brain barrier, and factors affecting cerebral blood flow.

4. Glick, J. H. and D. Glover. Oncologic emergencies. In G. Murphy, W. Laurence, and R. Lenhard (Eds.), *American Cancer Society Textbook of Clinical Oncology.* pp. 605–607. American Cancer Society, Atlanta. 1995.

   A section in the chapter about oncologic emergencies discusses the pathophysiology, clinical presentation, diagnosis, and treatment of brain metastases.

5. Guyton, A. C. and J. E. Hall. *Human Physiology and Mechanism of Disease.* W. B. Saunders Co., Philadelphia. 1997.

   This is a classic physiology text.

6. Hickey, J. V. *The Clinical Practice of Neurological and Neurosurgical Nursing.* J.B. Lippincott. Philadelphia. 1997.

   This book is an excellent reference concerning neuroscience nursing with chapters dedicated to neurological examination, assessment, and increased intracranial pressure.

7. Netter, F. H. *The CIBA collection of medical illustrations, Volume 1:* Nervous system. West Caldwell, NJ: CIBA-GIEGY Co. 1986.

   This book contains medical illustrations and radiographic images of brain tumors, infections, cerebral vascular disease, and hypoxic brain damage.

8. Ropper, A. H. Treatment of intracranial hypertension. In A. Ropper (Ed.), *Neurological and Neurosurgical Intensive Care.* pp. 29–52. Raven Press, New York. 1993.

   This chapter gives a summary of medical treatment for increased intracranial pressure.

9. Ropper, A. H. and M. A. Rockoff. Physiology and clinical aspects of raised intracranial pressure. In A. Ropper (Ed.), *Neurological and Neurosurgical Intensive Care.* pp. 11–28. Raven Press, New York. 1993.

   This chapter discusses the pathophysiology of increased ICP.

10. Sherwood, L. *Human Physiology: From Cells to Systems.* West Publishing Co., St. Paul, MN. 1989.

    This is a basic human physiology text.

11. Thapar, K. and E. R. Laws. Tumors of the central nervous system. In G. Murphy, W. Laurence, R. Lenhard (Eds.), *American Cancer Society Textbook of Clinical Oncology.* pp. 378–410. American Cancer Society, Atlanta. 1995.

    This text gives an overview of cancers, with a specific chapter dedicated to tumors of the CNS.

15B

B. Spinal Cord Compression

Diahann Kazierad

Cancer is the most common cause of spinal cord compression (SCC); approximately 95 percent of cases are due to metastatic spread, and the remaining 5 percent are caused by primary tumors of the spinal cord. Patients with solid tumors of the lung, breast, kidney, and prostate are at greatest risk for the development of SCC. Less commonly, hematologic malignancies such as lymphoma and multiple myeloma are involved. Patients with SCC present with neurologic dysfunction, and the degree of this dysfunction is the most powerful predictor of treatment outcome. Prompt intervention to relieve the SCC is required to prevent permanent disability. If motor function or sphincter control is lost, the majority of patients will not be able to regain this function.

PATHOPHYSIOLOGY

Spinal cord compression is classified by location and level, and its effects are summarized in Table 15B–1. Extradural tumors arise outside of the dura mater that lines the spinal cord in the vertebral bodies, paravertebral space, or epidural tissues. The majority of extradural lesions are within the vertebral bodies and are a result of metastatic spread. Intramedullary tumors occur within the cord itself and can be caused by gliomas or metastatic spread. Extramedullary tumors arise under the dura mater and occur within the meninges or subarachnoid space. The level of the lesion is either cervical, thoracic, or lumbosacral. Spinal cord compression caused by metastasis most commonly occurs at the thoracic level.

Compression of the spinal cord is a result of either collapse of the vertebrae from metastatic involvement or because of direct tumor extension. Both mechanisms apply pressure upon the cord. Based on postmortem findings and animal models of SCC, the compression causes circulatory disturbances within the arterial and venous microvasculature of the cord. Vascular congestion, increased vascular permeability, edema, ischemia, and infarction can occur. Complete transection of the spinal cord at any point will result in loss of sensory, motor, and autonomic function below the level of the lesion (i.e. quadriplegia, paraplegia). Partial or incomplete spinal cord transection will cause an unequal pattern of motor/sensory loss.

CLINICAL MANIFESTATIONS

Back pain is the most common symptom in patients with SCC. A typical history of the patient with acute SCC is one of progressive back pain that occurs up to six months prior to the diagnosis. The pain is described as either local or radicular. Local back pain is located close to the site of the actual compression and is constant, dull, and aching in nature. This type of pain is aggravated by lying supine, coughing, Valsalva maneuvers, sneezing, straining, or motion, and it is relieved by sitting. Radicular pain occurs along involved nerve roots of the spinal cord in a similar pattern to the dermatomes (Figure 15B–1). Patients might complain of intermittent, shooting pain. Bilateral band-like pain is characteristic of thoracic lesions, whereas unilateral pain is more common of cervical or lumbar lesions. Sudden, severe, agonizing pain, along with loss of motor and sensory function, indicates acute vertebral collapse, an oncologic emergency.

Some type of *sensory dysfunction* will occur with SCC. The specific deficit will depend on the level of the lesion, whether the lesion is partial or complete, and the sensory nerve tract (spinothalmic, posterior column) involved. In general, patients describe paresthesia, with numbness, tin-

Table 15B-1
Signs and Symptoms of Spinal Cord Compression by Vertebral Level

Location	Signs and Symptoms
Cervical—above C4	Respiratory compromise Weakness to paralysis from neck down Paresthesia Neck pain Occipital headache Cranial nerve VIII–XII dysfunction
Cervical—below C4	Shoulder and arm pain Paresthesias of upper extremities Weakness to paralysis from clavicles down Atrophy of upper extremity muscles associated with fasciculations of the muscles Horner's syndrome (ptosis, miosis, anhidrosis on the affected side) Hyperactive reflexes (occurs with upper motor neuron compression only)
Thoracic (T1–T12)	Chest/back pain Sensory deficits correspond with dermatomes Band-like hyperesthesia is often found above the level of the lesion Weakness to paralysis (remember landmarks T4 at nipple level and T10 at umbilicus) Positive Babinski Bowel and bladder dysfunction Sexual dysfunction
Lumbosacral (L1–S5)	Lower back pain which may radiate down legs and/or perineal area Weakness to paralysis of lower extremities Sensory loss of lower extremities Saddle anesthesia Bowel and/or bladder dysfunction Sexual dysfunction Diminished or absent lower extremity reflexes (occurs with compression of nerve roots off the cauda equina) Foot drop Atrophy of muscle groups

gling, and coolness of the extremity involved. Symptoms ascend from toes up to the level of the lesion in the spinal cord.

Motor dysfunction can occur at the same time or after sensory dysfunction. Weakness occurs in approximately 80 percent of patients and is the second most common symptom. Weakness will progress to paralysis as the SCC continues. Motor dysfunction depends on the level of the lesion, whether it is a partial or complete lesion, and which tract (corticospinal, extrapyramidal, cerebellar system) is involved. Patients might complain of heaviness of their

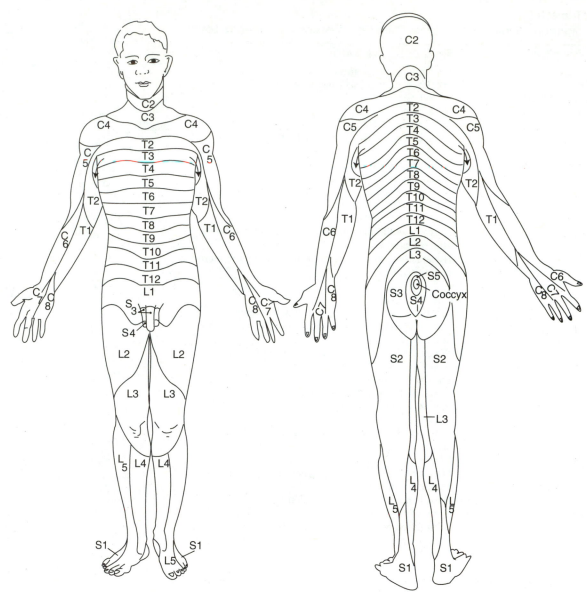

Figure 15B–1. Cutaneous distribution of spinal nerves (dermatomes).

extremities and report clumsiness and spasticity. The majority of patients with SCC who are unable to walk will not regain this function.

Reflexes will also be affected by SCC according to the location of the lesion. Direct compression on the upper motor neurons will cause hyperreflexia, whereas compression of the lower motor neurons will cause diminished to absent reflexes. Mixed upper and lower motor neuron compression will result in absent reflexes.

Symptoms of *bowel and bladder dysfunction* typically occur late in SCC and are associated with irreversible neurological damage. Bowel and bladder dysfunction presenting as the first signs of SCC could represent direct compression of the cauda equina or conis medullaris. Patients may complain of urethral, vaginal, and rectal numbness known as saddle anesthesia. Other symptoms include urinary hesitancy, frequency, urgency, retention, incontinence, constipation, and impotence.

ASSESSMENT

Assessment includes a thorough history of the patient's subjective complaints, eliciting specific information about onset, duration, and characteristics of symptoms. The patient should be asked about sensory changes, motor weakness, poor coordination, and any change in bowel and bladder habits, or change in sexual functioning. A complete neurological exam is performed initially to establish baseline function (see Chapter 11). Serial, focused neurological nursing assessments are done to monitor for subsequent changes in the patient's neurological function, understanding that SCC affects all function below the level of the lesion.

The patient with suspected SCC warrants immediate evaluation. In order to diagnose the level, location (e.g., intramedullary, extradural), size, and type (primary versus secondary) of the lesion within the spinal cord, several diagnostic studies can be performed, including magnetic resonance imaging and computerized tomography scans. Other diagnostic studies include lumbar puncture with CSF analysis, needle biopsy, and bone scans.

Vital Signs

Assessment of a patient's vital signs should focus on the ABCs: intact *airway*, effective *breathing* pattern, and adequate *circulation*. Patients with lesions of the cervical vertebrae are at risk for alterations in ventilation. A lesion at C4 or above can cause interruption of the innervation of the diaphragm, leading to respiratory compromise. Rate, depth, rhythm, and symmetry of respirations should be assessed. Neurogenic shock—characterized by severe orthostatic hypotension, bradycardia, and a low body temperature—is caused by sudden loss of peripheral sympathetic vasomotor control. Neurogenic shock occurs only as the result of acute, rapid spinal cord compression, such as might happen with rapidly growing tumors or acute vertebral collapse. Slow-growing tumors and metastasis will rarely cause neurogenic shock

Sensory Function

A complete sensory examination is detailed in Chapter 11. Beginning at the toes and moving upward bilaterally, both sides should be assessed in an orderly fashion to determine the level at which function is intact. Dermatomes can be used as anatomical landmarks to guide the assessment (Figure 15B–1). Just above the level of the spinal cord lesion, there might be a narrow band of hyperesthesia. In addition, vertebral percussion or palpation could elicit pain one or two vertebral bodies away from the level of compression. Touching the patient's skin with either light touch, pinprick, or a warm or cool object will test the spinothalamic tract. The patient's ability to identify where he or she has been touched will signify posterior column nerve function. It is important to assess the patient's level of pain, as increased intensity could indicate worsening SCC.

Motor Function

Assessment of the three motor tracts involves testing gait, coordination, strength, and muscle tone (Chapter 11). Observe the patient while walking to assess for ataxic gait. Observation of the patient performing activities of daily living (ADLs) will provide an assessment of fine and gross motor coordination. Assess for muscle strength and symmetry of movement:

0 = No muscle contraction
1 = Trace of a muscle contraction
2 = Active movement of the body part with gravity eliminated
3 = Active movement against gravity
4 = Active movement against gravity and some resistance
5 = Active movement against full resistance without evident fatigue.

Heel walking and toe walking can reveal subtle lower extremity weakness. Passive range of motion exercises are used to assess the patient for flaccid or spastic muscle tone. Flaccid muscles could indicate lower motor neuron damage, whereas muscles with increased tone and spasticity could indicate upper motor neuron damage. Assessment of cranial nerves VIII–XII might reveal motor dysfunction caused by a high cervical lesion.

Reflexes

Spinal reflexes are a function of both the sensory and motor systems (Table 15B–2). Reflexes are graded on a scale of 0 to 4+:

Table 15B–2
Spinal Reflexes

Reflex	Spinal Level
Plantar (Babinski)	Lumbar 5, Sacral 1
Ankle	Sacral 1
Patellar	Lumbar 2, 3, 4
Abdominal—upper	Thoracic 8, 9, 10
—lower	Thoracic 10, 11, 12
Biceps	Cervical 6, 7

4+ = Very brisk
3+ = Brisker than average
1+ = Diminished
0 = No response

Hyperreflexia occurs with upper motor neuron dysfunction. In addition, a positive Babinski sign, with fanning of the toes, indicates upper motor neuron damage. Absent reflexes indicate lower motor neuron dysfunction. Acute spinal cord injury can result in spinal shock, with temporary loss of all reflexes below the level of the lesion. Although spinal shock can last from hours to months, spinal neurons gradually regain excitability, and reflexes return.

Autonomic Function

Assessment of bowel and bladder control will indicate the extent of impairment. Patients presenting with bowel and / or bladder dysfunction will most likely not regain this function following treatment.

The patient should be assessed for bowel sounds, abdominal distention, anal reflex, and rectal tone. The anal reflex is elicited by stroking the skin near the anus, which causes puckering of the sphincter.

Assessment of the urinary system includes urine output over the previous 24 hours, time and amount of last voiding, and the presence of such symptoms as bladder distention, overflow, retention, dribbling, stress incontinence, frequency, urgency, and nocturia.

MEDICAL MANAGEMENT

The treatment of SCC should include a multidisciplinary approach involving oncology, neurology, neurosurgery, and radiation therapy. The goal of medical management is to relieve the compression as rapidly as possible in order to prevent further damage to the spinal cord, thereby preserving maximum function. Pain relief, prevention of local recurrence, and provision of spinal stability are additional goals of therapy. Patient prognosis is related to many pretreatment factors (see Table 15B–3).

The choice of treatment is dependent on the following factors: (1) tumor histology, (2) location (anterior versus posterior), (3) primary versus secondary tumor, (4) mechanism of compression, (5) initial neurological function prior to therapy, (6) speed of progression, (7) degree of spinal involvement, (8) prior radiation therapy to the area involved, and (9) expected patient survival. The average length of survival following diagnosis of SCC due to metastatic spread of cancer is three to four months.

Table 15B–3
Prognostic Indicators for Spinal Cord Compression

Indicator at Diagnosis	Improved Prognosis	Poor Prognosis
Pretreatment motor status	Ambulatory	Paralysis
Rapidity/severity of motor dysfunction	Slow onset/less severe symptoms	Fast onset/more severe symptoms
Duration of motor dysfunction, paralysis	Less than 24 hr	More than 48 hr
Sphincter control	Present	Absent, bladder involvement
Tumor location	Posterior, epidural space	Anterior, epidural space, extradural
Bony involvement of vertebral column	No structural loss, stable spine	Structural loss, unstable spine, vertebral collapse
General location of tumor	Lumbar, sacral	Cervical, thoracic
Primary cancer site	Breast, prostate, multiple myeloma lymphoma, neuroblastoma	Lung
	Responsive to RT	Unresponsive to RT

Adapted with permission from Bruckman, J. E., and W. D. Bloomer. Management of spinal cord compression. *Seminars in Oncology* 5 (2): 135–140. 1978.

Radiation

Radiation therapy (RT) is the mainstay of treatment for patients with SCC; the goal is to shrink the tumor compressing the spinal cord. It is indicated for radiosensitive tumors (lymphoma; seminoma; myeloma; neuroblastoma; cancers of the breast, prostate, lung), in conjunction with surgical intervention for SCC, and for slow onset SCC; it is instituted as soon as possible following diagnosis. In general the total dose of radiation therapy is 3000–4000 cGy to the cord over two to four weeks with a maximum tolerated dose of 4500 cGy. Radiation is often used concurrently with steroids. Recovery to baseline function after radiation therapy could be delayed for months.

Steroids

Dexamethasone is initiated immediately following the diagnosis of SCC to reduce edema of the cord around the tumor site and thereby reduce some of the effects of the cord compression. The dosage and schedule of administration are controversial and will vary among physicians and institutions. Usual doses are 10 mg followed by 4 to 24 mg every six hours, which is then tapered over several days to weeks. Higher doses of steroids could be used to provide pain relief in this setting. Steroids are often used in combination with radiation therapy and surgery.

Surgery

Surgery is indicated for patients with SCC of unknown histology, spinal instability, compression of the cord by bone fragments, progression of symptoms during radiation therapy, rapidly progressing SCC, recurrent SCC following RT, and extramedullary tumors. The significant morbidity associated with surgery for SCC, as well as the long postoperative convalescence, requires an estimated survival greater than two months and a reasonable general medical condition. Depending on the site of tumor, either a laminectomy (posterior cord) or decompression with mechanical stabilization (anterior cord) is performed. Radiation therapy might follow stabilization of the spinal cord.

Chemotherapy

The use of chemotherapy for the treatment of SCC is limited. Patients who are not candidates for radiation or surgery and who have tumors responsive to chemotherapy could benefit. Chemotherapy can also be used to supplement the effects of RT or surgery.

Pain Management

Steroid therapy, radiation, surgery, and chemotherapy can be effective in reducing pain caused by SCC. However, the patient will also require pharmacologic analgesic support (see Chapter 8A). Opioids are usually required to treat the pain caused by SCC. Special consideration should be given to the route of administration (PO, rectal, IV, SL), around the clock dosing, and breakthrough dosing. If opioids are given by continuous infusion, frequent assessment of respiratory status is necessary.

For each level of pain, adjuvant drugs and strategies can be used to provide relief. Non-opioids can be combined with the opioids to enhance pain relief. In addition, patients with SCC due to bone metastases might benefit from bisphosphonate compounds such as pamindronate, as bisphosphonates inhibit the bone destruction that occurs with vertebral metastases.

NURSING MANAGEMENT

Nursing management includes an individualized plan of care based on commonly recognized potential and actual problems that occur in acute SCC (Table 15B–4). Nursing actions center on preventing further damage to the spinal cord when suspected or documented vertebral instability is present. The nurse should consider the patient's spine unstable until proven otherwise. The objectives of care include early identification of neurological changes, maintenance of vital functions, pain control, management of sensory and motor deficits and their impact on ADLs, and management of bowel and bladder dysfunction (Chapter 12). Following stabilization of the patient, nurses must work collaboratively with physical therapy, occupational therapy, social services, home health care agencies, and the family to provide optimum care for this patient population.

Measurement of temperature, pulse, respiratory rate, blood pressure, and pulse oximetry should be obtained on admission. Cardiac monitoring may be necessary. The nurse must be aware of possible orthostatic changes due to neurogenic shock. Ongoing monitoring by the nurse at hourly intervals is warranted until the patient is stable. The risk of respiratory impairment is present with cervical and high thoracic lesions. Acute respiratory insufficiency could result, necessitating mechanical ventilation. Pulmonary hygiene should be instituted to prevent hypoventilation, atelectasis, and pneumonia (see Chapter 14).

Management of potential skin impairment begins on admission. A preventive approach is mandatory (see Chapter 10C).

Table 15B-4

Nursing Protocol for the Management of Acute Spinal Cord Compression

Factor	Intervention
Potential for vasomotor instability (from effects of CNS involvement)	Assess baseline vital signs (apical heart rate, pulse, respiratory rate, core temperature, extremity temperature, BP). Perform ongoing assessment hourly until stabilized. Diagram baseline sweating patterns. Neurogenic shock rare in this setting.
Potential for further injury to the spinal cord from unstable spinal column (increased risk with cervical and thoracic lesions)	Prevent rotation of the patient's head with cervical lesions (cervical collar, sandbags along either side of head, no pillows on the bed, support head and neck at all times). Prevent further movement of the spine if there is suspected or documented vertebral instability. Evaluate the need for a special neuro bed and/or stabilizing devices. Use a firm mattress. Maintain spinal alignment during turning and positioning (log-roll to turn, pull sheet on bed for moving the patient in bed). Use 2 people to turn patient. Advocate bed rest until instability is disproven or treatment is completed. Determine if an external brace is indicated (consult with the physician). Position the patient with spine in proper alignment (supine with footboard, no pillows). Assess movement, strength, and coordination q 8 hr. Document neuro check q 8 hr. Perform passive ROM to all extremities q 8 hr.
Potential alteration in comfort: pain related to tumor involvement of vertebral body and/or spinal cord	Provide ongoing pain assessment. Document methods used for pain control, and evaluate their effectiveness. Administer analgesics on a continuous schedule. Administer analgesics for break through pain. Explore alternative methods of pain control. See Chapter 8A.
Actual or potential alteration in skin related to motor and sensory impairment	Perform ongoing assessment of skin status q 2 hr. Provide skin care q 2 hr (turn and position q 2 hr, provide meticulous hygiene, massage bony prominences q 2 hr). Provide clean, dry, unironed, and unstarched bed linens. Provide nail and foot care. Provide a footboard on the bed to prevent foot drop. Monitor continually for irritants (e.g., heat, pressure, abrasion). See Chapter 10C.
Potential for ventilatory dysfunction related to impairment of intercostal and diaphragmatic muscles (increased risk with thoracic and cervical lesions)	Turn and position the patient q 2 hr. Perform pulmonary toilet q 2 hr (coughing, deep breathing, incentive spirometer [withhold percussion/vibration if spine is potentially unstable]). Suction as necessary. Provide ongoing assessment (need for ventilatory assistance [oxygen, IPPB, respirator, etc.], respiratory patterns and lung sounds, signs and symptoms of respiratory insufficiency, pulse oximetry). Maintain humidified environment. See Chapter 14.
Potential for alteration in bowel elimination related to loss of voluntary control, immobility, and sphincter dysfunction	Assess anal reflex and sphincter tone to monitor for progression of SCC or assess residual function after SCC is stabilized. Observe for signs and symptoms of paralytic ileus and impaction (check for abdominal distension, decreased or absent bowel sounds [hypotonic], nausea, and vomiting). Record and describe all stools. Perform digital examination on admission to determine if a stool is present in the rectal vault. Begin a bowel training program. See Chapter 12B.

Continued

Factor	Intervention
	Obtain a physician's order for laxative.
	Encourage liberal fluid intake (~3,000 ml/d).
	Encourage a high-fiber diet (5–10 g/d) and the use of natural laxatives (e.g., prunes, juices).
	Correct abdominal distension with antiflatulents, rectal tubes, and colon lavage.
	Provide ongoing assessment of bowel pattern with daily documentation of bowel sounds and stools.
Potential for alteration in urinary elimination related to overdistension of bladder and sphincter dysfunction from loss of voluntary control	Monitor urine output (check residual urine after each voiding, measure output q 1–2 hr, notify the physician if output is <60 ml/hr).
	Provide ongoing assessment (distension, retention, need for catheterization, signs and symptoms of urinary tract infection, laboratory values [BUN, creatinine, urinalysis]).
	Begin program of intermittent catheterization (see Chapter 12C).
	Encourage liberal fluid intake (~3000 ml/d).
Potential safety needs	Assess need for assistive devices.
	Provide assistive devices as indicated.
	Monitor environment for hazards as well as for potential adaptable changes.
Actual or potential rehabilitative needs	Assess functional impairments, degree of disability, and projected duration/prognosis.
	Teach patient to perform muscle-setting exercise (quadriceps and gluteal sets), leg exercises, upper extremity exercises.
	Plan for and practice progressive ambulation.
	Assess ability to assist, tolerance to activities.
	Obtain physical therapy and occupational therapy consult.
	Consider use of transfer techniques, teach patient same.
Potential complications from immobility	Consider use of venodyne boots or antiembolic stockings.
	See Chapter 11.
	Administer anticoagulants as ordered.
	Encourage ambulation as appropriate.
Potential autonomic dysreflexia (associated with lesions T8 and above) (Post-acute rehabilitation phase)	Continually assess for headache, acute increases in blood pressure, redness above the lesion level with pallor below, bradycardia, nasal congestion, sneezing, visual blurring, seizures, goose bumps.
	Monitor closely for distended bladder; promptly catheterize if necessary.
	Elevate head of bed 30–45 degrees.
	Lower foot of bed.
	Notify the physician promptly.
	Anticipate medication orders for short-acting antihypertensive medications and ganglionic blocking medications.
Lack of knowledge	Provide patient with information about SCC, its sequelae, and treatment.
	Teach patient to function within any residual disabilities.
	Provide opportunity for patient to learn techniques to aid in ADL.
	Assess ADL patterns and assist the patient to work toward methods of surmounting deficits.
	Assist patient to identify activities that can be attained, those that can be attained in the future, and those activities that are permanently unattainable.
	Assist patient to develop a daily activity plan that works toward agreed-upon goals.

IPPB, intermittent positive-pressure breathing; CNS, central nervous system; BP, blood pressure; ROM, range of motion; ADL, activities of daily living; SCC, spinal cord compression.

Loss of voluntary control of bowel and bladder function can result from the SCC. Often, paralytic ileus and abdominal distention occur, followed by constipation and impaction. The use of opioids to control pain can exacerbate bowel dysfunction. A bowel maintenance program should be initiated when these problems are identified (Chapter 12B). Loss of voluntary control of micturition can result in overdistention of the bladder, urine retention, and urinary tract infection. Ongoing observation to detect distention early and the use of catheterization if necessary to empty the bladder are effective preventative approaches. All patients should be checked for residual urine after voiding. If impairment is present, a schedule of intermittent catheterization can be instituted during the acute phase of SCC (Chapter 12C).

Following treatment for acute SCC, sexual functioning in both males and females with SCC might be impaired. Return of sexual function depends on prior functioning, level and duration of compression, extent of damage to the spinal cord, and status of the sacral reflex pathways. Loss of bowel and bladder control and persistent pain can interfere with the patient's sexual function. The nurse should direct the patient and his or her partner to appropriate sources for counseling and promote dialogue between the affected parties (Chapter 13).

FOLLOW-UP CARE

After discharge, this patient will require ongoing medical and nursing care. The patient should be assessed at regular intervals for signs of disease progression or recurrent SCC. Patients who suffer permanent neurological damage require more intensive nursing care to maintain quality of life. This can include referrals to home care agencies, physical and occupational therapy, and use of community resources. Common problems during this phase include altered coping and nutrition. The reader should refer to specific chapters in this book as well as other sources for the long-term care of the patient following spinal cord injury.

BIBLIOGRAPHY

1. Averbuch, S. D. New bisphosphonates in the treatment of bone metastases. *Cancer* 72: 3443–3452. 1993.

   The pathogenesis of skeletal metastases, conventional management, and the use of bisphosphonates are discussed. Clinical studies of bisphosphonates in a variety of cancers are presented.

2. Cherney, N. I., and K. M. Foley. Non-opioid and opioid analgesic pharmacotherapy of cancer pain. *Pain & Palliative Care* 10(1): 79–101. 1996.

   This article is a review of the pharmacotherapy effective in treating cancer pain.

3. Fisher, G., D. K. Mayer, and C. Struthers. Bone metastases: Part I—pathophysiology. *Clinical Journal of Oncology Nursing* 1(2): 29–35. 1997.

   The article discusses the normal bone physiology, the effects of metastatic spread, and clinical and diagnostic evaluation of the patient with bony metastases.

4. Fuller, B. G, J. Heiss, and E. H. Oldfield. Spinal cord compression. In V. DeVita, S. Hellman, and S. Rosenberg, eds. *Cancer: Principles and Practice of Oncology.* 2476–2486. Lippincott-Raven, New York. 1997.

   This authoritative chapter provides a comprehensive discussion about the pathophysiology and treatment of SCC for the advanced practitioner.

5. Glick, J. H., and D. Glover. Oncologic emergencies. In G. P. Murphy, W. Lawrence, and R. E. Lenhard, eds. *American Cancer Society Textbook of Clinical Oncology.* 600–603. American Cancer Society, Atlanta. 1997.

   This American Cancer Society text is an excellent starting place for nurses new to cancer care.

6. Held, J. L., and A. Peahota. Nursing care of the patient with spinal cord compression. *Oncology Nursing Forum* 20(10): 1507–1516. 1993.

   This article reviews the etiology, clinical presentation, assessment, treatment, and nursing care related to spinal cord compression.

7. Labovich, T. M. Selected complications in the patient with cancer: Spinal cord compression, malignant bowel obstruction, malignant ascites, and gastrointestinal bleeding. *Seminars in Oncology Nursing* 10(3): 189–197. 1994.

   A section of this article is dedicated to the epidemiology, pathophysiology, clinical presentation, treatment, and nursing implications for patients with SCC.

8. Mayer, D. K., C. Struthers, and G. Fisher. Bone metastases: Part II—nursing management. *Clinical Journal of Oncology Nursing* 1(2): 37–44. 1997.

   Clinical management of spinal cord compression, including surgery, radiation therapy, and medical therapies is the focus of this article. Pain control is addressed.

9. Portenoy, R. K. Adjuvant analgesic agents. *Pain & Palliative Care* 10(1): 103–119. 1996.

   Management of bone pain beyond standard analgesics and radiation therapy, including the bisphosphonate compounds, is presented.

10. Portenoy, R. K., R. B. Lipton, and K. M. Foley. Back pain in the cancer patient: An algorithm for evaluation and management. *Neurology* 37: 134–138. 1987.

    This article describes the use of a systematic approach in assessing cancer patients who present with back pain. The patients are separated into emergent and nonemergent groups. Recommendations are given for each patient group.

11. Raney, D. J. Malignant spinal cord tumors: A review and case presentation. *Journal of Neuroscience Nursing* 23(1): 44–49. 1991.

    Pathophysiology, diagnosis, treatment, and nursing implications are addressed in this article. A section of the article focuses on neurological assessment and nursing diagnoses for a malignant spinal cord tumor and includes a case presentation.

C. Superior Vena Cava Syndrome

Kristen Kreamer

The superior vena cava (SVC) is the major venous channel returning blood from the head, neck, upper extremities, and upper thorax to the right side of the heart. Obstruction of the SVC interferes with venous drainage, resulting in increased venous pressure, dilation of superficial veins, and the development of collateral circulation. Superior vena cava syndrome (SVCS) is a complex of symptoms and physical findings associated with obstruction of the superior vena cava.

PATHOPHYSIOLOGY

15c

The SVC is particularly vulnerable to obstruction because of its physical properties, location, and relationship to surrounding structures. The vessel walls are thin and venous pressure low, so that it collapses easily. Tightly locked within the right anterior superior mediastinum, the SVC is bounded by rigid structures: sternum, vertebral bodies, right main bronchus, and trachea. It is encircled by the mediastinal and paratracheal lymph nodes at the junction with the azygos vein (Figure 15C–1).

Malignant disease accounts for 80 to 97 percent of cases of SVCS; in a significant number of them (perhaps as many as 60 percent), it is the presenting condition that leads to a cancer diagnosis. Lung cancer is responsible for approximately 70 to 85 percent of SVCS cases, the majority of cases (about 44 percent) are small cell carcinoma, 26 percent are squamous cell, 16 percent adenocarcinoma, and 14 percent other bronchogenic histologies. Lymphoma, primarily non-Hodgkin's, accounts for an additional 5 to 15 percent of cases. Other cancers, either primary or metastatic to this anatomical site, account for 7 percent to 9 percent of cases of malignant origin. Benign diseases (e.g., thyroid goiter, pericardial constriction, mediastinal fibrosis, aortic aneurysm, or infectious diseases) produce obstruction in 3 to 11 percent of cases of SVCS. Overall, 3 to 5 percent of lung cancer patients will develop SVCS during the course of the illness.

Partial or total occlusion of the SVC can result from extrinsic compression of the SVC and associated tributaries by the malignant tumor itself or by metastatic disease in the mediastinal and paratracheal nodes; direct involvement of vessel walls by tumor; thrombus formation within the vessels secondary to inflammation, venous stasis, and platelet aggregation; and/or foreign body–induced fibrotic reactions. Any of these factors, alone or in combination, can produce SVCS. With increasing frequency (3 per-

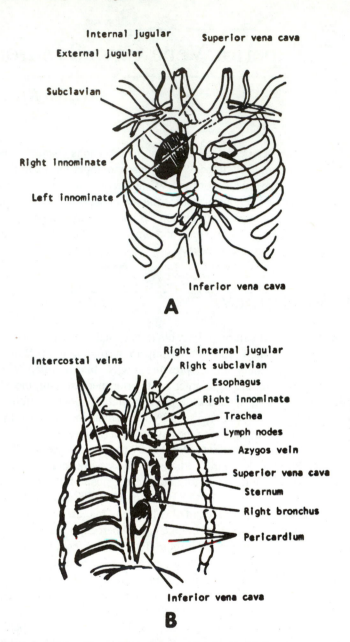

Figure 15C-1. Schematic representation of the frontal (A) and sagittal (B) sections of the thorax, showing the relationship of surrounding structures to the superior vena cava.

Reprinted with permission from Carabell, S. C., and R. L. Goodman. Superior vena cava syndrome. In DeVita, V. T., S. Hellman, and S. A. Rosenberg, eds. Cancer Principles and Practice of Oncology. J. B. Lippincott Co., Philadelphia. p. 1, 583. 1982.

cent to 5 percent of all cases) SVCS is associated with iatrogenic causes (e.g., thrombosis as a reaction to central venous and Swann Ganz catheters or pacemakers). One series of studies on central venous catheters and factors related to thrombus formation found a higher incidence with left-sided placement, particularly when the catheter tip lay in the innominate veins or in the upper half of the SVC.

CLINICAL MANIFESTATIONS

Symptoms of less than two weeks duration are reported by 20 to 30 percent of patients with SVCS, while about 35 percent give a history of between three and four weeks. Most frequently, patients complain of dyspnea, a sensation of fullness in the head, and of facial and neck swelling experienced as a "tight collar" feeling. The patient often notes swelling of the trunk and upper extremities, such that rings on fingers are tight. Chest pain, cough, and dysphagia are not uncommon. Central nervous system symptoms are relatively rare but could include headache, visual disturbance, anxiety, irritability, lethargy, or altered state of consciousness.

The clinician's suspicion of SVCS might be raised by a patient's report that symptoms are aggravated by lying down or bending over. Symptoms can also be more prominent in the morning and lessen as the day progresses and as gravity reduces the edema in the head and upper torso.

Physical findings on examination of the patient include thorax and neck vein distension, facial edema, and tachypnea of more than 30 breaths per minute. The face might become ruddy and edematous and achieve an appearance likened to that of a "purple frog." Cyanosis and edema of the upper extremities can be apparent. Interference with the cervical sympathetic nerve supply can result in hoarseness, because of paralysis of the true vocal cord, and/or in Horner's syndrome, a condition in which there is unilateral ptosis with a small, regular pupil and loss of sweating on the same side of the forehead. Table 15C–1 presents an organized approach to the nursing assessment of patients at risk for SVCS.

ASSESSMENT

Identification of SVCS will be facilitated by a complete and accurate review of the patient's subjective symptoms, along with the nurse's objective findings. Because SVCS frequently results from lung cancer, high-risk patients could be targeted by ascertaining whether there is a history of smoking or of exposure to environmental or occupational carcinogens. Strong suspicion of SVCS should be maintained for patients with already diagnosed malignancy, especially lung cancers and lymphomas.

The rapidity of onset of symptoms is a crucial factor in determining the patient's comfort and safety. More rapid onset precludes development

Table 15C-1
Nursing Assessment of Patients at Risk for Superior Vena Cava Syndrome

Factor	Assessment
Baseline	Vital signs
	Mental status
	Activity level
	Usual appearance
History	Malignant disease, particularly lung or lymphoma, or its predisposing factors (e.g., smoking)
	Duration of symptoms
	Presence of central venous catheter
	History of mediastinal RT
Presenting symptoms*	Dyspnea
	Facial and neck swelling (tightness of collar)
	Swelling of trunk and upper extremities (rings tight on fingers)
	Chest pain
	Cough
	Dysphagia
	CNS symptoms: headache, visual disturbances, anxiety, irritability, lethargy, altered state of consciousness
	Symptoms aggravated by lying down or bending over; symptoms greater in AM than later in the day
Physical findings*	Thorax and neck vein distension
	Facial edema
	Tachypnea (>30 breaths/min)
	Purple hue to face ("purple frog" look)
	Cyanosis and/or edema of upper extremities
	Hoarseness (caused by paralysis of true vocal cord)
	Horner's syndrome (unilateral ptosis with small, regular pupil and loss of sweating on same side of forehead)

*In order of most to least frequent.

of collateral circulation and can lead to greater circulatory compromise. The duration of symptoms tends to be longer for benign causes.

The diagnostic workup of a patient suspected of having SVCS includes a chest x-ray, which will be positive in approximately 80 percent of cases. Significant x-ray findings include evidence of mediastinal widening, a right superior mediastinal mass, mediastinal and paratracheal lymphadenopathy, and right-sided pleural effusion. A computerized tomography (CT) scan with IV contrast will be helpful when the chest x-ray is negative, and CT will also provide more detailed information about other critical structures such as the bronchi and spinal cord. Magnetic resonance imaging (MRI) will provide greater detail in multiple planes but costs more in time and money than CT. Radionuclide flow studies will be useful to pinpoint circulatory compromise; contrast venography could be done if surgical bypass is being considered.

Until the 1980s it was unanimously agreed that SVCS was a medical emergency, and treatment with radiation therapy (RT) was often initiated without a tissue diagnosis of malignancy. More recently, it has been recognized that a correct histologic diagnosis prior to instituting therapy is critical, because different modalities are effective and appropriate for different causes. Furthermore, RT before tissue sampling could make accurate histologic diagnosis more difficult, secondary to RT-induced tissue necrosis. In addition, the increasing incidence of benign causes of SVCS (for which RT is never helpful and potentially detrimental) requires diagnosis prior to treatment. Finally, contrary to previously held beliefs, SVCS itself is rarely fatal; it is recognized that poor outcome is related more to the underlying disease than to SVCS itself.

Procedures that can be undertaken to discover the histology of the lesion include biopsy obtained by bronchoscopy, CT-guided percutaneous fine needle aspiration, mediastinoscopy, lymph node biopsy of scalene or supraclavicular nodes, and cytologic examination of sputum, bronchial washings, or fluid obtained by aspiration from a pleural effusion. Thoracotomy would only be performed as a last resort. Diagnosis should be obtained with all reasonable speed with the goal of diagnosing and initiating treatment within 48 to 72 hours of presentation.

MEDICAL MANAGEMENT

The goals of medical therapy of SVCS are twofold: first, to relieve the symptoms, and second, to attempt to cure the underlying condition. When the underlying condition is a malignancy, cure is a realistic goal for small cell cancer of the lung (SCLC), lymphomas, and germ cell tumors.

Radiation therapy could be the treatment of choice for SVCS secondary to non–small cell lung cancer. It is also used in the rare instances in which a histologic diagnosis cannot be established or in cases in which the patient's clinical deterioration demands immediate treatment. Radiation can be given on either a high-dose or a conventional-dose schedule, with high doses initially resulting in more rapid relief of symptoms. On the high-dose schedule, the patient receives three to four daily doses of 300 to 400 cGy/dose, followed by smaller daily doses of 180 to 200 cGy until the total dose desired is reached. On the conventional-dose schedule, all daily doses are 180 to 200 cGy throughout therapy. The total dose required is determined by the type of tumor involved.

Chemotherapy is currently the primary therapy for SVCS in cases of SCLC or non-Hodgkin's lymphoma. Specific drugs and dosage schedules are determined by the type of tumor involved. In some cases RT can be added to chemotherapy in a combined approach to improve the chances of tumor cure or control.

Surgery is rarely used to treat these patients because it is of limited benefit and carries a high morbidity; however, venous bypass grafts using spiral vein, synthetic material, or autologous pericardium can be tried if other methods fail. Procedures such as balloon angioplasty might be attempted. Increasingly, expandable wire stents have been used effectively when the patient has received maximal RT to the area or when RT or chemotherapy fails to control the underlying disease and symptoms recur. These devices are placed under local anesthesia by interventional radiology through the femoral vein; the procedure takes about two hours. Stenting can also be employed when the patient is experiencing particularly acute symptoms, as relief is almost immediate after a successful stenting procedure. Although tumor invasion of the SVC is a contraindication to stent placement, the presence of thrombus is not. Thrombolysis can be attempted and continued up to, during, and after stent placement until the lumen is clear of all clot. Anticoagulation after stent placement, like prophylactic anticoagulation for central venous catheters, is a matter of continued controversy and might or might not be initiated, depending on individual clinical indicators.

Supportive medical management includes the prescription of oxygen for relief of dyspnea. Analgesics and tranquilizers could be ordered to decrease the patient's discomfort from chest pain and from the anxiety that often accompanies respiratory distress. Diuretics, particularly furosemide, could be ordered to provide rapid—though temporary—relief of the symptoms associated with fluid retention. In addition, sodium and fluid restriction could be instituted, although care must be taken to prevent dehydration, which can predispose to thrombus formation. There is also the risk of hypovolemia with impaired blood return to the heart secondary to vascular compromise.

Steroids, although of questionable efficacy, can be useful to treat respiratory compromise secondary to the inflammatory reaction associated with tumor and with RT. Anticoagulants might be indicated for SVCS associated with thromboses, but they could be problematic during invasive diagnostic procedures. When SVCS is catheter-induced, fibrinolytic drugs can be employed through the catheter itself as infusions over several hours to attempt to break up the clot. Streptokinase, urokinase, or tissue plasminogen activator could be used, but urokinase is the drug of choice because of its decreased incidence of allergenic and pyrogenic effects. If SVCS persists, the catheter might have to be removed, and anticoagulation with heparin and warfarin is initiated to prevent embolization. The use of low-dose warfarin (1 mg/day) as prophylaxis to prevent catheter-associated clots has been variously supported and refuted, and more research is needed to establish its efficacy.

For a majority of patients, symptoms improve. Good to excellent symptomatic relief has been reported by 95 percent of lymphoma patients and 70 percent of lung cancer patients. The length of time from initiation of therapy to noticeable improvement varies; some will get relief in three to four days, and approximately 50 to 70 percent of treated patients report improvement within two weeks.

Overall survival for patients treated for SVCS is poor, with only 10 to

20 percent living longer than two years. It must be kept in mind, however, that survival after SVCS depends on the type of malignancy involved and how responsive that malignancy is to current anticancer therapies. For instance, lymphoma patients, in general, live longer after developing SVCS than do lung cancer patients.

NURSING MANAGEMENT

Instituting measures for the relief of symptoms takes priority in the nursing care of patients with SVCS. The nurse should proceed quickly to relieve respiratory symptoms, arranging for the administration of oxygen, helping the patient to understand the role of gravity and positioning, discussing and implementing activity restrictions, and encouraging a calm, restful environment. For some patients, the body-image change, or "purple frog" appearance, is particularly distressing. The nurse should reassure the patient that the purplish color and edema will subside with successful therapy. The patient's objective response to medications, along with notable changes in physical findings, should be observed and documented.

The nurse must also monitor and educate the patient regarding possible complications of diagnostic procedures. Because of venous engorgement in the area, excessive bleeding can occur after invasive procedures; the nurse should assess the patient for signs of blood loss. Other postoperative care should be tailored to the specific procedure employed (e.g., the post-thoracotomy patient will have chest tubes and pleural drainage, whereas the postbronchoscopy patient should be evaluated for the return of the gag reflex).

The nurse should assess the patient for side effects of therapy and alleviate these when possible. The patient must be taught to recognize symptoms and to alert the nurse. The increasing use of combined modality treatment creates even greater challenges for nurses, who must educate patients experiencing potentiated side effects (e.g., more profound neutropenias with combined chemotherapy and RT).

Patients being treated with RT are likely to experience side effects, such as skin reaction, dysphagia, esophagitis, dry cough, fatigue, and nausea and/or vomiting. Suggestions for relief of these side effects are provided in Table 15C–2.

Side effects experienced by patients receiving chemotherapy depend largely on the particular agent employed (see Chapter 2C). In administering chemotherapy to SVCS patients, it is usually necessary to avoid the right arm as a phlebotomy or IV site, because there is likely to be increased venous pressure on the right side of the body, increasing the risk of bleeding after venipuncture. Furthermore, when the right arm is used for chemotherapy, decreased circulation could result in local accumulation of the drug, with poor absorption and local irritation. Some researchers and clinicians suggest that veins in the lower extremities be

Table 15C–2

Nursing Protocol for the Management of Superior Vena Cava Syndrome

Factor	Intervention
Respiratory compromise with hypoxia	
Dyspnea, orthopnea, tachypnea	Administer oxygen, monitor O_2 saturation.
	Vital signs q 4 hr till stable.
	Monitor for signs of increased respiratory distress (increased rate, increased use of accessory chest muscles, stridor, cyanosis, irritability, and restlessness).
	Position patient for maximal respiratory effort (probably orthopneic position, e.g., Fowler's).
	Limit activity by assisting with ADL.
Anxiety	Position call bell within reach and provide frequent reassurance of staff availability.
	Maintain a calm, restful environment.
	Assess need for and administer anxiolytics.
Circulatory compromise	
Venous stasis	Remove rings and restrictive clothing.
	Avoid right arm for venipuncture and for administration of parenteral medications.
	Monitor for excessive bleeding after invasive procedures in areas of venous engorgement.
	Elevate upper extremities on pillows to promote venous return.
	Assess skin integrity in edematous areas.
Side effects of anticoagulants and fibrinolytics	Observe for spontaneous bleeding, i.e., petechiae, ecchymoses, bleeding gums, epistaxis, melena, hematuria, headache, visual or mental status changes.
Metabolic/electrolyte disturbance	Weigh daily.
	Record intake and output.
Steroid therapy	Check urines for steroid-induced glycosuria.
	Evaluate for weakness of voluntary muscles.
	Assess for GI complaints of dyspepsia with hyperacidity.
	Be vigilant for focal signs of infection in absence of systemic complaints.
	Monitor for euphoria, mood swings, or other signs of CNS stimulation.
Diuretic therapy	Monitor for signs and symptoms of:
	hyponatremia: listlessness, mental confusion, loss of skin turgor, postural hypotension.
	hypokalemia: muscle weakness, decreased bowel sounds, depression, cardiac arrhythmias, tetany.
SIADH	See Chapter 16C.
Emotional/psychologic concerns	Provide brief, simple explanations of planned procedures and treatments.

Table 15C-2 *(Continued)*
Nursing Protocol for the Management of Superior Vena Cava Syndrome

Factor	Intervention
	Promote ventilation of concerns and feelings re: recent cancer diagnosis. Reassure that alterations in appearance will resolve with successful therapy.
Side effects of RT 　Skin reaction	See Chapter 2B. Do not remove purple marks indicating radiation ports. Wash area within marks with lukewarm water only; pat dry with towel. Do not use soaps, creams, ointments, or deodorants within radiation marks.
Dysphagia and esophagitis	Monitor quality and quantity of nutritional intake. Provide soft diet—avoid irritants such as alcohol, spices, extremes of temperature. Encourage small, frequent meals. Suggest antacids (carafate) for relief of burning on swallowing. Evaluate need for topical analgesia.
Dry cough	Increase humidity in room. Evaluate need for antitussives.
Fatigue	Assist patient in planning for periods of activity and rest.
Nausea and/or vomiting	Evaluate need for antiemetic 1/2 hr before therapy.
Side effects of chemotherapy	See Chapter 2C.

SIADH, syndrome of inappropriate antidiuretic hormone

used to administer medications; most, however, suggest central venous access when this is achievable, particularly for vesicants, in treating patients with SVCS.

The nurse must also monitor the patient for the side effects of drugs given for symptomatic relief; in particular, the nurse should be aware of the implications of steroid, anticoagulant, fibrinolytic, and diuretic therapy (see Table 15C–2). Hyponatremia and hypokalemia are relatively common side effects of diuretic drugs; in lung cancer patients, maintaining electrolyte balance can be complicated by syndrome of inappropriate antidiuretic hormone (SIADH), a metabolic oncologic emergency (see Chapter 16C).

The relatively rapid onset of symptoms and the intensity of the medical workup is especially distressing for those who previously had no idea that they had a malignant disease. Such patients and their families require additional support to deal not only with their immediate symptoms but also with the diagnosis of cancer. When diagnostic procedures and therapy are implemented without delay, there might not be enough time for thorough patient teaching. Nevertheless, each patient's need for information should be rapidly assessed and as much instruction provided as possible. Even a brief, simple explanation can alleviate the anxiety of patient and family.

More detailed information, along with continued reassurance and support, should be provided as part of the ongoing care of patients with SVCS. In most instances of SVCS, the patient can be treated entirely as an outpatient; therefore, both patient and family will need explicit yet understandable information with which they can monitor symptoms and report those that need attention. Preparing the patient and family for the integral role they will play in the management of this oncologic complication is one of the challenges facing the nurse caring for the patient with SVCS.

BIBLIOGRAPHY

1. Abner, A. Approach to the patient who presents with superior vena cava obstruction. *Chest* 103 (April): 394s–397s. 1993.

   This is a review of the pathogenesis, appropriate radiologic imaging, tissue diagnosis issues, and management of SVCS.

2. Jackson, J. and D. Brooks. Stenting of superior vena caval obstruction. *Thorax* 50 suppl 1: 531–536. 1995.

   This reviews practical aspects of stent insertion including types of stents, patient selection, and the role of thrombolysis and anticoagulation.

3. Mayo, D., D. Pearson, and M. Horne. Superior vena cava thrombosis associated with a central venous access device: A case report. *Clinical Journal of Oncology Nursing* 1(1): 5–10. 1997.

   This case report illustrates the typical presentation and treatment for superior vena cava thrombosis related to a venous access device. Excellent photographs clarify the SVC anatomy, and a Venous Access Device Flowsheet is provided.

4. Puel, V., M. Caudry, P. Metayer, J. Baste, D. Midy, C. Marsault, H. Demeaux, and J. Maire. Superior vena cava thrombosis related to catheter malposition in cancer chemotherapy given through implanted ports. *Cancer* 72(7): 2248–2251. 1993.

   This report studies on the relationship of catheter position to the development of catheter-related thromboses.

5. Stewart, I. Superior vena cava syndrome: An oncologic complication. *Seminars in Oncology Nursing* 12(4): 312–317. 1996.

   This reviews the clinical presentation, pathophysiology, diagnosis, treatment, and nursing care of SVCS.

D. Tracheal Obstruction

Sharon Dellinger
Lyn Sturdevant Davis

The trachea is a tube-like passageway through which air reaches the lungs. It is about 2.5 cm in diameter and 10–12.5 cm long and extends from the lower end of the larynx to the division of the right and left main bronchi. C-shaped rings cover the anterior part of the trachea; the trachea's posterior is contiguous with the esophagus.

Any reduction in tracheal lumen size (from tracheal stenosis, extrinsic compression, or a space-occupying luminal mass) compromises adequate gas exchange and respiratory functioning. Partial obstruction of the trachea impedes normal gas exchange, threatening life-sustaining respiratory and cardiovascular function. Without emergency intervention, complete obstruction of the trachea will rapidly lead to death.

PATHOPHYSIOLOGY

Primary tumors of the trachea are exceedingly rare. The most common types are squamous cell and adenoid cystic carcinomas. These tumors affect males twice as often as females and are frequently diagnosed late in their course. Tracheal obstruction with primary tumors results from intra-luminal tumor growth.

Secondary tumors involving the trachea are much more common than primary tracheal tumors. Those that occur most frequently are carcinomas of the larynx, lung, esophagus, and thyroid. Metastatic carcinomas of the head and neck, breast, and lymphomas can also involve the trachea. Tracheal obstruction from secondary tumors can result from direct tumor growth into the lumen or from encroachment and extrinsic compression from adjacent masses.

Tracheal obstruction because of secondary malignancies is sometimes caused by tumor growth in the mediastinum. This obstruction most often results from lesions developing in either the superior or the posterior medi-astinum (lymphomas and lung cancer). Lymphomas can cause impinge-ment and collapse of the tracheal wall, whereas lung cancers within the mediastinum often invade the trachea directly. Mediastinal tumor involve-ment is often associated with the development of superior vena cava syn-drome (SVCS) (see Chapter 15C).

Stenotic lesions resulting from a cuffed tracheostomy or endotracheal (ET) tube are the most common treatment-related cause of tracheal obstruction. A stenosis can develop at the tracheostomy site and/or at the inflatable cuff level. A *stomal stenosis* forms after the tracheostomy tube is removed and the margins unite in a fibrous scar. In a *cuff stenosis,* pressure that occurs between the inflated cuff and the tracheal wall leads to circumferential mucosal ulceration and tissue injury, with subsequent healing by concentric scar contracture. *Mechanical injury* from movement of the tube and cuff within the trachea is also believed to cause tracheal damage by abrading the mucous membrane, allowing bacterial colonization, tissue granulation, and scarring.

Because a tube will splint a cuff stenosis or potential stomal stenosis, symptoms of obstruction in nearly all cases appear after tube removal, usually within 90 days. In a small number of cases, however, obstructive symptoms have appeared as late as $1\frac{1}{2}$ years after extubation. Patients remain at risk for developing tracheal stenosis for at least two years after the tube is removed.

Stenotic lesions have been identified most frequently in patients who have received ventilatory assistance with cuffed tracheostomy or ET tubes; however, tracheal stenoses have also been seen in patients who have had cuffed tracheostomy tubes without ventilatory assistance. The advent of more aggressive management of cancer and its complications has resulted in increasing numbers of cancer patients who, as a result of intubation or tracheostomy, are at risk for stenotic lesions.

Radiation therapy (RT) is frequently employed to relieve malignant tracheal obstruction or to treat adjacent tumors before symptoms of obstruction appear. Within the first few days of treatment for tumors in the tracheal region, there might be local tissue swelling, presumably due to intracellular and extracellular edema resulting from cell damage. Therefore, the risk of tracheal obstruction and subsequent respiratory compromise can be accentuated during the initial phase of RT. Patients with chemotherapy-responsive tumors might also receive concomitant treatment with chemotherapeutic agents to augment radiation and surgical techniques.

CLINICAL MANIFESTATIONS

Reduction in tracheal lumen size, from whatever cause, impedes the normal flow of air to and from the lungs. The onset of obstruction can be acute, subacute, or chronic in nature. Patients with an acute onset of tracheal obstruction will seek medical assistance rapidly. Though the cause might not be apparent, the goal of immediate treatment is to relieve the obstruction through positioning, intubation, or tracheostomy. The onset of chronic obstruction is often subtle, allowing the patient time to compensate for a gradually worsening respiratory status. Symptoms are often unappreciated until the obstruction becomes subacute. At this time the airway is sufficiently compromised to cause hypercapnia with or without hypoxemia. The presence of respiratory acidosis complicates the management of these patients who still require urgent relief of obstruction.

Dysphonia and shortness of breath (especially with exertion) are early signs of upper airway obstruction. Wheezing, stridor, and orthopnea appear with progressive narrowing of the trachea. Cough is common, and hemoptysis might be present with primary tracheal tumors. Episodes of difficulty in clearing secretions can occur as the airway narrows. As airway obstruction progresses from mild to moderate to severe, level of consciousness deteriorates from normal to anxious or restless to lethargic and depressed.

ASSESSMENT

Diagnostic studies undertaken to evaluate tracheal obstruction include lateral films of the neck; posteroanterior, lateral, and oblique views of the chest; tracheal fluoroscopy; and tomography. Pulmonary function studies will confirm a high degree of airway obstruction in patients with lesions of the trachea. Bronchoscopy is usually deferred until preparations have been made for definitive treatment of the lesion, because post-bronchoscopy edema can precipitate complete obstruction.

When possible, the nurse obtains a history from the patient and/or family member regarding type, onset, and duration of symptoms, particularly shortness of breath, cough, and wheezing. Pulse oximetry is utilized to assess level of oxygenation. When airway obstruction is suspected, assessing for exercise-induced desaturation can precipitate distress and should be avoided. During physical assessment of the respiratory system, stridor could be present, as well as abnormal retraction of the interspaces and supraclavicular fossae during inspiration. Decreased breath sounds, rhonchi, and wheezes might be present on auscultation. Because patients with mediastinal malignancy are at risk for developing SVCS, the nurse should be alert for its associated signs and symptoms (see Chapter 15C).

MEDICAL MANAGEMENT

The most immediate concern in cases of tracheal obstruction is ensuring and maintaining a patent airway. Emergency or elective tracheostomy might be indicated before treatment of the cause is undertaken.

Primary Tumors of the Trachea

At present, surgical resection is the only potentially curative treatment for obstruction arising from primary tracheal carcinoma. Tracheal resection with end-to-end anastomosis is the recommended surgical approach. RT has been employed as an adjunct to surgical resection, either preoperatively or postoperatively, with variable results. Repeated endoscopic resections and RT are used as palliative methods of treatment for obstructing primary tracheal tumors.

Secondary Tumors

Secondary tumors involving the trachea are rarely amenable to tracheal resection, because in most cases the extent of disease precludes the potential for cure. Treatment aimed at the primary tumor utilizing chemotherapy and/or radiation therapy might relieve the obstruction. Endoscopic intubation—involving permanent placement of a small metal tube in the lower trachea—can be used emergently in acute respiratory obstruction and/or to provide long-term palliation for patients with malignant obstructing tracheal lesions. Because long-term stenting or use of tracheostomy tubes can injure normal tissue, self-sustaining stomas (flap-tracheostomy without tubes or stents) have been used in certain patients. Intraluminal brachytherapy using iridium 192, in varying doses, is used for palliation in lung cancer patients with obstructing lesions of the trachea and bronchus.

Tracheal obstruction associated with mediastinal tumor involvement or extrinsic tumor compression is often managed with chemotherapy and/or radiation therapy. Cure is possible when these modalities are utilized to treat responsive malignancies such as Hodgkin's disease. To reduce the potential for accentuating respiratory compromise during the initial phase of RT, oral steroids are administered before therapy begins and for the first days of treatment. In some cases, a tracheostomy can be performed before RT is started to avoid respiratory compromise from edema during the initial phase.

Postintubation Tracheal Stenosis

The preferred treatment for significant postintubation tracheal stenosis is resection and end-to-end anastomosis of the trachea. In less severe stenoses, or in cases in which surgery is not feasible, repetitive bronchoscopic dilations or dilation with intraluminal stenting (placement of an intraluminal tube, or stent, through the stenosis) can be used to maintain a patent airway. Retrograde tracheal bougienage has been employed to provide urgent relief of airway obstruction caused by tracheal stenosis. Endoscopic laser ablation of the stenosis is possible in early stage lesions with granulation tissue or in mature lesions with short segments of intraluminal fibrosis without cartilaginous skeletal involvement.

NURSING MANAGEMENT

Nursing intervention aimed at prevention or early detection of tracheal obstruction is outlined in Table 15D–1. The nurse should be alert to respiratory symptoms in patients with a history of tracheostomy or ET intubation. The early symptoms of airway obstruction (shortness of breath,

Table 15D–1
Nursing Protocol for Prevention and Early Detection of Tracheal Obstruction

Factor	Intervention
Malignancy Patients with metastatic/ advanced cancers of lung, larynx, head and neck, esophagus, breast, and thyroid; lymphomas and mediastinal tumor involvement.	Assess respiratory system. Obtain oxygen saturation. Evaluate for obstructive symptoms: shortness of breath, wheezing, difficulty clearing secretions, cough. Monitor for signs of obstruction: retraction of interspaces and supraclavicular fossae, abnormal lung sounds: decreased breath sounds, rhonchi, wheezes, and stridor. Educate regarding signs and symptoms requiring medical attention: shortness of breath, persistent cough, wheezing, difficulty clearing secretions.
Current treatment Patients intubated with ET or tracheostomy tubes.	Monitor cuff pressures Q shift using three way stopcock open simultaneously to cuff and manometer. Maintain at ≤20 mm Hg. Use minimal-leak or minimal-occluding-volume technique whenever possible. Prevent excessive tube movement: stabilize head position; stabilize tube and tubing. Limit transient cuff pressure elevations by judicious use of bagging and vibration; sedation as indicated to prevent "fighting" the ventilator. Use upright body position when possible to promote venous drainage and reduce edema in tracheal tissue.
Patients undergoing RT to obstructing tracheal tumors.	Monitor respiratory status closely (see Malignancy, above) especially during first 3 days of RT treatment. Observe for signs and symptoms of increasing obstruction. Educate regarding need to report to physician symptoms of increasing respiratory difficulty. Reinforce importance of taking oral steroids as prescribed.
Prior treatment Patients with prior history of ET or tracheostomy tube intubation, especially in conjunction with ventilatory assistance.	Assess respiratory system (see Malignancy, above). Evaluate for obstructive symptoms. Monitor for signs of obstruction. Educate regarding signs and symptoms requiring medical attention (see Malignancy, above), and importance of regular physician visits.
Patients with history of prior treatment (surgical resection, RT) for malignant obstruction.	Assess respiratory system (see Malignancy, above). Evaluate for obstructive symptoms. Educate regarding signs and symptoms requiring medical attention (see Malignancy, above) and importance of medical follow-up.

ET, endotracheal.

changes in activity tolerance, dysphonia, cough) can easily be overlooked or mistakenly attributed to other factors, such as preexistent disease, treatment effects, or smoking history.

Patients identified as being at risk for tracheal obstruction should be informed which respiratory symptoms require immediate medical attention. The nurse should educate patients who have obstructive tracheal tumors and are receiving pre-RT steroids about the importance of taking the medication as prescribed and reporting signs of increasing respiratory difficulty.

Supportive nursing interventions for patients with tracheal obstruction are aimed at maintaining a patent airway and allaying anxiety. The nurse should closely monitor the patient's respiratory status and immediately report changes that indicate hypoxia (such as restlessness and confusion) and increasing obstruction (e.g., wheezing, stridor, retraction of interspaces and supraclavicular fossae) to the physician. Because respiratory symptoms, such as dyspnea and difficulty clearing secretions, are often associated with high levels of anxiety, the nurse should try to reduce patient anxiety and promote a calm, restful environment.

BIBLIOGRAPHY

1. Chang, L. L., J. Horvath, W. Peyton, and S. Ling. High dose rate intraluminal brachytherapy in malignant airway obstruction of lung cancer. *International Journal of Radiation Oncology, Biology and Physics* 28(3): 589–596. 1994.

   The use of high-dose brachytherapy with iridium 192 to improve quality of life for patients with malignant lesions of the trachea, mainstem bronchus and lobar bronchus is described.

2. Clarke, D. B. Palliative intubation of the trachea and main bronchi. *J Thorac Cardiovasc Surg* 80(5): 736–741. 1980.

   This article presents a new method of endoscopic intubation of malignant tumors of trachea and main bronchi with a specially adapted esophageal tube.

3. Courrey, M. S. Airway obstruction the problem and its causes. *Otolaryngolic Clinics of North America* 28(4): 673–683. 1995.

   A comprehensive overview of the various causes of airway obstruction with a review of potential treatments. Photographs are used to augment narrative.

4. Decker, S. J. The patient with an obstructed airway. *Topics in Emergency Medicine* 8(4): 1–12. 1987.

   This article discusses signs, symptoms, and management of patients with airway obstruction due to any cause; anatomy is included.

5. Lokich, J. J. Pulmonary complications of malignancy. In Lokich, J. J., ed. *Clinical Cancer Medicine: Treatment Tactics.* G. K. Hall & Co., Boston. 144–164. 1980.

   This chapter contains a brief discussion of tracheal obstruction arising from mediastinal lesions and recommendations for management.

6. Portlock, C. S., and D. R. Goffinet. Tracheal obstruction. In Portlock, C. S., and D. R. Goffinet. *Manual of Clinical Problems in Oncology.* Little, Brown & Co., Boston. 1980.

This is a concise discussion of the management of tracheal obstruction from benign or malignant causes.

7. Raju, P., R. Tapan, R. McDonald, B. Harrison, C. Crim, T. Hyers, S. Marshall, J. Ohar, and K. Naunheim. IR-192, low dose rate endobronchial brachytherapy in the treatment of malignant airway obstruction. *International Journal of Radiation Oncology, Biology, and Physics* 27(3): 677–680. 1993.

This small study evaluates the use of after-loading catheters for the treatment of malignant airway obstruction utilizing low dose iridium 192. The results of the study indicate that low dose rate endotracheal brachytherapy provides excellent control of symptoms of dyspnea, hemoptysis, cough, and pneumonia with few complications.

8. Sise, J. G., and R. W. Crichlow. Obstruction due to malignant tumors. *Seminars in Oncology* 5(2): 213–224. 1978.

This article provides a brief but valuable summary of tracheal obstruction secondary to malignant tumors. Clinical presentation and diagnostic workup are well discussed.

9. Wanamaker, J. R. and I. Eliachar. An overview of treatment options for lower airway obstruction. *Otolaryngolic Clinics of North America* 28(4): 751–767. 1994.

This article discusses the potential causes of lower airway obstruction and reviews various treatments, including laser therapy, stent placement, and surgical techniques.

15E

E. Bowel Obstruction

Sharon Dellinger
Lyn Sturdevant Davis

SMALL BOWEL

One of the primary functions of the small bowel, or intestine, is to absorb the products of digestion (see Chapter 9). During this process, there is an enormous exchange of fluids and electrolytes across the small-bowel mucosa. Saliva and gastric, pancreatic, biliary, and intestinal secretions deliver about eight liters, or one-fifth of the total body water, to the small bowel in 24 hours. Most of this fluid is reabsorbed before it reaches the colon. Two unidirectional fluxes occur simultaneously in the small intestine. In *absorption,* fluids and electrolytes move from the intestinal lumen through the small-bowel mucosa to the interstitial fluid. Conversely, in *secretion,* fluids and electrolytes flow from the interstitial fluid to the intestinal lumen.

Pathophysiology

Mechanical bowel obstruction, the result of a physical block to the onward passage of intestinal contents, accounts for 90 percent of all bowel obstruction. *Functional* bowel obstruction is caused by a loss of propulsive peristalsis (e.g., paralytic ileus occurring after surgery). This discussion is focused on mechanical causes of bowel obstruction, which can be subdivided into three types:

- *Intraluminal* obstructions are caused by obstructing matter in the bowel lumen, such as fecal impaction or colon tumors.
- *Mural* obstructions can result from lesions of the bowel wall—such as stenosis from radiation injury, diverticulitis, ulcerative colitis, or colon carcinomas.
- *Extramural* obstructions are caused by external compression of the bowel wall—such as by hernias, masses, or adhesions.

Blockage within the small intestine forces secretions from the stomach, pancreas, and biliary tree, along with swallowed air, to pool above the obstruction causing distention of the small bowel. When distention occurs, venous return and the absorptive processes are impaired. The bowel wall becomes edematous and begins to secrete water, sodium, and potassium into the fluid pooled in the intestinal lumen. For reasons that are unclear, distention greatly stimulates the secretory activity of the gut but does not correspondingly increase the rate of absorption—accounting for the fluid and electrolyte imbalance seen with this type of obstruction.

The distension process extends proximally, involving successive loops of bowel and further impeding absorption. The pooling of fluid in the intestinal lumen depletes the body's circulating fluid volume. Without treatment, profound hypovolemic shock will ensue.

Distension of the small intestine can lead to pressure necrosis of the bowel wall and result in strangulation. Strangulating obstruction occurs when the blood supply of the bowel wall is impeded, causing the wall to become necrotic and liable to perforate. The complications of septic shock are then added to the effects of obstruction. If corrective surgery for strangulating obstruction is delayed beyond 36 hours, the mortality rate is greater than 25 percent.

Complete small-bowel obstruction is a life-threatening condition requiring immediate medical intervention. Fluid losses must be replaced to prevent hypovolemic shock, and close monitoring is necessary to permit early identification and treatment of strangulating obstruction.

Primary tumors of the small intestine are rare, constituting only 1 to 3 percent of all gastrointestinal (GI) tumors. Carcinoid tumors, adenocarcinoma, leiomyosarcoma, and lymphoma make up the great majority of primary small-bowel tumors. These malignancies can cause obstruction by progressive growth and occlusion of the lumen, kinking of the bowel, or intussusception. Carcinoid tumors are particularly prone to cause obstruction.

Secondary tumors involving the small intestine are the most common cause of small-bowel obstruction in cancer patients, occurring more than twice as frequently as obstruction caused by primary tumors. Small-bowel metastases can occur through direct extension of a primary tumor, by way of the lymphatic or blood vessels, or as the result of intra-abdominal carcinomatosis. Direct extension can occur from tumors originating in the pancreas, colon, or stomach. Small-intestinal metastases via the lymphatic and blood vessels can result from melanoma and cancers of the uterus, breast, and lung. Intra-abdominal carcinomatosis produces obstruction most frequently and is most commonly seen in ovarian, colonic, gastric, and pancreatic carcinomas. Metastases to the small bowel are often multiple. Obstruction results from the bulk of the growth, with angulation, fixation, and flattening of the bowel wall.

Bands of adhesions or *scar tissue* from abdominal operations can constrict the lumen if they encircle a loop of bowel, thus resulting in small-intestinal obstruction. Adhesions are the most common cause of small-intestinal obstruction (nearly 90 percent of all cases). Cancer patients frequently undergo abdominal surgery during diagnosis and treatment of their disease and are consequently at risk for developing small-bowel obstruction.

Abdominal and *pelvic radiation* can lead to late injury to the small bowel, commonly known as radiation enteritis. These late effects of radiation therapy (RT) can occur from months to 20 years after completion of treatment. Small-bowel obstruction is the most common presentation of severe late radiation injury to the small intestine. Tissue changes that occur include mucosal and submucosal ulcerations, atrophy of glandular mucosa, collagen degeneration, and vascular damage. The wall of the small intestine is usually thickened secondary to submucosal fibrosis, and there might be segments of bowel with narrowed lumens and proximal dilation. The mesentery might also be thickened, resulting in shortening of the bowel.

The incidence of late radiation injury appears to depend on the radiation dose and the volume of bowel radiated. The higher the dose of radiation and the larger the volume of bowel radiated, the greater the incidence of injury. Unfortunately, there is no reliable method for predicting the potential for long-term complications.

LARGE BOWEL

The major function of the large bowel (see Chapter 9) is absorption of water and electrolytes in the proximal half and storage of feces in the distal half until defecation occurs. Each day one to two liters of fluid are delivered to the large bowel from the small bowel. Of this fluid, all but 100 to 200 ml, which is excreted in the feces, is absorbed in the colon.

Pathophysiology

When the large bowel is obstructed, fluid and gas accumulation proximal to the obstruction occurs, but in comparison with small-bowel obstruction, intraluminal fluid accumulation is slight and the metabolic results of fluid loss are generally not as severe. The urgent nature of large-bowel obstruction is related to the potential for rupture and risk of intra-abdominal sepsis due to the large numbers of gram negative bacteria found in the large intestine. Perforation of the large bowel results in mortality rates greater than 50 percent. If, in cases of complete bowel obstruction, the ileocecal valve remains competent—thus preventing reflux of colonic contents—the escape of fluid and gas proximally is prevented. A closed-loop obstruction results. This type of obstruction causes a rapid increase in intraluminal pressure as the colon distends. The cecum, with its large diameter and thin walls, is predisposed to rupture. Prompt treatment of large-bowel obstruction is required to avoid perforation.

In cases in which the ileocecal valve permits reflux of colonic contents, small-bowel distension ensues, and the symptoms of small-bowel as well as large-bowel obstruction appear. Small-bowel distension often occurs with large-bowel obstruction. High intraluminal cecal pressure might be present in cases in which reflux occurs, so that immediate intervention is urgent.

Obstruction in the colon and rectum occurs with about half the frequency of small-bowel obstruction, but more than 50 percent of large-bowel obstructions are caused by a primary malignancy of the colon and rectum. It is estimated that one in five patients with colon carcinoma will present with obstruction as a significant feature, and that in half of this number, an emergency operation will be required.

Right-sided colonic carcinomas can obstruct with luminal tumor growth, although this is usually a late development because of the relatively large diameter of the right side of the colon. Other mechanisms of obstruction include intussusception and swelling and edema of the bowel wall secondary to tumor.

Left-sided colonic carcinomas are a common cause of large-bowel obstruction. Of obstructing lesions in the colon, 75 percent occur distal to the splenic flexure. Left-sided lesions tend to grow annularly, producing a "napkin-ring" constriction. Severe stenosis and obstruction can be produced as the carcinoma encircles the bowel completely. A partial obstruction can become complete if swelling and edema accompany the tumor or if solid fecal material lodges in the stenotic area.

Rectal carcinomas less commonly produce obstruction, because of the large diameter of the rectal ampulla, earlier recognition of symptoms, and the relative ease of diagnosis.

Occasionally, metastatic tumors could obstruct the colon or rectum by direct extension, usually from primary tumors arising in genitourinary (GU) organs, such as the ovary, cervix, uterus, or bladder. Metastases from distant primary tumors rarely obstruct the colon. When obstruction does occur, it usually arises from serosal deposits secondary to widespread metastatic carcinomas. Obstructive intestinal metastases can be seen with melanoma, soft-tissue, and Kaposi's sarcomas, as well as breast, stomach, pancreatic, lung, ovarian, and small bowel cancers. Rarely, retroperitoneal tumors (such as some soft-tissue sarcomas or lymphoma) will cause sufficient extrinsic pressure so that stenosis and obstruction result.

Late radiation injury to the large bowel, occurring months or years after treatment, is relatively uncommon. It generally presents as an obstruction or fistula of the rectosigmoid. Injury to the vascular and supporting tissues of the bowel is the presumed pathophysiologic cause.

The neurotoxicity of the vinca alkaloids, such as vincristine and vinblastine, or vinorelbine places patients at risk for the development of constipation and paralytic ileus. Severe constipation, with resultant large-bowel obstruction, has required surgical intervention in rare instances. Elderly patients and those receiving vinca alkaloids for prolonged periods have an increased risk for developing vinca alkaloid neurotoxicity. Concomitant usage of other constipating drugs, such as opioid analgesics, anticholinergics, and seratonin-inhibiting antiemetics (e.g., ondansetron, granisetron) further increases susceptibility to constipation (see Chapter 12B).

Constipation is a common symptom affecting cancer patients, and effective management is necessary to maintain quality of life and to avoid serious fecal impaction and bowel obstruction.

CLINICAL MANIFESTATIONS

Table 15E–1 presents a comparison of signs and symptoms for small- and large-bowel obstructions. Abdominal pain and vomiting are the most common symptoms in small-bowel obstruction. Episodes of cramping abdominal pain usually have a crescendo-decrescendo pattern, with a pain-free interval between attacks. Severe continuous pain could indicate strangulation. Vomiting occurs early and is profuse. Acid-base imbalances are common. Depending on the level of obstruction, vomiting can result in metabolic acidosis or alkalosis.

Table 15E-1

**Comparison of Clinical Presentations of Small-
and Large-Bowel Obstructions**

Factor	Small-Bowel Obstruction	Large-Bowel Obstruction
Onset	Rapid	Insidious
Abdominal pain	Severe: crampy, intermittent attacks	Generally less severe; usually crampy
Vomiting	Occurs early; frequent and profuse	Occurs late; sometimes never
Bowel habits	Obstipation once distal tract emptied	Diarrhea, narrowing of stools, eventual obstipation
Abdominal distension	Often present	Pronounced
Dehydration	Early, life-threatening	Late
Electrolyte and acid/base imbalances	Common	Rare

Characteristically, symptoms of large-bowel obstruction are insidious, developing over weeks or months. The most common complaint is abdominal pain or discomfort. The pain is usually crampy and generally milder than the pain associated with small-bowel obstruction. Abdominal distension is the most common physical finding and is frequently quite pronounced.

Assessment

Diagnostic studies undertaken in cases of suspected bowel obstruction include three-way abdominal x-rays and laboratory analysis. In instances of small-bowel obstruction, an abdominal flat plate classically demonstrates a ladder-like pattern of distended small-bowel loops with air-fluid levels. In the case of large-bowel obstruction, abdominal x-rays display a distended colon, often with an associated picture of small-bowel distension. Evaluation of large-bowel obstruction also includes proctosigmoidoscopy, barium enema, and pelvic examination for women. If perforation is suspected, barium enema should be avoided or performed with a water-soluble contrast material.

Required laboratory tests include a CBC and electrolyte studies. An elevated white blood cell (WBC) count (15,000–20,000 cells/mm^3) suggests strangulation. Elevated hematocrit (Hct) might reflect dehydration secondary to fluid shift. Hypochromic microcytic anemia might be seen in cases in which occult blood loss has occurred over the preceding weeks or months. Electrolyte imbalances—such as hypochloremia, hypokalemia, and hyponatremia—and acid-base disturbances are commonly present in small-bowel obstruction.

A GI history from the patient or family member might reveal such symptoms as anorexia, nausea, vomiting, abdominal distension, abdominal pain, change in bowel habits, constipation, obstipation, and GI bleeding.

On physical examination, gross distension is often observed with large-bowel obstruction. Distension could be great enough to raise the diaphragm and cause respiratory embarrassment. Waves of peristalsis in dilated loops of bowel are sometimes visible through the abdominal wall as the bowel attempts to propel its contents past the obstruction. High-pitched bowel sounds that occur in rushes during episodes of colic are frequently noted. If strangulation or long-standing obstruction is present, bowel sounds will be absent. Tympanitic percussion notes predominate because of gaseous distension. Localized tenderness on palpation suggests strangulation.

Medical Management

Small-bowel obstruction is usually managed by surgery. The compelling reason for surgery is that strangulation, associated with high morbidity and mortality, cannot be excluded with certainty so long as obstruction persists. The operation can be preceded by a period of careful preparation and close observation. In selected cases, surgery can be delayed or avoided. Surgery is generally avoided for patients who have had numerous prior operations for obstruction or who are in the terminal stage of illness. Operative mortality rates for patients with obstructing carcinomatosis have been reported as high as 50 percent, yet not correcting a complete small bowel obstruction has a mortality rate of 100 percent. Medical treatment, alone, can resolve some instances of partial small-bowel obstruction. During medical treatment, fluid and electrolyte imbalances are identified and corrected, and intubation with either a nasogastric or an intestinal tube for decompression is initiated. The patient is then closely monitored for signs of strangulation obstruction (elevated temperature, localized abdominal tenderness, elevated WBC count), which indicates the need for immediate surgery.

The management of obstruction arising from primary tumors of the small bowel is surgical resection. For cases of small-bowel obstruction secondary to metastatic tumor, surgery (consisting of side-to-side anastomosis) is usually indicated if there is no resolution of obstruction within a few days of medical management. Small-bowel obstruction secondary to RT injury is also treated surgically by side-to-side anastomosis if medical therapy is unsuccessful. Adhesive bands causing obstruction are lysed during laparotomy.

The management of *large-bowel obstruction* is also surgical. Immediate operation is required to avoid the life-threatening risk of cecal perforation. Surgery is delayed only long enough to correct any existing fluid and electrolyte imbalances. Preoperative intubation can be used to prevent vomiting and small-bowel distension, but it does not serve to decompress the large bowel.

The immediate goal of surgery for large-bowel obstruction is decompression of the obstructed segment. The secondary goal, when bowel obstruction is caused by primary carcinoma of the colon and rectum, is resection of tumor and the surrounding lymphatic. Tumor resection can be accomplished at the initial operation or planned as a second procedure two to three weeks after decompression of the proximal bowel. Table 15E–2 outlines surgical approaches in obstructive colorectal carcinomas. One-stage procedures have recently been recommended for left-sided obstructive colonic carcinomas; however, these are generally considered unduly hazardous, because of the technical difficulties of left-sided–colon reanastomosis in an obstructed bowel, as well as the increased potential for postoperative septic complications (Arnaud [1994] reports mortality rates for one and two-stage procedures of 50 percent and 31 percent respectively).

For metastatic cancers resulting in large-bowel obstruction, diversion by colostomy or bypass procedures such as enterocolostomy are the operations most frequently used. Selected patients might be considered candidates for radical surgery, such as pelvic exenteration. Rectosigmoid RT injuries that produce obstruction are usually managed by permanent end colostomy or low anterior resection (see Chapter 12A).

Nursing Management

Nursing interventions should be aimed at prevention and early detection of bowel obstruction. The importance of regular rectal examination, stool for occult blood, and sigmoidoscopy for persons over 40 years of age cannot be overemphasized. Digital-rectal examination can detect about

Table 15E–2
Surgical Approaches in Malignant Large-Bowel Obstructions

Carcinoma	Surgical Approaches
Right colon	One-stage procedure: resection with primary anastomosis.
Transverse colon	One- or two-stage procedure.
Left colon	One-stage procedure: decompression and resection. Two-stage procedure: preliminary diversion (cecostomy or transverse colostomy); definitive cancer surgery 2–3 weeks later.
Rectum	Two-stage procedure: proximal diversion (sigmoid loop colostomy); definitive cancer surgery.

Table 15E-3
Nursing Protocol for the Management of Bowel Obstruction

Factor	Intervention
During medical treatment*	
Potential for hypovolemic or septic shock	Observe for signs of shock: cool, clammy skin, diaphoresis. Monitor vital signs frequently: report increased pulse, decreased BP; elevated temperature (sign of strangulation). Monitor urinary output; report output <40 ml/hr. Monitor central venous pressure as applicable. Report localized abdominal tenderness and elevated WBC count (signs of strangulation). Plasma, blood, and antibiotics may be administered.
Potential/actual fluid deficit and electrolyte imbalance	Monitor serum electrolyte values as obtained. Monitor urinary output; maintain accurate intake and output measurements. Check urine sp gr: high sp gr may indicate inadequate fluid replacement. Monitor IV fluid and electrolyte replacement.
Alteration in GI functioning	Access GI system: abdominal pain; location, duration, character, abdominal distension; daily abdominal girths for prolonged medical treatment. Auscultate bowel sounds. Report abdominal tenderness. Check amount, consistency, guaiac of stools. Note volume, color, odor of emesis tube drainage. Nasogastric/intestinal decompression: Advance intestinal tube as prescribed. Maintain patency, irrigate as prescribed. Provide frequent mouth care, q 1–2 hr. Provide topical anesthetics for sore throat. Weigh patient daily; keep NPO. Eliminate noxious odors if possible.
Nutritional deficit	Parenteral nutrition often indicated (see Chapter 9). Use antiemetics as indicated.
Fear/anxiety	Provide clear, simple explanation of procedures, tests, treatments to patients and family members. Provide emotional support.
Alteration in comfort	Use opioids sparingly; may mask signs of obstruction and complications. Meperidine is preferred to morphine. Provide comfort measures (see Chapter 8A).
During Surgical Treatment	
Preoperative care	
Potential/actual fluid and electrolyte imbalance	Goal: stabilize physiologically. Monitor serum electrolyte values; administer fluid and electrolyte therapy as prescribed.
Potential anemia	Obtain CBC; blood transfusion may be indicated.

Continued

Table 15E–3 *(Continued)*
Nursing Protocol for the Management of Bowel Obstruction

Factor	Intervention
Potential infection/sepsis	Administer antibiotics as prescribed.
Need for information	Preoperative teaching for patient/family members when possible; give clear and simple explanations.
Fear/anxiety	Provide clear and simple explanations to patient and family members. Provide emotional support.
Postoperative care Potential infection	Administer antibiotics as prescribed. Monitor respiratory status; check lung sounds; decreased breath sounds, abnormal lung sounds; assist with turning, coughing, deep-breathing q 1–2 hr. Assess temperature q 4 hr. Observe for signs and symptoms of urinary tract infection: dysuria, frequency, cloudy, strong-smelling urine; avoid prolonged catheterization. Monitor for early signs of sepsis, especially hypotension.
Decreased mobility	Check for calf tenderness q 8 hr. Assist/instruct with leg exercises: flexion and extension, quadriceps setting, ankle turns q 2 hr. Promote self-care activities. Assist with progressive ambulation.
Alteration in GI functioning	Care for GI tube as above. Assess for abdominal distension; obtain daily abdominal girth as indicated; report increasing distension. Monitor return of GI functioning closely; check for return of bowel sounds and passage of flatus q 8 hr. Monitor for nausea and vomiting as diet is advanced.
Alteration in comfort: incisional pain	Administer analgesics to provide adequate pain relief. Assist/instruct in splinting incision. Provide comfort measures.
Nutritional deficit	Parenteral nutrition may be indicated. Consult with physician and dietician regarding need for oral supplements when bowel function returns.
Wound healing	Monitor for signs of infection: redness, tenderness, warmth, drainage, and impaired wound healing: poor approximation of wound edges. Provide meticulous wound care. Assess need for nutritional support as above.

sp gr, specific gravity.
*The medical management section applies primarily to patients with small-bowel obstruction who are receiving medical treatment. The majority of large-bowel obstructions require immediate surgical intervention.

one-half of all colonic cancers, and two out of three colorectal tumors can be visualized and biopsied with sigmoidoscopy. In asymptomatic patients with a positive test for occult blood who are found to have cancer, more than 80 percent have early lesions limited to the bowel. The nurse can play a valuable role in early detection by educating the public.

Patients at risk for developing bowel obstruction should be instructed to report symptoms such as vomiting, abdominal distension, and constipation. The nurse should be alert to GI complaints of patients with advanced malignancies and carefully evaluate symptoms that suggest possible bowel obstruction.

Supportive nursing interventions for patients with bowel obstruction are presented in Table 15E–3. Patients undergoing medical treatment for bowel obstruction must be closely monitored for signs of shock and strangulating obstruction. Careful attention to fluid and electrolyte status can help prevent dehydration or over-hydration.

During both medical and surgical management of bowel obstruction, the digestive tract cannot be used for an extended period of time. Consideration must be given to how a patient's nutritional needs will be met. Cancer patients (especially those with advanced disease) are often depleted nutritionally, and the stress of surgery further increases nutritional requirements (see Chapter 9). Parenteral nutrition might often be indicated until the enteral route is fully functional. During the postoperative period, special attention should be given to wound healing. Poor nutritional status and immunosuppression places many cancer patients at risk for wound infection and impaired healing. Meticulous wound care and adequate nutritional support can help prevent these complications. The use of parenteral nutrition in terminally ill patients with or without obstructive bowel symptoms is controversial. At this time, the American Nurses Association, the American Medical Association, and the American Dietetic Association agree that it is legally, ethically, and professionally acceptable to discontinue nutritional support for the terminally ill.

BIBLIOGRAPHY

1. Arnaud, J. P., and R. Berganaschi. Emergency subtotal/total colectomy with anastomosis for acutely obstructed carcinoma of the left colon. *Diseases of the Colon and Rectum* 37(7): 685–688. 1994.

   Results of an eight-year study indicate that emergency subtotal colectomy is an acceptable operation in patients with a reasonable operative risk, a resectable obstructing carcinoma, massively distended colon of dubious viability, signs of impending cecal perforation, masses suggesting synchronous colonic cancers, and a skilled surgeon.

2. Baker, A. Surgical emergencies. In V. T. DeVita, S. Hellman, and S. Rosenberg, eds. *Principles and Practice of Oncology*, 3d Ed. J. B. Lippincott Co., Philadelphia. 1993.

This chapter includes a brief discussion of the surgical management of intestinal obstruction in cancer patients.

3. Bryant, G. A. When the bowel is blocked. *RN* (January): 58–66. 1992.

   This is a basic presentation of the causes, presenting signs and symptoms, and nursing management of bowel obstruction.

4. Cheskin, L. J. Gastrointestinal bleeding. In Barker, L. R., J. Burton, and P. Zieve, eds. *Principles of Ambulatory Medicine*, 4th Ed. Williams & Wilkins, Baltimore. 1995.

   This chapter discusses tests utilized in the detection of blood in the stool, evaluation of patients who have gastrointestinal bleeding, and selected lesions that bleed.

5. Davis, S. Bowel obstruction. *Emergency Care Quarterly* 5(3): 57–63. 1989.

   An overview is offered of the causes, clinical presentation, and prehospital and medical/surgical management of small- and large-bowel obstruction.

6. Fainsinger, R. Integrating medical and surgical treatments in gastrointestinal, genitourinary, and biliary obstruction in patients with cancer. *Hematology/Oncology Clinics of North America* 10(1): 173–183. 1996.

   This article reviews the causes of various obstructive syndromes related to cancer, as well as discussing curative and palliative methods of treatment.

7. Kinsella, T. J., and W. D. Bloomer. Tolerance of the intestine to radiation therapy. *Surg Gynecol Obstet* 151(2): 273–284. 1980.

   This is a detailed description of acute and late effects of radiation to the bowel. It includes a discussion of small- and large-intestinal obstruction.

8. Lau, P. and T. Lorentz. Results of surgery for malignant bowel obstruction in advanced, unresectable, recurrent colorectal cancer. *Diseases of the Colon and Rectum* 36(1): 61–64. 1993.

   This is a retrospective study of 30 patients with unresectable intra-abdominal disease who have undergone laparotomy for relief of bowel obstruction.

9. Ripamanti, C. Management of bowel obstruction in advanced cancer. *Current Opinions in Oncology* 6(4): 351–357. 1994.

   This article reviews the causes of bowel obstruction as well as surgical, medical, and pharmacologic management of obstruction, focusing mainly on palliative efforts.

10. Spiro, H. M. *Clinical Gastroenterology*, 3d Ed. 429–500, 661–662. Macmillan, Inc., New York. 1983.

    The chapter on intestinal obstruction discusses pathophysiology, clinical features, diagnosis, and treatment of intestinal obstruction. It also contains a nice summary of small-bowel metastases.

11. Sykes, N. P. Current approaches to the management of constipation. *Cancer Surveys* 21: 137–146. 1994.

    The prevalence, compounded by the trivialization by the medical establishment, of constipation has rendered it more common than pain as a major distress for patients with cancer. Suggestions for safe and effective bowel regimens are provided.

F. Cardiac Tamponade

Sharon Sebold Kilbride

Cardiac tamponade is defined as a compression of the heart resulting from the accumulation of excessive fluid within the pericardial sac. Constriction of the pericardial sac by tumor will result in tamponade without fluid accumulation. In the cancer patient, the most common cause of pericardial effusion and tamponade is tumor invasion of the pericardium. This oncologic emergency can develop for a variety of reasons.

A series of studies have shown that approximately 20 percent of cancer patients have metastatic disease to the pericardium at autopsy. Tumors most often cited in reports of pericardial metastasis include lung, breast, leukemia, Hodgkin's and non-Hodgkin's lymphoma, and melanoma, with lung being the most prevalent. Primary tumors of the heart are rare and are usually mesothelioma or sarcoma. Lung and breast cancers are usually spread to the pericardium by direct extension of primary tumor or by lymphatic metastases. Lymphomas and leukemias are typically spread via hematogenous routes. Pericardial seeding by malignant cells alone is probably insufficient to cause tamponade, as concomitant lymphatic obstruction contributes greatly to the development of this oncologic emergency. Tumors that spread via hematogeneous routes or rarely spread to mediastinal nodes do not usually cause tamponade.

Radiation therapy of 4,000 cGy or greater to the mediastinum can result in acute pericarditis and pericardial effusion. Chronic constrictive pericarditis can lead to complications many years after completion of radiation therapy.

15F

PATHOPHYSIOLOGY

The pericardium encloses the heart and the roots of the great vessels (Figure 15F–1). It consists of two main parts: the parietal pericardium and the visceral pericardium The *parietal pericardium* is a dense fibrous sac attached at its base to the diaphragm and separated from the chest wall by the lungs, parietal pleura, and sternum. This strong exterior serves to protect the heart and helps to hold the heart in position. The *visceral pericardium* is a delicate serous membrane that lines the parietal pericardium and is contiguous with the heart. The pericardial space is created between the two layers where a small amount of serous fluid serves as a lubricant allowing the heart and pericardium to glide smoothly over each other dur-

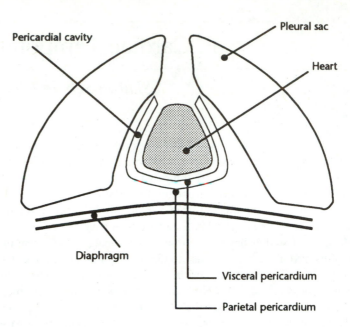

Figure 15F-1. Diagram showing the relationship of the heart to the pericardium and adjacent structures.

ing each heartbeat. This serous fluid, normally 10 to 50 ml, is produced primarily by the lymphatic channels that flow from the inner lining of the heart to the visceral pericardium.

Metastasis to the pericardium from lymphatic or hematogenous spread often results in the studding of the pericardium with dense tumor nodules. Diffuse tumor invasion can cause a thickened pericardium. The presence of tumor causes irritation and inflammation of the pericardial sac. As the body mounts its inflammatory response, it sends leukocytes, fibrin, platelets, and fluid to the area. During this process capillaries become more permeable, and additional exudate might leak into surrounding tissues and/or pericardial space. However, direct compression of the pericardial sac from adjacent primary tumors (e.g., breast and lung cancer) can cause significant constriction without fluid accumulation.

Hemodynamic consequences of cardiac tamponade are related to impairment of diastolic function of the heart. As fluid in the pericardial sac takes up space, it pushes on the heart and prevents it from fully expanding and filling during diastole. This results in reduced cardiac volume and cardiac output. Normally, ventricular filling is aided by pressure differences between the atria and ventricles. As intracardiac pressure rises with the accumulation of fluid, these differences abate and pressures begin to equalize in all chambers, resulting in a fall in arterial pressure and a rise in central venous pressure.

The body responds to a decrease in cardiac output with several compensatory mechanisms. The sympathetic branch of the autonomic nervous system releases catecholamines to increase heart rate and contractility. Selective vasoconstriction decreases venous pooling, increases venous pressure, and increases the blood return to the heart. Arterial vasoconstriction improves arterial tone and raises blood pressure. The kidneys compensate by releasing angiotensin II, a potent arterial vasoconstrictor. Decreased renal flow results in sodium and water retention, which increases intravascular volume.

When the cardiac chambers remain severely compressed, the compensatory mechanisms are overpowered and might even compound the problem. As the compensatory demands on the heart continue, increasing cardiac work load, so do the oxygen requirements of the myocardium. Tachycardia produces shorter diastole, and less time is available for the filling of the heart and for perfusion of coronary arteries. The increase in arterial resistance creates afterload so that the ventricle cannot overcome peripheral resistance and pump enough blood.

These compensatory mechanisms are most helpful in gradually developing effusions as the pericardium has time to stretch. In the event of acute tamponade, however, these mechanisms will not be able to overcome the rise in intracardiac pressures, and circulatory collapse will ensue.

CLINICAL MANIFESTATIONS

Pericardial effusions are difficult to detect by clinical examination unless the fluid accumulation is significant enough to interfere with normal hemodynamics. The symptoms that occur depend largely on the rate at which the pericardial fluid has accumulated. Slow accumulation allows the pericardium to stretch, so that intrapericardial pressures are not affected at first (see Table 15F–1).

The patient experiencing tamponade might exhibit symptoms of hoarseness, cough, and hiccoughs or difficulty swallowing because of compression of the nerves, trachea, or esophagus. Cardiac examination might reveal faint or muffled heart sounds, because sounds transmit poorly through pericardial fluid. A pericardial friction rub might also be heard. As diastolic filling is hindered by an unyielding pericardium, venous return is also impaired, resulting in engorgement of the jugular veins. Kussmal's sign, an exaggerated swelling of the neck veins during inspiration, is most often present.

As cardiac output decreases, systolic blood pressure decreases and diastolic pressure will rise with arterial constriction and systemic vascular resistance, causing a narrowing of pulse pressure. A characteristic sign of cardiac tamponade is the presence of a paradoxical pulse—a decline in systolic pressure during inspiration. Palpation of the carotid, femoral, and radial arteries is one method of assessing paradoxical pulse. If paradoxical pulse is present, the pulse amplitude will decrease or might even disappear on inspiration.

Table 15F–1
Clinical Manifestations of Cardiac Tamponade

Factor	Signs and Symptoms	Rationale
Decreased cardiac output	Tachycardia	Increased heart rate compensates for decreased cardiac output.
	Vasoconstriction Peripheral cyanosis	Attempts to increase cardiac output by increasing return of blood to heart.
	Tachypnea Use of accessory muscles	Restriction of lung expansion.
	Oliguria	Secondary to decreased kidney perfusion.
	Narrowing pulse pressure	As cardiac output decreases, systolic pressure falls; arteries constrict to maintain perfusion.
	Paradoxical pulse of >10 mm Hg	As tamponade constricts myocardium during inspiration, the diaphragm exerts additional pressure on the pericardial sac. The left ventricle receives less blood and cardiac output is decreased, resulting in a decrease in systolic blood pressure on inspiration.
	Anxiety, agitation, restlessness, confusion	Cerebral anoxia secondary to inadequate perfusion.
	Shock	Decompensation.
Compression of heart and adjacent structures	Dysphagia, cough, hoarseness, hiccoughs retrosternal chest pain	Fluid accumulation on heart and direct tumor invasion may cause compression of trachea, esophagus, and nerves in addition to heart.
Venous congestion, presacral edema	Peripheral edema Kussmal's sign (jugular venous distension on expiration) Nausea/vomiting Hepatomegaly Hepatojugular reflux	As ventricular filling is decreased, venous return is impaired, resulting in vascular congestion.
Distended pericardial sac	Dullness to percussion Distant or weak heart sounds Chest discomfort	Fluid in pericardial sac does not transmit sounds well.

The degree of paradoxical pulse can be obtained by sphygmomanometry, which is done by placing the cuff around the arm and inflating to a level above the systolic blood pressure. The cuff is then slowly deflated. The pressure reading where the first sound is heard is noted. This sound will occur during expiration and could disappear on inspiration. As the cuff continues to deflate, the pressure reading is noted where sounds are heard during inspiration and expiration. If the sounds are more than 10 mm Hg apart, paradox is present. It is important to note that in cases of extreme tamponade, paradoxical pulse might be absent if the systolic blood pressure is less than 50 mm Hg. In addition, patients with severe COPD, right ventricular infarction, hypovolemic shock, and pulmonary embolism might exhibit a paradoxical pulse in the absence of tamponade.

Systemic venous congestion can produce a variety of clinical symptoms. Peripheral and presacral edema might be noted. Occasionally facial plethora (redness and swelling) and a full neck will be present. Patients might complain of nausea, vomiting, and abdominal pain, probably due to intestinal congestion and hepatomegaly. Another characteristic sign of tamponade is the hepatojugular reflex. This can be demonstrated by having the patient lie down with head elevated to a position where jugular venous pulsations are easily observed. Continuous pressure is then placed over the right upper quadrant of the abdomen for 30 to 60 seconds. A positive reflex is present when jugular venous pulsations increase. The reflex is caused by an increase in vascular congestion due to the prolonged increase in central venous pressure.

Dyspnea is a common symptom of cardiac tamponade. Its severity depends on the degree of lung constriction caused by the pericardium. Although lung sounds are often clear on auscultation, severe tamponade can cause pulmonary edema as rising pulmonary vascular pressure causes fluid from pulmonary capillary beds to leak into alveoli. In this situation rhonchi, crackles, and frothy pink-tinged sputum may be present. The patient might use accessory muscles to aid breathing. Shallow breathing is often observed as the patient guards against pleuritic pain caused by deep breathing. A large effusion might even compress the base of the left lung, and tubular breath sounds might be auscultated.

Typically, patients experiencing cardiac tamponade will lean forward or sit in a knee-elbow posture in an attempt to alleviate chest pain and dyspnea. Patients might describe a vague distressing feeling in the chest. Extreme anxiety, restlessness, agitation, and confusion can be observed as symptoms of cerebral anoxia resulting from impaired perfusion.

DIAGNOSIS

If the clinician suspects cardiac tamponade, there are several diagnostic tests that can be ordered to confirm the diagnosis. A routine chest x-ray might reveal an enlarged cardiac silhouette or "water bottle heart." Large effusions (greater than 250 ml of fluid) within the pericardial sac are needed to enlarge the silhouette. The absence of cardiomegaly on a chest x-ray, however, does not rule out the presence of tamponade, which can be caused by a smaller amount of fluid that has accumulated rapidly.

Electrocardiogram is limited in its capability to demonstrate cardiac tamponade; nonspecific changes associated with pericardial effusions, such as sinus tachycardia, elevated ST segments, nonspecific T-wave changes, and decreased QRS voltage are common findings. However, the presence of total electrical alternans, which is the alteration of size and direction of P wave and QRS complexes on every other beat, is often found in patients with neoplastic cardiac tamponade. These EKG changes are caused by variations in the position of the heart at the time of electrical depolarization as it swings within the pericardial fluid.

Echocardiography is by far the simplest, most sensitive noninvasive method for diagnosing cardiac tamponade. When time is of the essence, it is the diagnostic test of choice because it can be performed at the bedside in approximately 30 minutes. Although the M-mode echocardiogram is sufficient for establishing the presence of pericardial effusion, two-dimensional echocardiography is more definitive, because it can assess the pericardium around the entire heart. Normal echocardiogram findings will show the anterior right ventricular wall in close proximity to the chest wall and the posterior left ventricle in contact with the posterior pericardium and pleura. Normally, a single echo will be seen moving with each heartbeat. In tamponade there are echo-free spaces separating the moving walls from the stiff pericardium, indicating the presence of fluid. Two echoes are seen, one from the pericardium and one from the posterior heart border. Although this technique cannot determine the cause of the effusion, it can be helpful in providing a gross estimate of fluid accumulation as well as for determining a site for pericardiocentesis. Detection of a thickened pericardium from radiation fibrosis is also possible with echocardiography.

Computerized tomography and magnetic resonance imaging can detect pericardial effusions with great sensitivity, identifying fluid collections as small as 50 cc. In addition the composition of the effusion (i.e., exudate, chyle, serous, or hemmorhagic) can be determined by these methods. Pericardial thickness can also be measured, aiding in the differential diagnosis of pericardial effusion versus radiation fibrosis. Both of these imaging techniques however have the disadvantage of requiring the patient to be transported to the scanner.

Cardiac catheterization can confirm the diagnosis of tamponade as well as determine the volume and exact location of the fluid. When tamponade is present, there will be increased intrapericardial pressure and the abnormal finding of nearly equal diastolic pressures in all chambers of the heart.

Patients who have received radiation therapy of 4,000 cGy or greater to a considerable area of the heart present a diagnostic dilemma. Pericardial injury can manifest as acute pericarditis during or shortly after the completion of therapy. Acute pericarditis is usually self-limiting and subsides without further sequelae. In its chronic form, radiation pericarditis can present up to 20 years after treatment. Chronic radiation pericarditis can lead to constriction, tamponade, and eventually death. Knowing how much radiation the heart has received can help determine whether the cause is radiation or progressive malignancy. Analysis of the pericardial fluid can be helpful, because a large percentage of cytology in malignant effusions will be positive.

MEDICAL MANAGEMENT

The primary goal in the treatment of neoplastic cardiac tamponade is to remove the fluid and relieve impending circulatory collapse. The long-term goal of therapy is the management of the underlying disease process. Decisions regarding therapy for malignant pericardial disease depend on the underlying condition of the patient and on previous treatment. Patients with widespread metastatic disease that is refractory to treatment might not be candidates for extensive diagnostic tests or aggressive treatment.

Pharmacologic Therapy

Mild tamponade might respond to treatment with steroids and diuretics, although this is usually a temporary measure. Typically, prednisone 40–60 mg daily, and a diuretic such as furosemide, 40 mg daily, or Aldactazide®, 25–200 mg daily are prescribed. This combination could alleviate the effusion and the need for pericardiocentesis. Patients experiencing mild tamponade from radiation pericarditis respond well to this therapy. Patients for whom surgical risks cannot be justified or who respond poorly to systemic or local therapies might gain some relief from steroid and diuretic therapy. Often when these drugs are discontinued, the effusion recurs, signaling the need for more aggressive treatment.

Pericardiocentesis

The only immediately effective treatment for tamponade is the removal of fluid. Aspiration of pericardial fluid should be performed when the patient exhibits signs of cyanosis, dyspnea, impaired consciousness, increasing central venous pressure, or shock-like syndrome. Pericardiocentesis, a technique used for both therapeutic and diagnostic reasons, involves introducing a large-bore needle into the pericardial space through a small incision under the xiphoid process. Echocardiography provides greatest assistance in locating the site for pericardiocentesis; EKG monitoring provides additional guidance during the procedure. EKG monitoring is employed by attaching the V lead directly to the hub of the needle. As the needle is advanced toward the left shoulder, a "pop" might be felt as the needle penetrates the fibrous pericardium. The QRS voltage will increase when the pericardium is touched. Acute elevation of ST or PR segments or development of premature atrial or ventricular contractions indicates that the needle has had contact with the myocardium and must be withdrawn.

Proper placement of the needle will yield a free return of straw-colored or serosanguinous fluid. Fluid will continue to be withdrawn over 10–30 minutes. Usually there will be a rapid improvement in the patient's hemodynamic status with the removal of as little as 50 cc of fluid. A flexible guide wire can be advanced through the needle and a drainage catheter subsequently substituted to provide further drainage or additional therapy.

Malignant effusions are often bloody and need to be tested immediately for hematocrit and fibrinogen to distinguish between a bloody effusion and penetration of the heart. Circulating blood has higher hematocrit and fibrinogen levels than do bloody effusions. Other tests routinely run on aspirated fluid include specific gravity, cell count, stains, cultures, and cytologic analysis. Cytologic examination is important to assist in diagnosis of the cause of the effusion and has an 80 percent to 90 percent sensitivity and specificity in metastatic cancer. This test, however, is less sensitive in lymphomas, sarcomas, Hodgkin's disease, and primary mesotheliomas.

Possible complications of pericardiocentesis include puncture of the right atrium or ventricle, arrythmias, infection, laceration of a coronary artery, bradycardia, or accidental introduction of air into chambers of the heart. The safety of the procedure depends on correct assessment of the amount and exact location of the fluid accumulation. In general there is less risk with larger effusions because of the increased distance between the pericardium and the heart, making it more difficult to come in contact with the heart inadvertently.

Pericardiocentesis will provide effective treatment of malignant effusions on an emergency basis. Unfortunately, fluid will usually reaccumulate within 24 to 48 hours. Multiple taps and placement of indwelling catheters are helpful in temporarily controlling fluid accumulation. Long-term catheter placement is contraindicated due to the high risk of infection. Therefore, local and/or systemic therapy should be initiated as soon as possible.

Percutaneous balloon pericardiotomy is a recently developed technique for the treatment of malignant pericardial effusions in the patient who is a poor surgical risk. This procedure is performed in a cardiac catheterization lab under local anesthesia. Using the subxiphoid approach, a guidewire is inserted into the pericardial space. Fluid is removed through a pigtail catheter. A balloon dilating catheter partially filled with contrast medium is then exchanged over the wire. The balloon catheter is withdrawn under fluoroscopic guidance until it straddles the pericardium. The balloon is then inflated until the "waisting" (or compression) produced by the parietal pericardium disappears. The balloon catheter can then be exchanged for a pigtail catheter, which is left in place for 24 hours to facilitate drainage directly into the mediastinum, pleural space, and peritoneum. Data available suggest a high success rate for this procedure. Although it is a less invasive alternative to surgery, it is still unknown whether this method is superior to subxiphoid pericardiectomy.

Chemotherapy

Chemotherapy is useful in the treatment of malignant pericardial effusions both locally and systemically. In a chemically sensitive tumor, systemic chemotherapy, as well as hormonal therapy and biotherapy, can produce disease regression and relief of fluid accumulation. For the 50 percent of patients whose effusion recurs after pericardiocentesis, a number of agents are available for instillation into the pericardial space via indwelling catheter. These agents are chosen based on their antitumor activity or their capability to cause sufficient irritation and inflammation to sclerose the pericardial space. Agents that have been used include tetracycline, bleomycin, cisplatin, mitomycin, mechlorethamine, teniposide, fluorouracil, thiotepa, quinacrine, gold, and radionuclides. Various success rates are reported, with an overall success rate of 80 percent. Sclerosing can cause symptoms of transient fever, chest pain, and nausea. Antimetabolites and alkylating agents have been reported to cause reactive effusion formation as well as cardiac arrythmias and bone marrow toxicity.

Surgery

Surgical procedures can provide prolonged palliation of recurrent neoplastic cardiac tamponade. The choice of surgical procedure depends primarily on the condition of the patient and the extent of metastatic disease. Subxiphoid pericardiotomy is a surgical technique performed using local anesthesia. A skin incision is made below the tip of the xiphoid, and tissues are removed and dissected until the pericardium is visualized. The pericardium is then incised and drained. Biopsy specimens of the pericardium can be obtained at this time. A thoracic catheter is left in place for continued drainage and/or instillation of cytotoxic or sclerosing agents.

A partial pericardiectomy or pericardial "window" is another surgical treatment option employing local anesthesia. Using the subxiphoid approach, a piece of the pericardium a few square centimeters in size is cut away, permitting drainage of fluid into the pleural space, where there is sufficient surface area to absorb it. This procedure has a 90 percent response rate, and the risks are acceptable. The major drawback is that adhesions can develop causing the window to close, leading to the recurrence of fluid accumulation. The procedure is also difficult to perform when tumor encases the heart or pericardium.

A total pericardiectomy involves removal of the visceral pericardium using general anesthesia. A median sternotomy is performed, which provides an excellent opportunity to view the pericardium and obtain biopsy samples. Large rectangular pieces of pericardium are removed to allow drainage. Following surgery chest tubes will be in place for several days. Total pericardiectomy is a more extensive surgery, but reaccumulation of fluid is rarely a problem. Total pericardiectomy is rarely justified in patients with widespread malignancy. It is most often recommended for treatment of the fibrotic effects of radiation-caused chronic constrictive pericarditis and for patients with a favorable prognosis.

Potential complications of these procedures are the risks associated with general anesthesia (if used), arrhythmias, hemothorax, infection, and bleeding.

Radiation Therapy

If gradually developing tamponade is caused by a radiosensitive tumor such as lung, breast, or hematopoietic malignancy, radiation therapy could be the treatment of choice. Generally 2,000 to 4,000 cGy is delivered to the heart, pericardial structures, and lower mediastinum. Cardiac tolerance is 3,500 to 4,000 cGy, beyond which the complication of pericarditis could develop. Studies have shown that lung and breast cancers exhibit significant improvement after 2,500 to 3,000 cGy. Lymphomas and leukemias might require lower doses.

To establish tissue tolerance, it is important to assess any previous radiation the patient might have received. Although external beam radiation is most often employed, internal therapy with agents such as radioactive phosphorous, yttrium, and gold have been instilled into the pericardial space.

NURSING MANAGEMENT

Nursing management of neoplastic cardiac tamponade begins with identifying patients at risk. Patients with lung, breast, and lymphomas are the most likely candidates. Early recognition and prompt diagnosis are key to the management of cardiac tamponade. Should the patient with cancer display signs of shortness of breath, fatigue, tachycardia, or hypotension, the nurse should be alert to the potential for cardiac complications. It is important to obtain a careful history and learn what symptoms the patient is currently experiencing. Nurses must be astute at physical assessment, including evaluation for presence or absence of paradoxical pulse, auscultation to assess intensity of heart sounds, and observation of neck veins for distention. A protocol for nursing management is described in Table 15F–2.

If cardiac tamponade is suspected, the nurse will be responsible for initiating supportive measures while a definitive diagnosis is made and preparations for pericardiocentesis are finalized. Close monitoring of vital signs is of utmost importance. Administration of volume expanders will be necessary to increase cardiac filling pressures to compensate for decreased cardiac output. Vasoactive drugs such as isoproterenol and dopamine might be ordered to increase cardiac output. The nurse will provide oxygen

Table 15F–2
Nursing Protocol for the Management of Neoplastic Cardiac Tamponade

Factor	Intervention
Circulatory Compromise Decreased cardiac output	Auscultate heart sounds. Monitor blood pressure for narrowing pulse pressure and paradox. Monitor EKG for ST segment changes, T-wave inversion, electrical alternans. Assist patient with all activities to reduce cardiac workload. Provide rest periods. Monitor electrolytes, especially Ca^{2+} and K^+, due to risk of arrhythmias.
Decreased tissue perfusion, temperature, and pulses	Assess extremities for color. Monitor I + O. Measure abdominal girth and note any ascites. Assess for positive hepatojugular reflux. Assess patient for respiratory difficulty, e.g., tachypnea, shortness of breath, air hunger. Position patient to assist with chest expansion. Administer O_2 as ordered. Monitor electrolytes, blood gases. Evaluate patient's level of consciousness and any changes. Provide analgesics as ordered to facilitate patient comfort.
Pericardiocentesis Supportive measures prior to procedure	Administer volume expanders as ordered, such as saline, fresh frozen plasma, blood, dextran, to increase cardiac filling pressures. Administer drugs, such as isoproterenol and dopamine, as ordered to increase cardiac output. Provide oxygen therapy as ordered. Monitor hemodynamic status. Have emergency equipment readily available.
Postpericardiocentesis	Monitor vital signs frequently. Assess for complications such as bleeding, pneumothorax, infection. Check catheter for patency. Use aseptic technique when handling catheter. Measure and record catheter drainage.
Instillation of sclerosing or antineoplastic agents	Evaluate need for antiemetic, analgesic, and antipyretic therapy. Maintain accurate records of catheter drainage.
Pericardiectomy	Monitor vital signs frequently. Assess for complications of bleeding and infection at surgical incision. Provide analgesics as ordered. Monitor and record chest tube drainage. Assess lung sounds for atelectasis and pulmonary edema.
Emotional/Psychological Concerns	Attempt to allay anxiety by clearly and concisely explaining diagnostic tests and procedures to patient and family members. Allow patient and significant others to discuss fears. Employ relaxation techniques. Administer antianxiety medications as ordered.
Education	Provide information on disease process and its effect on the heart. Educate patient/family about signs and symptoms of fluid reaccumulation. Stress importance of regular follow-up. Provide education on treatment for underlying disease.

as needed; however, intubation with positive pressure breathing should be avoided because it will further reduce venous return and increase intrapleural and intrapericardial pressures.

During pericardiocentesis the nurse continues to assess the patient's hemodynamic status. Electrocardiography monitoring is necessary to alert the team to any changes during the procedure that require additional intervention. The nurse must be aware of the potential complications of pericardiocentesis and provide frequent assessment of bleeding, respiratory function, and arrhythmias.

Should a catheter be left in place for further drainage or instillation of sclerosing or antineoplastic agents, the nurse maintains asepsis and patency of the catheter. The site is monitored for infection, and measurements of catheter drainage and vital signs are recorded accurately. Instillation of sclerosing or antineoplastic agents can result in pain, nausea, and fever. Medications will need to be administered as ordered to provide optimum comfort to the patient. Following pericardiocentesis the patient will require education on signs and symptoms to report should the fluid reaccumulate. Additional instruction regarding further treatment for the underlying disease process could also be warranted.

The patient experiencing tamponade will be extremely anxious and will require constant intervention to allay fears. Cancer by itself is emotionally trying, and the addition of a heart problem could prove to be overwhelming for these patients and their families. The nurse should offer information about the disease, diagnostic tests, and procedures. The patient and significant others should be encouraged to discuss their fears. Relaxation techniques could be employed, along with imagery, music, or anxiolytic agents as ordered.

The development of cardiac tamponade in the cancer patient is a grave prognostic sign. Survival depends on the variety and stage of malignancy, effectiveness of therapy, tumor responsiveness to chemotherapy and radiation therapy, severity of hemodynamic compromise, and the overall condition of the patient. Response rate for local therapies range from 50 percent to 90 percent with a remission of four to six months. The overall average survival, regardless of malignancy, is reported to be 16 months. Patients with Hodgkin's disease or breast cancer have been reported to survive for longer than two years, and those patients with radiation-induced effusion and tamponade could survive longer than any others. Regardless of discouraging statistics, aggressive treatment to remove fluid will provide a dramatic improvement in the patient's condition. It is important for the nurse to acknowledge the prognostic implications of tamponade development and provide support to patients and their families as they enter the terminal phase of the disease process.

As cancer treatment becomes more effective in prolonging patient survival, the incidence of pericardial metastasis could potentially become more common. Through careful assessment of the cancer patient, nursing can play a vital role in detecting signs and symptoms of cardiac tamponade before an actual emergency develops.

BIBLIOGRAPHY

1. Alcan, K. E., et al. Management of acute cardiac tamponade by subxiphoid pericardiotomy. *JAMA* 47: 1143–1148. 1982.

   Subxiphiod pericardiotomy used to treat cardiac tamponade from differing disease causes is discussed, including an excellent description of technique with diagram and some case reports.

2. Chong, H. H., and G. D. Plotnick. Pericardial effusion and tamponade: Evaluation, imaging modalites, and management. *Comprehensive Therapy* 21(7): 378–385. 1995.

   This article is a good presentation of imaging modalities with extra detail to echocardiography, with a summary of clinical findings and treatment modalities.

3. Consilus, E. M., and P. A. Bohachick. Cancer: Pericardial effusion and tamponade. *Cancer Nurs* 11(2): 391–397. 1984.

   This article provides a good description of the hemodynamic consequences of tamponade. A helpful figure illustrates the anatomy of the pericardial cavity. It offers clear discussion of clinical manifestations and a description of paradoxical pulse measurement.

4. Hankins, J. R., et al. Pericardial window for malignant pericardial effusion. *The Annals of Thoracic Surgery.* 30(5): 465–471. 1980.

   This contains a good description and diagnosis of technique used for creation of pericardial window using subxiphoid approach.

5. Joiner, G. A., and G. R. Kolodychuk. Neoplastic cardiac tamponade. *Crit Care Nurs Q* 11(2): 50–58. 1991.

   This provides a good summary of the etiology, pathophysiology, and clinical course of neoplastic cardiac tamponade. A comprehensive nursing care plan is provided.

6. Laham, R. J., et al. Pericardial effusion in patients with cancer: Outcome with contemporary management strategies. *Heart* 75: 67–71. 1996.

   This article reports a retrospective observational study of 93 patients with a cancer diagnosis and pericardial effusion in an attempt to determine the best management strategy. It includes discussion of results of analysis and recommendations.

7. Mangan, C. M. Malignant pericardial effusions: Pathophysiology and clinical correlates. *Oncol Nurs Forum* 19(8): 1215–1223. 1992.

   An overview of the pathophysiology is provided, including risk factors, stage of clinical dysfunction, medical management, and nursing interventions. It includes an excellent review of literature.

8. Muir, K. W., and J. C. Rodger. Cardiac tamponade as the initial presentation of malignancy: is it as rare as previously supposed? *Postgrad Med J* 70: 703–707. 1994.

   This article reports five cases of cardiac tamponade as initial presentation of malignancy. It includes a discussion of the importance of echocardiography to aid in diagnosis and a review of malignancies most commonly associated with pericardial effusion.

9. Otto, S. E. *Oncology Nursing.* 490–498. Mosby Year Book, St. Louis. 1991.

   This summarizes clinical features and diagnostic and treatment methods. Nursing management is well presented in a diagnosis-and-intervention format.

10. Palacios, I. F. et al. Percutaneous balloon pericardial window for patients with malignant pericardial effusion and tamponade. *Cathet Cardiovasc Diagn* 22: 244–249. 1991.

    This presents results of percutaneous balloon pericardial window performed on eight patients with malignant pericardial effusion and tamponade. It provides detailed description of procedure. Pictures of procedure as enhanced by contrast are included.

11. Pursley, P. Acute cardiac tamponade. *Am J Nurs* (October): 1414–1418. 1983.

    A good explanation is provided of clinical signs, pathophysiology, and compensatory mechanisms. An excellent figure illustrates the catastrophic effects of cardiac tamponade.

12. Sulzbach, L. M. Measurement of pulsus paradoxus. *Focus on Critical Care* 16(2): 142–145. 1989.

    This offers a detailed description and explanation of physiology and measurement of pulsus paradoxus.

13. Theologides, A. Neoplastic cardiac tamponade. *Seminars in Oncology* 5(2): 181–192. 1978.

    This is an excellent review of incidence and symptomatology. It describes diagnostic tests and treatment approaches.

14. Ziskind, A. A., et al. Percutaneous balloon pericardiotomy for the treatment of cardiac tamponade and large pericardial effusions: Description of technique and report of the first 50 cases. *J. Amer Coll Cardiol* 21(1): 1–5. 1993.

    This article describes technique in detail, clinical characteristics of population, and results. Comparisons are made with other forms of treatment in discussion section.

Metabolic Emergencies

A. Hypercalcemia

Joan Martin Moore

INTRODUCTION

Hypercalcemia is a common and potentially fatal complication of malignancy. A rise in the serum calcium level can occur slowly and go unrecognized until severe symptomatology develops, or it can occur swiftly, causing a crisis within a short period of time. Hypercalcemia is considered an oncologic emergency because it is potentially fatal yet is reversible with prompt, effective treatment. Fatal complications include renal failure, coma, and cardiac arrest. The prognosis depends on the degree of hypercalcemia, severity of symptoms, etiology, and the speed with which hypercalcemia is recognized and treated. Untreated hypercalcemia is associated with a 50 percent mortality.

Although the exact incidence of hypercalcemia is unknown, it is estimated to occur in approximately 10 percent to 20 percent of cancer patients. For certain breast and lung tumors, however, the incidence could be as high as 40 percent to 50 percent. Although any tumor type can cause hypercalcemia, multiple myeloma and tumors of the breast, lung, kidneys, head, neck, and esophagus are the most frequently associated malignancies (Table 16A–1). Estrogen and antiestrogen therapies used for metastatic disease can cause progression of hypercalcemia. Exacerbating nonmalignant conditions include primary hyperparathyroidism, thyrotoxicosis, prolonged immobilization, excessive vitamin A and D ingestion, renal failure, and thiazide diuretic therapy.

PATHOPHYSIOLOGY

Care of the patient at risk for hypercalcemia requires an understanding of the mechanisms of normal calcium regulation as well as the pathophysiology related to hypercalcemia in malignancy, its clinical manifestations, and the rationale for treatment.

16A

Table 16A-1
Malignancies Most Frequently Associated with Hypercalcemia

Breast
Lung
Renal
Head and neck
Multiple myeloma
Lymphoma

Normal Calcium Regulation

Calcium concentration in the body is maintained within a narrow range of 9–11 mg/dl under normal conditions. Three organ sites are involved in this process:

1. Bone, which contains 99 percent of the body's calcium;
2. The gastrointestinal (GI) tract, which absorbs ingested calcium or eliminates it in feces;
3. The kidney, which filters and reabsorbs ionized calcium (Ca^{2+}).

Hormonal Regulatory Mechanisms

Calcium homeostasis depends on sensitive regulatory mechanisms that are altered in response to the serum calcium level. These regulatory mechanisms include parathormone (PTH), vitamin D, and calcitonin. Their effects on calcium are outlined in Table 16A–2.

Parathormone is a hormone secreted by the parathyroid gland in response to low serum calcium levels that stimulate osteoclasts, cells that act to break down bone tissue. Calcium is thus moved from bone into the extracellular fluid. PTH also stimulates gastric and kidney reabsorption of calcium. The net result of PTH secretion is therefore an increase in serum calcium. Vitamin D secretion also increases serum calcium by enhancing gastric absorption of calcium and release of calcium from bones.

Conversely, calcitonin, a hormone secreted by the thyroid gland in response to high serum calcium, decreases serum calcium levels by inhibiting osteoclast activity. This reduces bone destruction and release of calcium into the bloodstream.

When hypercalcemia occurs, the body's effort to maintain homeostasis should result in suppression of PTH and vitamin D secretion and in enhanced calcitonin secretion. If these measures are inadequate, normal regulatory mechanisms fail and the hypercalcemic condition worsens.

Table 16A–2
Calcium Regulatory Mechanisms

Regulatory Mechanism	Effect on Calcium Level
Parathormone (PTH)	Increases Ca^{2+}
Vitamin D	Increases Ca^{2+}
Calcitonin	Decreases Ca^{2+}

Hypercalcemia in Malignancy

In the past decade, research has provided an increased understanding of the pathophysiology of hypercalcemia in malignancy. Previously, malignant hypercalcemia was primarily considered to result from tumor invasion into bone. Researchers recognized, however, that the extent of metastatic bone disease did not correlate with hypercalcemia. In addition, 15 percent of patients developed hypercalcemia without evidence of skeletal involvement with tumor, whereas several malignancies that frequently result in bone metastasis rarely result in hypercalcemia.

Malignancy associated hypercalcemia can be divided into two categories: humoral hypercalcemia of malignancy (HHM) and local osteolytic hypercalcemia (LOH). Categories of hypercalcemia in malignancy related to specific tumor types are described in Table 16A–3. Many tumors produce hypercalcemia by both humoral and local mechanisms.

It is now known that the most common form of hypercalcemia associated with solid tumors is humoral (factors circulating in the blood) hypercalcemia. Ectopic secretion of parathyroid hormone by tumors was previously considered to be the source of humoral hypercalcemia. Current evidence suggests that 80 percent of HHM is due to tumor production of parathyroid hormone related peptide (PTH-rP), which is normally undetectable; however, it is detectable in 80 percent to 90 percent of hypercalcemic cancer patients. Similar to parathyroid hormone, PTH-rP results in

Table 16A–3
Categories of Hypercalcemia in Malignancy Related to Specific Tumor Types

Category	Tumor Type

A. Humoral
    Calcitriol-mediated
	Epidermoid, renal, breast
	    Hodgkin's disease, non-Hodgkin's lymphoma

B. Local osteolytic	Lung, breast, myeloma

Table 16A–4
Osteolytic Cytokines Associated with Hypercalcemia

Cytokine	Action
Transforming growth factor alpha	Increases bone resorption. Produced by many tumor types.
Granulocyte macrophage colony stimulating factor	Stimulates immune cells to produce tumor necrosis factor and interleukin 1.
Tumor necrosis factor a+b	Increases osteoclast activation.
Interleukin 1	Increases osteoclast activation.
Interleukin 6	Increases recruitment and formation of osteoclasts. Produced by osteoclasts in response to stimulation by parathyroid hormone related peptide and interleukin 1.
Prostaglandin E	Increases bone resorption.
Procathepsin D	Activates osteoclasts directly.

increased serum calcium levels by stimulating osteoclastic activity and increasing bone resorption. Renal phosphate excretion is inhibited and renal tubular calcium reabsorption is enhanced.

Another type of HHM, which is rare, is that of calcitriol-mediated hypercalcemia. It is most commonly seen in patients with Hodgkin's disease and non-Hodgkin's lymphoma. Hypercalcemia results from ectopic production of 1,25 dihydroxyvitamin D, which causes increased gastrointestinal absorption of calcium. Cytokines have been implicated in modulating calcitriol-mediated hypercalcemia; however, the interactions are not yet fully understood.

The second category of malignancy-associated hypercalcemia, accounting for 20 percent of cases, is LOH. Hypercalcemia occurs as a result of increased bone resorption caused by activated osteoclasts in the area of metastatic bone sites. Several osteolytic cytokines have been implicated in this form of hypercalcemia and are identified in Table 16A–4. In addition to their roles in normal physiology, these humoral factors play a role in stimulating osteoclast activity. They can be released from or induced by malignant cells.

Role of Calcium in Metabolic Functions

Calcium plays a vital role in many metabolic functions. In addition to its role in maintaining bones, teeth, and normal clotting mechanisms, muscle contraction and nerve impulse transmission also depends on calcium. Cell membrane permeability is altered by changes in calcium levels. A decrease in extracellular calcium increases the excitability of nerve and muscle cells by decreasing the amount of depolarization needed to initiate changes in the cell membrane, which produces action potentials and results in contractile activity. Conversely, an increase in extracellular calcium decreases excitability. Because calcium is involved in a wide variety of metabolic functions, persons with abnormal calcium levels can exhibit a wide variety of symptoms. This varied symptomatology could contribute to confusion over the initial diagnosis of hypercalcemia discussed in the section "Clinical Manifestations."

ASSESSMENT

The initial step in the diagnostic workup is the laboratory serum calcium determination. To ensure accuracy, the following procedures have been recommended when obtaining serum calcium levels:

1. Clinician should make two determinations.
2. Specimens should be taken while patient is fasting to avoid postprandial changes.
3. Clinician should apply tourniquet no longer than two minutes. (A 10 percent increase in Ca^{2+} level could occur secondary to oxidation from increased venous pressure.) Urine calcium measurements are also recommended for symptomatic patients, because increases can be detected earlier in urine than in the serum.

Serum Calcium Levels

Serum calcium is normally maintained within a narrow range, approximately 9–11 mg/dl. The 1 percent of calcium not found in bone is reflected in a dynamic equilibrium between three forms: stored, albumin-bound, and ionized. Only the ionized portion of calcium is biologically active and therefore of clinical significance. Because laboratories generally measure the total serum calcium level, it is necessary when interpreting calcium levels to estimate changes in the ionized or active calcium, unless the laboratory reports the ionized calcium level. The normal ionized calcium level is 4.2–5.2 mg/dl.

It is especially important to interpret calcium levels in relation to serum proteins. For example, when serum albumin is reduced, less calcium is protein bound, which creates an increase in ionized calcium. A normal calcium level associated with a marked reduction in serum albumin should be considered hypercalcemia. Conversely, an abnormally low but asymptomatic calcium level might be found in a patient with hyperproteinemia, reflecting the increase in bound serum calcium. It is especially important to understand this relationship in the hypercalcemia of malignancy because many cancer patients have a low serum albumin. Recognition of the rela-

Table 16A–5
Rough Calculation to Correct Calcium Level
with Abnormal Low Albumin

0.8 mg/dl of Ca^{2+} for every 1.0 g/dl of albumin

Example: Laboratory reports

Calcium of 10.5 mg/dl
Albumin of 2.0 g/dl

3.5	normal albumin (low normal)
−2.0	reported albumin
1.5	corrected

to correct Ca^{2+} $\dfrac{0.8}{1.0} = \dfrac{x}{1.5}$

x = 1.2 mg Ca^{2+}

Corrected Ca^{2+}	10.5	reported
	+ 1.2	corrected
	11.7	corrected

Reprinted with permission from Raven Press, Ltd., from Mahon, S. M., Signs and symptoms associated with malignancy-induced hypercalcemia. *Cancer Nursing* 12(3): 153–160. 1989.

tionship between serum proteins and calcium is critical, particularly in the patient who has suspicious symptoms despite a normal calcium level. If hypoalbuminemia exists, the measured calcium concentration should be increased by .8 mg/dl for each 1.0 g/dl that plasma albumin concentration falls below normal. Sample calculations to correct the calcium level in the presence of low albumin are included in Table 16A–5.

Another important correlate in assessing calcium level is the phosphate level. Eighty-five percent of phosphate is combined with calcium in the skeleton. Because an inverse relationship exists between calcium and phosphate, factors that increase phosphate (PO_4^{3-}) levels will decrease calcium levels. This provides the rationale for the use of phosphates in the management of hypercalcemia.

Clinical Manifestations

Because of the role calcium plays in a wide variety of metabolic functions, the variety of possible signs and symptoms complicate the diagnosis. Further complicating the diagnosis are the variation in onset and the degree of severity of the presenting symptoms. Symptoms could be nonspecific and insidious in onset, such as anorexia, nausea, vomiting, constipation, and weakness. In other cases, symptoms of dehydration, renal failure, and coma could develop swiftly, corresponding to a very rapid rise in calcium, and result in a life-threatening hypercalcemic crisis. Not only can symptoms vary, but they might not correlate with serum calcium levels.

Table 16A–6 summarizes the degrees, signs, and symptoms of hypercalcemia. Many of the early symptoms of hypercalcemia, such as anorexia, nausea, vomiting, constipation, and abdominal pain, result from hypercalcemia's effect on smooth and skeletal muscle of the GI tract. Obstipation and ileus can occur as hypercalcemia progresses.

Neuromuscular and cardiac symptoms reflect interference with normal contractility of skeletal, smooth, and cardiac muscle along with altered nerve impulse transmission. Neurologic symptoms reflect the depressive effect of the hypercalcemia on central and peripheral nervous system functions. Alterations in mental status could manifest in slowed mentation, shortened attention span, reduced memory span, poor calculation, or inappropriate behavior and conversation. Confusion and somnolence can progress to coma and death. Hypotonicity of skeletal muscles is seen in de-

Table 16A–6
Degrees of Hypercalcemia: Signs and Symptoms*

Body System Affected	Mild (Less than 12 mg/dl)	Moderate (12–15 mg/dl)	Severe (Above 15 mg/dl)
Gastrointestinal	Anorexia, nausea, vomiting, vague abdominal pain	Constipation, increased abdominal pain, abdominal distension	Atonic ileus, obstipation
Neurologic	Restlessness, difficulty in concentrating, depression, apathy, lethargy, clouding of consciousness	Confusion, psychoses, somnolence	Coma → death
Muscular	Easily fatigued muscle weakness (generalized or involving shoulders and hips), hyporeflexia	Increased muscular weakness, bone pain	Profound muscular weakness, ataxia, pathologic fractures
Renal	Nocturia, polyuria, polydipsia	Renal tubular acidosis, renal calculi	Oliguric renal failure, renal insufficiency, azotemia
Cardiovascular	Hypertension (may or may not be present)	Cardiac dysrhythmias, EKG abnormalities (shortening of QT interval on EKG, coving of ST-T wave, widening of T wave)	Cardiac arrest → death

*Signs and symptoms regardless of serum calcium levels may vary from person to person.

Reprinted with permission from the Oncology Nursing Press. Poe, C. M. and Radford, A. I. The challenge of hypercalcemia in cancer. *Oncology Nursing Forum* 12(6): 31. 1985.

creased or absent deep tendon reflexes. Impairment in cardiac muscle conduction and contractility could be evident in EKG changes or arrhythmias. Initial EKG changes can suggest hypercalcemia but are rarely diagnostic. A lengthening of the PR interval, shortening of the QT interval, and widening of the T wave with a "cove-like" appearance can be seen. Cardiac arrest can occur with high calcium levels.

The acute renal effects of hypercalcemia, polyuria, and polydipsia result from renal compensatory mechanisms that increase urinary calcium absorption. Polyuria is caused by a defect in renal tubular function that leads to an inability to conserve water. Polyuria results in dehydration, causing polydipsia. Chronic hypercalciuria causes precipitation, resulting in nephrolithiasis and ultimately renal obstruction. These combined disorders lead to renal insufficiency and potential failure.

Hypercalcemic Crisis

A true emergency exists when hypercalcemia results in severe nausea and vomiting, dehydration, confusion, coma, and renal failure. As the calcium level rises, the effect of hypercalcemia on the kidneys exacerbates the problem. Figure 16A–1 illustrates the vicious cycles that develop.

The anorexia, nausea, vomiting, and polyuria caused by hypercalcemia result in dehydration, which accentuates the hypercalcemia by compromising renal function. The body strives to correct the dehydration by decreasing the glomerular filtration rate (GFR) and increasing sodium reabsorption. Both mechanisms result in water conservation. However, a reduced GFR also results in decreased excretion of calcium, whereas increased sodium reabsorption enhances calcium reabsorption. Thus the volume-depleted patient cannot adequately excrete calcium.

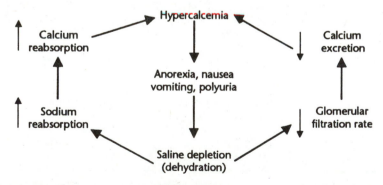

Figure 16A-1. Vicious cycles in hypercalcemia.

Reprinted with permission from Cunningham, S. E., Fluid and electrolyte disturbance associated with cancer and its treatment. Nursing Clinics of North America 17(4) (December 1982).

MEDICAL MANAGEMENT

All measures to control the hypercalcemia of malignancy will be futile if the tumor is not effectively controlled. Surgical removal of the tumor, effective radiation, chemotherapy, or hormonal manipulation is crucial.

Treatment of hypercalcemia related to malignancy is determined by the underlying disease, the degree of hypercalcemia, and the clinical presentation. Untreated hypercalcemia is progressive and ultimately fatal. In the presence of uncontrollable, advanced disease, the choice of treatment might be influenced by its implications for quality of life.

For an asymptomatic patient with a calcium level less than 13 mg/dl, tumor treatment might be the only therapy indicated. With new agents now available to decrease serum calcium levels, factors such as rapidity of response necessary and absence of contraindication can dictate the choice of treatment for symptomatic patients.

In the medical management of patients presenting with acute hypercalcemia, hydration with isotonic saline is the treatment first considered. Not only is dehydration corrected, but also the kidney's ability to excrete calcium is enhanced as sodium reabsorption is reversed. Fluid volumes range from five to eight liters per day initially to three liters per day for maintenance.

Diuretics such as furosemide or ethacrynic acid are often prescribed along with hydration. Furosemide promotes further diuresis of sodium by inhibiting the reabsorption of sodium in the proximal tubule of the kidney. Furosemide should not be given before the patient is adequately hydrated. Thiazide diuretics are contraindicated in this setting because they depress the urinary excretion of calcium. Medications with the potential to exacerbate hypercalcemia, such as estrogens and antiestrogens, should be discontinued.

Patients whose acute hypercalcemia resists these treatment methods and patients with impaired cardiac or renal function can be considered for hemodialysis if a rapid decrease in the calcium level is necessary to prevent heart block. In other cases, additional pharmacologic interventions can be employed (Table 16A–7).

A relatively new class of drugs, bisphosphonates, has become the treatment of choice in the management of moderate to severe hypercalcemia. Bisphosphonates inhibit osteoclastic bone resorption. Of the currently available bisphosphonates (etidronate, clodronate, and pamidronate), pamidronate seems to be the most potent. The onset of action is within 24–48 hours and the average duration of action is two to three weeks. The recommended dose of pamidronate in moderate hypercalcemia (corrected serum calcium of approximately 12–13.5 mg/dl) is 60–90 mg; in severe hypercalcemia (corrected serum calcium >13.5 mg/dl), it is 90 mg, given as an initial, single-dose intravenous infusion over 4–24 hours. If hypercalcemia recurs, it is recommended that seven days elapse before retreatment to allow for full response to the initial dose. At that time, retreatment with pamidronate can be administered in doses identical to initial therapy. The following adverse effects have been most commonly reported with pamidronate: mild transient fever and infusion site reaction (erythemia, swelling/induration, pain on palpation at catheter insertion site).

Table 16A-7
Drugs Utilized in Management of Hypercalcemia

Drug	Dosage	Administration	Side Effects
Diuretics			
Furosemide (Lasix®)	40–80 mg every 1–2 hrs	IV or PO	Potassium, sodium, and magnesium
Ethacrinic acid (Edecrin®)	20–40 mg every 1–2 hrs	IV	depletion
Bisphosphonates			
Etidronate (Didronel®)	7.5 mg/kg/d 3–7 days	IV 2–4 hr infusion	Gastric intolerance, diarrhea; contraindicated if serum creatinine >2.5 mg/dl
Pamidronate (Aredia®)	60–90* mg as single 24 hr infusion *90 mg recommended for severe hypercalcemia (serum Ca^{2+} > 13.5 mg/dl)	4–24 hr infusion	Transient fever or rash Mild fever, infusion site reaction, asymptomatic decreased PO_4^{3-}, K^+, and Ca^{2+}
Clodronate (Bonefos®) (Clastoban®) (Loron®) (Ostac®)	1.5 g	IV 4 hr infusion	Acute renal failure with rapid infusion
Calcitonin (Calcimar®)	4 IU/kg every 6 hrs for 2 days	IM or SC	Mild nausea, facial flushing, urticaria, potential allergic reaction
Glucocorticoids			
Prednisone	30–60 mg/d	PO	Hyperglycemia, gastric distress, increased infection risk, Cushingoid symptoms, emotional disturbances, osteoporosis, hypertension
Hydrocortisone	100 mg every 6 hrs	IV	
Gallium nitrate (Ganite®)	200 mg/m²/d for 5 days	IV 24 hr infusion	Nephrotoxicity Contraindicated if serum creatinine >2.5 mg/dl
Plicamycin	15–25 mcg/kg body weight every 24–48 hrs	IV	Clotting abnormalities, renal and hepatic toxicity, nausea, local tissue necrosis if extravasated
Oral Phosphates			
Fleet Phosphosoda®	6.7 ml/d	PO	Diarrhea, soft-tissue calcification
Neutra-Phos®	250 mg, 4 times daily	PO	

Hypophosphatemia, hypomagnesemia, hypokalemia, and hypocalcemia, all asymptomatic, have been reported. Therefore, close monitoring of laboratory values is indicated.

Another bisphosphonate, clodronate, is also highly effective in achieving normal calcium levels. Intravenous clodronate has an onset of action between 2 and 3 days that lasts 10–12 days. Lowest calcium levels occur at day 5 or 6. The present dose recommendations are 1.5 g as a single dose over four hours or 300 mg daily for up to 10 days.

Etidronate appears to bind to the bone surface and prevent osteoclast resorption. Etidronate is administered at 7.5 mg/kg/day in a two-hour infusion for three to seven days. At this dose it is free of significant toxicity when administered to patients without renal failure (creatinine <2.5 mg/dl). Serum calcium levels begin to decline within two days, with the lowest level reached within seven days of administration.

There is evidence to suggest that response to treatment with bisphosphonates is dependent on the mechanism responsible for the hypercalcemia. Patients with hematological malignancies respond more favorably than those with humoral hypercalcemia. It has been hypothesized that the lack of effect of bisphosphonates on the kidney is responsible for the variability of the response and is an area of continued investigation.

Oral bisphosphonates are currently available for maintenance use when the serum calcium has normalized. However, these agents are very poorly absorbed from the GI tract, significantly limiting their use. Research with this class of drugs involves exploring the possibility of preventing bone metastases and its associated morbidity. Development of new bisphosphonates with improved bioavailability will greatly enhance this effort.

Calcitonin, a hormone that causes hypocalcemia by inhibiting osteoclast activity and thereby reducing bone depletion, has been utilized in the treatment of acute hypercalcemia because of its rapid onset of action and minimal toxicity. Dramatic decreases in calcium levels can be seen two to three hours after the drug is administered; however, the decrease in serum calcium is transient, lasting only one day. The usual starting dose is 1–4 IU/kg subcutaneously or by intramuscular injection every six hours for a maximum of eight consecutive doses. Using salmon calcitonin (Calcimar®), side effects are mild and infrequent, with approximately 10 percent of patients experiencing mild nausea and vomiting. Facial flushing, urticaria, and local dermatologic reactions can occur. Side effects can be minimized by administering injections at night. Calcitonin can be used in addition to pamidronate when rapid decrease in serum calcium is desired.

Steroids are indicated for the rare occurrence of hypercalcemia due to increased production of 1,25 dihydroxyvitamin D or if the malignancy is steroid responsive. Glucocorticoids, such as prednisone, have been used in hypercalcemia management. The efficacy of this treatment could be due to an antitumor or antivitamin D effect. They have been most effective for hypercalcemia due to multiple myeloma, non-Hodgkin's lymphoma, and breast carcinoma. The disadvantages of using glucocorticoids include the seven- to ten-day period required for response and the well-known side effects that occur when they are used over extended periods of time (see Table 16A–7). Glucocorticoids have also been used in conjunction with calcitonin in attempts to prolong the hypocalcemic effect.

Gallium nitrate (Ganite®) is one of the most recently approved agents for hypercalcemia management. Although ineffective as the antineoplastic for which it was developed, this agent was discovered to be very effective for treating bone conditions associated with bone resorption. Gallium nitrate inhibits bone resorption by inhibiting PTH-induced calcium resorption. The recommended dose is 200 mg/m^2 daily, administered as a 24-hour infusion for five days. Serum calcium concentrations decrease within 48 hours. Normocalcemia is achieved in four to seven days and lasts six to eight days or longer. Nephrotoxicity occurs in 8 percent to 15 percent of patients. This adverse effect is reversible with vigorous hydration and maintaining a urine output of 2L/day. Concurrent use of nephrotoxic agents such as amphotercin B and aminoglycosides should be avoided. This agent is contraindicated in patients with renal insufficiency (creatinine >2.5 mg/dl). The use of gallium nitrate for hypercalcemia has been limited by its adverse effects, necessary duration of therapy and cost.

Plicamycin, an antibiotic with cytotoxic activity, has been shown to produce hypocalcemia, presumably by blocking PTH. It can also inhibit bone resorption. In doses of 15–25 mcg/kg, its maximal effect is demonstrated in 24–72 hours and lasts four to six days. No antitumor effect is seen with this dosage. Its use has been limited by potential side effects, which include thrombocytopenia, hemorrhage, azotemia, and hepatocellular necrosis. Therefore, it is contraindicated for thrombocytopenic patients and not recommended for patients with clotting, renal, and liver function abnormalities.

Oral phospates are rarely administered for chronic hypercalcemia. Doses of 30–60 ml daily inhibit bone resorption. Caution is indicated if the serum phosphate level is high, because calcium precipitation can result in renal or soft-tissue calcification. Diarrhea is a common, bothersome side effect that patients often find intolerable. Indomethacin and aspirin, though once popular in treating hypercalcemia, are now rarely used because they cause variable and inconsistent decreases in serum calcium. More effective therapy is available.

Because immobilization enhances bone resorption, nonpharmacological management emphasizes mobilization to minimize bone depletion. Calcium intake need not be restricted, because gastric absorption of calcium is decreased in hypercalcemia due to malignancy. A rare exception that might require restriction is when increased intestinal absorption of calcium is known to be exacerbating the problem. Excessive ingestion of vitamin A and D should be avoided

In the palliative care setting, withholding treatment for malignant hypercalcemia has frequently been advocated. The coma resulting from hypercalcemia was believed to reduce terminal suffering and avoid futile measures. That position is being reconsidered by clinicians for two reasons. First, the symptoms of nausea, anorexia, vomiting, constipation, confusion, and sedation, which result from hypercalcemia, are very distressing. Second, effective, well-tolerated treatment for hypercalcemia, involving intravenous medication followed by oral maintenance medication, is available with biphosphonates. Bisphosphonate therapy has also been shown to decrease bone pain and pathological fractures, an added benefit for terminally ill patients with skeletal metastases.

NURSING MANAGEMENT

Although hypercalcemia might not be preventable, early recognition enables the patient to avoid a crisis state with serious sequelae. Nurses need to recognize the population at risk and distinguish early signs of hypercalcemia from disease symptoms or treatment-related toxicity. Patients and their families should be taught the signs and symptoms of hypercalcemia that could develop. Home health nurses must also be made aware of the risk so the patient can be monitored at home for early signs and symptoms. Table 16A–8 outlines the nursing protocol for the prevention and early detection of hypercalcemia.

The need and rationale for mobilization should be stressed. Because pain and weakness often interfere with ambulation, pain medication and rest periods before and after walking can help patients to meet this goal. Patients with multiple metastases to the bone are at risk for pathological fractures, a risk that must be considered in efforts to mobilize the patient. If a bony area is noted to be painful, x-ray evaluation is indicated and, if necessary, stabilization measures or radiation therapy should be undertaken before further attempts at mobilization. Although weight bearing is required

Table 16A–8
Nursing Protocol for the Prevention and Early Detection of Hypercalcemia

Problem	Nursing Intervention
Tumor type	Recognize population at risk for hypercalcemia (Table 16A–1) and those with bone metastasis. At each visit, check serum Ca^{2+}, $PO_4{}^{3-}$, and albumin. Evaluate for symptoms of anorexia, nausea, vomiting, constipation. Monitor pulse, BP, muscle strength, and mental status.
Immobility	Emphasize importance of mobility to patient/family. Ambulate patient TID if possible. Evaluate for pathological fracture if bone pain occurs.
Dehydration	Emphasize need to maintain hydration in high-risk patients.

to prevent demineralization, isometric exercises while on bed rest will help maintain muscle tone so that weight bearing can be achieved as soon as possible. When mobilization can be achieved safely, it has the twofold benefit of minimizing bone destruction and helping to prevent constipation.

The importance of maintaining hydration cannot be overemphasized. Any condition leading to dehydration, such as nausea and vomiting, decreased fluid intake, or diarrhea, must be reported. Family members are taught to recognize the early signs of hypercalcemia (e.g., anorexia, constipation, nausea, lethargy). If they are adequately prepared, their familiarity with the patient enables them to discern early mental status changes. Early recognition will result in prompt treatment before a crisis occurs. The nursing protocol for the supportive management of hypercalcemia focuses on the problems of altered mental status, fluid and electrolyte balance, GI disturbances, effects of treatment, and potential cardiac as well as renal changes (see Table 16A–9). The mental status of these patients ranges

Table 16A-9
Nursing Protocol for the Supportive Management of Hypercalcemia

Problem	Nursing Intervention
Altered mental status	Record baseline mental status and neurological exam. Monitor for increasing fatigue, confusion, stupor, loss of consciousness. Provide protective environment.
Fluid balance	Correct dehydration by IV saline administration. Maintain accurate I&O. Observe for signs of fluid overload—increased BP, shortness of breath. Administer diuretics and record response.
GI disturbance	Administer antiemetics to minimize nausea and vomiting. Correct constipation with stool softeners and laxatives as needed.
Electrolyte balance	Monitor electrolytes, especially K^+. Correct hypokalemia with IV potassium chloride.
Effect of treatment for hypercalcemia	Evaluate response to hypercalcemia treatment by monitoring serum Ca^{2+}, PO_4^{3-}, albumin. Administer specified drugs to induce hypocalcemia and observe for side effects (Table 16A–6). Observe for symptoms of hypocalcemia—seizures, tetany.
Potential cardiac changes	Monitor for arrhythmias, bradycardia, tachycardia, cardiac arrest. Observe EKG for widening QT intervals. Reduce doses of digoxin administered, monitor closely. Observe for signs of CHF.
Potential renal failure	Observe for oliguria, anuria. Monitor BUN, creatinine. Prepare for temporary hemodialysis.

CHF—congestive heart failure; I&O—intake and output; K^+—potassium

from confused and lethargic to fully comatose. The baseline mental status is documented and assessed frequently as treatment is undertaken. Attention is given to providing a protective environment until mental status returns to normal.

As normal saline is administered in large volumes to correct dehydration, the patient is observed for signs of fluid overload or congestive heart failure. This is especially critical for patients with cardiac impairment. Because of the possibility of cardiac damage, caution is indicated for patients who have received doxorubicin and daunorubicin. Strict intake and output records are maintained, noting the response to diuretics. Renal function is monitored in this manner along with serum BUN and creatinine.

Serum calcium levels are monitored frequently to determine response to therapy. Potent drugs with rapid onset of action that are used to reduce hypercalcemia could induce hypocalcemia. Patients should be observed for signs of hypocalcemia, including increased cardiac and neuromuscular irritability. Evidence of tetany can be demonstrated by positive Chvostek's and Trousseau signs. Phosphate and albumin levels are monitored in conjunction with serum calcium for accurate interpretation.

Plicamycin is a potent tissue irritant that can cause local necrosis if infiltration occurs. Therefore, the intravenous site must be observed carefully throughout the infusion for signs of infiltration. Clotting abnormalities and abnormal liver functions can result from the administration of plicamycin. Platelet status, clotting parameters as indicated by prothrombin and partial thromboplastin time, and liver function tests must be monitored for patients receiving plicamycin for acute or chronic hypercalcemia.

As noted previously, patients with very high calcium levels are at risk for cardiac arrest. Therefore, monitoring for arrhythmias and EKG changes is critical. The risk of tachyarrhythmias is increased if the patient becomes hypokalemic from hydration combined with furosemide diuresis. Because both hypercalcemia and hypokalemia increase cardiac irritability, monitoring electrolytes, including potassium, is essential. In addition to cardiac irritability, hypercalcemia also potentiates the inotropic and toxic effects of such cardiac glycosides as digitalis. Caution is indicated when administering these drugs to the hypercalcemic patient. Lowering the dose with careful monitoring is recommended.

When the acute hypercalcemia has been brought under control, patients whose underlying disease is not well controlled might require continuous or intermittent medication to keep their calcium levels within a normal range.

Both patients and families must understand the dosage and importance of prescribed medication for hypercalcemia and report when the patient is unable to take the medication. If the medication, like the oral phosphates, causes diarrhea, patients and family need to be aware of such side effects and how to manage them, so they will not discontinue the drug.

In the past, hypercalcemic patients were taught to avoid excessive calcium intake. Because the excess of calcium in the body comes from bone and not dietary intake, calcium restrictions are unnecessary and could cause further eating difficulties for anorexic patients.

In conclusion, hypercalcemia is a commonly encountered problem in patients with malignancy. The need to maintain hydration has been stressed throughout this section. Patients who are taught the simple measures of maintaining hydration, mobilization, and early recognition and reporting of symptoms will more likely seek and receive medical attention early, preventing an acute hypercalcemic state.

BIBLIOGRAPHY

1. Body, J. J, R. E. Coleman and M. Piccart. Use of bisphosphonates in cancer patients. *Cancer Treatment Reviews.* 22(4): 265–287. 1996.

   This article outlines use of bisphosphonates for hypercalcemia as well as prevention of bone metastasis.

2. Chisholm, M. A., A. L. Mulloy, and A. T. Taylor. Acute management of cancer-related hypercalcemia. *The Annals of Pharmacotherapy* 30(5): 507–513. 1996.

   This article contains useful algorithms for hypercalcemia management and cost analysis.

3. Kaplan, M. Hypercalcemia of malignancy: A review of advances in pathophysiology. *Oncol Nurs Forum* 21(6): 1039–1046. 1994.

   This is an excellent review of hypercalcemia with emphasis on recent advances in pathophysiology and nursing management.

4. Kovacs, C. S., S. M. MacDonald, C. L. Chik, et al. Hypercalcemia of malignancy in the palliative care patient: A treatment strategy. *Journal of Pain and Symptom Management.* 10(3): 224–232. 1995.

   This article outlines hypercalcemia management in the palliative care setting.

5. Seymour, J. F. and R. F. Gagel. Calcitriol: The major humoral mediator of hypercalcemia in Hodgkin's disease and non-Hodgkin's lymphomas. *Blood* 82(5): 1383–1394. 1993.

   This provides an excellent overview of calcitriol, a humoral mechanism of hypercalcemia of malignancy.

6. Takai, E., T. Yano, H. Iguchi, et al. Tumor-induced hypercalcemia and parathyroid hormone-related protein in lung carcinoma. *Cancer* 78(7): 1384–1387. 1996.

   Prognostic implications of tumor-induced hypercalcemia in lung cancer are discussed.

7. Vinholes, J., C. Guo, O. P. Purohit, et al. Evaluation of new bone resorption markers in a randomized comparison of pamidronate or clodronate for hypercalcemia of malignancy. *Journal of Clinical Oncology* 15(1): 131–138. 1997.

   This article reports a clinical trial comparing two bisphosphonates, demonstrating superiority of pamidronate.

8. Walls, J., N. Bundred and A. Howell. Hypercalcemia and bone resorption in malignancy. *Clinical Orthopaedics and Related Research* 312: 51–63. 1997.

This article outlines the role of parathyroid hormone-related protein and other osteolytic cytokines along with new biochemical markers to monitor response to treatment.

9. Watters, J., G. Gerrard and D. Dodwell. The management of malignant hypercalcemia. *Drugs* 52(6): 837–848. 1996.

This article reviews pharmacologic agents available in current practice for hypercalcemia management.

B. Tumor Lysis Syndrome

Joan Martin Moore

INTRODUCTION

Tumor lysis syndrome (TLS) is a disorder characterized by the development of specific metabolic and electrolyte abnormalities. These abnormalities include hyperphosphatemia, hyperkalemia, hyperuricemia, and hypocalcemia. The consequences of hyperkalemia and acute renal failure can be life-threatening.

This syndrome is primarily an iatrogenic complication of effective chemotherapy regimens. Tumor lysis syndrome occurs when rapidly growing tumors are treated with chemotherapy. As cells die and lyse following chemotherapy, large amounts of intracellular electrolytes and chemicals enter the bloodstream. Massive cell necrosis can also occur after radiation therapy and result in TLS. The syndrome can also be found when malignancies characterized by rapid cell growth, such as leukemia and lymphomas, are accompanied by an increased breakdown of nucleic acids.

It is important to recognize that TLS is not limited to those receiving therapy with antineoplastic agents. Any treatment for cancer that results in rapid cellular destruction, or a disease process that produces significant cell proliferation, can induce TLS. This syndrome has been reported in patients receiving high doses of corticosteroids without concomitant chemotherapy. It has also been reported following intrathecal methotrexate administration.

PATHOPHYSIOLOGY

The mechanism of TLS is more easily understood by considering the physiology involved in rapid cell growth and rapid cell destruction (Table

16B

16B–1). A review of the electrolyte composition of cells will facilitate understanding of the specific metabolic and electrolyte abnormalities that result from TLS.

The electrolyte concentration within cells differs from extracellular fluid content in that sodium and chloride dominate the fluid outside of cells while potassium and phosphorus dominate the fluid within the cell. Therefore, when cells lyse and release their contents, the result is increased serum potassium and phosphorus.

Another factor that contributes to hyperphosphatemia in TLS is the destruction of circulating lymphoblasts by chemotherapy. Because lymphoblasts contain more phosphorus than mature lymphocytes, the destruction of these immature forms results in increased serum phosphorus. As discussed in the section on hypercalcemia, an inverse relationship exists between phosphorus and calcium. An increase in serum phosphorus results in decreased serum calcium. This accounts for the hypocalcemia that develops in TLS. In addition to hypocalcemia, hyperphosphatemia also results in calcium-phosphate precipitation in various soft tissues, which can diminish the function of organs, especially the kidney.

Cells undergoing rapid growth and division contain high concentrations of nucleic acids. When rapid growth is accompanied by increased catabolism of nucleic acids, the result is increased uric acid formation and hyperuricemia. Chemotherapy-induced cell destruction also causes hyperuricemia as a result of nucleic acid degradation. Because uric acid is relatively insoluble in body fluids, small increases can result in precipitation. Urate crystals then form in renal tubules and collecting ducts, causing renal insufficiency and failure. The incidence of severe uric acid nephropathy after chemotherapy can be as high as 10 percent in patients with acute lymphoblastic leukemia.

The degree of TLS has been correlated with actual tumor mass estimated by clinical staging and serum LDH levels. Rapidity of cell turnover and responsiveness to chemotherapy are also factors in determining risk of

Table 16B–1
Mechanism of TLS

Etiological Factors	Electrolyte/Metabolic Abnormality
Lysis of cells results in intracellular K^+ release	$\uparrow K^+$
Lysis of cells results in intracellular PO_4^{3-} release	$\uparrow PO_4^{3-}$
Inverse relationship between Ca^{2+} and PO_4^{3-}	$\downarrow Ca^{2+}$
Increased cell destruction increases uric acid formation	$\uparrow$ Uric acid

TLS. Burkitt's lymphoma is an example of a rapidly dividing tumor (doubling time less than 66 hours) that is highly sensitive to chemotherapy. There have been reports of TLS caused by spontaneous necrosis unrelated to treatment in both hematologic and nonhematologic malignancies.

The duration of the metabolic disorders of TLS is related to tumor burden and renal function. Phagocytosis, hepatic metabolism, and renal excretion are all involved in clearing the products of tumor cell destruction. As the tumor burden is lessened through effective chemotherapy, the metabolic disorders of TLS are brought under control.

Excretion of uric acid, potassium, and phosphate depends on adequate renal function. If the body cannot clear the products of tumor lysis, the syndrome worsens. As would be expected, patients with compromised renal function are at higher risk for developing TLS and experience more severe symptomatology.

Assessment

The clinical manifestations of TLS are listed in Table 16B–2. Signs and symptoms of TLS vary depending on which metabolic imbalance predominates. If evidence for hyperphosphatemia (>2.6 mEq/L), hyper-

Table 16B–2
Clinical Manifestations of Tumor Lysis Syndrome

TLS	GI	Renal	Cardiac	Neuromuscular
Hyper-phosphatemia		Oliguria Anuria Azotemia		
Hyperkalemia			EKG changes Bradycardia Cardiac arrest	Muscle weakness Flaccid paralysis
Hyperuricemia	Nausea Vomiting	Oliguria Anuria Azotemia Acute renal failure		Lethargy
Hypocalcemia			EKG changes Ventricular arrhythmias Heart block	Twitching Cramping Digital and perioral paresthesia Tetany Convulsions

kalemia (>5 mEq/L), hyperuricemia (>8 mg/dl), and hypocalcemia (<9 mg/dl) are not sought together, confusion could arise over the etiology of a specific metabolic imbalance, which obscures the diagnosis. The physical exam focuses on an evaluation of cardiac, neurological, gastrointestinal (GI), and renal status as well as a determination of muscle strength. Pulse and EKG are monitored for changes in rate and/or rhythm.

MEDICAL MANAGEMENT

The primary treatment goals in the management of TLS are (1) to prevent renal failure and (2) to prevent severe electrolyte imbalance. Whenever cytotoxic treatment is undertaken in patients with leukemia, lymphoma, or bulky disease, prophylactic treatment to prevent uric acid formation is essential. Vigorous intravenous hydration is administered for one to two days before chemotherapy and continued for several days after to decrease uric acid concentration in the urine and to enhance renal excretion. Diuretics can be used to sustain output.

Prophylactic diuresis is one of the primary measures to prevent uric acid nephropathy. In addition to enhancing renal function, treatment is also aimed at preventing electrolyte imbalance. Diuretics such as furosemide, while inducing diuresis, also cause excretion of potassium. Thus, they are especially useful when TLS has resulted in hyperkalemia. However, such diuresis can result in hypomagnesemia and hypokalemia. Therefore, frequent electrolyte monitoring with correction of imbalances is warranted.

Allopurinol is the drug most commonly used to decrease uric acid concentration and prevent acute renal failure. Allopurinol prevents the formation of uric acid by inhibiting xanthine oxidase, the enzyme essential for the conversion of nucleic acids to uric acid.

Despite the use of allopurinol, renal failure could still occur in some patients. Patients with preexisting renal compromise are at high risk for renal failure. Although its efficacy is controversial, an alkaline diuresis could be added to the treatment. This is generally accomplished by administering 5 percent dextrose intravenously plus 50–100 mEq of sodium bicarbonate per liter. Urine pH is then maintained at 7.0 or greater. As the urine becomes more alkaline, uric acid becomes more soluble, minimizing precipitation and stone formation. Urine alkalinization is associated with potential complications. First, if the patient is hyperphosphatemic, it can cause increased calcium phosphate deposits in kidney tubules; second, if systemic alkalosis occurs, hypocalcemia is exacerbated.

Management of hyperkalemia consists of restricting potassium and avoiding pharmacologic agents that cause potassium retention. Acidosis is corrected because it exacerbates hyperkalemia. Administration of 50–100 grams of Kayexalate® as a retention enema is recommended. Measures designed to shift potassium into cells is of limited value in this situation and should only be used in conjunction with other potassium reduction measures.

Hyperphosphatemia is managed by limiting dietary phosphate and administering oral phosphate-binding antacids (aluminum hydroxide orally, 30 to 60 ml every four to six hours). Constipation is a common complication. Lowering the serum phosphate level is the most effective treatment for hypocalcemia. In case of ureteral obstruction, cystoscopy with alkaline lavage of the ureters has been recommended.

If all previous measures fail to increase the urine output, hemodialysis can be used to reduce hyperkalemia and serum uric acid and improve azotemia. Daily hemodialysis might be required to reduce the metabolic toxins, control volume, and manage uremia. Limitations of hemodialysis in TLS have been rebound hyperkalemia and poor control of serum phosphorus. Continous arteriovenous hemodialysis has been utilized as a more effective hemodialysis technique.

NURSING MANAGEMENT

Of primary importance in preventing TLS is recognition of the population at risk by home care as well as acute care nurses. One such group comprises patients with large, rapidly growing tumors, lymphomas, leukemias, small cell carcinoma of the lung, metastatic breast carcinoma, testicular carcinoma, and metastatic medulloblastoma. Allopurinol is prescribed for this high-risk group and administered before and during chemotherapy. Patients and families are taught the importance of allopurinol in preventing hyperuricemia. The second population at high risk to develop TLS includes patients with preexisting renal insufficiency (creatinine >1.6 mg/dl, uric acid >8 mg/dl). Maintaining hydration for both groups of patients is critical; urine alkalinization could be indicated.

In addition to conventional cytotoxic drugs, agents such as prednisolone, tamoxifen, and alpha interferon have been associated with the complication of TLS. Therefore, it is important to observe for signs of TLS when unconventional agents are used as well.

Lastly, due to the combination of metabolic disorders that characterize the onset of TLS, patients at risk to develop TLS and their families are taught to report signs of hyperphosphatemia, hyperuricemia, hyperkalemia, and hypocalcemia. The nursing protocol for the prevention and early detection of TLS is summarized in Table 16B–3.

The supportive nursing management in acute TLS focuses on maintaining fluid balance, monitoring electrolyte and metabolic imbalances, and observing for signs of renal insufficiency (Table 16B–4). While vigorous intravenous hydration is being administered along with the diuretics, the patient's weight, intake, output, and response to diuretics are carefully monitored. Observing for signs of fluid overload is critical, particularly in patients with preexisting or potential cardiac damage.

Due to the combined metabolic and electrolyte disorders found with TLS, electrolytes, calcium, and phosphorus are monitored daily, and more

Table 16B–3
Nursing Protocol for the Prevention and Early Detection of Tumor Lysis Syndrome

Factor	Nursing Intervention
Tumor type	Recognize population at risk for TLS: patients with large, rapidly growing tumors; lymphomas; leukemias; small cell lung carcinoma; metastatic breast carcinoma, and metastatic medulloblastoma.
Disease extent	Aggressive lymphomas (Stage C—abdominal tumor or Stage D—abdominal tumor with extra-abdominal sites). Increased pretreatment LDH levels. Obtain prescription for allopurinol and administer before and during chemotherapy. Maintain hydration with PO or IV fluids.
Renal insufficiency	Recognize high-risk patients—those with baseline creatinine >1.6 mg/dl and uric acid >8 mg/dl.
Early detection	Recognize combination of metabolic disorders that represent the onset of acute TLS.

often at first, depending on the clinical status of the patient. Patients are observed for signs of hyperkalemia: weakness, flaccid paralysis, EKG changes, and cardiac arrest. It is important to note that the effects of hyperkalemia on the heart are more severe in hypocalcemic patients. Symptoms of renal insufficiency related to hyperphosphatemia, such as oliguria and anuria, are noted. Patients are also observed for symptoms related to hypocalcemia, such as increased cardiac and neuromuscular irritability. Low serum calcium levels could be misleading in the presence of hypoalbuminemia (see chapter 16A). Hyperuricemia may be asymptomatic and evidenced only by an elevated uric acid level, or it could be accompanied by nausea, vomiting, lethargy, and signs of renal insufficiency.

To prevent uric acid formation, allopurinol is administered in doses of 600–800 mg daily either orally or intravenously, before and for several days after chemotherapy. Side effects from this agent are uncommon. Hypersensitivity reactions do occur and are manifested by skin rash, fever, abnormal liver function tests, eosinophilia, and acute renal failure. Allopurinol could potentiate the action of mercaptopurine and azathioprine; therefore, doses of these drugs are decreased when used in conjunction with allopurinol.

Urine alkalinization is accomplished by intravenous administration of sodium bicarbonate. Urine pH is continually monitored to maintain a value greater than seven. Patients are monitored for systemic alkalosis, which can enhance hypocalcemia.

Observing patients for signs of renal insufficiency and failure is critical. Daily BUN and creatinine are monitored. Any decrease in urine output or anuria is reported. Failure to respond to hydration and diuretics by in-

Table 16B–4
Nursing Protocol for the Supportive Management of Tumor Lysis Syndrome

Problem	Nursing Intervention
Fluid balance	Administer IV hydration. Monitor weight, I&O response to diuretics. Observe for signs of fluid overload, especially in patients with potential or preexisting cardiac damage.
Electrolyte balance	Monitor electrolytes qd or q 6–12 hrs as indicated. Correct imbalances as prescribed. Observe for signs of hyperkalemia: weakness, flaccid paralysis, EKG changes, cardiac arrest. Limit potassium intake. Avoid potassium-retaining drugs. Prepare for medical management of hyperkalemia, e.g., glucose and insulin, calcium sodium bicarbonate, cation-exchange resin.
Potential renal failure	Monitor Ca^{2+}, $PO_4{}^{3-}$, uric acid, BUN, and creatinine daily for the 5- to 7-day period of cytolysis. Maintain hydration especially if preexisting renal insufficiency (creatinine >1.6 mg/dl, uric acid >8 mg/dl). Administer allopurinol 600–800 mg IV or PO qd. Monitor urine pH—maintain >7 by administering IV $NaHCO_3$ as prescribed. Report decreased urine output, anuria. Observe for nausea, vomiting, lethargy. Prepare to manage patient on temporary hemodialysis.
Potential cardiac irritability	Monitor lab values for hyperkalemia and hypocalcemia. Check pulse rate and rhythm frequently. Report irregularity. Observe for EKG changes, cardiac arrest.
Potential neuromuscular irritability	Monitor serum Ca^{2+} level. Observe for symptoms of hypocalcemia: muscle cramps, paresthesia, tetany, positive Chvostek's and Trousseau signs, seizures. Institute seizure precautions if indicated. Limit dietary phosphates. Administer phosphate-binding antacids. Minimize constipation with stool softeners. Administer calcium gluconate as prescribed.
Potential effects of drug therapy	Observe for side effects and hypersensitivity from allopurinol: skin rashes, eosinophilia, abnormal LFTs, renal failure. Decrease doses of 6-MP and azathioprine if given concurrently with allopurinol.

LFT—liver function test; $NaHCO_3$—sodium bicarbonate; 6-MP—mercaptopurine

creased output could indicate an obstructive problem due to precipitation of calcium phosphate or uric acid crystals in the kidney. In either event, hemodialysis will be undertaken to rapidly correct the metabolic imbalances that are potentially lethal if uncontrolled. Nursing management then centers on care of the patient undergoing temporary hemodialysis.

The daily monitoring of renal function as well as electrolyte and metabolic imbalances is continued for five to seven days, the time of greatest cytolysis and therefore the time of greatest risk to the patient.

In conclusion, TLS can be a serious and potentially fatal complication for patients undergoing cytotoxic chemotherapy. The combination of electrolyte and metabolic disorders places the patient at high risk for renal failure and/or cardiac arrest. Adequate measures to prevent hyperuricemia and to manage the signs and symptoms of TLS effectively are essential to minimize the risk. Extremely close monitoring by the medical and nursing staff is indicated to prevent serious or fatal complications until the TLS subsides.

BIBLIOGRAPHY

1. Arrambide, K. and R. D. Toto. Tumor lysis syndrome. *Seminars in Nephrology* 13(3): 273–279. 1993.

   This is review of TLS with an emphasis on the presentation of renal failure and the importance of dialytic management.

2. Hoffman, V. Tumor lysis syndrome: Implications for nursing. *Home Healthcare Nurse* 14(8): 595–600. 1996.

   This article describes the population at risk for TLS to assist home care nurses with early identification and intervention of symptoms.

3. Malik, I. A., S. Abubakar, F. Alam, et al. Dexamethasone-induced tumor lysis syndrome in high-grade non-Hodgkin's lymphoma. *Southern Medical Journal* 87(3): 409–411. 1994.

   This case study demonstrates the rare occurrence of TLS following dexamethasone.

4. Miaskowski, C. Body fluid composition, alteration in: Tumor lysis syndrome. In McNally, J. C., E. T. Somerville, C. Miaskowski, and M. Rostad, eds. *Guidelines for Oncology Nursing Practice.* 408–412. W.B. Saunders Company, Philadelphia. 1991.

   A detailed nursing care plan is offered for patients with TLS.

5. Pinchette, V., M. Leblanc, A. Bonnardeaux., et al. High dialysate flow rate continuous arteriovenous hemodialysis: A new approach for the treatment of acute renal failure and tumor lysis syndrome. *American Journal of Kidney Disease* 23(4): 591–596, 1994.

   This article contains description of dialysis technique that more efficiently reduces hyperphosphatemia without rebound hyperkalemia.

6. Simmons, E. D. and K. A. Somberg. Acute tumor lysis syndrome after intrathecal methotrexate administration. *Cancer* 67: 2062–2065. 1991.

   This case study illustrates unrecognized potential complication of intrathecal methotrexate induced–TLS.

7. Stucky, L. A. Acute tumor lysis syndrome: Assessment and nursing implications. *Oncol Nurs Forum* 20(1): 49–59. 1993.

This presents a detailed but clear pathophysiology of TLS, medical management, and nursing diagnoses/orders. A lengthy review of the literature is also provided.

8. Warrell, R. P. Metabolic emergencies. In DeVita, J., et al., eds. *Cancer Principles and Practice of Oncology*. 2128–2141. J.B. Lippincott Company, Philadelphia. 1993.

This section includes a complete description of hyperuricemia as a result of cell destruction following chemotherapy. Development of acute hyperuricemia nephropathy and treatment options are discussed.

C. Syndrome of Inappropriate Antidiuretic Hormone Secretion

Joan Martin Moore

INTRODUCTION

The syndrome of inappropriate antidiuretic hormone secretion (SIADH) is a disorder characterized by continuous secretion of antidiuretic hormone (ADH). Approximately 1 percent to 2 percent of patients with cancer will develop SIADH. For these patients, the result is fluid retention, inability to excrete dilute urine, and dilutional hyponatremia. The syndrome can be an oncologic emergency because of associated seizures, coma, and possible death. Because the most common etiology of SIADH is malignancy, oncology nurses should be aware of the population at risk in order to facilitate early detection. Knowledge of the pathophysiology of SIADH, as well as its clinical manifestations and available treatment options, is essential.

PATHOPHYSIOLOGY

Understanding SIADH depends on understanding how the body regulates water and the role that ADH plays in that regulation. The body constantly regulates water by either conserving or excreting it. ADH, which is released from the posterior pituitary gland, controls the balance. The distal renal tubules and collecting ducts of the kidneys are its site of action. As suggested by the word "*antidiuresis*" in its name, water is conserved when

16c

ADH is released. This conservation is achieved by increased reabsorption of water from the kidney.

There are two mechanisms by which the brain regulates ADH secretion. First, baroreceptors detect increases or decreases of the blood pressure in the left atrium. Increased atrial pressure stimulates the baroreceptors, sending impulses to the hypothalamus and posterior pituitary to limit the secretion of ADH. Conversely, decreased atrial pressure results in less baroreceptor stimulation so that more ADH is secreted. Thus, hypervolemic and hypovolemic states or changes in extracellular volume can be corrected appropriately by an increase or decrease in ADH secretion.

The other major control of ADH secretion is determined by extracellular osmolality. Receptors exist that are sensitive to extracellular osmolality. These osmoreceptors are located in the hypothalamus, where an increase in serum osmolality (or a more concentrated serum) causes increased ADH secretion and water conservation, producing a more dilute serum and more concentrated urine. If the serum osmolality decreases, ADH secretion is inhibited, which results in more dilute urine as excess water is excreted. Normal serum osmolality is 275–295 mOsm/kg.

In SIADH the normal osmolar response of the osmoreceptors malfunctions. As serum osmolality decreases, urine osmolality is concentrated, indicating hyperosmolality, rather than being diluted.

The factors known to stimulate ADH release are listed in Table 16C–1. In addition to changes in extracellular volume—i.e., hypovolemic states (fluid or blood loss)—and increased serum osmolality, stress is known to increase ADH secretion. As part of the body's stress response, mechanisms to conserve water are necessary in case of hemorrhage or sweating. This could account for why pain, surgery, and trauma also result in ADH secretion. Lastly, medications such as opioids, barbiturates, anes-

Table 16C–1
Factors Stimulating ADH Release

Clinical Condition	Medication
Hypovolemia	Opioids
Hypotension	Barbiturates
Increased serum osmolality	Anesthetics
Hyponatremia	Tricyclic antidepressants
Stress	Thiazide diuretics
Pain	Antineoplastics
Surgery	Cyclophosphamide
	Vincristine
	Vinblastine
	Cisplatin

thetics, tricyclic antidepressants, as well as some cancer chemotherapeutic agents, have been found to stimulate ADH release.

ETIOLOGY OF SIADH

Causes of SIADH are either secondary to a clinical disorder or pharmacologically induced (Table 16C–2). Clinical disorders causing SIADH fall into three categories: malignancy, pulmonary disease, and central nervous system disorders. Tumors with ectopic production of ADH are by far the most common cause of SIADH. Of the malignancies, lung carcinoma, especially of the small- or oat-cell carcinoma type, has the highest incidence. As many as 80 percent of these small cell lung cancer patients demonstrate some impairment in water excretion that is related to the extent of disease. The malignant lung cells of patients with SIADH have the capacity to synthesize, store, and release ADH. Laboratory research has shown that the ADH produced by neoplasms is identical to that produced by the posterior pituitary. Other tumor types associated with SIADH are listed in Table 16C–2.

Table 16C–2
Etiology of SIADH

Clinical Disorders	Pharmacologic Agents

1. Malignancy
  A. Lung, especially small cell
  B. GI: duodenal, colon, pancreatic, esophageal
  C. Head and neck
  D. Thymoma
  E. Diffuse large cell lymphoma of bone
  F. Hodgkin's and non-Hodgkin's lymphomas
  G. Adrenal cortex
  H. Brain tumors
  I. Bronchial carcinoids
	1. Chemotherapeutic Agents
	  A. Cyclophosphamide
	  B. Vincristine
	  C. Vinblastine
	  D. Cisplatin
	  E. Melphalan (high dose)

2. Central Nervous System
  A. Meningitis
  B. Encephalitis
  C. Brain abscesses
  D. Cranial trauma
  E. Brain tumors
	2. Miscellaneous Drugs
	  A. Chlorpropamide, antipsychotic tranquilizers
	  B. Tricyclic antidepressants
	  C. Narcotics, analgesics
	  D. General anesthetics
	  E. Barbiturates
	  F. Thiazide diuretics
	  G. Beta adrenergics
	  H. Clofibrate (Atromid-S®)
	  I. Diabinese®
	  J. Tobacco

3. Pulmonary
  A. Tuberculosis
  B. Aspergillosis
  C. Pneumonia	

The second major group of disorders associated with SIADH are those of the central nervous system. Meningitis, encephalitis, brain tumors and abscess, cranial trauma, and subarachnoid hemorrhage can all be accompanied by SIADH. It has been hypothesized that the mechanism responsible for SIADH is stimulation of the hypothalamic and posterior pituitary systems.

Hyponatremia and SIADH are associated with many pulmonary disorders. SIADH has been found in conjunction with many infections and inflammatory conditions such as aspergillosis, tuberculosis, lung abscess, asthma, and both viral and bacterial pneumonia. It is believed that benign pulmonary tissue also has the capacity to synthesize and secrete ADH.

Many drugs utilized in medical treatment can also cause SIADH. Certain drugs could increase hypothalamic production and release of ADH; others might exert the direct action on renal tubules that potentiates ADH. Particularly relevant to oncology is the fact that some commonly used cancer chemotherapeutic agents have been shown to induce SIADH by stimulating release of ADH from the posterior pituitary. Cyclophosphamide, vincristine, vinblastine, and cisplatin have all been implicated in SIADH. To minimize toxicity to the bladder and kidneys, vigorous hydration is required for the administration of cyclophosphamide and cisplatin; this further exacerbates the problem of water retention. Cyclophosphamide, vincristine, and cisplatin are commonly used for lung cancer; so the additional risk of SIADH for these patients becomes apparent.

Several pharmacologic agents known to increase ADH levels or potentiate the action of ADH are summarized in Table 16C–2. Other contributing factors in the pathogenesis of SIADH include stress, pain, and fear, which increase ADH production; and nausea, which stimulates ADH release.

ASSESSMENT

A classic feature of this syndrome is the existence of hyponatremia as a result of the dilution of body fluids. Normally the serum sodium is 140 mEq/L. In SIADH, serum sodium levels can fall below 120 mEq/L. Edema does not usually occur because the hypervolemia that results from the excess water stimulates volume receptors that cause an increase in urinary sodium excretion with concentrations in excess of 20 mg/L.

The presenting signs and symptoms of SIADH include weight gain, lethargy, weakness, irritability, and confusion. Anorexia, nausea, and vomiting can occur. If untreated, the serum sodium concentration continues to drop below 120 mEq/L, neurological abnormalities develop, and symptoms progress to convulsions and coma. Table 16C–3 illustrates the clinical presentation of SIADH.

Table 16C–3
Clinical Presentation of SIADH

Hyponatremia	Neurological	Gastrointestinal	Muscular	Renal
130	Normal	Normal	Normal	Normal
MILD 120	Fatigue Headache Altered sensorium Confusion	Anorexia	Muscle cramps Weakness	Weight gain
MODERATE 110	Lethargy Decreased deep tendon reflexes Personality changes	Nausea Vomiting Diarrhea Abdominal cramps	Weakness	Oliguria Anuria
SEVERE 100	Seizures Coma Death			

*(Left margin label, read vertically: **SERUM SODIUM**)*

The history and physical examination include evaluation of neurological and hydrational status. Early mental status changes could be subtle and require astute observation. An assessment of gastrointestinal function is made because anorexia, nausea, and vomiting can occur.

The clinical manifestations of SIADH consist of hyponatremia with corresponding hypo-osmolality in the absence of clinical evidence of hypovolemia. Laboratory data generally suggest water retention and hemodilution (Table 16C–4). Hyponatremia is the most striking of the electrolyte disorders. Serum sodium and serum osmolality will be decreased; urine sodium concentration and urine osmolality will be increased. BUN, creatinine, and albumin levels tend to be low or within normal range. In SIADH, the T3, T4, and adrenocorticoid hormone levels are normal. Calcium and potassium can be low secondary to dilution.

To make a confident diagnosis of SIADH, adrenal insufficiency and hypothyroidism must be ruled out, because both can increase ADH secretion. Pain and hypotension must be corrected because both can result in

Table 16C–4
Laboratory Values in SIADH

Decreased	Increased
Serum Na$^+$ <130 mEq/L	Urine Na$^+$ >220 mEq/24 hrs
Serum osmolality <275 mOsm/kg	Urine osmolality >1,200 mOsm/kg water

further ADH secretion despite hypo-osmolality. Dilutional hyponatremia can exist with congestive heart failure, renal failure, and liver disease with ascites. Thus, the coexistence of these states can complicate the diagnosis.

Determining the individual's response to a water load helps establish the diagnosis of SIADH. An oral water load is administered over a 15- to 20-minute period. The patient is then monitored for water excretion and urine osmolality. Normally, 80 percent of water is excreted within five hours, and the urinary osmolality falls to less than 100 mOsm/kg. In the presence of SIADH, water excretion is less than 40 percent by five hours and urine is less than maximally dilute. This procedure can be very dangerous if the serum sodium is not corrected to at least 125 mEq/L prior to the water load.

MEDICAL MANAGEMENT

Fluid restriction is the initial treatment in the management of SIADH. When symptoms are mild to moderate (serum sodium 125–134 mEq/L), fluid restriction to approximately 800–1,000 ml daily is adequate. Response is determined by increases in serum sodium and osmolality accompanied by weight loss.

When symptomatology is severe (coma, seizures, sodium less than 120 mEq/L), more aggressive therapy is indicated. Three percent saline is administered at a rate of 1–2 ml/kg per hour to raise the serum sodium no faster than 1–2 mEq/L per hour. Hypertonic saline must be administered via an infusion pump while patients are closely monitored for symptoms of hypernatremia. The risk of heart failure in patients who are volume overloaded and receiving 3 percent saline is significant. The addition of large doses of furosemide helps to improve symptomatology rapidly. Patients are then carefully monitored for potential electrolyte imbalances. Rapid fluctuation in the serum sodium can result in cerebral edema and seizures. Generally, until the serum sodium is normal, fluid intake should equal urine output. Fluid is restricted to 500 ml/day. Hyponatremia, when corrected, will recur if fluid restriction is not maintained. Any drugs that could contribute to water retention are withheld.

Drugs used in the management of SIADH include demeclocycline, furosemide, and lithium carbonate. Demeclocycline is the treatment of choice; however, an average of three days is required to increase the serum sodium level to >130 mEq/L. Demeclocycline, an antibiotic that decreases the renal response to ADH, has been shown to improve diuresis and hyponatremia when doses of 900–1,200 mg/day are administered; it is more effective than lithium. The major side effects have been azotemia, which promptly reverses when the drug is withdrawn, and the risk of superinfection. In addition, use of this agent in SIADH patients with cirrhosis has resulted in renal failure.

Furosemide, at 40 mg/day orally, could be useful for patients tolerant to demeclocycline. Salt must be replaced in the diet of those on oral furosemide therapy. Monitoring is also required to prevent alkalosis from a hypokalemic-hypochloremic state. Table 16C–5 lists drugs used in the management of SIADH and their nursing implications.

Lithium, an established ADH inhibitor, has been used with some success in treating both acute and chronic forms of SIADH. However, the use of this agent is limited by toxic side effects, manifested by sluggishness, drowsiness, tremors or muscle twitching, gastrointestinal disturbances, cardiac irritability, and thyroid dysfunction. Serum lithium levels are required to monitor toxicity levels.

When symptoms are brought under control, successful treatment of the disease process responsible for the syndrome must be initiated. Surgery, chemotherapy, radiation therapy, or a combination of these treatment modalities could be started. Absence of SIADH is an indicator of successful treatment. In the face of advanced disease, therapy might be palliative in order to reduce the need for fluid restriction, which might increase discomfort and reduce the quality of life for the cancer patient with SIADH.

Table 16C–5
Drugs Used in SIADH Management with Nursing Implications

Drug	Dose	Side Effects	Nursing Implications
Demeclocycline	900–1,200 mg/d PO	Azotemia Superinfection potential	Monitor urine output and renal function. Monitor for signs and symptoms of infection. Administer no less than 1 hour before meals and no sooner than 2 hours after meals. Milk- and calcium-containing products impair drug absorption.
Furosemide	40 mg/d PO	Hypokalemia Hypochloremia	Monitor electrolytes, especially potassium. Replace salt in diet. Monitor for alkalosis.

NURSING MANAGEMENT

Preventing SIADH might not be possible, but serious consequences can be avoided through early detection. A nursing protocol for early detection of SIADH is outlined in Table 16C–6. Early detection of weight gain, low urine output, hyponatremia, and mental status changes is essential. Symptoms of lethargy, weakness, weight gain, nausea, and irritability might not coincide. Therefore, the cause of these symptoms might be overlooked or attributed to the malignancy itself, unless one maintains a high index of suspicion, especially with patients at high risk. Lung cancer patients, particularly those with the small cell type, are monitored carefully for symptoms that suggest SIADH. Patient and family are taught to report those signs and symptoms to their caregivers. The importance of daily weights is emphasized. Attention is given to reducing factors that contribute to the release of ADH.

After the diagnosis of SIADH has been established, the focus of supportive nursing care is fluid balance (Table 16C–7). Restricting fluids to specified limits is essential. Weight, intake, and the quantity and concentration of output are carefully monitored. Water retention places the patient at risk for fluid overload and congestive heart failure. Patient with known cardiac disease, or those who have received doxorubicin, daunorubicin, and other anthracyclines with potential cardiac impairment, should be closely observed for shortness of breath, hypertension, and dependent edema.

Electrolytes are continually monitored for hyponatremia and hypokalemia. Seizure precautions are indicated if the serum sodium falls below 120 mEq/L. Hypokalemia often results when high doses of

Table 16C–6
Nursing Protocol for the Early Detection of SIADH

Problem	Nursing Intervention
Early detection	Recognize population at risk: patients with small cell lung carcinoma.
	Recognize presenting symptoms: weight gain, low urine output, hyponatremia, mental status changes, especially lethargy and drowsiness.
	Teach patients to report early signs and symptoms to health care team.
	Explain factors that stimulate ADH secretion (e.g., stress, smoking) and identify ways to minimize or eliminate them.
	Emphasize importance of daily weight and teach correct technique.

Table 16C–7
Nursing Protocol for the Supportive Management of SIADH

Problem	Nursing Intervention
Altered fluid balance	Restrict fluids to specified limits, monitor compliance. Determine amount of fluid PO/IV to be given every shift. Use infusion pump to avoid inadvertent IV fluid overload. Provide dietary consultation. Choose dietary fluids high in sodium. Assess skin turgor, mucous membranes. Obtain daily weights: same time, scale, clothes. Record careful I&O, monitor serum and urine osmolality and urine specific gravity. Perform frequent lung auscultation. Monitor for signs/symptoms of fluid overload. Administer antiemetics, antidiarrheals as prescribed.
Altered electrolyte balance	Monitor electrolytes frequently, especially sodium and potassium. Observe for hypokalemia. Monitor pulse, rate and rhythm, EKG for arrhythmias. Institute seizure precautions if serum sodium <120 mEq/L. Monitor for hypernatremia secondary to overcorrection: thirst, dry mucous membranes, lethargy, irritability, seizures.
Altered mental status	Obtain history and PE to include neurological exam with evaluation of mental status. Observe and report changes—confusion, irritability, weakness, lethargy, hyporeflexia, coma. Ensure protective environment for confused or comatose patient.

Altered comfort secondary to fluid restriction	Provide fluids within restriction.
	Provide frequent mouth care.
	    Avoid commercial mouthwash.
	    Provide artificial saliva PRN.
	Emphasize importance of fluid restriction and need for compliance.

Potential for immobility and altered skin integrity	Assess skin integrity every shift with special attention to bony prominences. Assess need for pressure-alternating mattress. Monitor and document signs/symptoms of pressure injury.

Potential effects of drug therapy	Observe for side effects related to drug therapy:
	    Demeclocycline: decreased urine output, azotemia, signs of infection.
	    Avoid administering demeclocycline at meal time.
	    Urea: abdominal pains, contraindicated for patients with ulcers.
	    Furosemide: hypokalemia, hypochloremia, replace salt in diet, and monitor for alkalosis.
	Document response to treatment: weight loss, increased serum sodium, increased serum osmolality.

Lack of response to therapy	Examine factors contributing to ADH release. Minimize pain, stress, and nausea. Limit use of opioids, barbiturates, tricyclic antidepressants. Examine compliance with fluid restriction.
Knowledge deficit regarding SIADH management	Teach patient/family to report early signs and symptoms: weight gain, lethargy, weakness, nausea, mental status changes. Teach patient/family the importance of compliance with fluid restriction as well as the dose, side effects, and rationale for prescribed medications.

ADH—antidiuretic hormone; I&O—intake and output; PE—physical exam

furosemide are being administered; close monitoring for cardiac irritability is required. Hypernatremia can result from overcorrection secondary to treatment efforts.

The patient's mental status can range from fully alert to comatose, depending on the degree of hyponatremia. Frequent evaluation of mental status is essential as cytotoxic therapy begins and progresses. Mental status changes, evidenced early by lethargy, are frequently seen as the serum sodium drops to approximately 125 mEq/L (see Table 16C–3).

Severe fluid restrictions can be a source of considerable discomfort to patients. Nursing interventions are aimed at relieving thirst and ensuring that patients receive their allowed fluids. If patients and families understand the rationale for restriction, greater compliance will most likely result. Dietary consultation is helpful.

Patients confined to bed are at increased risk for the skin effects that result from immobility due to water retention. Nursing efforts are directed at monitoring and maintaining skin integrity (see Chapter 10C).

Pain and stress are known to increase ADH secretion. Successful efforts to relieve pain and minimize stress should have a therapeutic effect. When possible, the use of opioids, barbiturates, and tricyclic antidepressants should be minimized because they are also known to enhance ADH secretion.

When drugs such as demeclocycline and furosemide are being used in SIADH management, patients are evaluated for side effects, adverse effects, and response to the therapy (Table 16C–5). Patients responding favorably to drug therapy will demonstrate weight loss, a rising serum sodium, and increasing serum osmolality. Failure to respond to therapy requires a review of compliance with fluid restriction as well as further examination of factors influencing ADH release.

As stated previously, SIADH can only be permanently controlled by effective antitumor therapy. If effective tumor control cannot be achieved, the patient and family must learn to manage chronic SIADH. Their ability to manage the syndrome and enhance the quality of life for the patient depends to a large extent on how carefully they are taught about SIADH and their ability to understand and accept the treatment.

BIBLIOGRAPHY

1. Batcheller, J. Syndrome of inappropriate antidiuretic hormone secretion. *Critical Care Nursing Clinics of North America* 6(4): 687–692. 1994.

   This is an excellent review of SIADH treatment and nursing implications.

2. Bunn, P. A., and E. C. Ridgway. Paraneoplastic syndromes. In DeVita, V. T, S. Hellman, and S. A. Rosenberg, eds. *Cancer: Principles and Practice of Oncology,* 4th Ed. 2026–2071. J.B. Lippincott, Philadelphia. 1993.

   This chapter details the diagnosis of ectopic AVP production and the SIADH syndrome along with frequency and treatment.

3. Kratcha-Sveningson, L. Body fluid composition, alteration in: Syndrome of inappropriate antidiuretic hormone (SIADH). In McNally, J. C., et al. *Guidelines for Oncology Nursing Practice.* 402–407. W.B. Saunders Company, Philadelphia. 1991.

This provides a detailed nursing care plan according to degree of hyponatremia.

4. Maesaka, J. K. An expanded view of SIADH, hyponatremia and hypouricemia. *Clinical Nephrology* 46(2): 79–83. 1996.

This article addresses differential diagnosis of hyponatremia and SIADH.

5. Mayer, D. K. Inappropriate antidiuretic hormone syndrome. In Baird, S. B. *Decision-Making in Oncology Nursing.* 198–199. B.C. Decker, Inc. Toronto, Ontario. 1988.

Useful clinical outlines for SIADH management are provided.

6. Poe, M., and L. M. Taylor. Syndrome of inappropriate antidiuretic hormone: Assessment and nursing implications. *Oncol Nurs Forum* 16(3): 373–381. 1989.

This is an excellent overview of SIADH pathophysiology with detailed tables outlining diagnosis and treatment.

7. Schafer, S. L. Oncologic complications. In Otto, Shirley E., ed. *Oncology Nursing.* 519–523. Mosby Company, St. Louis. 1991.

This detailed review of etiology, risk factors, pathophysiology, and nursing management of SIADH includes a case report of the use of lithium carbonate, a known inhibitor of ADH in the treatment of SIADH.

8. Sorensen, J. B., M. K. Andersen, and H.H. Hansen. Syndrome of inappropriate secretion of antidiuretic hormone (SIADH) in malignant disease. *Journal of Internal Medicine* 238: 97–110. 1995.

This article presents a thorough review of the literature of SIADH and includes a concise discussion of pathophysiology and treatment.

16D

D. Anaphylaxis

Kristen Kreamer

INTRODUCTION

The immune system is one of the human body's basic defenses against foreign substances. Normally, the immune system mounts a protective and beneficial response to antigen assault by inactivating the antigen and rendering it harmless. In the case of a hypersensitivity response, however, the immune system is excessively stimulated, and tissue damage to the host can result.

There are four classes of hypersensitivity response (HSR): Types I, II, III, and IV. Types II, III, and IV, though not benign, develop only after time has elapsed. Examples of these reactions include hemolytic anemia (Type II), serum sickness (Type III), and contact dermatitis (Type IV). Type I reactions, in contrast, are immediate hypersensitivity reactions (IHSRs); they include urticaria, allergic rhinitis, allergic asthma, and anaphylaxis.

PATHOPHYSIOLOGY

Immediate hypersensitivity reactions are labeled anaphylactic or anaphylactoid depending on whether the reaction is IgE mediated. An *anaphylactic reaction,* which is IgE mediated, develops in two phases. During the first phase, sensitization, complementary IgE antibodies are formed in response to contact with the antigen. These IgE antibodies become fixed to mast cells in tissue and basophils in circulation. During the second phase, hypersensitivity response, subsequent exposure to the antigen results in the reaction of that antigen with the already fixed IgE antibodies. This reaction triggers degranulation within the mast cells and basophils. These cells store granules, known as vasoactive mediators, which are released and are thought to be responsible for the symptoms associated with Type I IHSRs.

Anaphylactoid reactions occur without prior sensitization and can happen on first exposure to a drug antigen. Although indistinguishable from anaphylactic reactions in type and severity of signs and symptoms, anaphylactoid reactions are not IgE mediated but result from antigens binding directly to cell surfaces with consequent direct release of vasoactive substances.

The mediator that is probably most central to the pathogenesis of IHSRs in humans is histamine. Other mediators believed to be implicated are the leukotrienes, chemotactic factors, platelet-activating factor, neuropeptides, prostaglandins, and proteases. Research continues into the exact role of each of these mediators in IHSRs; their presumed biologic effects are detailed in Table 16D–1.

Because mast cell concentrations are highest in skin, lungs, heart, and gastrointestinal tract, signs and symptoms of IHSRs are most dramatic in these organ systems. In general, symptoms begin within seconds or minutes of exposure but can be delayed for up to an hour or more. Anaphylaxis is characterized by the following:

Subjective symptoms:
1. Pain or tightness in chest, dyspnea;
2. Inability to speak;

3. Generalized itching;
4. Complaints of uneasiness, agitation, warmth, or dizziness;
5. Feeling of impending doom;
6. Nausea, crampy abdominal pain;
7. Desire to urinate or defecate.

Objective signs:

1. Respiratory embarrassment with or without wheezing, stridor;
2. Sneezing, coughing;
3. Local or generalized urticaria and/or erythema;
4. Angioedema of face, eyelids, hands, or feet;
5. Hypotension, tachycardia, or arrhythmia;
6. Cyanosis;
7. Disorientation, unconsciousness;
8. Vomiting and/or diarrhea;
9. Incontinence.

Not all of these signs and symptoms must be present to make a diagnosis of anaphylaxis. Furthermore, it is recommended that immediate treatment be instituted in the face of a reasonable suspicion because, in severe cases, death can ensue rapidly because of respiratory failure, cardiac arrhythmia, or complete vascular collapse.

Table 16D-1
Mediators of the Anaphylactic Response

Mediator	Response
Histamine	Vasodilation
	Contraction of smooth muscle
	Increased vascular permeability
	Stimulation of sensory nerve endings
	Increased mucous secretion
Leukotrienes	Increased vascular permeability
	Contraction of smooth muscle
Chemotactic factors	Eosinophil attraction
	Neutrophil attraction
Platelet-activating factor	Aggregation and degranulation of platelets
	Increased vascular permeability
Neuro peptides	Degranulation of mast cells in skin
Prostaglandins	Contraction or relaxation of smooth muscle
	Increased vascular permeability
Proteases	Increased vascular permeability

ANAPHYLAXIS AND THE CANCER PATIENT

It is imperative to remember that the person with cancer is subject to the same risks of anaphylaxis as any other patient. For example, a cancer patient can experience a Type I anaphylactic response to an antibiotic or to other agents commonly used as adjuncts in cancer treatment and care (e.g., radiocontrast dye, antiemetics, opioids). However, most anaphylactic and anaphylactoid reactions in cancer patients are caused by antitumor chemotherapeutic agents.

Some of these reactions are anaphylactic. The drug most frequently cited in this regard is asparaginase, for which anaphylaxis is a major dose-limiting toxicity. Other IHSRs to chemotherapeutic agents are thought to be anaphylactoid, with many chemotherapeutic agents able to act as direct histamine releasing agents. Chemotherapeutic agents with a greater than 5 percent incidence of IHSRs in the literature include L-asparaginase, paclitaxel, cisplatin, teniposide, procarbazine, melphalan (IV), mechlorethamine (topical), and the anthracycline antibiotics (e.g., doxorubicin, daunorubicin). Additional drugs with reported cases of IHSRs are carboplatin, docetaxel, etoposide, cyclophosphamide, ifosfamide, chlorambucil, fluorouracil, mitoxantrone, bleomycin, cytarabine, methotrexate, trimetrexate, mitomycin, dacarbazine, pentostatin, and diaziquone. Although nearly every antitumor agent has been implicated in at least one report of IHSRs, these reports have not all been well documented.

In general, certain factors can contribute to an increased risk of anaphylactic or anaphylactoid response. The intravenous route of administration is more likely to cause anaphylaxis than the oral or topical route. Drugs derived from bacteria, such as asparaginase, are more likely to cause exaggerated immunologic reactions than are drugs from inorganic sources. Crude preparations of drug are more likely to be highly antigenic; these are more common in the early stages of investigational use, before refinement and isolation techniques have been perfected. There is also the possibility of contaminants or unrefined elements in the diluent, e.g., Cremophor in paclitaxel. Certain combinations of drugs can alter the risk of IHSRs; e.g., asparaginase given with prednisone and vincristine decreases the risk of a hypersensitivity response, but the risk is increased when mitomycin is administered along with vinblastine. Recently, it has been suggested that increased risk of IHSRs could relate to drugs given in protocols that combine chemotherapy with immunotherapy. The scheduling of doses could also be a factor, with repeated interrupted courses more likely to induce IHSRs than uninterrupted treatment. Finally, although the risk of anaphylaxis increases with repeated administration, it is important to remember that anaphylactoid reactions occur in persons with no known prior exposure to that particular drug.

ASSESSMENT

To identify patients at increased risk, the nursing history should include a thorough review and documentation of prior allergic episodes, including the agent thought to be responsible and a precise description of the episode. There is no conclusive evidence that a history of allergic response in general predisposes a person to anaphylaxis; however, it is important to identify persons who report previous allergic reactions to antitumor drugs, because there is evidence of cross-reactivity within classes of chemotherapeutic agents. It is also important to determine persons with prior reactions to drugs commonly used supportive to treatment, such as antiemetics. For example, there are case reports of IHSRs involving the 5-HT$_3$ serotonin receptor antagonists (e.g. ondansetron, granisetron). Additionally, a complete list of current patient medications should be obtained. There is evidence that beta-adrenergic blocking agents (e.g. propanolol) appear to increase the likelihood and severity of anaphylaxis and that angiotensin-converting enzyme inhibitors (e.g. enalapril) may also increase risk for IHSRs.

MEDICAL MANAGEMENT

Prevention

Preventive medical measures include a change in drug or route and premedication with steroids and H$_1$ and H$_2$ blocking agents (e.g., diphenhydramine and cimetidine, respectively). Test doses are unreliable predictors, yielding many false negatives and false positives and are increasingly thought to be worthless. The physician might change to another preparation of drug; for instance, although cross-reactivity has been noted, asparaginase derived from Erwinia crysanthemia could be substituted for asparaginase derived from E. coli. More recently, drugs have been formulated that avert IHSRs by attaching peptide polymers to "hide" the chemotherapy agent from the immune system (e.g., pegaspargase). If possible, the route of administration of a drug may be switched from intravenous to intramuscular or oral. In addition, the physician could order premedication. Hydrocortisone or dexamethasone, diphenhydramine, ephedrine, and cimetidine are frequently used as a precaution against anaphylaxis.

The question of retreatment after an IHSR is a difficult one and can only be answered on an individual basis. How critical the particular drug is to the patient's successful treatment, as well as the severity of the IHSR, must be taken into account. If the reaction was characterized by hypotension, bronchospasm, and a slow response to restorative measures, the patient should probably not be rechallenged. If retreatment is attempted, measures include increasing the dilution, lengthening the infusion time, and maximizing premedication by initiating steroid prophylaxis one to two days prior to retreatment. In the near future, patients could benefit from compounds currently under development, such as mast cell suppressants, which interfere with mediators of the anaphylactic response.

Support

Medical support measures consist of maintenance of a patent airway, administration of epinephrine, correction of hypotension through fluid administration, and administration of antihistamines and steroids. Mainte-

Table 16D-2
Nursing Protocol for the Management of Anaphylactic Shock

Factor	Intervention
Prior to drug administration	Nursing history: Elicit specific information regarding previous allergic responses, especially to cancer chemotherapeutic agents.
	Educate patient in need to report subjective symptoms of allergic response.
	Ensure that emergency equipment is available.
	Secure baseline data: pulse, respiration, BP.
	Prepare IV site to expose complete course of vein.
Evidence of anaphylactic response	Stop flow of drug and replace IV bag and tubing to keep line open with saline.
	Rapidly evaluate signs and symptoms.
	Call for medical attention and/or emergency services.
	If anaphylaxis is suspected, proceed to:
	Administer epinephrine (solution strength 1:1,000); repeat after 5–15 min if inadequate response.
	— Adults: 0.3–0.5 mg SC (smaller dose in elderly or those of slight build). IV dosing only for refractory hypotension requiring CPR
	— Children: 0.01 mg/kg SC (maximum single dose of 0.5 ml)
	Maintain patent airway: Suction and/or oropharyngeal intubation may be required.
	Administer oxygen.
	Administer other supportive drugs as ordered (e.g., nebulized beta agonists).
	Place patient in supine position, with feet elevated, unless contraindicated by respiratory distress.
	Administer IV NS to support BP.
	Monitor pulse, respiration, BP.
	Maintain close observation; symptoms may recur.
	Reassure patient.

CPR—cardiopulmonary resuscitation; NS—normal saline
Adapted with permission from the Oncology Nursing Press. Kreamer, Kristen. Anaphylaxis resulting from chemotherapy. *Oncology Nursing Forum* 8(4): 13–16, 1981.

nance of patent airway might require simple repositioning, suction, or oropharyngeal intubation. In extreme cases with glottic edema, tracheostomy could be performed. Epinephrine is the drug of choice for IHSRs and is administered for its bronchodilator and vasoconstrictive effects. A dose is given immediately and repeated in 5–15 minutes if required (Table 16D–2). A key physiologic change during anaphylaxis is altered vascular permeability, which results in fluid shift and hypotension. Rapid fluid replacement might be required to counter the drop in blood pressure. H_1 blocker antihistamines (e.g., diphenhydramine) are administered to control urticaria and could also prevent cardiac arrhythmias and peripheral vasodilatation. Glucocorticoids (e.g., methylprednisolone) are given to control abnormal vascular-wall permeability. These latter drugs do not contribute to the resolution of the life-threatening emergency but are instrumental in managing later symptoms. Nebulized beta agonists (e.g., albuterol) can be administered to control wheezing.

NURSING MANAGEMENT

Prevention

The nurse has two main responsibilities in preventive care for anaphylaxis: preparing the setting and preparing the patient. The former includes ensuring that emergency drugs and equipment are readily available. How this is done will depend on whether the drug is being administered in a hospital, outpatient clinic, private physician's office, or the home. If in the home, the nurse should be sure that emergency services for the area have been identified and that relevant phone numbers have been obtained.

Baseline data on pulse, respiration, and blood pressure should be obtained and recorded. When preparing the intravenous site, the nurse should ensure that the entire course of the vein along the extremity can be seen, unobstructed by clothing or tape. This area should be observed for localized urticaria or erythema.

The patient should remain under observation for at least 30 minutes after the dose of drug. In addition, it is of critical importance that the patient be instructed in the subjective symptoms of anaphylaxis. Although the nurse should be careful not to alarm the patient, it is essential that the patient be aware that such symptoms, if experienced, need to be reported immediately.

Support

A nursing protocol for anaphylaxis is presented in Table 16D–2 as a general guideline, which should be adjusted to the specific institution or setting where chemotherapy is administered.

If no physician is immediately available in a case of suspected anaphylaxis, the nurse should not delay in instituting supportive treatment. As the protocol indicates, the nurse must stop the flow of drug, rapidly evaluate the patient's objective signs and subjective symptoms, and, when indicated, administer epinephrine. Although other conditions can be mistaken for anaphylaxis, the subcutaneous administration of epinephrine in correct dosage is not likely to be hazardous.

Finally, the nurse should be sensitive to the patient's need for reassurance should a hypersensitivity reaction occur. The symptoms experienced by the patient can be alarming. The situation requires a nurse who, while acting quickly, maintains a calm attitude and supports the patient through verbal reassurance and physical contact. In the oncologic emergency of anaphylaxis, as in all other medical emergencies, the patient's need for psychologic safety must be a primary concern.

BIBLIOGRAPHY

1. Heywood, G., S. Rosenberg, and J. Weber. Hypersensitivity reactions to chemotherapeutic agents in patients receiving chemoimmunotherapy with high-dose Interleukin 2. *Journal of the National Cancer Institute* 87(12): 915–922. 1995.

   This is a report of apparent IL-2 induced hypersensitivity to chemotherapy agents.

2. Marquardt, D. and S. Wasserman. Anaphylaxis. In E. Middleton, C. Reed, E. Ellis, N. Adkinson, J. Yunginger, and W. Busse, eds. *Allergy: Principles and Practice.* 1525–1535. Mosby, St. Louis, 1993.

   This is a detailed description of the etiology, clinical findings, and treatment of anaphylaxis.

3. Oncology Nursing Society. *Cancer Chemotherapy Guidelines and Recommendations for Practice.* Oncology Nursing Press, Inc., Pittsburgh, PA. 1996.

   The Oncology Nursing Society's clinical practice committee and other experts detail clinical guidelines for the recognition and collaborative management of anaphylaxis.

4. Rowinsky, E., E. Eisenhauer, V. Chaudhry, S. Arbuck, and R. Donehower. Clinical toxicities encountered with paclitaxel. *Seminars in Oncology* 20(4) suppl. 3: 1–15. 1993.

   This article is a discussion of paclitaxel side effect assessment and management, including the presentation and treatment of anaphylaxis.

5. Sullivan, T. Drug allergy. In E. Middleton, C. Reed, E. Ellis, N. Adkinson, J. Yunginger, and W. Busse, eds. *Allergy: Principles and Practice.* 1726–1743. Mosby, St. Louis, 1993.

   This chapter is a discussion of risk factors for drug allergy and management of acute allergic reactions.

6. Weiss R. Hypersensitivity reactions. *Seminars in Oncology* 19(5): 458–477. 1992.

   This is a comprehensive review of hypersensitivity reactions to chemotherapy agents.

E. Septic Shock

Jeanne M. Erickson

INTRODUCTION

Infectious complications of cancer and cancer therapy remain a leading cause of mortality in the oncology population. Invasive cancer treatments, which increase the patient's susceptibility to infection, and the prevalence of drug-resistant organisms continue to make management of infections a challenge for clinicians today. Sepsis is the systemic response to infection and is reported to be the most common cause of death in noncoronary intensive care units.

Clinicians have recently developed a new framework to define sepsis and related processes in an effort to improve detection and interventions and to guide research (see Table 16E–1). These definitions are linked to the physiologic changes and clinical manifestations in the patient and represent a continuum of clinical severity.

PATHOPHYSIOLOGY

The sepsis cascade begins with an active infectious process in the patient, caused by bacteria, fungi, viruses, or other pathogens. Common portals of entry for microorganisms are through the integumentary, genitourinary, gastrointestinal, and respiratory systems. When viable microorganisms enter the bloodstream, a systemic inflammatory response occurs.

Endotoxin from gram-negative bacteria as well as toxins released from other pathogens initiate an inflammatory response through effects on white blood cells and other tissues. Endotoxins stimulate release of various immune mediators, such as tumor necrosis factor (TNF), interleukin 1 (IL-1), and interleukin 6 (IL-6). These substances activate the coagulation cascade and complement systems, resulting in increased endothelial permeability, relaxation of smooth muscle, and inhibition of platelet aggregation. The generalized vasodilation causes decreased circulating blood volume and increased oxygen demand.

In response to inflammation, neutrophils increase, aggregate, and eventually occlude the microvasculature, compromising circulation and tissue perfusion. Progressive hypoperfusion causes cells to shift to anaerobic metabolism, and various alterations in organ function begin to occur. Several mediators, including TNF, directly cause myocardial depression

16E

Table 16E-1
Newer Definitions of Sepsis and Related Conditions

Infection	Microbial phenomenon characterized by an inflammatory response to the presence of microorganisms or the invasion of normally sterile host tissue by those organisms.
Bacteremia	The presence of viable bacteria in the blood.
Systemic inflammatory response syndrome (SIRS)	The systemic inflammatory response to a variety of severe clinical insults. Manifested by two or more of the following conditions: Temperature >38°C or <36°C Heart rate >90 beats/min Respiratory rate >20 breaths/min or $PaCO_2$ <32 mm Hg White blood cell count >12,000 cells/mm^3, <4000 cells/mm^3, or >10% immature (band) forms
Sepsis	The systemic response to infection, manifested by two or more of the following conditions as a result of infection: Temperature >38°C or <36°C Heart rate >90 beats/min Respiratory rate >20 breaths/min or $PaCO_2$ <32 mm Hg White blood cell count >12,000 cells/mm^3, <4000 cells/mm^3, or >10% immature (band) forms
Severe sepsis	Sepsis associated with organ dysfunction, hypoperfusion, or hypotension. Hypoperfusion and perfusion abnormalities may include but are not limited to lactic acidosis, oliguria, or an acute alteration in mental status.
Sepsis-induced hypotension	A systolic blood pressure <90 mm Hg or a reduction of >40 mm Hg from baseline in the absence of other causes for hypotension.
Septic shock	Sepsis induced with hypotension despite adequate fluid resuscitation along with the presence of perfusion abnormalities, that may include but are not limited to lactic acidosis, oliguria, or an acute alteration in mental status. Patients who are receiving inotropic or vasopressor agents may not be hypotensive at the time that perfusion abnormalities are measured.
Multiple organ dysfunction syndrome (MODS)	Presence of altered organ function in an acutely ill patient such that homeostasis cannot be maintained without intervention.

Reprinted with permission from Bone RC, Balk RA, Cerra FB, et al. Definitions for sepsis and organ failure and guidelines for the use of innovative therapies in sepsis. *Chest* 101:1644–1655. 1992.

and decreased cardiac output. If uncontrolled, the process eventually results in progressive failure of several interdependent organ systems.

Patients who present with a systemic infection usually are febrile, with tachycardia and tachypnea. The skin might be warm and flushed, and peripheral edema could be present. Clinical features of severe sepsis include hypoperfusion abnormalities, such as lactic acidosis, oliguria, and mental status changes. Patients with septic shock develop hypotension in addition to signs of organ hypoperfusion. Progressive pulmonary, hepatic, and renal failure—as demonstrated by symptoms of adult respiratory distress syndrome (ARDS), disseminated intravascular coagulation (DIC), and electrolyte abnormalities—characterize the late stages of multiple organ dysfunction syndrome.

ETIOLOGY

A detailed discussion of the causes of infection in patients with cancer is included in Chapter 10A. Numerous factors related to the disease process predispose the cancer patient to infections that could lead to septic shock. Because cancer is by definition an invasive disease, malignancies can erode mechanical barriers, allowing pathogens to enter through skin and mucous membranes. Obstructive tumors allow overgrowth of normal resident flora. A variety of malignancies affect host defenses by interfering with bone marrow function. Severe granulocytopenia (granulocyte count <500 cells/mm^3) often results from leukemia and other cancers involving the bone marrow. Lymphoproliferative disorders, such as lymphoma, cause defects in cell-mediated and humoral immunity.

Cancer therapy is also responsible for increasing the patient's susceptibility to infection. Numerous chemotherapeutic agents cause profound bone marrow suppression, and administration of chemotherapy, as well as surgery and radiation therapy, can affect skin integrity. Other therapies that disrupt mechanical barriers include the placement of urinary catheters, intravenous catheters, and drainage devices. Impaired nutritional status, often associated with cancer and its treatment, causes immunologic deficiencies as well as delayed skin healing. Finally, the hospital environment introduces the patient to a variety of potentially more virulent and resistant microorganisms than would otherwise be encountered.

When a patient becomes granulocytopenic as a result of cancer and/or its treatment, sources of infection are commonly the patient's endogenous flora. *Escherichia coli, Pseudomonas* species, and *Klebsiella* species are gram-negative aerobic bacilli associated with a high incidence of sepsis among granulocytopenic patients. The incidence of infection by *Staphylococcus* species and other gram-positive bacteria has also recently increased and could account for up to one-half of all cases of sepsis. *Candida* species are common causes of sepsis in patients with prolonged periods of granulocytopenia. Viruses, other fungi, and protozoa can also infect the patient.

The incidence of septic shock has increased 140 percent over the past two decades, with the greatest increases in persons over 65 years of age, a rapidly growing proportion of our population. Overall estimates suggest that shock develops in about 40 percent of patients with sepsis. Episodes of septic shock are associated with gram-negative, gram-positive, and viral and fungal infections, in descending order. The presence of shock dramatically affects mortality due to infection. According to studies by Bone (1991), the sepsis syndrome without shock results in 13 percent mortality, the sepsis syndrome presenting with shock leads to 28 percent mortality, and shock developing after the sepsis syndrome claims 43 percent of patients. Other studies report mortality from septic shock of up to 90 percent.

ASSESSMENT

The patient can deteriorate unpredictably through the stages of septic shock over a course of days or in a matter of hours. Furthermore, the symptoms of septic shock might not always progress in an orderly fashion. Because the treatment of septic shock is most effective in the early stage, identification of patients at risk for sepsis and septic shock and prompt recognition of the early symptoms of shock are imperative for patient recovery.

Nursing measures to prevent septic shock begin with an assessment of the patient's susceptibility to infection (see Chapter 10A). Patients should be educated about their risk of infection and taught to report early symptoms. Granulocytopenic patients must be closely monitored, because the classic signs of inflammation could be absent or limited to only local tenderness and/or fever.

Mouth, nasopharynx, skin, lungs, perineum, and intravenous sites of susceptible patients should be inspected daily for signs of infections. Vital signs should be checked every four hours. Fever is defined as an oral temperature greater than 38.5°C at a single reading or as three readings greater than 38.0° in a 24-hour period. For all granulocytopenic patients, patients with known or suspected infections, and patients who have undergone pelvic or abdominal surgery, nurses should be alert for the signs and symptoms of early septic shock: tachycardia, tachypnea, vasodilation, decreased oxygen saturation, and/or hypotension before, during, or following a febrile episode. The first sign of infection should be immediately discussed with the physician and treatment initiated.

Frequent assessment of the patient with signs of sepsis should include monitoring of vital signs, mental status, tissue perfusion, and oxygen saturation. Assessment of mental status should include the patient's level of consciousness, orientation, memory, and cognitive functioning. Tissue perfusion is evaluated by checking the color of lips, nailbeds in hands and feet, skin temperature, and quantity of urine output. Oxygen saturation can be assessed by pulse oximetry. Laboratory tests might include a complete blood count, chemistry panel, urinalysis, and arterial blood sampling.

Blood cultures from two separate sites should be obtained at once, with other regional cultures (urine, sputum, drainage, and catheters), and x-rays completed as a priority.

MEDICAL MANAGEMENT

Early recognition and aggressive treatment of sepsis are imperative to increase a patient's chance for survival. The basic goal of medical therapy is to support the patient's cardiovascular system until the infectious process is controlled.

Antimicrobial therapy must be prescribed to control the infection, but at the time of shock, the treatment will not be sufficient to save the patient's life. A careful history and physical examination should be made to identify the source of infection, with particular attention to the nasopharynx, lungs, perineum, wounds, and sites of any invasive device. Urinalysis and chest x-ray—as well as routine bacterial and fungal cultures of throat, sputum, urine, stool, blood, and any drainage—should be obtained to identify the organism and guide the choice of antimicrobial drugs. Any obviously contaminated device should be removed.

Antimicrobial therapy is generally instituted immediately after blood cultures are obtained. A broad-spectrum antibiotic regimen, consisting of an aminoglycoside and a beta-lactam antibiotic, is usually necessary to cover the commonly infecting gram-negative bacilli. This regimen can be adjusted after culture results are known or if surveillance cultures have been done and indicate an unusual colonizing organism. If a patient remains febrile or has symptoms of sepsis while already on broad-spectrum antibiotics, the drug regimen can be expanded to cover staphylococcal organisms (e.g., vancomycin) and fungi (e.g., amphotericin B).

For the patient with septic shock, fluid therapy to restore circulating blood volume and maintain cardiac output is the most rapidly effective measure for improving tissue perfusion and vital signs. Fluids are administered incrementally with close monitoring to prevent the complications of fluid overload. Fluid boluses of 100 ml at 10- to 15-minute intervals are recommended and should be repeated until vital signs, urine output, and mental status improve. If there is no initial response to fluid therapy, a pulmonary artery catheter should be inserted to monitor cardiac and pulmonary function. Controversy exists about whether fluid replacement should be administered as a colloid or crystalloid solution. Crystalloid solutions, including normal saline and Ringer's lactate, are inexpensive but rapidly diffuse into the interstitial space, causing edema. Colloids, such as 5 percent albumin or 6 percent hetastarch, are more expensive but remain intravascular and are more effective at expanding the blood volume. When a patient is anemic, blood products are the most effective way to increase blood volume and enhance oxygen delivery.

If the patient does not improve with fluid therapy, an inotropic agent is prescribed to improve oxygen delivery and maintain an adequate perfusion pressure. Dopamine is frequently used in septic shock because of its flexibility. At low doses (3 mcg/kg/min), dopamine improves splanchnic, mesenteric, and renal circulation, and at moderate doses (3 to 5 mcg/kg/min), it increases cardiac output by increasing heart rate and stroke volume. At 10 mcg/kg/min, dopamine supports blood pressure through vasoconstriction. Dobutamine could also be prescribed to increase cardiac output, provided adequate fluid resuscitation has occurred. Norepinephrine can also be used to achieve adequate blood pressure.

All patients in septic shock have an increased demand for oxygen because of increased metabolism and ensuing hypoperfusion. Oxygen therapy should be administered early to maintain oxygen saturation above 90 percent. If adequate oxygenation and ventilation cannot be maintained, mechanical ventilation is indicated.

The hypoperfusion in septic shock leads to anaerobic metabolism and lactic acid production, resulting in metabolic acidosis. Aggressive oxygen delivery often reduces lactic acidosis, and serum lactate levels can be followed to monitor patient response.

Disseminated intravascular coagulation (DIC) can develop from excessive tissue damage and blood pooling and contributes to high mortality (see Chapter 16F). Administration of fresh-frozen plasma, platelets, and packed red blood cells may be prescribed if hemorrhage or other signs of DIC occur, although DIC secondary to sepsis is not readily reversed.

Renal damage and fluid overload can also complicate recovery from septic shock. If adequate blood pressure and tissue perfusion have been attained but urine output remains low, a cautious trial of diuretics can be instituted. Serum electrolytes should be monitored and replaced as needed. Dialysis might be indicated for irreversible renal failure.

New therapies directed against key mediators in the sepsis sequence continue to be investigated. Monoclonal antibodies to endotoxin (E5 and HA-1A) have been developed and tested in large multicenter randomized trials, but current results are inconclusive. Research with anti-TNF antibodies and IL-1 antagonists are underway. Nitric oxide is being studied as a regulator of systemic and pulmonary vascular tone, and new methods to monitor laboratory and physiological parameters are being examined.

NURSING MANAGEMENT

Nursing measures to prevent and detect infection in susceptible cancer patients, as outlined in Chapter 10A, can prevent sepsis and its sequelae. When signs and symptoms of infection are documented in the patient, nurses become involved in controlling the infectious process. If the patient presents with progressive sepsis, nursing interventions are directed toward reversing the hypotension and organ failure. Table 16E–2 outlines a protocol for the nursing care of patients in septic shock.

Because a patient in septic shock requires immediate medical and nursing interventions with hemodynamic monitoring, an intensive care setting might be indicated until the patient's condition has stabilized. Even after successful treatment, however, the patient remains at risk for complications and will continue to need frequent assessment. Rehabilitation with the goal of restoring normal activities will be necessary following the in-

Table 16E-2
Nursing Protocol for Management of Septic Shock

Problem	Intervention
Susceptibility to infection	Identify patients at risk for infection. Institute measures to prevent infections in susceptible patients. Inspect mouth, nasopharynx, skin, lungs, perineum, and IV sites of susceptible patients.
Sepsis	Obtain blood cultures at once, regional cultures and appropriate x-rays. Institute prescribed antibiotics at once and maintain on strict schedule. Check patient's drug allergies. Know and monitor for side effects.
Inadequate tissue perfusion	Assure IV access with 1–2 large gauge catheters. Infuse fluids as prescribed. Insert urinary catheter. Record intake and output hourly. Assess for effectiveness of fluid therapy: increased BP, urine output >20 ml/hr, improved mental status, and improved tissue perfusion. Anticipate insertion of pulmonary artery catheter with continued fluid therapy. Manage administration of vasoactive drugs (dopamine, dobutamine, norepinephrine) if prescribed for persistent hypotension.
Inadequate oxygenation	Prescribe bedrest. Monitor oxygen saturation with pulse oximetry. Notify physician if SaO_2 <90%. Monitor results of arterial blood samples. Notify physician if pH <7.35 or PaO_2 <60 mm Hg.
Abnormal body temperature	Monitor temperature q 30 minutes until stable. Administer antipyretics as prescribed. Use cooling blankets as indicated.
Bleeding from DIC	Monitor for signs of bleeding. Monitor results of coagulation profile. Be alert for elevated PT and PTT, elevated D-dimers, decreased fibrinogen and platelet values. Apply pressure to sites of active bleeding. Administer blood products as prescribed.
Fluid overload	Assess for signs of fluid overload: pulmonary rales, dyspnea, wet cough, edema, weight gain. Assess baseline BP, tissue perfusion, and electrolytes before administering diuretics. Administer diuretics as prescribed.
Patient/family fear and anxiety	Explain need for intensive monitoring and intervention. Provide frequent, calm verbal and physical contact with patient and family.

DIC—disseminated intravascular coagulation; PaO_2—partial pressure of arterial oxygen; PT—prothrombin time; PTT—partial thromboplastin time; SaO_2—saturation of arterial oxygen

tensive therapy required for sepsis. Because septic shock can develop in any patient with an infection, oncology nurses must be knowledgeable and skilled in monitoring and supporting the patient's cardiovascular and respiratory functions during this emergency.

BIBLIOGRAPHY

1. Bone, R. The pathogenesis of sepsis. *Ann Intern Med* 115(6): 457–469. 1991.

   This summarizes the mediators that play a role in sepsis and their reported effects.

2. Bone, R. et al. Definitions for sepsis and organ failure and guidelines for the use of innovative therapies in sepsis. *Chest* 101(6): 1644–1655. 1992.

   This article presents the consensus committee's report on the new clinical framework to define sepsis and its continuum.

3. Brown, K. Septic shock: How to stop the deadly cascade. *Am J Nurs* 94(9): 20–26. 1994.

   Part 1 presents a case study of sepsis and outlines pathophysiology as well as early medical and nursing interventions for septic shock.

4. Brown, K. Critical interventions in septic shock. *Am J Nurs* 92(10): 20–25. 1994.

   Part 2 describes the late sequelae and interventions for a patient with shock.

5. Rackow, E. and M. Astiz. Pathophysiology and treatment of septic shock. *JAMA* 266(4): 548–554. 1991.

   This article reviews the pathophysiology and medical treatment of septic shock.

6. Toney, J. and J. Parker. New perspectives on the management of septic shock in the cancer patient. *Inf Dis Clin N Am* 10(2): 239–253. 1996.

   This article discusses the clinical approach to septic shock in the patient with cancer.

F. Coagulopathies

Anne R. Bavier

Normal hemostatic functioning is a delicate system that prevents both excessive hemorrhage and excessive clot (thrombus) formation. A change in the system, tipping the balance to either extreme, can cause diffuse venous thrombosis or its acute form, disseminated intravascular coagulation (DIC), either of which can be life-threatening. Nursing actions for cancer patients at risk for developing a coagulopathy are designed to promote normal coagulation and clot lysis.

NORMAL PHYSIOLOGY

To understand hemostasis, it is necessary to recognize the interrelationships among vasoconstriction, platelet plug formation, and blood clot formation. Vasoconstriction attempts to minimize blood loss by decreasing blood flow. Vascular spasm occurs immediately after a blood vessel is cut, thus reducing the blood loss from the wound. Nervous reflexes and local myogenic spasm initiate this vascular constriction. The degree of constriction is directly proportional to the extent of trauma to the vessel. The spasm lasts for up to one-half hour, during which time the other processes of coagulation occur: platelet plug formation and blood coagulation leading to fibrin formation.

The platelet plug is a loose collection of platelets that acts as the base for the formulation of a stable clot. Vessel wall damage stimulates platelet aggregation by exposing the underlying collagen layer and releasing adenosine diphosphate (ADP). The platelets themselves release ADP, serotonin, and an enzyme that forms thromboxane A. Serotonin is a vasoactive substance that can enhance hemostasis by constricting small arteries and veins. Together, these chemicals attract additional platelets, which adhere to the mass and become the plug. The platelet plug is effective only in stopping blood loss through small rents in vessel walls, which are continually occurring naturally. The absence of adequate platelet supplies to mend such small tears is noted in thrombocytopenic patients who develop petechiae.

Vasoconstriction and platelet plug formation contain the blood initially; then blood coagulation begins to provide a stable clot and promote vascular healing. The general mechanism of blood coagulation has three parts: (1) formation of prothrombin activator; (2) conversion of prothrombin to thrombin by the activator; and (3) conversion of fibrinogen to fibrin with thrombin as initiator and subsequent formation of solid fibrin strands.

There are two catalysts to the formation of prothrombin activator: the intrinsic and extrinsic pathways. The intrinsic pathway is initiated by trauma to the blood itself or contact by blood with a surface, such as collagen. An alteration of any blood component, such as the platelets, can initiate the intrinsic pathway. Tissue or vessel injury is required to initiate the extrinsic pathway, which begins with exposure of blood to tissue factor (tissue thromboplastin) released by traumatized tissue.

Within the blood are clotting factors that are utilized in sequence to reach the prothrombin activator stage. Clotting factors, which are referred to by Roman numeral (e.g., factor V, factor VIII), are inactive forms of proteolytic enzymes that become activated and, in turn, cause the next factor to be activated. The process requires nonenzyme cofactors to produce this cascading sequence. Vascular or tissue injury initiates the formation of

16F

tissue factor and tissue phospholipid and uses factor VII in the extrinsic pathway to prothrombin activation.

The intrinsic and extrinsic pathways converge at the formation of the prothrombin activator, and the rest of the coagulation process follows a common pathway. To succeed, these steps require adequate serum calcium levels.

The blood clot itself is composed of all blood-cell forms and plasma products caught in a mesh of fibrin threads, which holds the clot to the vessel walls. The action of factor XIII on fibrin results in cross-links between the fibers, further stabilizing the clot.

Clot retraction, the next event, is very important because it pulls the edges of the vessel closer together to promote healing. The fibrin strands contract, squeezing out the blood serum. Platelet secretion of fibrin-stabilizing factor is largely responsible for this vital phenomenon. Consequently, severely thrombocytopenic patients might be unable to mount this response; so vessel healing is deterred, and a less stable clot is formed.

It is important to note that the absence of any of the components of clot formation jeopardizes the patient. The danger is massive hemorrhage. Patients might have a genetic condition (such as classic hemophilia A, in which factor VIII levels are inadequate) or an acquired condition (such as massive trauma that has exhausted the supply of clotting factors, or severe calcium depletion).

Balancing the clot formation process is clot lysis. Plasmin, or fibrinolysis, digests the fibrin strands and consumes coagulation factors. The fibrinogen degradation products that result from fibrinolysis act to prevent thrombin formation. Thus, the process of clot lysis also includes a mechanism that limits new clot formation. Usually, the relatively small quantities of these fibrinogen degradation products only limit local expansion of the clot, because the entire body's capability to form thrombin is not affected.

Clot formation and lysis exist in a delicate balance that maintains blood flow through the vessels. This balance responds rapidly to changes and has remarkable capacity to intensify or restrain activities. The speed of the normal responses underscores the need for nurses to recognize that harmful changes can occur rapidly in cancer patients. Either or both mechanisms can become altered in cancer patients. Excessive clot formation, resulting in the blockage of vessels, occurs primarily as diffuse venous thrombosis. Chronic DIC also is associated with excessive clotting. Ineffective clotting, resulting in major hemorrhage episodes, is the acute form of DIC, an oncologic emergency. Each condition is discussed in the following sections.

THROMBOTIC DISORDERS

Pathophysiology

The term *prethrombotic state* gradually is replacing the term *hypercoagulation* in recognition of the multiple, and interacting, causes of thrombus formation: blood flow, vessel wall characteristics, and blood composition. Although platelet plugs are a normal part of the clotting process, a thrombus is a plug that occurs at the wrong place or the wrong time. Two dangers exist: impairment of local/regional tissue perfusion, and embolization of a portion of the clot to another part of the body. Either can cause tissue death. If embolization occurs to a vital organ, such as the lungs, the patient can die. Cancer patients could be at increased risk due to alteration in any or all of the causes of thrombus formation (see Table 16F–1).

A major challenge is that it is hard to predict which patients are most likely to develop thrombosis. Risk factors for venous thromboembolism include previous venous thromboembolism, congestive heart failure, and stroke. Surgery is a major risk factor among cancer patients as well as advanced cancer, and specific tumors: mucin-secreting adenocarcinomas of the gastrointestinal (GI) tract and lung; tumors of the pancreas, ovary, brain, and liver; and acute myelogenous leukemia, especially promyelocytic and monocytic forms. Data do not support an increased risk among prostate cancer patients, although anecdotal information suggests an association. Approximately 15 percent of cancer patients exhibit clinical thrombosis, and a higher incidence is evident in autopsy studies. Although typical laboratory data for cancer patients often indicate abnormal coagulation, a relationship between the abnormal values and risk of thrombosis has not been established. Comorbid conditions that increase risk include smoking, hypertension, diabetes, and use of oral contraceptives.

The presence of the prethrombotic state increases the risk that events associated with treatment can cause thrombus formation. Intravenous catheters and heparin administration are common procedures that can result in thrombosis.

Chemotherapy and hormonal therapies warrant special vigilance. Chemotherapy is often associated with thrombosis, although the mechanisms are unclear. Breast cancer patients receiving chemotherapy and hor-

Table 16F–1
Potential Causes of Thrombus Formation in Cancer Patients

1. Abnormalities in blood flow
   Immobilization (e.g., bed rest)
   Vascular compression from tumors
   Hyperviscosity of blood (e.g., Waldenström's macroglobulinemia, IgG or IgA multiple myeloma, or high concentration of leukocytes in leukemias)

2. Abnormalities of the vessel wall
   Direct tumor invasion of wall
   Hypercortisolism
   Increased vascular tone associated with reduced plasminogen activator (postulated)

3. Abnormalities of blood composition
   Elevated serum levels of coagulation factors
   Increased circulating activated coagulation factors (e.g., in liver failure due to tumor invasion of the liver)

monal therapy have experienced thrombotic events, usually deep vein thromboses and pulmonary emboli. Superficial thrombophlebitis (e.g., in a brachial artery) also has been reported in this group. L-asparaginase has been associated with thrombosis or bleeding problems, usually in the central nervous system. Occlusion of veins in the liver has been associated with several drugs (e.g., acute myelocytic leukemia patients treated with thioguanine and daunomycin with or without cytarabine). Cisplatin, bleomycin, vinca alkaloids, and mitomycin have been associated with thrombotic microangiopathy. Bleomycin, with or without vinblastine, has been associated with Raynaud's phenomenon.

ASSESSMENT

Traditional coagulation studies are not useful in predicting or evaluating the prethrombotic state, primarily because the tests measure bleeding propensity rather than thrombosis. Radioimmunoassays are being developed to detect by-products associated with thrombus formation; these could become available for general clinical services.

Typically, the thrombus develops in a large vein, often in the legs. Patients experience erythema and edema from blocked venous flow. In addition, severe pain associated with tissue death occurs. When initial symptoms are observed, it is prudent to assess the originally affected limb as well as other body parts because the obstruction can gradually involve larger areas, expanding the affected region. For example, edema of the lower leg can spread throughout the leg and lower abdomen.

All body systems must be assessed for obstructive symptoms because of the propensity for embolus formation (Table 16F–2). Pulmonary embolism is a common cause of death. Other similar complications are CNS infarcts, microangiopathic hemolytic anemia, and nonbacterial thrombotic endocarditis.

In addition, less common thrombotic complications can occur. Gastrointestinal cancers, especially pancreatic, are associated with migratory superficial thrombophlebitis (Trousseau's syndrome). Typically, sites are multiple, and the superficial vasculature of the arms, forearms, and chest is blocked. They appear to resolve spontaneously, but serious complications can develop when patients are shifted from heparin to oral anticoagulants. Careful assessment and documentation are critical to ensure that anticoagulation is managed appropriately.

Nonbacterial thrombotic endocarditis has been associated with mucin-producing tumors. These aseptic vegetations grow in the heart and can embolize, causing strokes, myocardial infarction, or ischemic necrosis of peripheral organs. Evidence of any embolizing situation (e.g., heart murmurs) warrants further diagnostic evaluation, typically echocardiography or nuclear magnetic resonance imaging.

Table 16F–2
Ongoing Assessments of Patients in the Prethrombotic State

Body Part	Nursing Observation
Skin	Color changes, especially redness. Calf tenderness: note any increase. Vascular filling: check speed of return of normal color to nailbeds after compression. Vascular size/fullness: look for localized abnormal areas of enlarged veins (e.g., over lower extremity).
Lungs	Breathing patterns: note changes to more labored, shallow breathing and changes to more vertical posture, onset of coughing, symmetry of chest expansion, use of accessory muscles. Pain: note sudden onset of shooting or stabbing pain and its location, especially if concurrent with temperature elevation. Quality of gaseous exchange in each lobe: look for rales, wheezing, absence of breath sounds. Hemoptysis is uncommon.
Extremities	Measure girth at standardized point, noting gradual increase in size and differences between extremities. Pulses: check for unequal, decreased, or absent pulses. Assess for pain.
Neck	Check veins for distension.

Hepatic vein thrombosis (Budd-Chiari syndrome) and portal vein thrombosis are associated with myeloproliferative disorders, hepatomas, and renal cell and adrenal carcinomas. Patients complain of abdominal pain, and physical examination reveals ascites and hepatomegaly. Other frequent findings are distension of superficial abdominal veins and splenomegaly. The most useful diagnostic procedure is venogram through the inferior vena cava and hepatic vein. In portal vein thrombosis, ascites is less common, occurring acutely in patients with liver disease.

MEDICAL MANAGEMENT

Anticoagulants are given to control diffuse venous thrombosis (Table 16F–3); however, withdrawal of the drugs frequently causes the return of symptoms. Successful treatment appears to be more directly related to control of the tumor than to anticoagulant therapy.

Initial therapy can be either continuous intravenous infusion or 12-hour high-dose subcutaneous (SC) administration of unfractionated heparin. Patients might require long-term SC heparin therapy while receiving antitumor treatments. Control of coagulation by drugs is a delicate process, and adjustments of dose will be based upon laboratory reports of blood co-

Table 16F–3
Therapy in Diffuse Venous Thrombosis

Drug	Administration/Comments
Unfractionated Heparin	IV, begin with 5,000 U bolus then approximately 30,000 U/24 hrs (adjusted based on activated partial thromboplastin time [APTT] 1.5 to 2 times control). SC, 20,000 U twice daily. Adjusted doses can be used for maintenance to prevent recurrence.
Low Molecular Weight Heparin	Dose based on patient's weight.
Warfarin (Coumadin®)	Adjust oral dose to prothrombin time.
Streptokinase*	IV, begin with 250,000 U over 30 minutes, then 100,000 U/hr for 72 hrs.
Urokinase*	IV, begin with 4,400 U/kg over 10 minutes, then 4,400 U/kg/hr for 12 hrs.

*At the end of streptokinase or urokinase therapy, treat with continuous IV heparin.

agulation. Patients might be switched to oral anticoagulants within 24 hours of initial heparin therapy, with administration of both agents for three to four days. However, long-term anticoagulant therapy might not be possible due to the risk of hemorrhage and recurrent venous thromboembolism. Low-dose SC heparin can be used when oral anticoagulants cannot be continued. Low molecular weight heparin (LMWH) is being considered for its potential to further reduce recurrence over standard oral anticoagulants. LMWH offers advantages over traditional unfractionated heparin, including better bioavailability and subcutaneous administration based on the patient's weight without requiring laboratory tests to adjust dosages and achieve effects. Inferior vena cava filter devices can be used to prevent pulmonary embolism.

Nurses should be alert for bleeding, which indicates excessive medication. Furthermore, the antidotes for both heparin and warfarin (Coumadin®) should be available. Vitamin K (phytonadione) should be administered to counteract warfarin, and protamine sulfate to counteract heparin.

The principal danger of all medical management approaches, whether anticoagulation or fibrinolytic therapies, is hemorrhage. Such catastrophic events generally occur at the sites of known vascular defects. Nurses should closely monitor arterial puncture sites, surgical incisions, and anatomic regions where tumors have invaded blood vessels. Table 16F–4 lists conditions that pose increased risk of hemorrhage in the presence of thrombosis.

Table 16F–4
Increased Risk of Hemorrhage in Thrombotic Patients

Any intracranial lesions

Active bleeding

Recent surgery

Gastrointestinal lesions prone to bleeding; esophagitis due to candida or herpes simplex virus

Underlying bleeding diathesis; thrombocytopenia, DIC

NURSING MANAGEMENT

All nursing care measures have the common goal of reducing the risk of embolization by maintaining a consistent venous pressure that is low (Table 16F–5). Low venous pressure encourages additional aggregation at a thrombus site, which deters further bleeding. However, if there is a subsequent increase in pressure, the loosely attached elements can dislodge, becoming emboli.

Hydration poses a special challenge. Ideally, intake of large volumes (2,000 to 3,000 ml/24 hr) is encouraged. The goal is to keep the blood diluted sufficiently so that the blood components are unlikely to contact each

Table 16F–5
Protocol for Nursing Management in Thrombotic Patients

Alteration in venous pressure	Bed rest initially; when ambulation allowed and sitting permitted, encourage frequent position change. Use elastic hose or extremity supports cautiously because excessive edema may cause device to actually constrict. No massages. Elevate affected extremities.
Alteration in fluid balance	Maintain accurate intake and output records. Encourage fluid intake to 2,000–3,000 ml/24 hr, unless other physiologic conditions prevail (e.g., congestive heart failure).
Potential for bleeding complications	Avoid invasive procedure (e.g., arterial puncture, line placement). Have available antidotes for heparin and warfarin, if used. Have available cryoprecipitate or plasmin to correct hypofibrinogenemia. Have E-aminocaproic acid (EACA) available.

other or the existing thrombus, thus preventing expansion or creation of additional thrombi. Maintaining a consistent hydration level promotes a consistent venous pressure. These patients, however, who are often critically ill, might not be able to tolerate large fluid volumes because of other physiologic conditions, such as congestive heart failure. Although maximum hydration might be impossible, nurses should be alert to prevent dehydration, which would promote contact among the blood's elements and alter venous pressure.

DISSEMINATED INTRAVASCULAR COAGULATION

Pathophysiology

Disseminated intravascular coagulation (DIC) is the term commonly used to describe an aberrant hemostatic mechanism. Other terms are *acute intravascular coagulation* and *consumption-coagulation*. The condition appears to develop as a result of thrombin formation, which depletes the supply of fibrinogen and other coagulant proteins. It can be initiated by injury to either the vascular epithelium or tissue. It is important to note that macrophage clearance decreases, making more activated clotting factors available to aggravate the initial thrombin formation process and complicate resolution.

The most common presentation of DIC in cancer patients is in association with manifestations of thrombi. Minor localized bleeding associated with the tumor site or postoperative state can also be the presenting sign. Finally, severe, diffuse hemorrhage occasionally occurs.

In the chronic phase (also called compensated or low grade DIC), DIC resembles the diffuse venous thrombosis described previously. The chronic phase can culminate in the acute phase (or fulminant phase) of active bleeding. It is believed that the chronic process eventually consumes all the clotting factors, making active bleeding inevitable. The precise mechanism for initiating this coagulation remains unknown.

Assessment

DIC in cancer patients is most often associated with acute promyelocytic leukemia and adenocarcinomas; other cancers associated with DIC include acute myelomonocytic leukemia, lung, prostate, colon, breast and any metastatic cancer. The patient who develops unexplained or unexpected bleeding should be evaluated carefully (Table 16F–6). Nurses can detect subtle changes in patient status and greatly facilitate early diagnosis and intervention. Particular attention should be given to

Table 16F–6
Ongoing Assessment for Blood Loss

Body Site/ System	Nursing Observations
Renal	Check urine for red color. Check for occult blood.
GI	Check for occult blood (guaiac test). Observe for presence of bleeding hemorrhoids, which may respond to local measures. Check emesis for bright red (fresh) blood or dark brown (old) blood. Check emesis for consistency: stickiness and clots with red color or coffee-ground consistency with dark-brown color.
Skin/mucous membranes	Check blood loss around invasive devices: IV lines, venipuncture sites, surgical sites. Check blood loss on dressings. Measure loss by: removing dressing and weighing; marking saturated area of dressing and rechecking area hourly; removing dressing and estimating blood loss as extent of saturation (e.g., $\frac{1}{2}$ saturation of 4x4-in gauze square). Check color (pale) and condition (oozing blood or irritation) of gingival tissue. Observe for ecchymosis. Observe for petechiae.
Cardiovascular	Observe for tachypnea. Observe for orthopnea. Observe for tachycardia. Observe for angina, indicating deficit in myocardium.
Neurologic	Monitor mentation, especially for confusion or irritability. Observe for changes in consciousness: less conscious, more difficult to arouse, decreased awareness of light touch, changing responses to painful stimuli only. Check for headaches.
Eyes	Assess for changes in vision (e.g., blurred, spots in visual field). Check for retinal hemorrhage by asking about pain in eyes, visual disturbances, and by use of ophthalmoscope to see vessels and bleeding.
Abdominal	Check for tenderness associated with palpation, indicating increasing fluid in abdomen or inadequate perfusion. Measure girth at consistent place, noting any gradual increase.

cancer patients who experience other conditions associated with the development of DIC, specifically sepsis, volume deficits, and transfusion reactions.

Although early, subtle changes in patients might be noted, it is often sudden dramatic changes that cause people to seek help. Patients might note small changes (e.g., decreasing ability to perform customary activities, petechiae) or dramatic events (e.g., frank bleeding). The urinary and GI systems are frequent sites of acute blood loss.

Diagnosis is made through evaluation of laboratory values and clinical assessment. The most critical laboratory tests are prothrombin time, partial thromboplastin time, platelet count, thrombin time, and fibrin and fibrinogen split products. The D-dimer assay, for fibrin degradation products/fragments, is also useful. Consumption of platelets is reflected in markedly decreased platelet counts ($<20,000$ cells/mm^3). As supplies of factor V and VII and prothrombin are exhausted, the prothrombin time and partial thromboplastin times are prolonged. Fibrinogen degradation products appear as fibrolysis proceeds. The hematocrit falls because of acute blood loss.

Medical Management

As in diffuse venous thrombosis, treatment of DIC is aimed at the underlying tumor or other precipitating factor. If symptoms are not present, specific therapy can be directed not at the DIC but rather at the underlying tumor. However, chemotherapeutic agents that induce cell lysis can change the delicate balance by releasing procoagulant enzymes. Heparin at 1,000 U/hour might offset this change. For severe hemorrhage, patients might receive coagulation factors through transfusion with cryoprecipitate and fresh-frozen plasma. Red blood cell (RBC) transfusions can be administered, as well as fluids to replace lost volume.

The use of heparin (300 to 600 U/kg/24 hr) is controversial, except in the case of leukemic patients and as noted previously. The rationale is that by its antithrombin effect heparin could interrupt the coagulation mechanism. Heparin prevents the formation of prothrombin activator by factors V, activated X, Ca^{2+}, and phospholipid via the intrinsic pathway when the concentration of these procoagulants is low. It can be used when there is clinical evidence of severe bleeding while treatment of the precipitating cause or tumor is initiated. Heparin use is contraindicated in patients with open wounds, intracranial hemorrhage, or recent surgery. When heparin is administered, the patient's concurrent medications should be scrutinized for drug interactions (e.g., digitalis, nicotine, tetracycline, and antihistamines deter heparin's effect, so increased heparin doses are often required). Insulin's effects may be promoted by heparin.

Nursing Management

Nurses who care for patients with DIC must be aware of three major problems: massive blood loss, altered fluid balance, and decreased oxygen-carrying capacity (Table 16F–7). The patient's inability to form a stable clot means that seemingly minor nursing acts can have major hemorrhagic consequences. Efforts to prevent blood loss should be initiated when DIC is suspected, by such actions as using a small-gauge needle to obtain blood samples. Awaiting confirmation of the diagnosis should not delay precautionary measures.

Table 16F–7
Nursing Protocol for the Management of DIC

Problem	Intervention
Potential for massive hemorrhage	Avoid medications that affect coagulation (e.g., aspirin-containing products).
	Avoid medications that interact with heparin (when it is used).
	Minimize trauma to patient: have patient wear slippers; pad side rails for restless, bedridden patient.
	Use smallest-gauge needles for fewest possible punctures of skin.
	Decrease trauma to gums by brushing gently.
	Apply direct pressure to any puncture site.
	Suction carefully.
	Minimize use of BP cuffs: do not inflate much above previous reading and release pressure quickly.
	Use existing infusion lines whenever safe.
	Avoid use of straight razors, IM and SC injections.
	Monitor for blood loss (see Table 16F–6).
	Count and weigh dressings saturated with blood.
	Calculate blood loss through suction devices.
Altered fluid balance	Use flow-control devices whenever possible, especially for heparin.
	Include volume of blood products in intake calculations.
Decreased oxygen-carrying capacity	Minimize requests for patient to move, perform self-care, etc.
	Provide supplemental oxygen, when prescribed.
	Provide slow pace and rest periods during any patient activity.
Patient need for information	Provide patient and family with information on symptoms related to alterations in hemostasis caused by either excessive clotting or bleeding; swelling of arms, legs, abdomen, or neck; change in color of the skin anywhere; pain in swollen areas; change in the ability to perform customary activities (e.g., excessive fatigue or trouble breathing); frank bleeding from any injection site, nose, mouth, rectum, or urinary tract; development of petechiae.

Fluid volumes can fluctuate between too much and too little. Blood products as well as intravenous solutions may be administered. Too much replacement volume can cause fluid overload, resulting in additional complications such as congestive heart failure. With significant blood loss, however, hypovolemia can become a problem. Quantifying actual blood loss whenever possible and keeping accurate cumulative records of fluid intake that include all fluid types are important deterrents to such problems.

Inadequate oxygenation can manifest as tachycardia and dyspnea. These conditions represent the body's attempt to maximally oxygenate the remaining blood and to move it throughout the system. RBC transfusions and supplemental oxygen might be indicated. Caregivers can help patients conserve energy and oxygen by doing whatever is necessary for them.

The great potential for abnormal coagulation, whether bleeding or thrombus formation, requires that nurses monitor and report early subtle changes in patients. Moreover, patients and families need to recognize common symptoms for which they must seek professional help. In addition to the symptoms of bleeding caused by inadequate platelet production, a common side effect of many anticancer regimens, patients should be aware of the symptoms that indicate abnormal coagulation problems.

BIBLIOGRAPHY

1. Chaplin, M. Disseminated intravascular coagulation: A multisystem problem. *Dimensions of Critical Care Nursing* 3(2): 76–83. 1984.

    A thorough analysis of nursing interventions and their rationale is presented in a systematic and detailed fashion.

2. Colman, R. W., and R. N. Rubin. Disseminated intravascular coagulation due to malignancy. *Seminars in Oncology* 17(2): 172–186. 1990.

    This article provides a good discussion of DIC in the context of cancer management.

3. Gensini, G. F., D. Prisco, M. Falciani, M. Comeglio, and A. Colella. Identification of candidates for prevention of venous thromboembolism. *Seminars in Thrombosis and Hemostasis* 23(1): 55–67. 1997.

    A good review of medical and surgical risks for venous thromboembolism is presented.

4. Gray, W. J., and W. R. Bell. Fibrinolytic agents in the treatment of thrombotic disorders. *Seminars in Oncology* 17(2): 228–237. 1990.

    This article offers a good review of trials and uses of these agents.

5. Guyton, A. C., and J. E. Hall. *The Textbook of Medical Physiology, 9th Ed.* W.B. Saunders, Philadelphia. 1996.

    This classic text provides exceptionally clear information and relevant illustrations.

6. John, W. J., K. A. Foon, and R. A. Patchell. Paraneoplastic syndromes. In De-Vita, V. T., S. Hellman, and S. A. Rosenberg, eds. *Cancer: Principles and Practices of Oncology, 5th Ed.* Lippincott-Raven Publishers, Philadelphia. 1997.

The comprehensive, sophisticated description of DIC medical management contained in this chapter focuses on several conditions.

7. Levine, M., and J. Hirsh. The diagnosis and treatment of thrombosis in the cancer patients. *Seminars in Oncology* 17(2): 160–171. 1990.

Issues of heparin and oral anticoagulant use are well outlined.

8. Luzzatto, G., and A. I. Schafer. The prethrombotic state in cancer. *Seminars in Oncology* 17(2): 147–159. 1990.

A clear perspective is given on the origin of the problem and medical management issues.

9. Monreal, M. Heparin in patients with venous thromboembolism and contradictions to oral anticoagulant therapy. *Seminars in Thrombosis and Hemostasis* 22(1): 69–75. 1997.

This very clear review covers the treatment issues and new trends in medical management.

10. Shuey, K. M. Platelet associated bleeding disorders. *Seminars in Oncology Nursing.* 12(1): 15–27. 1996.

This useful article covers in-depth discussion of physiological disorders in the context of cancer nursing care.

11. Valentine, K. A., R. D. Hull, and G. Pineo. Low molecular weight heparin therapy and mortality. *Seminars in Thrombosis and Hemostasis* 23(2): 173–178. 1997.

This article contains good explanations of current thinking on low molecular weight heparin.

17

Infiltrative Emergencies

A. Carotid Artery Erosion and Rupture

Diahann Kazierad
Karen Kane McDonnell

INTRODUCTION

Cancers of the head and neck comprise 4 percent of all cancers diagnosed in the United States. Forty percent are of the oral cavity; 25 percent, the larynx; 15 percent, in the oro/hypopharynx; 7 percent, the major salivary glands; and the remaining 13 percent are from other sites. At the time of initial diagnosis, 40 percent to 60 percent of patients have advanced disease. Cancers of the head and neck grow aggressively and invade adjacent structures. Treatment options include surgical resection, radiation therapy, and chemotherapy. Both treatment and characteristics of the disease can damage the carotid arterial system leading to erosion and rupture. Mortality from carotid artery rupture is reported at 40 percent, and 25 percent of those who survive will suffer neurologic complications. The role of the nurse is to identify patients at risk for carotid erosion, early signs and symptoms of erosion, and appropriate emergency interventions.

ANATOMY

The carotid arterial system includes the common carotid artery, which divides into the internal and external carotids. The internal carotids feed the ophthalmic artery and join the cerebral circulation at the Circle of Willis. The external carotids supply the musculoskeletal structures of the face, the dental structures, and the dura mater covering the brain.

The walls of the carotid artery receive 80 percent of their blood supply from a capillary network called the vasa vasorum. There are three distinct layers to the arterial wall: the adventitia, media, and intima (Figure 17A–1). The outermost, or adventitial, layer is composed of connective tissue; the medial layer is smooth muscle; and the intima is both connective and endothelial tissues. The arterial system is subject to a great deal of stress during cardiac contraction. These vessels must allow for stretch during systole of the heart.

17A

751

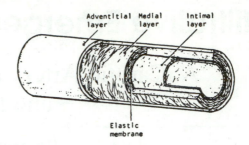

Figure 17A-1. Cross-sectional view of an artery.

PATHOPHYSIOLOGY

The incidence of carotid rupture in the surgical patient with head and neck cancer is 3 percent to 4 percent. The etiology of carotid erosion includes (1) local tumor invasion from recurrent or persistent disease, (2) radiation therapy, (3) radical surgery, and (4) postoperative complications. Each of these mechanisms has the potential to weaken and destroy the vascular walls, particularly the advential layer. The weakened carotid arteries are not able to withstand the force of the systolic arterial pressure, and rupture occurs. Frequently more than one of these mechanisms of carotid erosion occurs simultaneously.

A characteristic of cancer cell growth is that it does not respect the boundaries of neighboring cells. Cancers of the head and neck aggressively invade the surrounding structures such as the carotid system. The vessel walls lose their elasticity and integrity as a result of tumor invasion.

A late effect of radiation therapy can be destruction of the vasa vasorum, thereby robbing the adventitial layer of the carotid of its blood supply. The wall of the carotid artery becomes ischemic and weakens, because of the loss of the blood supply from the vasa vasorum. In addition, the soft tissue in the radiation field loses its vascularity. These soft tissues are more susceptible to trauma, infection, and irritation because of a decrease in blood flow. Radical surgical procedures also affect the adventia and the vasa vasorum. Often, this layer and its capillary system are stripped away. The vessel wall becomes unstable, and ischemia occurs.

Delayed wound healing following surgical resection of head and neck tumors places the patient at risk for carotid exposure and subsequent rupture. Complications such as infection, tissue necrosis, and fistula formation can occur. Preoperative radiation (>6000 cGy) has been identified as a significant risk factor for poor wound healing, because of decreased soft tissue perfusion. Inadequate perfusion can lead to abscess formation, infection, and necrosis. Infection can also be caused by closure of a contaminated wound, prolonged surgical procedure, hematoma formation, and the development of salivary fistulas.

Still other factors have been implicated in poor wound healing. Malnutrition, including vitamin and protein deficiencies, adversely affects wound healing and host immunity. Age is inversely related to rate of wound healing. Steroids or chemotherapy given during the first seven to ten days postoperatively have a negative effect on wound recovery. Comorbidities—such as diabetes mellitus, alcoholism, tobacco use, atherosclerosis, and hypothyroidism—have been implicated in poor wound healing.

If the wound is not healing, the artery becomes exposed to the atmosphere. It is hypothesized that the adventitial layer becomes fragile if subject to drying. Eschar develops because the wound cannot be closed by epithelialization. The eschar eventually separates from the wound by a process known as *sloughing*. When this occurs, the underlying medial layer is exposed and undergoes the same process. The remaining fragile intimal layer is then the only tissue containing the vascular flow. At this point rupture is inevitable.

CLINICAL MANIFESTATIONS

Carotid rupture can present in three ways: (1) an exposed carotid, (2) impending carotid rupture, and (3) acute carotid rupture. Breakdown of a surgical wound exposes the carotid artery to the atmosphere. In this situation the carotid artery is clearly visible; however, no bleeding has occurred. With impending carotid rupture, episodic bleeding which can be controlled by pressure occurs. A pseudoaneurysm is the source of the initial bleed. In this situation the carotid vessels are very fragile. With acute carotid rupture, massive hemorrhage followed by rapid deterioration in the patient's status occurs. The patient might present with hemoptysis, hematemesis, bleeding from the mouth, nose, or surgical incision.

ASSESSMENT

Assessment begins by identifying patients who are at high risk for carotid rupture. Risks include a diagnosis of recurrent head and neck cancer, surgery to a previously radiated area, radical surgery, open surgical wounds, salivary fistulae, skin flap necrosis, and wound infection. Other factors to consider are advanced age of the patient, poor nutritional status, steroidal therapy, chemotherapy, and comorbidities.

Ongoing assessment of the surgical site, with documentation of any change, is necessary to detect evidence of post-operative complications (Table 17A–1). A change in color from red to pale or black, a change of skin temperature from bilateral warmth to unilateral coolness, or the presence or increase of edema signifies impaired circulation. Progres-

Table 17A–1
Assessment of Wound and Surrounding Skin

Factor	Assessment
Color	Erythema, pallor, black.
Temperature	Warm, cool, unilateral temperature changes.
Edema	Presence, absence, or changes.
Lesion	Location, size, shape, type.
Thickness	Inspect for level of repair or tumor invasion.
Turgor	Taut, mobile.
Moisture	Dryness, sweating, oiliness, drainage.
Odor	Odorless, malodorous.
Texture	Roughness, smoothness.
Vascularity	Evidence of bleeding and/or bruising, pulsations, arterial exposure.

Adapted from Bates, B. *A Guide to Physical Assessment*. 6th Ed. Lippincott-Raven Publishers, Philadelphia. 1995.

sively compromised blood supply to the vessel and surrounding area will result in continued deterioration. Normally, wounds will change in shape in response to skin tensions at the wound site. A change in turgor, as indicated by an increase in size and a change in the shape of the wound, will occur as tension at the site relaxes, resulting in wound deterioration. Changes in the type, amount, or odor of any drainage present will aid in recognizing infection. Redness and tenderness could accompany infection. Obviously, it is important to observe evidence of bleeding, pulsations, or arterial exposure.

Few warnings of carotid artery rupture are noted in the literature. Some patients will complain of sternal or high epigastric pain several hours before rupture. A small prodromal or "sentinel" bleed might be noted at the wound site 24 to 48 hours before. Ballooning of the carotid artery suggests that a rupture will occur within hours. Because forewarnings are either lacking or inconsistent, ongoing assessment of the wound is the most accurate predictor of arterial erosion. When the artery is exposed or invaded by tumor, the patient and family should be made aware. An unexpected hemorrhage can be a horrifying event. Informing the patient and family that it might occur and what will be done to prevent and manage it might lessen their anxiety. The staff should also be alerted.

PREVENTION

Prevention of carotid artery erosion and rupture must focus on promoting wound healing. Preoperative evaluations should assess the patient for presence of risk factors. Prophylactic antibiotics and stable hemodynamics should be maintained to promote healing in the perioperative phase. Post operatively, the incision should be covered with a moist dressing such as bacitracin ointment. Drainage of the wound must be maintained. (See the "Nursing Management" section and Table 17A–2.) Adequate nutrition should be provided; enteral feeding is preferred over parenteral.

MEDICAL AND SURGICAL MANAGEMENT

An exposed carotid artery requires emergent intervention, including local wound care, debridement of necrotic tissue, optimal wound drainage, cultures, topical antibiotic dressing to keep it covered and moist, and intravenous antibiotics if the patient is febrile. Hyperbaric oxygen therapy has been used to promote wound healing. Frequent assessment of the response of the wound to these measures is necessary. If the wound improves, it can be covered by a vascularized skin flap. Wounds that do not improve require elective surgical or endovascular intervention.

In the event of an impending rupture, a vascular consultation can help identify the site as well as the timing and type of therapeutic intervention. In many situations, an impending hemorrhage can be treated by elective ligation of the eroded arterial ends, ligation of the involved vessel, or endovascular occlusion techniques. Prior to any procedure, a complete neurologic evaluation should be performed to document baseline neurologic function. Surgical ligation is not without significant morbidity and mortality. The greatest morbidity is related to neurologic sequelae. These include contralateral hemiplegia, hemianesthesia, aphasia, and dysarthria, likely to occur within 24 hours of surgery as a result of cerebral hypoxemia. The placement of detachable balloons (balloon embolization) for carotid artery occlusion has been used in patients at risk for rupture who are not candidates for surgery or whose vascular disease is not amenable to ligation, or when carotid bleeding sites are not surgically accessible. As there is less morbidity and mortality associated with balloon occlusion than with ligation, this technique might replace surgical ligation.

Emergency medical management of carotid rupture includes securing an airway, applying external pressure and/or packing the nares and pharynx, securing at least two large bore intravenous lines, and hydration. Hypotension is the most accurate predictor of outcome in acute carotid rupture. Measures should be directed at keeping the systolic blood pressure greater than 110 mm Hg. Rapid infusion of crystalloids, colloids, and blood is indicated. The patient needs intensive care monitoring, which should include an arterial line for blood pressure monitoring, continuous cardiac monitoring, central venous access, and a pulmonary artery catheter to assess volume resuscitation. If the patient can be stabilized, the previously described surgical or endovascular procedures can be performed.

Following either procedure, the patient should be monitored in the intensive care unit for signs of neurologic changes caused by cerebral ischemia or emboli. The patient who undergoes a vascular procedure is at risk for thromboembolus. Therefore, it is recommended that the patient receive anticoagulation to decrease this risk.

Nursing Management

An important role of the multidisciplinary team is to help the patient and family make decisions about aggressive or supportive care options. The nurse, as a member of the team, must know that the patient and family understand the prognosis and what their desires for treatment are. The goals of nursing care will vary, depending on the expectations for care.

A plan of preventive action should be developed after the patient is identified (Table 17A–2). Preventive wound care requires strict aseptic technique. The dressing should support the wound, protect it from trauma and contamination, absorb drainage, and/or provide an aesthetic cover for what could be a necrotic, malodorous, and fungating neck mass. Wound healing might not be a realistic goal for the patient. If not, the goal of wound care is to prevent drying and infection.

The optimal dressing material is fine-mesh gauze because it inhibits the interweaving of granulation tissue into the dressing material. A nonadherent dressing soaked in normal saline or topical antibiotic solutions can be used to ensure constant moisture, prevent debridement of healthy tissue, and absorb wound drainage. A nonocclusive dressing will prevent growth of fungi, particularly yeast, which thrive in dark, moist, warm environments. Using porous tape to secure the dressing will allow circulation of air in the area. If tape cannot be used, an isolation mask tied around the neck can provide a snug bandage. Dressings should be changed frequently to reduce bacterial growth and odor. Anti-odor agents (baking soda, Hexon®, balsam of Peru) can be applied to the outside dressing. If excessive drainage makes frequent dressing changes necessary, remove only the external dressing and reinforce the inner layer of gauze. The dressing should be removed cautiously. Normal saline can be applied to loosen it without causing debridement, which could result in the unnecessary exposure of the underlying tissue layers to the atmosphere.

If the wound does not heal normally, the risk for infection is increased due to loss of the normal skin barrier against bacterial invasion. All identifiable zones of necrosis, inflammation, and infection should be cultured.

Any factor that increases physical stress on the wound can interfere

Table 17A-2
Nursing Protocol for the Preventive Management of Carotid Artery Rupture

Factor	Intervention
Wound/incision care	Schedule dressing changes (based on amount of drainage and need for continuous nursing assessment of the area). Sample nursing orders: Change dressing q 8 hr (11 AM, 7 PM, 3 AM) or more frequently if excess drainage soils dressing. Initially document color, shape, mobility, skin temperature, tenderness, presence or absence of edema, thickness and odor of wound, vascularity. Document changes as they occur.
Prevention of debridement	Remove dressing cautiously using normal saline applications to loosen dressing if necessary. Use a nonadherent dressing material (fine-mesh gauze).
Prevention of infection	Culture suspicious areas for infection and take appropriate isolation measures. Use nonocclusive dressing.
Maintain adequate nutritional and hydration status	Perform a baseline assessment. Intervene as appropriate.
Wound stressors Respiratory efforts	Explore ways to minimize strenuous respiratory effects: reposition the patient; teach and encourage deep, sustained inhalations; consult the physician concerning the need for oxygen therapy or respiratory therapy treatments.
Coughing	Determine the etiology of the coughing. If pulmonary secretions are present, suction can be used. A cough suppressant may be indicated.
Vomiting	Assess the etiology of the vomiting. Administration of an antiemetic or nasogastric intubation may be necessary.
Constipation	Determine factors that cause constipation. Plan should be designed reflecting patient's ability/desire to eat and drink fluids, level of activity, and use of medications.
Emotional factors	Explore potential sources of emotional stress. Promote an atmosphere conducive to the expression of feelings, fears, and questions.

with the healing of wounds of the head and neck area. Strenuous respiratory efforts, coughing, vomiting, and straining at defecation are common stressors for the hospitalized cancer patient. Hypertension also increases the risk of carotid rupture, and when the vessel is thin and fragile, the blood pressure need not be excessive to cause rupture. Identification of hypertension and the administration of anti-hypertensives can protect the patient from carotid rupture.

Strenuous respiratory efforts call upon muscles not ordinarily used. Included in this group of accessory muscles are the sternomastoid and trapezius of the neck. The proximity of these contracting muscles to the wound and to the carotid arteries renders them a source of stress. Depending on the underlying disease and the patient's condition, positioning the patient in a Fowler's or semi-Fowler's position; encouraging deep, sustained inhalations; and the administration of oxygen can help minimize strenuous efforts.

Vigorous coughing increases intrathoracic pressure, which can create cardiovascular and wound complications for the patient with a head and neck tumor. To reduce the excess pressure generated by coughing, nasotracheal, tracheal, or oropharyngeal suction can be used to remove pulmonary secretions. The stress produced by intermittent suction might be lower and the treatment more satisfying than a continuous unproductive cough. Suctioning should be done with caution to prevent trauma and only after the presence of secretions has been documented.

The contraction of the diaphragm and abdominal muscles that accompanies vomiting raises intra-abdominal pressure, which in turn increases intrathoracic pressure, further stressing the wound site. Appropriate management to prevent vomiting depends on accurate determination of the etiology. Whether the treatment is the administration of an antiemetic or nasogastric intubation, prompt treatment is required to avoid contamination of the neck wound with gastric contents.

The hospitalized patient is also prone to constipation (see Chapter 12B). Patients with constipation strain excessively when trying to expel feces. The Valsalva maneuver, achieved by forced expiration against a closed glottis, causes maximum intrathoracic pressure. Management of this problem involves the patient's ability to eat, his or her level of activity, and the use of a stool softener and laxative as appropriate. A fiber diet and/or appropriate fluid intake can assist in preventing this complication.

Emotional stress is another important factor. The hospital setting itself, the location of the patient's room, visiting hour restrictions, fear of death, and fear of isolation are but a few of the emotional concerns shared by many patients. The nurse's recognition of emotional stress and its physical consequences is an obvious and important aspect in the care of these patients.

Nursing Management of a Carotid Rupture

The goals of nursing intervention are to (1) maintain an airway and prevent aspiration, (2) minimize blood loss, (3) provide circulatory support, and (4) provide physical and emotional comfort to patient and family.

Anticipation of this emergency will allow for the maintenance of peripheral venous access with a large-bore needle. A central venous access device might be preferred. Precautions should be taken to avoid delay in blood product replacement. If an arterial rupture occurs, the normal blood volume must be restored before surgical ligation is attempted. Updated typing and cross-matching and the availability of several units of blood products are important. Supplies at the bedside should include several packages of sterile 4 × 4 gauze, vascular clamp, suction and resuscitation equipment, complete intravenous setup, central line kits, several bags of one-liter normal saline solution, emergency oxygen therapy setup, cuffed Shiley tracheostomy tube, an arterial blood gases kit, gloves, disposable gowns, goggles, and absorptive dressing materials.

Placement of the patient at risk near the nurses' station will facilitate close observation. If a tracheostomy tube is place, the cuff should remain inflated to prevent aspiration of blood from the wound. Cuff pressures should be monitored at least every eight hours. This is also true if the patient has a stoma from a laryngectomy procedure. A cuffed laryngectomy or tracheostomy tube should be inserted and remain inflated.

When sudden hemorrhage occurs (Table 17A–3), the patient is placed in a head-down position and pressure is applied to the bleeding area. This positioning should not increase blood loss if pressure is applied properly. If blood descends the oropharynx and no tracheostomy is in place, an oral airway should be inserted. Suctioning around the airway might help remove blood and secretions from the oro- and hypopharynx. Oxygen might be needed.

To prevent cardiovascular collapse, intravenous fluids should be rapidly infused and blood product transfusions initiated. Vital signs should be monitored frequently to assess further changes in the patient's status.

Table 17A–3
Nursing Protocol for the Aggressive Management of Carotid Artery Rupture

Factor	Intervention
Airway maintenance	Inflate cuff of tracheostomy or laryngectomy tube to prevent aspiration of blood. Insert oral airway if patient does not have a tracheostomy. Suction aspirated blood. Administer oxygen.
Minimizing blood loss	Put patient in Trendelenburg's position to minimize cerebral hypoxemia. Determine site of bleeding. Apply digital pressure with gauze or dressing material to the bleeding site. Notify other caregivers of the emergency situation.
Stabilization of cardiovascular status	Maintain rapid infusion of IV fluids. Initiate blood-product transfusion. Monitor vital signs.
Comfort	Reassure patient and family that everything is being done. Act in a calm, organized manner. Administer analgesics as prescribed.

Providing support to the patient and family will be important during this crisis situation. Reassuring them and explaining the procedure being done can help lessen their anxiety.

When aggressive treatment has failed or is not possible or appropriate, easing suffering becomes the primary focus of patient care (Table 17A–4). The goals of nursing intervention are to (1) maintain an airway and prevent aspiration, (2) relieve discomfort and distress, and (3) provide psychological support to patient and family.

Supplies that will be needed for supportive care during a carotid rupture should be placed at the bedside beforehand, including suction equipment, gloves, absorptive dressing materials, and parenteral medication with anxiolytic/analgesic properties.

Maintenance of airway might not be possible. If hemorrhage occurs externally, the patient can be positioned supine with the head turned to the affected side or laterally to facilitate drainage and prevent aspiration. Absorptive dressing materials can be used to suppress a pulsatile discharge from the site, even though control of bleeding might not be achieved. If hemorrhage occurs internally, nothing can be done to prevent aspiration. To ease the patient's discomfort, suction can be used in an attempt to remove blood that ascends into the oral cavity or through a tracheostomy.

The nurse at the bedside should remain aware of the family's presence and their needs. Allowing the family members the opportunity to leave the bedside might lessen the shock of this sudden death. Treating the patient with gentle respect will have a calming effect on both the patient and family during the crisis of carotid artery rupture.

An important role for the nurse at this time is to give appropriate drugs to alleviate the patient's anxiety and alter the sensitivity to pain.

Table 17A–4
Nursing Protocol for the Supportive Management of Carotid Artery Rupture

Factor	Intervention
Airway maintenance	Tracheostomy tube cuff or laryngectomy tube cuff should be inflated. Position patient supine with head turned toward the affected side or laterally to facilitate drainage. Absorb bloody discharge with dressing materials. Suction to remove blood from oral cavity or tracheostomy/laryngectomy.
Comfort	Administer appropriate drugs to relieve anxiety and alter sensitivity to pain. Provide emotional support to patient and family. Allow family members the opportunity to leave the bedside. Do not leave the patient alone.

Drugs that are effective against pain and anxiety must be parenteral, rapid-acting, and available at the bedside for prompt administration. Morphine is often the drug of choice.

Many times the patient dies in the absence of family. The patient, realizing that death is near, might be apprehensive and should not be left alone. Reassuring the patient that he or she is not alone and explaining procedures might provide comfort.

CONCLUSION

A small portion of patients with cancers of the head and neck are at risk for carotid erosion and rupture. Radiation therapy prior to surgery has been identified as the most common cause of poor wound healing leading to carotid rupture. It is important that patients at risk for carotid rupture be identified. Preventative measures should focus on wound care and healing. Other factors known to further increase the risk of erosion and rupture should be minimized. Nursing staff should also be prepared for this catastrophic event. A specific plan of care should be followed that is consistent with the wishes of the patient and family. Lastly, resources should be mobilized to support the patient and family during all phases of cancer treatment.

BIBLIOGRAPHY

1. Bumpous, J. M., and J. T. Johnson. The infected wound and its management. *Otolaryngologic Clinics of North America*, 28(5): 987–1001. 1995.

   Infection prevention, preoperative assessment, patient factors, tumor factors, and treatment factors are addressed prior to surgery in head and neck cancers. Perioperative antibiotics, surgical techniques, postoperative care, and infected wound management are discussed following surgical treatment.

2. Citardi, M. J., J. C. Chaloupka, Y. H. Son, S. Ariyan, and C. T. Sasaki. Management of carotid artery rupture by monitored endovascular therapeutic occlusion (1988–1994). *Laryngoscope*, 105: 1086–1092. 1995.

   Eighteen patients with carotid artery rupture received endovascular therapeutic occlusion as management of their bleeding. The technique is described. Risk factors related to these patient's carotid rupture as well as the outcomes of treatment are presented. The discussion section focuses on risk factors, management of this patient population, and the endovascular procedure.

3. Goodman, M. Head and neck cancer. In S. L. Groenwald, M. H. Frogge, M. Goodman, and C. H. Yarbro, eds. *Cancer Nursing, Principles and Practice* 1199–1234. Jones & Bartlett, Boston. 1997.

   Anatomy, pathophysiology, and pretreatment/postoperative concerns of the head/neck cancer patient are described. Carotid artery rupture is identified as a major postoperative complication. A listing of equipment needed for carotid precautions is included.

4. Groenwald, S. L., M. H. Frogg, M. Goodman, and C. H. Yarbro, eds. *Comprehensive Cancer Nursing Review*. Jones & Bartlett, Boston. 1995.

In an outline format, cancers of the head and neck including epidemiology, risk factors, and pathophysiology are discussed. Cancers at each anatomic site with treatment modalities and nursing management are contained in the text.

5. Horn, D. B., G. L. Adams, and D. Monyak. Irradiated soft tissue and its management. *Otolaryngologic Clinics of North America* 28(5): 1003–1019. 1995.

Radiation therapy for head and neck cancers and its early and late effects to soft tissue are presented.

6. Koopmann, C. F. Jr. Cutaneous wound healing: An overview. *Otolaryngologic Clinics of North America* 28(5): 835–845. 1995.

Phases of wound healing and positive and negative factors effecting wound healing are the topics of this journal article.

7. Lesage, C. Carotid artery rupture. *Cancer Nursing* 9(1): 1–7. 1986.

Prediction, prevention, and nursing preparation in the event of carotid rupture are presented in this article.

8. Morrissey, D. D., P. E. Andersen, G. M. Nesbit, S. L. Barnwell, E. C. Everts, and J. I. Cohen. Endovascular management of hemorrhage in patients with head and neck cancer. *Archives of Otolaryngolic Head and Neck Surgery* 123:15–19. 1997.

This article presents a retrospective chart review of 12 patients selected for endovascular embolization as a therapeutic alternative to surgical ligation in the management of carotid hemorrhage. The cause of hemorrhage and the location of the bleeding is identified. The risks of this procedure are discussed. Four case studies are included.

9. Shaha, A. R., and E. W. Strong. Cancer of the head and neck. In G. P. Murphy, W. Lawrence, & R. E. Lenhard, Eds. *American Cancer Society Textbook of Clinical Oncology* 355–377. American Cancer Society, Atlanta. 1995.

Cancers of the head and neck—including epidemiology, risk factors, natural history of disease, diagnostics, staging, and treatment—are discussed.

B. Leukostasis

Diahann Kazierad
Karen Kane McDonnell

INTRODUCTION

Leukostasis is a syndrome of intravascular sludging that can occur in patients with acute or chronic leukemia. The syndrome is present when the leukocyte count is greater than 100,000 cells/mm^3, when a high percentage of these cells are myelo- or lymphoblasts. The result is capillary obstruction, tissue ischemia, tissue infarction, and organ dysfunction. Although any organ can be affected, it is most life-threatening when the pulmonary or central nervous system (CNS) is involved. Acute respiratory distress and intracerebral hemorrhage are the most common and lethal manifestations of this complication. Emergency treatment is necessary to prevent death. Nursing responsibilities include collaborating with physicians to recognize patients at risk for leukostasis, observation for early signs and symptoms of organ dysfunction, and monitoring the prescribed medical treatment.

PATHOPHYSIOLOGY

The exact mechanism underlying the development of leukostasis syndrome is not clearly understood. It is known that myeloblast and lymphoblast cells are larger, more rigid, and have an increased mean cell volume when compared with normal mature leukocytes (Figure 17B–1). Myeloblasts are, on average, larger and less distensible than lymphoblasts; therefore, the leukostasis syndrome is more common with myeloid leukemias than lymphoid leukemias. When these cells are present in abnormally large numbers, they can cause an increase in blood viscosity, stagnation of blood flow, and mechanical obstruction of small capillaries. As a result, the tissues that are fed by these capillary beds are deprived of oxygen. Capillary endothelial damage occurs due to (1) release of toxic cellular enzymes from the blast cells, (2) poor tissue perfusion caused by capillary obstruction, and (3) high oxygen consumption by the blast cells, which further robs the tissues of desperately needed oxy-

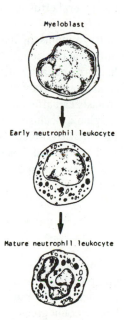

Myeloblast

Early neutrophil leukocyte

Mature neutrophil leukocyte

Figure 17B–1. Three stages in the development of a myelogenous leukocyte.

17B

gen. The capillary walls leak and eventually weaken to the point of rupture and hemorrhage.

In the pulmonary vasculature capillary, obstruction with endothelial damage causes fluid to leak into the alveolar space. The flooded alveoli cannot diffuse oxygen across their membranes, and hypoxemia and respiratory distress follows (see Chapter 14). On post-mortem examination, patients with acute nonlymphocytic leukemia (ANLL) who died of leukostasis syndrome, white thrombi consisting of blasts were found within the distended and obstructed pulmonary vasculature. The alveolar membranes were damaged causing pulmonary interstitial edema and pleural effusions. Small hemorrhagic infarcts and parenchymal leukemic infiltration also were found.

In the CNS, capillary obstruction is followed by capillary leak, leukemic infiltration, and small vessel rupture. Cerebral infarction, increased intracranial pressure, herniation of the brain, and death can occur rapidly (see Chapter 15A).

CLINICAL MANIFESTATIONS

Signs and symptoms of *pulmonary* leukostasis include fever, acute onset of shortness of breath, tachypnea, shallow breathing, diffuse pulmonary crackles, stridor, decreased oxygen saturation (SaO_2), decreased partial pressure of oxygen (PaO_2) in the absence of hypercapnia, and increased oxygen requirement. Pulmonary hemorrhage could additionally cause blood-streaked sputum or hemoptysis. Radiographic findings include diffuse pulmonary infiltrates, pleural effusions, vascular engorgement, and cardiomegaly.

Neurological signs and symptoms of leukostasis include dizziness, acute visual changes, tinnitus, ataxia, confusion, delirium, stupor, and coma. With intracerebral hemorrhage, acute deterioration in mental status, cranial nerve dysfunction, and motor dysfunction occur (see Chapter 15A).

Less commonly, leukostasis can affect other organ systems and cause coronary artery occlusion, splenic occlusion, vascular insufficiency, and priapism. Signs and symptoms of coronary artery occlusion mimic an acute myocardial infarction. Patients with splenic occlusion might present with an acute, rigid abdomen from infarcted bowel. Vascular insufficiency and priapism cause severe and acute pain in the affected areas.

ASSESSMENT

Persons who present with a markedly elevated white blood cell count require a full leukemia workup to diagnose their disease. Those who are at risk for leukostasis are identified by laboratory examination of peripheral blood, which shows a leukocyte count greater than 100,000 cells/mm^3 with a high percentage of immature cells.

When these patients have been identified, the primary role of the nurse is to observe for signs and symptoms of pulmonary or neurological compromise. Patients who present with leukostasis remain at risk during the early induction treatment period even as the leukocyte count is lowered. This increased risk can be caused by preexisting endothelial damage and the effect of rapid cell lysis.

Initial neurological and pulmonary assessments will establish a baseline. Neurological assessment should include level of consciousness, cranial nerve function, motor function, and vital signs (see Chapters 11, 15A). Pulmonary assessment includes observation of (1) respiratory rate, pattern, and work of breathing; (2) percussion of lung fields; (3) auscultation of breath sounds; and (4) pulse oximetry and arterial blood gas analysis. Frequent follow-up assessment is indicated until it is determined that therapy has significantly reduced the risk of vessel occlusion and/or hemorrhage.

MANAGEMENT

Medical Management

Emergency treatment of a patient with leukostasis is necessary to prevent serious organ dysfunction and/or hemorrhage. Therapy is initiated immediately to lower the circulating myeloblast/lymphoblast count.

Antineoplastic chemotherapy is one modality used to reduce the total blast count. Hydroxyurea inhibits DNA synthesis and causes a rapid fall in the leukocyte count within 24–48 hours. The drug is administered in pill form, often in one of two schedules: (1) 3 g/m^2 daily for two days, or (2) 50 to 100 mg/kg daily until the leukocyte count is <100,000 cells/mm^3. Intravenous single-dose cyclophosphamide is sometimes used in place of hydroxyurea to rapidly lower the leukocyte count. This alkylating agent primarily causes a defect in DNA replication. A recommended dose range is 20–30 mg/kg. In patients with acute nonlymphocytic leukemia, the leukocyte count is often rapidly reduced using a combination of the anthracycline antibiotic daunorubicin and the antimetabolite cytarabine. Both of these drugs work by interfering with DNA and RNA synthesis.

Additional therapies can help to reduce the leukocyte count and the risk for fatal complications. The delivery of cranial radiation (400–600 cGy) over one to three days will destroy intracerebral leukostatic aggregations. Leukapheresis and exchange transfusions are temporary measures that rapidly remove excess circulating leukocytes, but they have no effect on established foci of leukostasis.

Acute tumor lysis syndrome can result when large numbers of cells are killed in a short period of time (see Chapter 16B). This is characterized by acute hyperuricemia, hyperkalemia, hyperphosphatemia, hypocalcemia, and/or renal failure. The degree of metabolic imbalance depends on renal function because uric acid, phosphorus, and potassium are excreted primarily in the urine. Acute precipitation of uric acid or phosphate crystallization can occur, causing kidney damage.

Allopurinol, the anti-gout xanthine oxidase inhibitor, is given to reduce serum uric acid concentrations. Allopurinol decreases uric acid levels by interfering with purine metabolism. It inhibits the enzyme xanthine oxidase, which is needed to convert xanthine and hypoxanthine to uric acid. Absorption of allopurinol is excellent when administered by the oral route. The usual adult dose is 300 mg daily, yet more than 800 mg/day can be prescribed for a patient at great risk of uric acid nephropathy. Allopurinol can cause a skin rash within seven days of the initial dosage, requiring palliative measures to relieve discomfort. Vigorous intravenous hydration is also necessary during tumor lysis.

This patient population will also require complex supportive care. When patients present, they are often anemic and thrombocytopenic; their course might be complicated by coagulopathy and infection. Transfusions of packed red blood cells (PRBCs) should not be given until after cytoreductive therapy has begun, as the PRBCs will increase the viscosity of the blood and exacerbate leukostasis syndrome. Thrombocytopenia and coagulopathy place these patients at extremely high risk for bleeding. Transfusions of platelets, plasma, and other coagulation factors might be necessary. Lastly, the patient will need cultures and broad spectrum antibiotic coverage in the face of fever and neutropenia.

Nursing Management

The major life-threatening complications of leukostasis are respiratory failure and intracranial hemorrhage. The goals of nursing intervention are to (1) identify respiratory decompensation, (2) identify changes in mental status, (3) monitor for acute tumor lysis syndrome, (4) provide supportive care as ordered, and (5) support the patient and family during a life-threatening medical crisis (Table 17B–1).

Frequent assessments of pulmonary status are necessary in order to intervene before respiratory failure occurs. The nurse should assess the patient for tachypnea (>28 breaths per minute), dyspnea, stridor, and tachycardia. Pulse oximetry is a noninvasive technique used to monitor the SaO_2 of hemoglobin and indirectly the patient's respiratory function. A SaO_2 of 90 percent correlates to a PaO_2 of 60 percent, which is critical for tissue oxygenation. Supplemental oxygen therapy might be indicated for SaO_2 less than 90 percent. In addition, periodic arterial blood gas analysis can be performed to measure the PaO_2, $PaCO_2$, and the patient's acid-base balance. Acute decompensation of respiratory function with or without intrapulmonary hemorrhage will require mechanical ventilation.

Symptoms of intracranial hemorrhage might be insidious in onset. Frequent neurological assessments are indicated to identify CNS alter-

Table 17B–1
Nursing Protocol for the Management of Leukostasis

Factor	Intervention
Pulmonary function	Monitor vital signs q 2–4 hrs including pulse oximetry. Assess breath sounds q 2–4 hrs. Assess pulmonary secretions. Monitor the administration of oxygen. Monitor blood gases. Assist patient to the Fowler's position to decrease work of breathing. Teach and encourage patient to use incentive spirometer hourly while awake.

Neurological function	Assess neurological status q 2–4 hrs (see Chapters 11, 15A).
	   —level of consciousness
	   —cranial nerve function
	   —motor function

Acute tumor lysis	Serial electrolyte monitoring. Monitor renal function and urine output. Monitor for EKG changes ($\downarrow$ potassium: peaked T waves, widened QRS, V-tach and/or V-fib, cardiac arrest; $\downarrow$ calcium: prolonged QT interval).
Fever	Monitor for temperatures >100.5°F. Panculture for source of infection. Initiate antibiotics if indicated.
Bleeding	Monitor serial CBC and coagulation studies as ordered. Transfuse blood products as ordered. Limit invasive procedures. Heme test all stool, vomitus, and urine daily.

Coping	Consult social services.
	Assess supports for the patient and family members.
	Assess the coping style.
	Assess amount of information patient and family require, and provide information regarding diagnosis, treatments, test, procedures, and results of the tests and procedures.
	
	Assess stressors to patient and family.
	   —diagnosis
	   —financial
	   —role (career, family)
	
	Provide emotional support.
	
	Mobilize resources.
	   —Medicaid and insurance assistance
	   —transportation
	   —child care
	   —care of the household
	   —lodging

ations early (see Chapter 15A). Changes in mental status might require radiological tests such as computerized tomography and magnetic resonance imaging. Rapid intervention, including platelet transfusions, is indicated to prevent permanent neurological damage from acute hemorrhage.

In the patient with leukocytosis, normal cell death, even prior to cytoreductive therapy, can cause acute tumor lysis syndrome (Chapter 16B). Serial laboratory analysis of electrolytes, uric acid, and renal function should be performed during the cytoreductive phase of treatment, and until the blast count is reduced.

Patients presenting with leukemia and leukostasis are acutely ill. This situation can be frightening and frustrating for the patient and family. An important role of the nurse will be to help the patient and family identify the major stressors, degree of support systems, and the educational needs and readiness regarding disease (see Table 17B–1). With the assistance of social services and/or spiritual care, the nurse can provide support and information to the patient and family. Resources in the community might be available to the patient and family for support in coping with life stressors exacerbated by the disease (see Chapter 7).

CONCLUSION

Patients with acute or chronic leukemia can present with leukostasis syndrome. This group of patients has a higher mortality during induction therapy due to the risk of respiratory failure and acute cerebral hemorrhage. Nursing assessment and intervention should focus on changes in pulmonary or/and neurological function as well as acute tumor lysis syndrome.

BIBLIOGRAPHY

1. Baer, M. R. Management of unusual presentations of acute leukemia. *Hematology/Oncology Clinics of North America* 7(1): 275–291. 1993.

   The clinical manifestations and treatment of leukocytosis are discussed.

2. Dutcher, J. P., C. A. Schiffer, and P. H. Wiernik. Hyperleukocytosis in adult acute nonlymphocytic leukemia: Impact on remission rate and duration, and survival. *Journal of Clinical Oncology* 5(9): 1364–1372. 1987.

   The clinical course of 353 patients with ANLL is described including the clinical features at presentation, causes of early death, response to treatment, and long-term survival. The group with leukocyte counts > 100,000/μL had significantly more deaths in the first week of therapy, with CNS hemorrhage as the primary cause. This patient group also had a shorter duration of complete remission.

3. Gerson, S. L., and H. M. Lazarus. Hematopoietic emergencies. *Seminars in Oncology* 16(6): 532–542. 1989.

   This article presents a good discussion of the clinical presentation, disease specific symptoms, and treatment of leukostasis.

4. Lester, T. J., J. W. Johnson, and J. Cuttner. Pulmonary leukostasis as the single worst prognostic factor in patients with acute myelocytic leukemia and hyperleukosytosis. *The American Journal of Medicine* 79: 43–48. 1985.

   The remission induction and median survival rates are compared in patients with CNS and/or pulmonary leukostatis and those patients without leukostasis. Pulmonary leukostasis was found to be the worst prognostic factor.

5. Lichtman, M. A., and J. M. Rowe. Hyperleukocytic leukemias: Rheological, clinical, and therapeutic considerations. *Blood* 60(2): 279–283. 1982.

   Pathophysiology, clinical manifestations, and treatment of hyperleukocytosis are discussed.

6. Myers, T. J., S. R. Cole, A. U. Klatsky, and D. H. Hild. Respiratory failure due to pulmonary leukostasis following chemotherapy of acute nonlymphocytic leukemia. *Cancer* 51: 1808–1813. 1983.

   Four patients with acute nonlymphocytic leukemia and at risk for pulmonary leukostasis, with leukocyte counts greater than 200,000/mm³, experienced respiratory distress within 10 to 48 hours after initiation of chemotherapy. The pathophysiology of pulmonary leukostasis and potential treatment modalities are discussed.

7. Van Buchem, M. A., T. E. Velde, R. Willemze, and P. J. Spaander. Leukostasis, an underestimated cause of death in leukemia. *Blut* 56: 39–44. 1988.

   This is a retrospective clinicopathological study on the causes of death in 52 patients with AML. Forty percent of patients had pulmonary leukostasis. Other organs affected included the heart, brain, and testes. A review of the literature follows.

8. Wujcik, D. Leukemia. In S. L Groenwald, M. H. Frogge, M. Goodman, and C. H. Yarbro, eds. *Cancer Nursing, Principles and Practice.* 1235–1259. Jones and Bartlett, Boston. 1997.

   An overview of leukemia is presented. Leukostasis is identified as one of four complications specific to the leukemic process.

U N I T **IV**

APPENDICES

Appendix A Tumor Type and Metastatic Spread

Appendix B Tumor Type and Oncologic Emergency

Appendix C Staging of Cancer

A

B

C

Tumor Type and Common Sites of Metastatic Spread

Primary Disease	Common Sites of Metastases													
	Bone	Bone Marrow	Skin	Lung	Liver	Bowel/Rectum	Nodes	Spleen	Kidney/GU	Brain	Serosa	Other Pelvic Organs	Meninges	Adrenal Glands
Bladder							X		X			X		
Brain													X	
Breast	X			X	X		X			X			X	
Cervix	X			X	X	X	X		X			X		
Colon				X	X		X				X			
Esophagus	X			X	X		X							X
Head/neck			X	X			X							
Hepatoma	X			X			X							
Kidney	X			X	X		X			X				X
Lung	X	X			X		X		X	X			X	
Melanoma	X		X	X	X	X	X		X	X			X	
Mycosis fungoides		X	X				X	X						
Ovary				X	X	X	X				X	X		
Pancreas				X	X	X	X							
Prostate	X			X	X		X							

Primary Disease	Common Sites of Metastases													
	Bone	Bone Marrow	Skin	Lung	Liver	Bowel/Rectum	Nodes	Spleen	Kidney/GU	Brain	Serosa	Other Pelvic Organs	Meninges	Adrenal Glands
Sarcoma				X			X							
Stomach	X			X	X		X							
Testes	X			X	X		X							
Thyroid	X			X			X							
Uterus				X							X	X		

Tumor Type and Potential Oncologic Emergency

Tumor Type	Increased Intracranial Pressure	Spinal Cord Compression	Superior Vena Cava Syndrome	Tracheal Obstruction	Bowel Obstruction	Hypercalcemia	Tumor Lysis Syndrome	Syndrome of Inappropriate Antidiuretic Hormone	Sepsis†	Disseminated Intravascular Coagulation	Thrombosis	Cardiac Tamponade	Carotid Artery Rupture	Leukostasis	Other
Bladder					X										Renal failure
*Bone		X				X									Pathologic fracture
*Brain	X							X			X				
Breast		X				X	X			X	X				
Colon/rectum					X			X		X	X				Hemorrhage
Esophagus			X	X		X		X							Hemorrhage
Head/neck				X									X		
Kidney		X				X									Renal failure
Leukemia							X		X	X	X	X		X	
Lung		X	X	X		X	X	X	X	X	X	X			
Lymphoma		X	X			X	X	X	X			X			
Melanoma												X			
Myeloma		X				X	X								
Ovary					X						X				

Tumor Type	Increased Intracranial Pressure	Spinal Cord Compression	Superior Vena Cava Syndrome	Tracheal Obstruction	Bowel Obstruction	Hypercalcemia	Tumor Lysis Syndrome	Syndrome of Inappropriate Antidiuretic Hormone	Sepsis†	Disseminated Intravascular Coagulation	Thrombosis	Cardiac Tamponade	Carotid Artery Rupture	Leukostasis	Other
Pancreas					X			X		X	X				Hyperglycemia
Prostate		X							X	X					
Testes							X		X						
Thyroid				X											
Uterus					X										

*Risk for oncologic emergency exists for patients with either primary or metastatic disease in these sites.

†Risk for oncologic emergency exists for any patient experiencing bone marrow depression from chemotherapy or radiation therapy.

Staging of Cancer

Marion E. Morra

Staging is a method used by health professionals to classify cancers based on anatomical site, natural course of the disease, and apparent spread in the body. Using clinical and histologic determinants, staging helps in planning and evaluating treatment options, determining eligibility of patients for individual clinical trials, giving an indication of prognosis, and comparing worldwide statistics. In addition, by condensing detailed descriptions into a manageable classification system, it eases communication between health professionals.

There is now a worldwide system of staging. Both the American Joint Commission on Cancer (AJCC) and the TNM Committee of the International Union Against Cancer (UICC) use uniform definitions and stage groups of cancer for all anatomic sites.

The AJCC classification is based on the premise that cancers of similar histology or similar site of origin share similar patterns of growth and extensions. The system for describing the anatomic extent of disease assesses three components: T, the extent of the primary tumor; N, the absence or presence and extent of regional lymph node involvement; and M, the absence or presence of distance metastasis. Numbers from zero (0) to four (4) are added to these letters to show progressive increase in tumor size or involvement (e.g., T1, N2, M0).

Four classifications are available for each site: *clinical*, based on evidence acquired before treatment; *pathologic*, based on the evidence acquired before treatment and supplemented or modified by the additional evidence acquired from pathologic examination of a resected specimen; *retreatment*, used after a disease-free interval and when further definitive treatment is planned; and *autopsy*, done after the death of a patient. However, classification by anatomic extent of disease, as determined clinically and histopathologically (a qualitative assessment characterizing the tumor according to the tissue or cell type it mostly closely resembles), is the classification to which the AJCC and the UICC are primarily directed.

The following TNM symbols normally have the same meaning regardless of cancer site and, unless there are other special explanations needed, are not repeated in the tables that follow:

TX Tumor cannot be assessed
T0 No evidence of primary tumor
TIS Carcinoma in situ
NX Regional lymph nodes cannot be assessed
N0 No regional lymph node metastasis

MX Metastasis cannot be assessed
M0 No known distant metastasis
M1 Distant metastasis present

Staging systems for seven of the most common tumors are included alphabetically. The tables are based on information from the PDQ database of the National Cancer Institute.

REFERENCES

1. Murphy G. P., W. Lawrence, and R. E. Lenhard. *American Cancer Society Textbook of Clinical Oncology*. American Cancer Society, Atlanta. 1995.

2. National Cancer Institute. *PDQ Treatment Information for Health Professionals*. Bethesda, MD. 1997.

Breast Cancer

Stages are defined by the TNM classification.

Table AC-1
Staging Classification—Breast Cancer

TNM		Explanation
TIS		Carcinoma in situ; intraductal carcinoma, lobular carcinoma in situ or Paget's disease of the nipple with no tumor.
T1		Tumor 2.0 cm or less.
	T1a	Tumor .5 cm or less.
	T1b	Tumor more than .5 cm or not more than 1 cm.
	T1c	Tumor more than 1 cm but not more than 2 cm.
T2		Tumor more than 2 cm but not more than 5 cm.
T3		Tumor more than 5 cm.
T4		Tumor of any size with direct extension to chest wall or skin (T4d-inflammatory carcinoma).
NX		Regional nodes not assessable.
N0		No regional node metastases.
N1		Metastases to one or more movable ipsilateral axillary nodes.
N2		Metastases to one or more movable ipsilateral axillary nodes fixed to one or another or to other structures.
N3		Metastases to ipsilateral internal mammary lymph nodes.
MX		Presence of distant metastases not assessable.
M0		No distant metastasis.
M1		Distant metastasis (including metastases to one or more ipsilateral supraclavicular nodes.

Table AC–2
Stage Groupings—Breast Cancer

Stage	TNM
Stage 0	TIS, N0, M0
Stage I	T1, N0, M0
Stage IIA	T0–T1, N1, M0 or T2, N0, M0
Stage IIB	T2, N1, M0 or T3, N0, M0
Stage IIIA	T0–T2, N2, M0 or T3, N1–N2, M0
Stage IIIB	Any T, N3, M0 or T4, any N, M0
Stage IV	Any T, any N, M1

Cervical Cancer

The staging of cervical cancer is based on the TNM or FIGO (International Federation of Gynecology and Obstetrics) classification systems. The systems are comparable.

Table AC–3
Staging Classification—Cervical Cancer

FIGO	TNM	Explanation
Stage 0	TIS	Carcinoma in situ; intraepithelial carcinoma.
Stage I	T1, N0, M0	Carcinoma is confined to the cervix.
Stage II	T2, N0, M0	Carcinoma extends beyond the cervix but has not extended to the pelvic wall. The carcinoma involves the vagina but does not extend as far as the lower third.
Stage IIIA	T3, N0, M0	Tumor involves lower third of vagina; tumor has not extended to pelvic wall.
Stage IIIB	T3, N0-N1, M0	Carcinoma has extended to pelvic wall or hydronephrosis or nonfunctioning kidney.
Stage IV	T4, NX-N1, M0 or any T, any N, M1	The carcinoma has extended beyond the true pelvis or has clinically involved the mucosa of the bladder or rectum.

Colon Cancer

Colon cancer stage usually is defined by the TNM system with treatment decisions made in reference to the Dukes' or the Modified Astler-Coller (MAC) classification systems.

Table AC-4
TNM Staging Classification—Colon Cancer

TNM	Explanation
TIS	Carcinoma in situ; intraepithelial or invasion of the lamina propria.
T1	Tumor invades submucosa.
T2	Tumor invades muscularis propria.
T3	Tumor invades through muscularis propria into subserosa or into nonperitoneal pericolic tissues.
T4	Tumor directly invades other organs or structures and/or perforates the visceral peritoneum.
N1	Metastasis in 1–3 pericolic lymph nodes.
N2	Metastasis in 4 or more pericolic lymph nodes.
N3	Metastasis in any lymph node along named vascular trunk and/or metastasis to apical node.

Table AC-5
Staging Grouping—Colon Cancer

Stage	Classification	TNM	Explanation
Stage I	Dukes' A MAC A or B1	T1–T2, N0, M0	Tumor limited to bowel wall.
Stage II	Dukes' B2 MAC B2 or B3	T3–T4, N0, M0	Tumor has spread to extramural tissue.
Stage III	Dukes' C MAC C1–C3	Any T, N1–N3, M0	Regional nodes involved.
Stage IV	Dukes' D	Any T, any N, M1	Any degree of regional disease involved.

Endometrial Cancer

The surgical staging for endometrial cancer is based on the FIGO (International Federation of Gynecology and Obstetrics) classification system.

Table AC–6
Staging-Endometrial Cancer

FIGO	Explanation
Stage 0	Carcinoma in situ or atypical hyperplasia.
Stage I	Carcinoma confined to corpus uteri.
Stage II	Cancer has invaded corpus and cervix but has not extended outside of uterus.
Stage III	Cancer has extended outside the uterus but confined to true pelvis.
Stage IV	Cancer involves the bladder or bowel mucosa or has metastasized.
Grade	Endometrial cancer can be grouped according to degree of differentiation of adenocarcinoma.
G1	5% or less of nonsquamous or nonmorular solid growth pattern.
G2	6%–50% of nonsquamous or nonmorular solid growth pattern.
G3	More than 50% nonsquamous or nonmorular solid growth pattern.

Lung Cancer

The AJCC endorsed a new staging system for lung cancer in 1986. Unless the choice of treatment is affected by stage, small cell lung cancer is usually staged by a simple two-stage system developed by the Veterans Administration Lung Cancer Group.

Table AC-7
Staging Classification—Lung Cancer

TNM	Explanation
TX	Primary tumor cannot be assessed; or tumor proven by presence of malignant cells in sputum or bronchial washings but cannot be seen by imaging or bronchoscope.
T1	A tumor 3.0 cm or less in greatest diameter.
T2	A tumor more than 3.0 cm in greatest diameter or any size tumor that involves the main bronchus (2.0 cm or more distal to the carina) or invades the pleura or has associated atelectasis or obstructive pneumonitis extending to the hilum.
T3	Any tumor that extends into an adjacent structure; or that involves a main bronchus less than 2.0 cm distal to the carina; or that is associated with atelectasis or obstructive pneumonitis of an entire lung.
T4	Any tumor with pleural effusion or that invades the mediastinum, heart, great vessels, trachea, esophagus, vertebral body, or carina.
N1	Metastasis in ipsilateral peribronchial or ipsilateral hilar lymph nodes, or both.
N2	Metastasis in ipsilateral mediastinal or subcarinal hilar lymph nodes, or both.
N3	Metastasis in contralateral mediastinal, contralateral hilar, ipsilateral or contralateral scalene or supraclavicular lymph nodes.
M0	None.
M1	Distant metastasis present.

Table AC–8
Stage Groupings—Lung Cancer

Stage	TNM
Occult carcinoma	TX, N0, M0
Stage 0	TIS, N0, M0
Stage I	T1–T2, N0, M0
Stage II	T1–T2, N1, M0
Stage IIIA	T1–T2, N2, M0 or T3, N0–N2, M0
Stage IIIB	Any T, N3, N0 or T4, any N, M0
Stage IV	Any T, any N, M1

Table AC–9
Staging—Small Cell Lung Cancer

Stage	Explanation
Limited stage	Tumor confined to hemithorax of origin, mediastinum, and supraclavicular nodes. Tumor is encompassed within a "tolerable" radiation therapy port.
Extensive stage	Tumor is too widespread to be staged as limited.

Lymphoma: Adult Hodgkin's Disease

The staging classification used for Hodgkin's disease was adopted at the Ann Arbor Conference held in 1971, with modifications from the Cotswolds meeting in 1989.

Table AC-10
Staging Classification—Adult Hodgkin's Disease

Stage*	Explanation
Stage I	Involvement of a single lymph node region (I) or localized involvement of a single extralymphatic organ or site (IE).
Stage II	Involvement of two or more lymph node regions on the same side of the diaphragm (II) or localized involvement of a single associated extralymphatic organ or site and its lymph nodes with or without involvement of other lymph node regions on the same side of the diaphragm (IIE).
Stage III	Involvement of lymph node regions on both sides of the diaphragm (III). There can also be localized involvement of an associated extralymphatic organ or site (IIIE), involvement of the spleen (IIIS), or both (IIIE+S).
Stage III(1)	Involvement limited to the upper abdomen above the renal vein.
Stage III(2)	Involvement of pelvic and/or para-aortic nodes.
Stage IV	Disseminated (multifocal) involvement of one or more extralymphatic organs, with or without associated lymph node involvement, or isolated extralymphatic organ involvement with distant (nonregional) nodal involvement.

*Each stage is divided into an A or B category: A, asymptomatic; B, fever, night sweats, weight loss >10% of body weight in prior six months.

Lymphoma: Adult Non-Hodgkin's Disease

There are several histopathologic classifications in use through the world, including the Rappaport system, which was the one most widely reported. A conference held in 1982 resolved the differences between the classifications, resulting in the working formulation, including a modified Rappaport classification for the categories. The Ann Arbor staging system is commonly used.

Table AC-11
Working Formulation and Rappaport Classifications

Working Formulation	Rappaport Classification
Low Grade	
Small lymphocytic, consistent with chronic lymphocytic leukemia (SL)	Diffuse lymphocytic lymphoma, well-differentiated (DLWD)
Follicular, predominately small cleaved (FSC)	Nodular lymphocytic poorly differentiated (NPDL)
Follicular, mixed small cleaved cell and large cell (FM)	Nodular mixed, lymphocytic and histiocytic (NM)
Intermediate Grade	
Follicular, predominantly large cell (FL)	Nodular histiocytic (NH)
Diffuse, small cleaved cell (DSC)*	Diffuse lymphocytic, poorly differentiated (DLDP)
Diffuse mixed, small and large cell (DM)	Diffuse mixed, lymphocytic and histiocytic (DM)
Diffuse, large cell cleaved or noncleaved cell (DL)	Diffuse histiocytic (DH)
High Grade	
Immunoblastic, large cell (IBL)**	Diffuse histiocytic (DH)
Lymphoblastic, convoluted or nonconvoluted cell (LL)	Diffuse lymphoblastic (DL)
Small noncleaved cell, Burkitt's or non-Burkitt's (SNC)	Diffuse undifferentiated, Burkitt's or non-Burkitt's (DU)

*frequently managed as a low grade lymphoma

**frequently managed as diffuse, large-cell (DL) lymphoma and also include Ki-1 antigen-positive anaplastic large cell lymphoma

Table AC-12
Staging Classification—Adult Non-Hodgkin's Lymphoma

Stage*	Explanation
Stage I	Involvement of a single lymph node region (I) or localized involvement of a single extralymphatic organ or site (IE).
Stage II	Involvement of two or more lymph node regions on the same side of the diaphragm (II) or localized involvement of a single associated extralymphatic organ or site and its regional lymph nodes with or without involvement of other lymph nodes regions on the same side of the diaphragm (IIE).
Stage III	Involvement of lymph node regions on both sides of the diaphragm (III). There can also be localized involvement of an extralymphatic organ or site (IIIE), involvement of the spleen (IIIS), or both (IIIE+S).
Stage IV	Disseminated (multifocal) involvement of the one or more extralymphatic sites, with or without associated lymph node involvement or isolated extralymphatic organ involvement with distant (nonregional) nodal involvement.

*Each stage is divided into an A or B category: A, asymptomatic; B, fever, night sweats, weight loss >10% of body weight in prior six months.

Prostate Cancer

The American Urological Association staging which consists of ABCD stages has been translated into the TNM classification by the AJCC and the UICC. In addition, Gleason pathologic grades are used to report the degree of differentiation.

Table AC-13
Staging Classification—Prostate Cancer

TNM		Explanation
T1		Tumor not palpable or visible by imaging.
	T1a	Tumor incidental histologic finding in 5% or less of tissue resected.
	T1b	Tumor incidental histologic finding in more than 5% of tissue resected.
	T1c	Tumor identified by needle biopsy (e.g., performed because of elevated PSA).
T2		Tumor confined within the prostate.
	T2a	Tumor involves half of a lobe or less.
	T2b	Tumor involves more than half of a lobe but not both lobes.
	T2c	Tumor involves both lobes.
T3		Tumor extends through the prostatic capsule.
	T3a	Unilateral extracapsular extension.
	T3b	Bilateral extracapsular extension.
	T3c	Tumor invades seminal vesicle(s).
T4		Tumor is fixed or invades adjacent structures other than seminal vesicles.
	T4a	Tumor invades bladder neck, external sphincter, or rectum.
	T4b	Tumor invades levator muscles and/or is fixed to pelvic wall.
N1		Metastasis in single lymph node, 2 cm or less.
N2		Metastasis in single lymph node, more than 2 cm but not more than 5 cm or multiple lymph nodes metastases, none more than 5 cm.
N3		Metastasis in lymph node more than 5 cm.
M1		Distant metastasis (M1a, nonregional lymph nodes; M1b bone(s); M1c, other site(s).

Grade

G1 = Well differentiated, slight anaplasia
G2 = Moderately differentiated, moderate anaplasia
G3–4 = Poorly differentiated or undifferentiated, marked anaplasia

Table AC-14
Stage Grouping—Prostate Cancer

Stage	TNM/Jewett
Stage I	T1a, T1b or T1c, N0, M0 Stage A1, A2
Stage II	T2a, T2b, T2c, N0, M0 Stage B1, B2
Stage III	T3, N0, M0 Stage C
Stage IV	T4a, N0 M0; any T, N1–3, M0; any T, any N, M1 Stage D1, D2

Index

Italic page numbers indicate figures; page numbers with an t indicate tables.

A

Abdominal hernias, 539
Absorption, 379–382, 662
    impaired, 385–388
Accelerated fractionation, 41
Accumulation-depletion model on
    fatigue, 361
Acid-base imbalances, 665
Acid phosphatase, 253
Actinic keratosis, 463
Activated lymphocyte therapy,
    111–112
Activities of daily living (ADLs),
    636
Acute intravascular coagulation,
    744
Acute nonlymphocytic leukemia
    (ANLL), 764
Acyclovir, 477, 504–505
Adaptation phase of illness,
    294–295
Addiction, 326
Adjuvant chemotherapy, 46, 88t,
    95
Adjuvant medications, 326, 327t,
    328
Adjuvant therapy, studies of, 223
Adrenal corticosteroids, 93–94
Adult respiratory distress syndrome
    (ARDS), 146
Agency for Health Care Policy and
    Research, standards for pain
    management, 334
Airflow obstruction, 601, 603
    nursing protocol for management
    of, 603, 605–609t
Airway obstruction, 612
Alcohol and increased risk for
    cancers, 244, 245
Alkaline urine, 543
Alkylating agents, 14
    in chemotherapy, 68–69, 69t

Allogeneic transplantation, 131–132
Allopurinol, 706, 708
    for leukostasis, 766
Alopecia, 472
    management of, 481, 484t
    as side effect in chemotherapy,
        100
Alpha-fetoprotein (AFP), 253
Altered fractionation schedules, 45t
Ambulatory pumps, 197–199
    assessment of, 199, 199t
Amenorrhea, 68
American Brain Tumor
    Association, 280
American Cancer Society, 277–278
    "I Can Cope" course, 270
American Nurses' Association,
    Position Statement on Promotion
    of Comfort and Relief of Pain in
    Dying Patients, 330
Amifostine, 521
Amitriptyline (Elavil®), 326
Amplification, 422
Amsacrine (m-AMSA), 90
Anaerobic glycolysis, 389
Analgesics, 505
    ladder approach to pain
        management, 318, 322
    opioids, 313–316
Anaphylactic reactions, 722
Anaphylactoid reactions, 722
Anaphylaxis, 721–728
    assessment, 725
    and cancer patients, 724
    medical management, 725–727
    nursing management, 727–728
    pathophysiology, 722–723
Anaplasia, 9
Anemia, 417, 428
    and constipation, 550
    medical management of, 433
Anesthetic interventions into
    cancer pain, 329

Angiogenic factors, 15–16
Ankle-foot orthoses, 518
Anorexia, 384–385
    as side effect of chemotherapy,
        99
    as side effect of radiation
        therapy, 392
Anthracenedione in chemotherapy,
    91
Anthracyclines in chemotherapy,
    91
Anticoagulant citrate dextrose
    (ACD), 139
Antidepressants, 355
Antiemetic agents, 504
    in treating gastric side effects of
        chemotherapy, 97–99, 98t
Antihistamines, 355
    in managing nausea, 406
Antimetabolites in chemotherapy,
    89
Antimicrobials, 504–505
    in treating septic shock, 733
Antimicrotubule agents, 89–90
Antineoplastic agents, 46
    local reaction to, 172
Antineoplastic chemotherapy, 765
Antioxidants, 14
Antitumor antibiotics, 90–91
Anxiolytic antidepressants, 504
Apheresis, 138–139
    complications associated with,
        139
Apoptosis, 4
Appearance, difference in cell, 7, 8f
Area Under the Curve (AUC) in
    drug dose calculations, 95, 97
Arrest, 17–18
Asbestos, 15
    carcinogenic potential of, 15
Ascending colostomy, 528
Ascites, 475, 486, 488
    nursing protocol for management
        of, 488t
Aseptic necrosis
    as complication for bone marrow
        transplantation, 168
    as complication of bone marrow
        transplantation, 168
Aspiration biopsy, 25t

Assessment for tracheal
    obstruction, 657
Ataxia telangiectasia, 12
Ataxia-telangiectasia, 13
Autologous marrow and peripheral
    stem cell transplantation,
    132–134
Autologous transplants, frequency
    of, 127
Autonomic function, 637
Autonomic nervous system, 518
Autoregulation, 618
Azoospermia, 68

B

Babinski reflex, 517
Babinski sign, 637
Bacillus Calmette-Guerin (BCG)
    therapy, 564
Baclofen, 326
Bacterial carcinogenesis, 13
Bacterial infections, 475–476
Bactrim™, 504–505
Balloon angioplasty for superior
    vena cava syndrome, 650
Bands of adhesions, 663
Barrier therapy, 579
Basal cell carcinoma (BCC), 463
Basement membrane, invasion of,
    16
Behavioral approaches of treating
    nausea and vomiting, 406,
    407–408t 408
Benign neoplasms, 9
Benzene, 14
Benzodiazepines, 354–355
Betatron, 47
Bile, 382
Biochemical alterations in cancer
    cells, 10
Biochemistry, cell differences in,
    10
Biologicals, effect of, on mucosa,
    449
Biologic response modifiers (BRMs)
    nursing care of patients
        receiving, 113, 114–124t
    routes of administration and
        known side effects, 114–116t

Biopsy, 253
   endometrial, 590
   surgical techniques for, 24, 25*t*
Biotherapy, 105–124, 501, 503
   agents used in, 106–107,
      108–111*t,* 110–113
   effect of, on tissue, 472
Bisphosphonates, 695–697
Bladder
   functional alterations of,
      557–581
      assessment, 565–570
      medical management, 570,
         572–576
      nursing management, 576,
         577–578*t,* 578–581
      pathophysiology, 561–565
      physiology, 558–561
   retraining, 576
Bladder dysfunction, 635
Bleeding, 427
Blood-brain barrier (BBB), 617
Blood cell lineages
   granulocytes, 419–424
   monocytes, 419–424
Blood cells
   formation of, 417
   normal laboratory values for, 421*t*
Blood drawing, use of venous
   access devices (VADs) for,
   187–189
Blood pressure, 624
Bloom syndrome, 12
B-lymphocytes, 421
Body surface area (BSA) in drug
   dose calculations, 95
Bolus, 48
Bone marrow, 417–438
   anatomy and physiology, 417,
      418, 419
   and blood cell lineages, 419–424
Bone marrow depression (BMD),
   417
   assessment of patients at risk for,
      428–429
   complications of, 426–428, 428*t*
   medical management
      anemia, 433
      granulocytopenia, 429–432
      thrombocytopenia, 432–433

nursing management, 434–437*t*
   437–438
   pathophysiology of, 424–428,
      425*t,* 426*t*
Bone marrow suppression, 101
Bone marrow transplantation
   (BMT), 127–169, 473–474, 473*t*
   acute complications, 142,
      143–144*t*
      cardiac, 148
      gastrointestinal toxicity, 142,
         144
      graft-versus-host disease, 145
      hematologic, 144–145
      hemorrhagic cystitis, 146
      infection, 148
      neurologic, 147–148
      pulmonary, 146–147
      renal, 145–146
      veno-occlusive disease, 146
   cryopreservation, 140
   discharge from hospital, 148
      community practice, 158
   donor selection, 137–138
   history, 128–129
   late complications of, 158
      aseptic necrosis, 168
      chronic graft-versus-host
         disease, 166
      dental effects, 168
      gonadal dysfunction, 166–167
      graft failure, 168
      graft-versus-host disease,
         164–165, 166
      growth and development, 167
      neurological, 168
      nursing care of, 159–163*t*
      quality of life, 169
      relapse, 167
      second malignancies, 168–169
   late effects of, 149–157*t*
   versus peripheral blood stem
      cell transplantation, 129–131,
      130*t*
   pre-transplant conditioning
      regimens, 140–142
   pretransplant evaluation and
      preparation, 134–137
   stem cell harvest, 138–139
   types of, 131–134

Bowel
dysfunction of, 635
functional alterations of, 545–546
assessment, 547–549
medical and surgical treatment,
549–550
medical management, 550–554
nursing management,
554–556, 555*t*
pathophysiology, 546–547
management of, in preventing
constipation, 627
Bowel obstruction, 661–671
assessment, 666–667
clinical manifestations, 665–666
large, pathophysiology, 664–665
medical management, 667–668
nursing management, 668–670*t*,
671
small, 661–664
pathophysiology, 662–663
Bowen's disease, 463
Brachytherapy, 46, 50
and painful bladder disorder, 565
remote afterloading, 50–51
in treating brain metastases, 497
Brain stem functioning and cranial
nerves, 621, 623
Brain tumors, 496–497, 498*t*, 499*t*
Brain volume, 617–618
BRCA1, 246
BRCA2, 246
Breakthrough pain, 308–309
Breast cancer, 599
prevention and early detection of,
258
stage groupings, 779*t*
TNM classification of, 778*t*
Breast self-examination (BSE), 254,
255
Budd-Chiari syndrome, 741
Bulk producers, 551–552
Burkitt's lymphoma, 13, 245, 705
Burst forming unit—erythroid
(BFU-E), 422
Burst forming unit-megakaryocyte
(BFU-Mega), 422
Butyrophenes in managing nausea,
406

C

Cachexia, 383
Calcitonin, 688, 697
Calcium
normal regulation of, 688
regulatory mechanisms, 689
role of, in metabolic functions,
690–691
serum levels of, 691–692
Cancer. *See also* Breast cancer;
Cervical cancer; Colon cancer;
Colorectal cancer; Lung cancer;
Ovarian cancer; Prostate cancer
causes of, 10–15
decline in mortality from, 21
diagnosis of, 24
risk factors and common signs
and symptoms for common,
251*t*
staging of, 777–788
breast, 778*t*, 779*t*
cervical, 779*t*
colon, 780*t*
endometrial, 781*t*
lung, 782*t*, 783*t*
lymphoma
adult Hodgkin's disease, 784*t*
adult non-Hodgkin's disease,
785*t*, 786*t*
prostate, 787*t*, 788*t*
summary of second cancers
following initial, 250*t*
systemic metabolic alterations of,
388–391
Cancer cachexia, 384
Cancer Care, Inc., 280–281
Cancer cells
appearance of, 7, 8f
biochemistry of, 10
differentiation of, 8–9
gene structure, 10
growth patterns of, 3–7
surfaces of, 9
Cancer centers, 286–287
Cancer Information Service (CIS),
278
Cancer metastasis, 15–19
CancerNet, 279

CancerNet™, 236, 279
Cancer pain
  nonpharmacological treatment
    of, 328
  nurse's role in management of,
    312
  pharmacological treatment of,
    313
Cancer patient, information needs
  of, 263–266
Cancer-suppressor genes, 3, 12
Cancer treatment, 21–22. *See also*
  Biotherapy; Chemotherapy;
  Parenteral therapy; Radiation;
  Surgery
  complications caused by,
    501–504
  nutritional consequences of,
    391–392, 393*t,* 394*t*
  radiation, 36–63
  surgery, 22–33
Cancer treatment studies
  clinical research, ethical
    considerations for nurses in,
    233–235
  clinical trials, 220
  drug development, 219–220
  nursing in clinical research,
    223–233
    data management, 233
    follow-up, 227, 233
    response, 227, 232*t*
    roles, 224
    study initiation and eligibility,
      224–226
    toxicities, 227, 230–232*t*
    treatment, 226, *228–229*
  Phase I trials, 220–221
  Phase II trials, 222
  Phase III trials, 222–223
  Phase IV trials, 223
  resources, 235–236
Candida, fungal invasion with, 444
Candlelighters Childhood Cancer
  Foundation, 281
Cannabinoids in management of
  vomiting, 405
Carbohydrate metabolism, altered,
  389

Carcinoembryonic antigen (CEA),
  253
Carcinogenesis
  bacterial, 13
  chemical, 14
  definition of, 10
  dietary, 13–14
  familial, 12–13
  phases of, 11
  physical, 14–15
  viral, 13
Carcinogens, 11
Carcinomatosis, leptomeningeal,
  500
Cardiac catheterization in diagnosing
  cardiac tamponade, 678
Cardiac complications, from bone
  marrow transplantation, 148
Cardiac tamponade, 673–684
  clinical manifestations, 675–677
  diagnosis, 677–679
  medical management, 679–682
  pathophysiology, 673–675
Carmustine, 172
Carotid artery erosion and rupture,
  751–761
  anatomy, 751
  assessment, 753–754
  clinical manifestations, 753
  medical and surgical
    management, 755–756
  nursing management, 756–761,
    757*t,* 759*t,* 760*t*
  pathophysiology, 752–753
  prevention, 755
Case-finding, 254, 256
Catheters
  nontunneled, 178
  tunneled, 178–179
CathFinder™ Catheter Tracking
  System, 180
CathLink, 180
Celiac plexus blocks for pancreatic
  cancer, 329
Cells
  appearance of normal, 7, 8f
  comparison with cancer cells,
    3–10, 5, 5f, *8,* 8f
  control of division of, 3

Cells (cont'd)
    differences in growth of, 3–7, *5*
    differences in surface of, 9
    growth of normal, 3–7, *5*
    phases of cycle, 5–6, 5f
Cell-surface glycoproteins, 18
Cellular nutrition model on fatigue,
    361–362
Cellular proliferation, 4–6
Cellular radiosensitivity, 39, 39*t*, 40*t*
Cellulitis, 475
Centigray (cGy), 41
Central-peripheral model on
    fatigue, 361
Cerebellar dysfunction
    management of, 511–512
    signs/symptoms of, 511*t*
Cerebellar nervous system,
    assessment, 507, 510
Cerebral dysfunction, management
    of, 514
Cerebral edema, vasogenic, 617
Cerebral function, assessment,
    512–513
Cerebrospinal fluid (CSF), 618–619
Cerebrovascular disease, 506
Cervical cancer
    prevention and early detection of,
        258
    TNM classification, 779*t*
Challenge appraisals, 290
Chemical carcinogenesis, 14
Chemoprevention, 246, 247*t*
Chemoreceptor trigger zone (CTZ),
    388
Chemotherapeutic and/or biological
    agents, administration of, 176
Chemotherapy, 66–104
    adjuvant, 88*t*, 95
    agents used in
        alkylating, 68–69, 69*t*
        antimetabolites, 89
        antimicrotubule, 89–90
        antitumor antibiotics, 90–91
        hormones and hormone
            antagonists, 84–87*t*, 92–94
        miscellaneous, 91–92
        new formulations, 92
        topoisomerase I and II
            inhibitors, 90

    antineoplastic, 765
    for cardiac tamponade, 681
    combination, 94
    drug dose calculation in, 95–97
    effect of
        on bone marrow, 425–426
        on mucosa, 442–444, 445–449*t*
        on tissue, 469, 470–471*t*, 472
    intrathecal, 501
    long-term effects of, 102–103
    neoadjuvant, 94–95
    nursing care of patients
        receiving, 97–103
        cutaneous and mucosal
            toxicity, 100
        gastrointestinal side effects,
            97–99, 98*t*
        hematologic toxicity, 101
        hepatic effects, 102
        immunosuppression, 102
        pulmonary effects, 102
        renal effects, 102
    nutritional consequences of,
        392–393, 395*t*
    and painful bladder disorder, 564
    potential damage from, 172*t*
    for spinal cord compression,
        639–640
    for superior vena cava syndrome,
        649
    systemic, 212–213, 501
    and urinary system distress, 565
Chemotherapy-induced
    granulocytopenia (GCP), 424
    fever in patient with, 429
Children's Hospice International,
    281
Chloral hydrate, 355
Chlorpromazine (Thorazine®), in
    managing nausea, 406
Choline magnesium trisalicylate
    (Trilisate®), 313
Chronic graft-versus-host disease
    as complication of bone marrow
        transplantation (BMT), 166
Chronic insomnia, 337
Chronic radiation encephalopathy,
    503
Circadian rhythm, 345
Circle of Willis, 751

Cisplatin, 520
  and vomiting as side effect of, 405
Cladribine, 89
Clinical research
  ethical considerations for nurses
    in, 233–235
  nursing in, 223–233
  principles of, 219–236
Clinical Trials, 220
  Cooperative Group Program, 287
  home page, 236
Clodronate, 697
Clonazepam (Klonopin®), 326
Coagulopathies, 736–748
  assessment, 740, 741t
  disseminated intravascular
    coagulation, 744, 745t,
    746–748, 747t
  medical management, 741–742,
    742t, 743t
  normal physiology, 737–738
  nursing management, 743–744,
    743t
  thrombotic disorders, 738–739
Cobalt 60 machines, 47
Codeine, 314
Collagen, 460
Colon cancer
  left-sided, 664–665
  right-sided, 664
  staging groupings, 780t
  TNM classification, 780t
Colony forming unit—erythroid
  (CFU-E), 422
Colony stimulating factors (CSF),
  423
Colorectal cancer, prevention and
  early detection of, 260
Colostomies
  ascending, 528
  left transverse, 527
  placement of, 527
  transverse, 527
Combination chemotherapy, 94
Combined Health Information
  Database, 280
Comfort
  fatigue, 360–372
  pain, 305–335
  sleep, 336–358

Common variable
  immunodeficiency, 13
Community Clinical Oncology
  Program (CCOP), 287
Computerized tomography in
  diagnosing cardiac tamponade,
  678
Consciousness, level of, 621
Constipation, 546
  affecting cancer patients, 665
  after bowel diversion, 535
  bowel management to prevent,
    627
  definition of, 547
  primary, 547–548
  as side effect in chemotherapy,
    99
Consumption-coagulation, 744
Contact inhibition, 4
Continent bladder, constriction of,
  543
Continent ileostomy, 539
Continent reservoir, 539
Coping with cancer, 289–303
  adaptation phase, 294–295
  initial phase, 291–293
  nursing care management of
    patients and families
    assessment, 297–299
    management, 299, 300–301t
      302–303
  recurrent phase, 295–296
  stress, 289–290
  terminal phase, 296–297
Core needle biopsy, 25t
Corticosteroids, 174
Cranial nerves, 518, 519–520t
  and brain stem functioning, 621,
    623
  management of dysfunctions,
    520–521
Cryopreservation, 129, 140
Cuff stenosis, 656
Cunningham clamp, 573–574
Cutaneous melanoma, 464
Cutaneous metastasis, 466
Cutaneous paraneoplastic
  syndromes, 466, 467–468t, 468
Cutaneous T-cell lymphoma
  (CTCL), 465–466

Cutaneous toxicity in
  chemotherapy, 100
Cyclophosphamide, 129, 138
  and vomiting as side effect of,
    405
Cyclosporine, 505
Cyclotrons, 47
Cystitis
  hemorrhagic, 146
  radiation-induced, 564
Cytokines, 106–107, 129
  multilineage, 127
Cytology, 253
Cytomegalovirus (CMV), 477

D

Dacarbazine, 172
  and vomiting as side effect of,
    405
Dactinomycin, 172
  and vomiting as side effect of,
    405
Daunomycin (DaunoXome®), 92
Daunorubicin, 172
  in chemotherapy, 91
D-dimer assay for fibrin
  degradation products/fragments,
    746
Defecation, 382, 546–547
Defecation reflex, 546
Delirium, 513
Delta-9-tetrahydrocannabinol
  (THC), 99
Demargination, 420
Demeclocycline for syndrome of
  inappropriate antidiuretic
  hormone (SIADH), 717
Dementia, 513
Density-dependent growth, 4
Dental effects as complication of
  bone marrow transplantation, 168
Desipramine, 326
Desquamation as side effect in
  chemotherapy, 100
Detection, early, 254
Detrusor instability, 561, 562
Detrusor stability, 558–560
Dexamethasone, 405
Diagnosis of cancer, 24

Diarrhea, 386
  and colostomies, 535
  management of problems related
    to, 401, 403, 404t
  pathophysiology of, 387t
  as side effect in chemotherapy,
    99
Dietary carcinogenesis, 13–14
Dietary deficiency or excess in
  cancer causation, 244
Dietary history and intake in
  nutritional assessment, 397
Diethylstilbestrol (DES), 93, 245
Differentiation, cell differences in,
  8–9
Digestion, 379–382
  impaired, 385–388
Dimenhydrinate (Dramamine®),
  323
  in managing nausea, 406
Dimethylsulfoxide (DMSO), 140,
  174
Diphenhydramine (Benadryl®),
  174, 355
  in managing nausea, 406
Direct effect, 38
Discharge planning, 31, 32
Disease-related causes of skin
  impairment, 463–466
Disseminated intravascular
  coagulation (DIC), 734, 744,
  745t, 746–748, 747t
Dissemination, 16
Diuresis, prophylactic, 706
DNA
  interaction of ionizing radiation
    with target, 38
  structure and chemotherapy, 68
DNA viruses, 13
Docetaxel, 89–90
Doll-eye movements, 623
Double-blinded study, 220
Doubling time, 7
Doxepin, 326
Doxorubicin, 172
  in chemotherapy, 91
Drug development process,
  219–220
Drug dose calculation in
  chemotherapy, 95–97

Drug-induced lung disease (DILD), 601
Dukes' classification for colon cancer, 25
Duodenum, 380
Dysgeusia, 385
Dysphonia, 657
Dysplasia, 9
Dysplastic nevi, 463
Dysplastic nevus syndrome, 12
Dyspnea, 600–601, 601, 677
Dyspraxia, 513
Dyssynergia, 562–563

E

Early detection, 241, 254
  considerations in, 246–248
Echocardiography in diagnosing cardiac tamponade, 678
Edema, 475
  intracellular, 617–618
  nursing protocol for management of, 488*t*
  vasogenic cerebral, 617
Education. *See* Patient education
Ejaculation dysfunction, 588
Electrocardiogram, 677–678
Electromagnetic radiation, 38
Electrostimulation in management of voiding dysfunction, 570
Elimination, anatomical alterations
  common problems, 532–540
  fecal diversion, 527–532
  management of other draining wounds, 544
  urinary diversion, 540–543
Emission dysfunction, 593
Emission failure, 588
Emotional support, patient's need for, 32
En bloc dissection, 26–27
EncorePlus, 281–282
Endocarditis, nonbacterial thrombotic, 740
Endometrial biopsy, 590
Endometrial cancer, surgical staging, 781*t*
Endo-reduplication, 422
Enemas, 554

Enriched stem cell product, 139
Enteral nutrition, 408, 409*t*, 410–411, 412*t*
Enteritis, radiation-induced, 450
Epidermis, 459–460
Epidermolysis as side effect in chemotherapy, 100
Epidural therapy, 206–207
Epirubicin, 172
Epstein-Barr virus (EBV), 13, 245, 477
Erythema, 472
Erythrocytes/red blood cells, 422–423
Erythropoietin (EPO), 423
Estramustine, 172
Estrogens and cancer risk, 245–246
Ethacrynic acid, 695
Etidronate, 697
Etopophos®, 90
Etoposide phosphate, 90
Etoposide (VP-16), 90, 172
Excisional biopsy, 25*t*
Excretion, 382
Expanding tissues, 6
External nutrient losses, 387–388
External radiation, 46
  equipment, 47
  treatment, 49–50
  treatment planning, 48–49
Extracellular matrices, invasion of, 16
Extramural obstructions, 662
Extraocular movements (EOMs), 623
Extrapersonal stressors, 289–290
Extraurethral incontinence, 563
  management of, 574
Extravasation, 18
Extravasation treatments, 174–176, 175*t*

F

Familial carcinogenesis, 12–13
Familial polyposis, 12
Fanconi's anemia, 12
Fat, 383
Fat-free mass, 383

Fatigue, 359–372
  clinical assessment of, 366–369
  and constipation, 550
  medical management of, 369
  nursing management of, 369,
    370–371t, 372
  pathophysiology, 361–366
  as side effect of radiation
    therapy, 392
Fat metabolism, 391
Fecal consistency, 527
Fecal diversion, 527–532
  management, 528–529
  pathophysiology, 527–528
  procedure, 529–532
Feeding center, 378
Fertility
  assessment of, 590
  problems of, 588
Fibrin-platelet clot, 17
Flow sheet, 226, 228–229
Fludarabine, 89
Flutamide, 93
Folic acid, anticancer effects of, 67
Follicle-stimulating hormone
  (FSH), 590
Follow-up care in spinal cord
  compression, 643
Food and Drug Administration
  (FDA), filing of investigational
  new drug application with, 67
Fractionation, 41
Frenkel exercises, 512t
Functional bowel obstruction, 662
Functional incontinence, 563
  nursing management of, 579–580
Fungal infections, 477–478
Furosemide, 695, 717

G

Gabapentin (Neurontin®), 326
Gallium nitrate, 698
Gastrocolic reflex, 546
Gastrointestinal side effects in
  chemotherapy, 97–99, 98t
Gastrointestinal toxicity as
  complication of bone marrow
  transplantation, 142, 144
Gemcitabine, 89

Genes
  cancer-suppressor, 12
  cell differences in, 10
Gene therapy, 112
Genetic predisposition to cancer,
  246
Glasgow Coma Scale, 622
Glucocorticoids, 405
Gonadal dysfunction as
  complication of bone marrow
  transplantation, 166–167
G_0 phase, 5–6, 5f
G_1 phase, 5–6, 5f
G_2 phase, 5–6, 5f
Graft failure as complication of
  bone marrow transplantation
  (BMT), 168
Graft-versus-host disease (GVHD)
  as complication of bone marrow
    transplantation, 145, 164–165,
    166
  complications of chronic,
    164–165, 166
  improvements in management,
    129
Granisectron (Kytril®) 5-HT_3, in
  managing nausea, 406
Granisetron (Kytril®), 323
Granulocyte colony-stimulating
  factor (G-CSF), 127
  in reducing side effects from
    chemotherapy, 101
Granulocyte erythrocyte monocyte
  megakaryocyte (CFU-GEMM),
  419
Granulocyte macrophage (CFU-
  GM), 419–424
Granulocyte macrophage—colony-
  stimulating factor (GM-CSF),
  127, 420
  in reducing side effects from
    chemotherapy, 101
Granulocytes, 419–424, 441
  functions of, 420–421, 420t
Granulocytopenia, 417
  and constipation, 549
  medical management of,
    429–432
Gray (Gy), 41
Groshongs, 178, 179

Growth factors, 4
Growth fraction, 7

H

Haloperidol (Haldol®), 323, 504
Harm appraisals, 290
Healthfinder, 279–280
*Healthy People 2000: National
  Health Promotion and Disease
  Prevention Objectives,* 249
Heel walking, 636
Helicobacter pylori, 13
Help for Incontinent People, 282
Hematologic complications, from
  bone marrow transplantation,
  144–145
Hematologic toxicity in
  chemotherapy, 101
Hematopoiesis, 417, *418*
Hematopoietic growth factors
  (HGFs), 419, 423–424
Hematopoietic inductive
  microenvironment (HIM), 417
Hematopoietic progenitor cells,
  127
Hemorrhage, risk for spontaneous,
  427–428
Hemorrhagic cystitis, from bone
  marrow transplantation, 146
Heparin in management of
  disseminated intravascular
  coagulation (DIC), 746
Hepatic effects in chemotherapy,
  102
Hepatic vein thrombosis, 741
Hepatitis B virus (HBV), 13
Hepatocellular carcinoma, 13
Hepatojugular reflex, 677
Hereditary nonpolyposis Colorectal
  cancer, 12
Hernias, abdominal, 539
Herniation, 619–620
Herpes virus, 476
Herpes zoster, 506
Heterogeneity, 10
Hickman-type catheters, 179
High-efficiency particulate (HEPA)
  filters, 129
High-tech pain management, 333

HIV-related skin cancers, non-
  Kaposi's sarcoma, 465
Hodgkin's disease, 13, 245
Hormonal regulatory mechanisms,
  688
Hormone-secreting tumors, 386
Hormones in chemotherapy,
  84–85t, 92–94
Horner's syndrome, 647
Hospice Link, 282
Human chorionic gonadotropin
  (HCG), 253
Human Genome Project, 246
Human hematopoietic growth
  factors, 110–111
Human leukocyte antigen (HLA),
  128
Human papillomaviruses (HPV),
  13
Human T-cell leukemia-lymphoma
  virus (HTLV-1), 13
Humoral hypercalcemia of
  malignancy, 689
Hyaluronidase, 174
Hydromorphone (Didaudid®), 315
Hydroxine (Vistaril®, Atarax®),
  355
Hypercalcemia, 687–702
  assessment, 691–694
  and constipation, 548
  in malignancy, 689–690
  medical management, 695–699
  nursing management, 699–702,
    699t, 700t
  pathophysiology, 687–691
Hypercalcemic crisis, 694
Hyperchromatic cells, 7
Hypercoagulation, 738
Hyperfractionation, 41
Hyperkalemia, management of, 706
Hyperphosphatemia, 704
  management of, 707
Hyperpigmentation as side effect in
  chemotherapy, 100
Hyperplasia, 9
Hyperreflexia, 637
Hypersensitivity reactions,
  cutaneous manifestations of, 472
Hyperthermia, 43t, 625
  effect of, on tissue, 472

Hyperuricemia, 102
Hyperventilation, 625
Hypogeusia, 385
Hypokalemia, 653
Hyponatremia, 653, 714
Hypothermia, 625
Hypoventilation, 601, 612
    prevention of, 612
Hypoxia, 601, 612
    prevention of, 612

I

I Can Cope, 282
Idiopathic pneumonia, 147
Ileum, 380
Illness
    adaptation phase of, 294–295
    initial phase of, 291–293
    recurrent phase, 295–296
    terminal phase of, 296–297
Immune surveillance theory, 106
Immunocompetence, 422
Immunologic response, 17
Immunosuppressed patients,
    infection in, 505
Immunosuppression
    in chemotherapy, 102
    related skin cancers
        HIV, 465
        non-HIV, 465
Incisional biopsy, 25t
Incontinence, 478
Increased intracranial pressure,
    617–630
    assessment, 620–625
    clinical manifestations, 620
    medical and surgical
        management, 625–626
    nursing management, 626–627,
        628–629t, 630
    pathophysiology
        blood volume, 618
        brain volume, 617–618
        cerebrospinal fluid, 618–619
        herniation, 619–620
Indirect effect, 38
Indomethacin (Indocin®), 313
Infection from bone marrow
    transplantation, 148

Infiltrative emergencies, 751–761
    carotid artery erosion and
        rupture, 751–761
        anatomy, 751
        assessment, 753–754
        clinical manifestations, 753
        medical and surgical
            management, 755–756
        nursing management,
            756–761, 757t, 759t, 760t
        pathophysiology, 752–753
        prevention, 755
    leukostasis, 762–768
        assessment, 764–765
        clinical manifestations, 764
        medical management, 765–766
        nursing management, 766,
            767t, 768
        pathophysiology, 763–764
Information
    needs of cancer patient, 263–266
    obtaining, 293
    resources of, 277–287
Information seeking behaviors,
    267–268
Informed consent, 270–273
    and clinical research, 235
Infusaid pump, 198
Ingestion, 378–379
    inadequate, 384
Initial insomnia, 337
Initial phase of illness, 291–293
Initiator, 11, 243
Insomnia
    chronic, 337
    definition of, 336–337
    initial, 337
    intermittent, 337
    mild, 337
    moderate, 337
    terminal, 337
Instability reflex incontinence,
    medical management of, 572
Integrins, 16
Interferons, 106, 107
Interleukin-1 (IL-1), 729
Interleukin-2 (IL-2), 107, 111t
Interleukin-3 (IL-3), 420
Interleukin-6 (IL-6), 729
Interleukins, 107

Intermittent insomnia, 337
Internal radiation, 46, 50–53, 51*t*
International Association for the
  Study of Pain, 305–306
International Association of
  Laryngectomies, 282
International Bone Marrow
  Transplant Registry (IBMTR),
  127
International Federation of
  Gynecologists and Obstetricians
  (FIGO), 25
Interpersonal stressors, 289
Interstitial brachytherapy, 504
Interstitial implants, 50
Interstitial pneumonia, 147
Intestinal obstruction, 385–386
Intra-arterial therapy, 192–196
  assessment, 193, 194–195*t*
  management, 193, 195–196
Intracavitary implant, 50
Intracavitary management of
  pleural effusions, 212–214, 213*t*,
  214*t*, 215*t*
Intracellular edema, 617–618
Intracranial hemorrhage, symptoms
  of, 766, 768
Intraluminal obstructions, 662
Intraoperative radiotherapy
  (IORT), 43–44*t*
Intraperitoneal catheters, 210*t*
Intraperitoneal therapy, 207–212
  agents used for, 209*t*
Intrapersonal stressors, 289
Intrathecal chemotherapy, 501
Intraventricular subcutaneous
  reservoirs, 200–201
  assessment, 202, 202*t*
  management, 202–205
Investigational new drug (IND)
  application, filing with Food and
  Drug Administration (FDA),
  67
Ionizing radiation, 14
  interaction with target DNA,
  38
Irinotecan (Camptosar®), 90
Irritants, 172–176, 172*t*, 175*t*
Isoproterenol (Isuprel®), 174
Isotonic sodium thiosulfate, 174

J

Jaundice, 478
Jejunum, 380

K

Kaposi's sarcoma, 245, 465
Karnofsky Performance Scale, 169,
  507, 508*t*
Ketocanazole, 93
Ketorolac (Toradol®), 313
Kussmal's sign, 675
Kwashiorkor, 383

L

Laminar air-flow (LAF) rooms, 429
Laminar air-flow (LAF) units, 129
Large-bowel obstruction,
  management of, 667–668
Large intestine, 381
Laser surgery, 28–29
L-asparaginase in chemotherapy,
  91
Laxatives
  osmotic, 552–553
  saline, 552–553
  stimulant, 553
  surfactant, 553
Learning needs, assessment of,
  31–33
Left-sided colonic carcinomas, 664
Left transverse colostomy, 527
Leptomeningeal carcinomatosis,
  500
Leukemias, 673
Leukemia Society of America, 283
Leukoencephalopathy, 504
Leukopheresis, 129
Leukostasis, 762–768
  assessment, 764–765
  clinical manifestations, 764
  medical management, 765–766
  nursing management, 766, 767*t*,
    768
  pathophysiology, 763–764
Level of consciousness, 621
Levorphanol (Levo-Dromoran®),
  315
Lhermitte's' syndrome, 503

Li Fraumeni syndrome, 12
Linear accelerators, 47
Liposomal doxorubicin (Doxil®), 92
Lithium, 717
Liver, 382
Local excision, 26
Local osteolytic hypercalcemia (LOH), 689
Look Good, Feel Better, 283
Loss appraisals, 290
Lubricants, 552
Lung cancer, 599, 645
    prevention and early detection of, 259
    small-cell staging, 783*t*
    stage groupings, 783*t*
    TNM staging classification, 782*t*
Luteinizing hormone (LH), 590
Lymphedema, 475
    nursing protocol for management of, 488*t*
Lymphocytopenia, 417
Lymphokines, 106
Lymphomas, 599, 645, 673
    adult Hodgkin's disease, TNM staging classification, 784*t*
    adult non-Hodgkin's disease TNM staging classification, 785*t*, 786*t*
        working formulation and Rappaport classifications, 785*t*
    stage groupings, 788*t*
Lymphoproliferative cancers, 14

M

Macrophages, 460
Macular rashes as side effect in chemotherapy, 100
Magnetic resonance imaging (MRI), in diagnosing cardiac tamponade, 678
Malignant lesions, 463
Malignant melanoma, prevention and early detection of, 259
Malignant neoplasms, 9
Malignant pleural effusions, 599

Malnutrition, 383–384
    protein-calorie, 383
Man to Man, 283
Marasmus, 383
Marrow transplantation versus peripheral blood stem cell transplantation, 129–131, 130*t*
Mass effect, 619
Mass movements, 546
Mazepine (Tegretol®), 326
Mechanical bowel obstruction, 662
Mechlorethamine, 172
    anticancer effects of, 66
    and vomiting as side effect of, 405
Medical management
    of constipation, 549–550
    for fatigue, 369
    for tracheal obstruction, 657–658
    for voiding dysfunction, 570, 572–576
Melanoma
    cutaneous, 464
    treatment of, 464–465
Mendelian dominance, 12–13
Menopause, premature, 588
Meperidine (Demerol), 316
Mercaptopurine, 89
Metabolic emergencies
    anaphylaxis, 721–728
        assessment, 725
        and cancer patient, 724
        medical management, 725–727
        nursing management, 727–728
        pathophysiology, 722–723
    hypercalcemia, 687–702
        assessment, 691–694
        medical management, 695–699
        nursing management, 699–702, 699*t*, 700*t*
        pathophysiology, 687–691
    septic shock, 729–736
        assessment, 732–733
        etiology, 731–732
        medical management, 733–734
        nursing management, 734–736, 735*t*
        pathophysiology, 729, 731

syndrome of inappropriate
antidiuretic hormone secretion,
711–720
pathophysiology, 711–713
syndrome of inappropriate
antidiuretic hormone (SIADH)
assessment, 714–716
etiology of, 713–714, 713*t*
medical management, 716–717
nursing management,
718–719*t,* 720
tumor lysis syndrome, 703–710
assessment, 705–706
medical management, 706–707
nursing management, 707–710
pathophysiology, 703–705
Metabolic encephalopathy, 505
Metals, 14
Metaplasia, 9
Metastasis
cutaneous, 466
neovascularization and growth
of, 18–19, 19f
treatment of, 28
Methadone, 316
Methotrexate, 89
anticancer effects of, 67
Methylprednisolone, 405
Metoclopramide (Reglan®), 323,
405, 504
Metronidazole, 505
Mid-arm muscle circumference
(MAMC), in nutritional
assessment, 397
Mild insomnia, 337
Misoprostol (Cytotec®), 313
Mitomycin, 172
Mitotic index, 440
Mitoxantrone in chemotherapy,
91
Moderate insomnia, 337
Mohs micrographic surgery, 27
Monoclonal antibodies (MAbs),
112
Monocyte—colony stimulating
factor (M-CSF), 420
Monocytes, 419–424
functions of, 420*t,* 421–422
Monokines, 106

Mood changes, 513
Morphine, 314
Motility disorders, 548
Motor capability, 623–624
Motor dysfunction, 633–634
assessment of, 516–517
management of, 517–518
Motor function, 636
M phase, 5–6, 5f
Mucosa-associated lymphoid tissue
(MALT) lymphoma, 13
Mucosal neuromas, 13
Mucosal toxicity in chemotherapy,
100
Mucous membranes, 440–457
anatomy and physiology,
440–441
assessment
esophagus, 453
oral cavity, 451–452
rectal area, 453
management, 453, 454–455*t,*
455–457, 456*t*
pathophysiology, 441–442
biologicals, 449
chemotherapy, 442–444,
445–449*t*
nutritional status, 450
primary malignancies,
450–451
radiation therapy, 449–450
Multileaf collimators, 48
Multilineage cytokines, 127
Mural obstructions, 662
Mycosis fungoides (MF), 465
Myelosuppression, 101

N

Nabumetone (Relafen®), 313
Naloxone (Narcan®), 314
2-Naphthylamine, 14
Nasopharyngeal carcinoma, 13,
245
National Alliance of Breast Cancer
Organizations (NABCO), 283,
288
National Brain Tumor Foundation,
284

National Cancer Institute (NCI), 236
  Cancer Information Service
    (CIS), 264
  Cancer Prevention Awareness
    Program, 254
  program for drug development, 67
National Coalition for Cancer
    Survivorship, 284
National Hospice Organization,
    284
National Kidney Cancer
    Association, 284–285
National Library of Medicine, 279
National Lymphedema Network,
    285
National Marrow Donor Program
    (NMDP), 132, 285
Nausea and vomiting
  management of problems related
    to, 403, 405–406, 407–408t,
    408, 409t, 410–411, 412t, 413,
    414t
  as side effect in chemotherapy,
    97–99
Neoadjuvant chemotherapy, 46,
    94–95
Neo-bladder
  constriction of, 543
  construction of, 564
Neoplasia, 9
Neovascularization and growth of
    metastasis, 18–19, 19f
Nephrostomy, 541
Neurofibromas, 13
Neurofibromatosis, 12
Neurologic complications, 495–525
  in autonomic nervous system,
    518
  from bone marrow
    transplantation, 147–148
  in bone marrow transplantation,
    168
  in cranial nerves, 509–510t, 518,
    520–521
  pathophysiology, 495, 496t
  in peripheral nervous system,
    514–518
  prevention of, 521
  secondary, 505–506

Neurologic dysfunctions
  assessment, 507, 508t, 509–510t
  malignant causes of, 496–500
  nonmalignant causes of, 501,
    502t, 503–505
  nursing management of common,
    522–524t
Neuropathic pain, 306–308
Neurostimulatory interventions of
    cancer pain, 329
Neurosurgical interventions of
    cancer pain, 329
Neutropenia, 417
Nitrosoureas in chemotherapy,
    69
Nociceptive pain, 306
Nonbacterial thrombotic
    endocarditis, 740
Non-Kaposi's sarcoma, 465
Nonopioid analgesics, 313
Nonpharmacological treatment of
    cancer pain, 328
Nontunneled catheters, 178
Normothermia, 626
Nortriptyline (Pamelor®), 326
NREM sleep, 337–338
Nursing assessment
  of ambulatory pumps, 199–200,
    199t
  of epidural therapy, 207
  of extra-arterial therapy, 193,
    195–196
  of fatigue, 369, 370–371t, 372
  for intraperitoneal therapy,
    208–212, 209t, 210t
  for intraventricular subcutaneous
    reservoirs, 202–205, 202t
  of sleep disorders, 358
Nursing care
  in cancer pain management, 312
  to cancer patients, 29–33
  in clinical research, 223–233
  issues in radiation therapy, 53,
    54–56t, 57, 58–62t
  of late effects of bone marrow
    transplantation, 159–163t
  of patients receiving biologic
    response modifiers (BRMs)
    therapy, 113, 114–124t

of patients receiving
  chemotherapy, 97–103
  cutaneous and mucosal
    toxicity, 100
  gastrointestinal side effects,
    97–99, 98t
  hematologic toxicity, 101
  hepatic effects, 102
  immunosuppression, 102
  pulmonary effects, 102
  renal effects, 102
Nursing care management of
  patients and families
  assessment, 297–299
  management, 299, 300–301t,
    302–303
Nursing management, 593, 594t,
  734–736, 735t
  for ambulatory pumps, 199–200,
    199t, 200
  for anaphylaxis, 727–728
  assessment, 593, 595–596
  for bowel obstruction, 668–670t,
    671
  for bowel program, 554–556, 555t
  for cardiac tamponade, 682, 683t,
    684
  for carotid artery erosion and
    rupture, 756–761, 757t, 759t,
    760t
  counseling, 596
  education, 596
  for epidural therapy, 207
  for extra-arterial therapy, 193,
    195–196
  for hypercalcemia, 699–702,
    699t, 700t
  for intraperitoneal therapy,
    208–212, 209t, 210t
  for intraventricular subcutaneous
    reservoirs, 202–205, 202t
  for irritant and vesicant drugs,
    173–174, 175t, 176
  for leukostasis, 766, 767t, 768
  for obstructive emergencies,
    626–627, 628–629t, 630
  for patient with bone marrow
    depression (BMD), 434–437t,
    437–438

referral, 597
  for sexuality, 593, 594t
  for superior vena cava syndrome,
    651, 652–653t, 653–654
  for syndrome of inappropriate
    antidiuretic hormone (SIADH),
    718–719t, 720
  for tracheal obstruction, 659–660,
    659t
  for tumor lysis syndrome,
    707–710
  for urinary incontinence, 576,
    577–578t, 578–581
Nutrition, 377–414
  assessment of adult with cancer,
    394–397, 398–399t, 400, 401,
    401t
  changes in status, 383
  consequences of cancer, 383–391
  consequences of cancer
    treatment, 391–392, 393t, 394t
  enteral, 408, 409t, 410–411, 412t
  management of problems related
    to
    diarrhea, 401, 403, 404t
    nausea and vomiting, 403,
      405–406, 407–408t, 408,
      409t, 410–411, 412t, 413,
      414t
  parenteral, 411, 413, 414t
  and physiology, 377–382
  and wound healing, 474–475
Nutritional-deficiency stomatitis,
  450
Nutritional status
  effect of, on mucosa, 450
  and primary malignancies,
    450–451

O

Obstructive emergencies
  assessment, 620–625
  medical and surgical
    management, 625–626
  nursing management,
    626–627, 628–629t, 630
  bowel obstruction, 661–671
    assessment, 666–667

Obstructive emergencies (cont'd)
    clinical manifestations,
        665–666
    large, pathophysiology,
        664–665
    medical management, 667–668
    nursing management, 668–670t
        671
    small, 661–664
        pathophysiology, 662–663
    cardiac tamponade, 673–684
        clinical manifestations,
            675–677
        diagnosis, 677–679
        medical management, 679–682
        nursing management, 682,
            683t, 684
        pathophysiology, 673–675
    clinical manifestations, 620
    increased intracranial pressure,
        pathophysiology, 617–618
    spinal cord compression, 631
        assessment, 635–637
        clinical manifestations,
            633–635
        medical management, 637–640
        nursing management, 640,
            641–642t, 643
        pathophysiology, 632, 633t
    superior vena cava syndrome,
        645–654
        assessment, 647–649
        clinical manifestations, 647
        medical management, 649–651
        nursing management, 651,
            652–653t, 653–654
        pathophysiology, 645–647
    tracheal obstruction
        assessment, 657
        clinical manifestations,
            656–657
        medical management, 657–658
        nursing management, 659–660
        pathophysiology, 655–656
Oligospermia, 68
Ommaya reservoir, 200–201
Oncogenes, 3
Oncology Nursing Society, 235
    establishment of patient
        education standards by, 269

Oncology patients, sleep problems
    in, 344–345
Ondansetron (Zofran®), 323
    in managing nausea, 406
Open-label study, 220
Opioids, 313–316
    as cause of constipation, 549
    dose, route, and scheduling, 316,
        317t, 318–321t, 322
    side effects of, 322–323, 324t
Oral cavity, mucous membranes in,
    451
Oral intake, 408, 409t, 410–411,
    412t, 413, 414t
Oral mucositis, 441, 442–444
    treatment of, 445–449t
Organic disease as source of
    constipation, 548–549
Osmotic diuresis, 625–626
Osmotic laxatives, 552–553
Osteoradionecrosis, 450
Ovarian cancer, 599
Ovarian failure, 588
Oxycodone (Roxicodone®, Oxy
    IR®, OxyContin®), 314–315

P

p170, 94
Paclitaxel, 89–90
Paget's disease, 466
Pain, 305–335
    assessment of, 309–312
    breakthrough, 308–309
    definition of, 305–306
    neuropathic, 306–308
    nociceptive, 306
    in person with cancer, 306–309
    visceral, 306
Painful bladder disorders, 557–558,
    564–565
    medical management of, 574
    nursing management of, 580–581
Pain management in spinal cord
    compression, 640
Palliative surgical treatment, 27
Pamidronate, 695–696
Pancreas, 381–382
Pancreatic polypeptide, 382
Pap smear, 258

Paraneoplastic syndromes, 506
Parathormone, 688
Parenteral nutrition, 411, 413, 414*t*
Parenteral therapy, 171–216
  ambulatory pumps, 197–199
  intra-arterial, 192–196
  intracavitary management of pleural effusions, 212–214, 213*t*, 214*t*, 215*t*
  intraperitoneal, 207–212
  intraventricular subcutaneous reservoirs, 200–201
  irritant and vesicant drugs, 172–173, 172*t*
  management, 173–174, 175*t*, 176
  venous access devices, 176–177, *177, 178*
    patient education, 189, 190–191*t*, 192
Parietal pericardium, 673
Partial pericardiectomy, 681
Particulate radiation, 39
PAS-port™, 180
Patient
  available information resources for, 270
  information seeking behaviors of, 267–268
Patient education, 268–269
  and clinical research, 235
  for patient with bone marrow depression (BMD), 438
  and sexuality, 596
  on venous access devices, 189, 190–191*t*, 192
Patient-Generated Global Assessment (PG-SGA), 400*t*, 401
Pegasparagenase (Oncaspar®), in chemotherapy, 91, 92
Pelvic descent, 563
Pentostatin, 89
Percocet®, 314
Percutaneous balloon pericardiotomy, 680
Percutaneous central venous catheters (CVCs), 178
Pericardial friction rub, 675

Pericardiectomy
  partial, 681
  total, 681–682
Pericardiocentesis, pharmacologic therapy for cardiac tamponade, 679
Peripheral blood stem cell transplantation (PBST), 127
  evolution of, from bone marrow transplantation, 129
  versus marrow transplantation, 129–131, 130*t*
Peripherally inserted central venous catheters (PICC), 178
Peripheral nerve injury, 515
Peripheral nervous system
  assessment of motor dysfunction, 516–517
  assessment of sensory dysfunction, 514–515
  management of motor dysfunction, 517–518
  management of sensory dysfunction, 515–516
Peripheral neuropathy, 514
Peripheral scalp hypothermia, 481
Peripheral stem cell reinfusion, complications of, 141*t*
Perirectal abscesses, 549
Peristalsis, 380–381
Pharmacological treatment
  accountability, 333–335
  anesthetic and neurosurgical interventions, 329
  of cancer pain, 313
    addiction, 326
    adjuvant medications, 326, 327*t*, 328
    dose, route, and scheduling of opioids, 317*t*, 318–321*t*, 322
    nonopioid analgesics, 313
    opioid analgesics, 313–316
    physical dependence, 325
    pseudoaddiction, 325–326
    side effects of opioids, 322–323, 324*t*
    tolerance, 325
  for cardiac tamponade, 679
    pericardiocentesis, 679

Pharmacological treatment (cont'd)
managing pain at end of life,
330–332
neurostimulatory interventions,
329
nonpharmacological, of cancer
pain, 328
physiatric interventions, 329–330
psychological interventions, 330
use of placebos in pain
management, 333
Phase I trials, 220–221
Phase II trials, 222
Phase III trials, 222–223
Phase IV trials, 223
Phenothiazines, 405–406
Pheochromocytomas, 13
Phosphate, 89
Photons, 38
Photosensitivity, 469
as side effect in chemotherapy,
100
Physiatric interventions of cancer
pain, 329–330
Physical activity in preventing
cancer, 245
Physical carcinogenesis, 14–15
Physical care, 32–33
Physical dependence, 325
Physical well-being, 362–364
Physician's Data Query (PDQ),
236
Piper Fatigue Scale (PFS), 366–367
Piper's Integrated Fatigue Model,
367
Placebos in pain management, 333
Pleomorphic cells, 7
Pleural effusions
definition of, 212
intracavitary management of,
212–214, 213t, 214t, 215t
malignant, 599
Plicamycin, 698, 701
Pneumonia, 599
cytomegaloviral (CMV), 147
idiopathic, 147
interstitial, 147
Pneumonitis, radiation, 600–601
Postintubation tracheal stenosis, 658
Prednisone, 93

Premalignant lesions, 463
Premature menopause, 588
Preoperative assessment, 31
Pressure ulcers, 478–479, 480t,
488–491
nursing protocol for management
of, 489t
Prethrombotic state, 738–739
Pre-transplant conditioning
regimens, 140–142
Prevention, 248–249
chemoprevention, 246, 247t
conceptual considerations, 241
considerations, 243–246
early detection, 249–250.253,
254
epidemiologic considerations,
242–243, 242t, 243
nursing protocol for, 255t
primary, 241
secondary, 241
tertiary, 241
Primary hepatocellular carcinoma,
245
Primary peristalsis, 379–380
Primary prevention, 241
Prochlorperazine (Compazine®),
323, 504
in managing nausea, 406
Promethazine (Phenergan®), 355
Promoters, 11
Promotion, 11
Promotor, 243–244
Pronator drift, 517
Prophylactic diuresis, 706
Prophylactic surgery, 24
Prostate cancer
prevention and early detection of,
258–259
TNM staging classification, 787t,
788t
Prostate specific antigen (PSA),
253
Proteases, 9
Protective mechanisms. See Bone
marrow; Mucous membranes
Protein-calorie malnutrition, 383
Protein metabolism, 390–391
Proton beam delivery, 504
Proto-oncogene, 10

Pruritus, management of, 481, 484

Pseudoaddiction, 325–326

Psychiatric conditions, effect on gastrointestinal tract, 548

Psychological interventions of cancer pain, 330

Psychological well-being, 364

Psychotropic drugs, 504

Pulmonary complications, from bone marrow transplantation, 146–147

Pulmonary edema, 146

Pulmonary effects in chemotherapy, 102

Pulmonary fibrosis, 601

Pulmonary function, 599–613
    assessment, 603, 604t
    management, 603, 605–611t, 611–613
        pathophysiology and presentation, 599–601, 600t, 602t

Pulmonary function tests (PFTs), 601, 657

Pulse, 624

Purine analogues, 89

Pustular rashes as side effect in chemotherapy, 100

Pyrimidine analogues, 89

Q

Quality of life, 29, 30t
    as complication of bone marrow transplantation, 169
    impact of fatigue on, 363t

R

Radiation and painful bladder disorder, 564–565

Radiation damage to normal lungs, 600

Radiation enteritis, 663

Radiation-induced cystitis, 564

Radiation-induced enteritis, 450

Radiation myelopathy, 503

Radiation necrosis, 503

Radiation pneumonitis, 600–601, 612

Radiation therapy
    biology of, 38–39, 39t, 40t, 41, 42–45t, 46
    for cardiac tamponade, 682
    as cause of neurologic dysfunction, 503–504
    definition of, 36–37
    and diarrhea, 403
    effect of
        on mucosa, 449–450
        on tissue, 468–469, 469t
    effect on bone marrow, 425–426
    goals of treatment, 37–38, 37t
    induced skin changes in, 486, 487t
    methods of treatment, 46–53, 51t
    nursing care issues, 53, 54–56t, 57, 58–62t
    nutritional consequences of, 392, 394t
    for spinal cord compression, 639
    for superior vena cava syndrome, 649
    for tracheal obstruction, 656
    for treating brain metastases, 497
    for treating spinal cord tumors, 499–500
    and urinary system distress, 565

Radicular pain, 632

Radioimmunotherapy, 45t

Radiopharmaceutical therapy, 51–52

Radioprotectors, 41, 44t, 46

Radiosensitivity of normal tissues, 40t

Radiosensitizers, 41, 44t, 46

Radio-surgery (SRS), 42t, 504

Randomization, 220

Reach to Recovery, 285–286

Rectal area, mucous membranes in, 453

Rectal carcinomas, 665

Recurrent phase of illness, 295–296

Reflexes, 635

Reflex incontinence, 562–563
    nursing management of, 578

Regional perfusion, 192

Rehabilitation, 33

Rehabilitative surgery, 28

Relapse as complication of bone marrow transplantation, 167

Remote afterloading
brachytherapy, 45*t*, 50–51
REM sleep, 338, 340
deprivation of, 346
Renal complications, from bone
marrow transplantation, 145–146
Renal effects in chemotherapy, 102
Renewing cell populations, 6
Resection of metastases, 28
Respirations, 625
Respiratory failure, 601, 612–613
nursing protocol for management
of, 611*t*
Retinoblastoma, 12
Retrograde ejaculation, 588
Rhabdosphincter, 560
Right-sided colonic carcinomas, 664
Romberg test, 517
Rosenstock's Healthy Belief
Model, 248–249

S

Saline laxatives, 552–553
Saliva, 440–441
functions of, 441
Salivary glands, 440
Satiety center, 378
Scalp tourniquet, 481
Scar tissue, 663
Scopolamine, 323
Screening, 254, 256–257
Sebaceous glands, 460
Secondary neurologic
complications, 505–506
Secondary peristalsis, 380
Secondary prevention, 241
Second malignancies as
complication of bone marrow
transplantation, 168–169
Secretion, 662
Secretion clearance, 601, 612
nursing protocol for management
of, 609–610*t*
Sedatives, 504
Self-care management, 270
Senescence, 4
Sensory dysfunction, 632–633
assessment, 514–515
management of, 515–516

Sensory function, 637
Sensory loss, 515
Septic shock, 729–736
assessment, 732–733
etiology, 731–732
medical management, 733–734
nursing management, 734–736,
735*t*
pathophysiology, 729, 731
Serosal seeding, 16
Serotonin antagonists in managing
nausea, 406
Sexuality, 585–597
guidelines in discussing, 595*t*
medical management, 588,
590–591, *592, 593*
nursing management, 593,
594*t*
pathophysiology, 585–586,
587*t*, 588, 588*t*, 589–590*t*
Sexual response cycle, 586, 587*t*
disease-related causes of
disruptions to, 588*t*
treatment-related causes of
disruption to, 588–589*t*
Sezary's syndrome, 465–466
Shortness of breath, 657
Simulation, 48
Simulator, 48
Simulator films, 48
Skin, 459–492
anatomy and physiology, 459
dermis, 460
epidermis, 459–460
function o, 460–461
assessment, 479–480, 479*t*,
480*t*
management of disease and
treatment-related
manifestations
products, 482*t*
symptom, 481, 483–484*t*, 484,
485*t*, 486, 487*t*, 488–492,
488*t*, 489*t*, 490*t*, 491*t*
pathophysiology, 462–463
cutaneous paraneoplastic
syndromes, 466, 467–468*t*,
468
disease-related causes of
impairment, 463–466

other treatment and disease-related factors affecting, 474–479
treatment-related causes of impairment, 468–469, 470–471t, 472–474
tissue injury and wound repair, 461–462, 461t
Skin Cancer Foundation, 285
Skin cancer treatment, 464–465
Sleep, 336–358
assessment, 347–348
definition of, 336
deprivation of, 345–346
disturbances related to sleep cycles, 345–346
educational and behavioral interventions, 348
nursing assessment and intervention, 358
over the life span, 346–347
pharmacologic treatment, 348, 352, 354–355, 356–357t
physiology, 337–347, 339–340t, 341–342t, 343t
problems in oncology patients, 344–345
Small-bowel obstruction, management of, 667
Small-bowel ostomy, 528
Small intestine, 379–380
primary tumors of, 663
secondary tumors, 663
Social well-being, 364–365
Sodium bicarbonate, 174
Solar keratosis, 463
S phase, 5–6, 5f
Sphincter deficiency, 563
Sphygmomanometry, 676–677
Spinal cord compression, 631
assessment, 635–637
clinical manifestations, 633–635
medical management, 637–640
nursing management, 640, 641–642t, 643
pathophysiology, 632, 633t
Spinal cord tumors, 499–500
Spinal reflexes, 636–637, 637t
Spiritual well-being, 365–366
Squamous cell carcinoma, 463–464

Staging, 24–25, 26t
of cancer, 777–788
breast, 778t, 779t
cervical, 779t
colon, 780t
endometrial, 781t
lung, 782t, 783t
lymphoma
adult Hodgkin's disease, 784t
adult non-Hodgkin's disease, 785t, 786t
prostate, 787t, 788t
Static tissues, 6
Stem cell harvest, 138–139
Stem cells, 127
Stenotic lesions, 655–656
Stereotactic radiation therapy, 42t, 504
in treating brain metastases, 497
Steroids, 504
for hypercalcemia, 697–698
for spinal cord compression, 639
for superior vena cava syndrome, 650
Stimulant laxatives, 553
Stoma, 527
complications, 532–540
dilation of, 533
structuring of, 532–533
viability of, 532
Stomach, 380
Stomal stenosis, 656
Stoma prolapse, 533
Stoma retraction, 533
Stomatitis, 441
nutritional-deficiency, 450
Stratification, 222
Streptozocin, 172
and vomiting as side effect of, 405
Stress, 289–290
Stress incontinence, 563
Stressors
appraisal of, 290
extrapersonal, 289–290
interpersonal, 289
intrapersonal, 289
Stress urinary incontinence (SUI), 561
management of, 572–574
nursing management of, 578–579

Subcutaneous venous access
     devices, 179–180
Subjective Global Assessment
     (SGA), 401
Subscapular skin-fold thickness
     (SST), in nutritional assessment,
     397
Superior vena cava syndrome,
     645–654
     assessment, 647–649
     clinical manifestations, 647
     medical management, 649–651
     nursing management, 651,
          652–653t, 653–654
     pathophysiology, 645–647
Supportive care, 27
Support medications, 504
Suppositories, 554
Surfactant laxatives, 553
Surgery
     for cardiac tamponade, 681–682
     and constipation, 549–550
     effect of, on tissue, 473
     nutritional consequences of, 392,
          393t
     preparation for, 31–32
     for spinal cord compression, 639
     for superior vena cava syndrome,
          649–650
     wound management in,
          490–491t, 491
Surgical decompression in treating
     spinal cord tumors, 499–500
Surgical oncology
     approaches in, 23–29, 23t, 25t,
          26t
     evolution of, 22–23
     nursing considerations in, 29–33
     and quality of life, 29, 30t
Survival rates, increase in, 21
Swallowing, 379
Syndrome of inappropriate
     antidiuretic hormone (SIADH),
     618, 653, 711–720
     assessment, 714–716
     etiology of, 713–714, 713t
     medical management, 716–717
     nursing management, 718–719t,
          720
     pathophysiology, 711–713

Systemic chemotherapy, 212–213,
     501
Systemic metabolic alterations of
     cancer, 388–391
Systemic venous congestion,
     677

T

Tamoxifen, 93
Taxanes in chemotherapy, 89–90
T-cell growth factor, 107, 111t
Telomere, 4
Temperature, 625
Tenckhoff catheter, 208–209,
     211
Teniposide (VM-26), 90, 172
Terminal insomnia, 337
Terminal phase of illness, 296–297
Tertiary prevention, 241
Testicular biopsy, 590
Testicular self-examination (TSE),
     254, 256
Testosterone, 590
Therapeutic intent, 21
Thiethylperazine (Torecan®,
     Norzine®), 323
Thioguanine, 89
Thoracentesis, 212, 213, 213t, 214t,
     215t
Threat appraisals, 290
Thrombocytes/platelets, 422
Thrombocytopenia, and
     constipation, 549
Thrombocytopenia (TCP), 417,
     424, 427, 444
     medical management of,
          432–433
Thrombotic disorders, 738–739
Thrombus formation, potential
     causes of, 739t
Tissue hypoxia, 423
Tissue injury and wound repair,
     461–462, 461t
Tissues, radiosensitivity of normal,
     40t
T-lymphocytes, 421
TNF-alpha (TNF-α), 110
TNF-beta (TNF-β), 110
TNM, 25

Tobacco
  association of, with lung cancer, 14
  and risk of lung cancer, 245
Toe walking, 636
Tolerance, 325
Topoisomerase I and II inhibitors
  in chemotherapy, 90
Topotecan (Hycamtin®), 90
Total body irradiation (TBI),
  42–43*t*, 129
Total pericardiectomy, 681–682
Total protective environment
  (TPE), 429
Toxicities in clinical research, 227,
  230–232*t*
Trachea
  primary tumors of, 655, 657–658
  secondary tumors of, 655, 658
Tracheal obstruction, 655–660
  assessment, 657
  clinical manifestations, 656–657
  medical management, 657–658
  nursing management, 659–660,
    659*t*
  pathophysiology, 655–656
Tracheal stenosis, postintubation,
  658
Transdermal fentanyl, 315–316
Transient hypocalcemia, 139
Transvaginal or transrectal
  electrostimuation, 576, 578
Transverse colostomies, 527
Treatment-related causes of skin
  impairment, 468–469, 470–471*t*,
  472–474
Triceps skin-fold thickness (TSF)
  in nutritional assessment, 397
Tricyclic antidepressants, 504
True vomiting center (TVC),
  387–388
Tubulin, 89
Tumor-associated antigens, 9
Tumor growth and
  neovascularization, 15–16
Tumor lysis syndrome, 703–710,
  765–766
  assessment, 705–706
  medical management, 706–707
  nursing management, 707–710
  pathophysiology, 703–705

Tumor markers, 253
Tumor necrosis factor (TNF), 107,
  110, 729
Tumor progression, 7, 10, 11
Tumors, 6
  brain, 496–497, 498*t,* 499*t*
  growth of, 6–7
  hormone-secreting, 386
  relative sensitivity of, 39, 39*t*
  spinal cord, 499–500
Tumor types
  and common sites of metastatic
    spread, 773–774*t*
  and potential oncologic
    emergency, 775–776*t*
Tunneled catheters, 178–179
24-Hour recall approach in
  nutritional assessment, 397
Tylenol #3®, 314
Tylox®, 314

U

Ulcers, pressure, 478–479, 480*t*
Ultraviolet radiation, 14
United Ostomy Association, 286
Ureterostomy, 540–541
Urethral barrier devices, 573
Urge incontinence, 562
Urinalysis, 570
Urinary continence, 558
Urinary diversion, 591
  common problems, 542
  management, 541–542
  pathophysiology, 540–541
  procedures, 542–543
Urinary dysfunction, diagnostic
  tests for, 571*t*
Urinary incontinence, 557,
  561–563
Urinary retention, 557, 563–564
  assessment of, 570
  management of, 574
Urinary system distress, 558, 565
  management of, 574, 578
  nursing management of, 581
Urine, alkaline, 543
Urine alkalinization, 708
US TOO, International, Inc.,
  286

V

Vaccine therapy, 113
Valproate (Depakene®), 326
Valsalva maneuver, 627, 758
Varicella-zoster virus, 476
Vasa vasorum, 751
Vascular disorders, 506–507
Vasogenic cerebral edema, 617
Veno-occlusive disease, from bone marrow transplantation, 146
Venous access devices (VADs), 176–177, *177, 178*
  assessment, 181, 182*t*
  complications associated with, 176–177
  management, 181–182, 183*t,* 184–189
  nontunneled catheters, 178
  nursing assessment of patient with, 181–182, 183*t,* 184–189
  subcutaneous, 179–180
  tunneled catheters, 178–179
Ventriculostomy, 626
Vesicants, 172–176, 172*t,* 175*t*
Vesicostomy, 540
Vesicourethral reflux, nursing management of, 581
Vicodin®, 314
Vinblastine, 89, 172
Vincristine, 172
Vindesine, 89, 172
Vinorelbine, 89
Vinyl chlorides, 14

Viral carcinogenesis, 13
Viral infections, 476–477
Viral interference, phenomenon of, 106
Viral mucosal infections, 444
Viruses and cancer risk, 245
Visceral pain, 306
Visceral pericardium, 673
Vital signs, 624–625, 635
Vitamin D secretion, 688
Voiding diary, 568, *569,* 570
Voiding dysfunction, 557
von Hipple-Lindau syndrome, 12

W

Weight for height in nutritional assessment, 397
Wilms' tumor, 12
Winningham's Psychobiologic Entropy Model, 367
Wiskott-Aldrich syndrome, 13
Wound healing, phases of, 461–462, 461*t*

X

Xeroderma pigmentosum, 12
Xerosis, management of, 484, 486*t*
Xerostomia, 449–450

Z

Zolpidem (imidazophyridine), 355

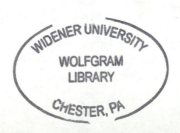